HEART AND HEART–LUNG TRANSPLANTATION

HEART AND HEART-LUNG TRANSPLANTATION

Edited by

John Wallwork

Department of Cardiothoracic Surgery
Papworth Hospital
Cambridge, England

W. B. SAUNDERS COMPANY
Harcourt Brace Jovanovich, Inc.
Philadelphia · London · Toronto
Montreal · Sydney · Tokyo

W. B. SAUNDERS COMPANY
Harcourt Brace Jovanovich, Inc.

The Curtis Center
Independence Square West
Philadelphia, PA 19106

Library of Congress Cataloging-in-Publication Data

British Library Cataloguing-in-Publication Data

Heart and heart–lung transplantation.
1. Man. Heart. Transplantation 2. Man.
Lungs. Transplantation
I. Wallwork, John, *1946–*
617′.4120592

ISBN 0-7216-2787-0

To the late Professor Philip Caves. His untimely death 10 years ago precipitated the events which led to my involvement in transplantation. Fifteen years following his introduction of endomyocardial biopsy to detect rejection, we are still searching for a better way—a testimony to the value of his all too brief contribution to cardiac transplantation.

Contributors

F. Baud, Service de Chirurgie CardioVasculaire, Hôpital de la Pitié, Paris, France
William A. Baumgartner, Division of Cardiac Surgery, The Johns Hopkins Medical Institutions, 600 N. Wolfe Street, Baltimore, MD 21205, USA
D. W. Bethune, Department of Cardiothoracic Surgery, Papworth Hospital, Papworth Everard, Cambridge, CB3 8RE
James R. Bonner, Department of Cardiothoracic Surgery, University of Alabama Hospital, School of Medicine, University Station, Birmingham, AL 35294, USA
V. Bors, Service de Chirurgie CardioVasculaire, Hôpital de la Pitié, Paris, France
Marguerite Brown, Donor Coordinator, Stanford University School of Medicine, Stanford, CA 94305, USA
M. J. Buxton, Health Economics Research Group, Brunel University, Uxbridge, Middlesex, UB8 3PH
C. Cabrol, Service de Chirurgie CardioVasculaire, Hôpital de la Pitié, Paris, France
Noreen Caine, Senior Research Associate, Department of Community Medicine, University of Cambridge, Papworth Hospital, Papworth Everard, Cambridge, CB3 8RE
N. Cavarocchi, Department of Cardiovascular Surgery, Temple University Hospital, 3401 N. Broad Street, Philadelphia, PA 19140, USA
J. D. Cooper, Division of Cardiothoracic Surgery, Washington University School of Medicine, St. Louis, MO 63110, USA
Jack G. Copeland, Department of Surgery, Health Sciences Center, University of Arizona, Tucson, AZ 85724, USA
Margaret J. Dallman, Nuffield Department of Surgery, University of Oxford, John Radcliffe Hospital, Oxford
P. Dalous, Service de Chirurgie CardioVasculaire, Hôpital de la Pitié, Paris, France
Robert W. Emery, Department of Surgery, Health Sciences Center, University of Arizona, Tucson, AZ 85724, USA
M. Arisan Ergin, Department of Surgery, The Mount Sinai Medical Center, New York, NY, USA
I. Gandjbakhch, Service de Chirurgie CardioVasculaire, Hôpital de la Pitié, Paris, France
Randall B. Griepp, Department of Surgery, The Mount Sinai Medical Center, New York, NY, USA

Bartley P. Griffith, Department of Surgery, University of Pittsburgh School of Medicine, 1084 Scaife Hall, Pittsburgh, PA 15261, USA

M. Hakim, Mayo Clinic, Rochester, MN 55905, USA

I. Hardy, Department of Cardiothoracic Surgery, Papworth Hospital, Papworth Everard, Cambridge, CB3 8RE

Tim Higenbottam, Department of Respiratory Physiology, Papworth Hospital, Papworth Everard, Cambridge, CB3 8RE

Sharon A. Hunt, Department of Cardiology, Stanford University Medical Center, Stanford, CA 94305, USA

J. A. Hutter, Senior Transplant Fellow, Papworth Hospital, Papworth Everard, Cambridge, CB3 8RE

Timothy B. Icenogle, Department of Surgery, Health Sciences Center, University of Arizona, Tucson, AZ 85724, USA

Stuart W. Jamieson, Department of Cardiovascular and Thoracic Surgery, Minnesota Heart and Lung Institute, University of Minnesota, Minneapolis, MN 55455, USA

Michael P. Kaye, Department of Cardiovascular and Thoracic Surgery, Minnesota Heart and Lung Institute, University of Minnesota, Minneapolis, MN 55455, USA

Bernhard M. Kemkes, Department of Cardiac Surgery, University of Munich, Marchioninistrasse 15, D-8000, Munich 70, Federal Republic of Germany

James K. Kirklin, Department of Surgery, University of Alabama Hospital, School of Medicine, University Station, Birmingham, AL 35294, USA

J. Kneeshaw, Department of Cardiothoracic Surgery, Papworth Hospital, Papworth Everard, Cambridge, CB3 8RE

Steven L. Lansman, Department of Surgery, The Mount Sinai Medical Center, New York, NY, USA

R. D. Latimer, Department of Cardiothoracic Surgery, Papworth Hospital, Papworth Everard, Cambridge, CB3 8RE

David C. McGiffin, Department of Cardiothoracic Surgery, Prince Charles Hospital, Rode Road, Chermside, Brisbane, Queensland 4034, Australia

Peter J. Morris, Nuffield Department of Surgery, University of Oxford, John Radcliffe Hospital, Oxford

David C. Naftel, Department of Surgery, University of Alabama Hospital, School of Medicine, University Station, Birmingham, AL 35294, USA

Virginia O'Brien, Transplant Patient Adviser, Papworth Hospital, Papworth Everard, Cambridge, CB3 8RE

A. Oduro, Department of Cardiothoracic Surgery, Papworth Hospital, Papworth Everard, Cambridge, CB3 8RE

G. A. Patterson, Department of Cardiothoracic Surgery, Toronto General Hospital, Eaton Building, 10th Floor, Toronto, Canada, M5G 1L7

A. Pavie, Service de Chirurgie CardioVasculaire, Hôpital de la Pitié, Paris, France

D. Glenn Pennington, Department of Surgery, St. Louis University, 1325 South Grand, St. Louis, MO 63104, USA

Ariela Pomerance, Department of Histopathology and Cytology, Harefield and Mount Vernon Pathology Laboratories, Mount Vernon Hospital, Northwood, Middlesex, HA6 2RN

B. A. Reitz, Department of Cardiothoracic Surgery, The Johns Hopkins Hospital, 618 Blalock Building, 600 N. Wolfe Street, Baltimore, MD 21205, USA

E. Solis, Service de Chirurgie CardioVasculaire, Hôpital de la Pitié, Paris, France

Susan Stewart, Department of Pathology, Papworth Hospital, Papworth Everard, Cambridge, CB3 8RE

Edward B. Stinson, Department of Cardiology, Stanford University Medical Center, Stanford, CA 94305, USA.

P. G. I. Stovin, Department of Histopathology, Papworth Hospital, Papworth Everard, Cambridge, CB3 8RE

Mark E. Thompson, Division of Cardiology, University of Pittsburgh School of Medicine, Pittsburgh, PA 15261, USA

John Wallwork, Department of Cardiothoracic Surgery, Papworth Hospital, Papworth Everard, Cambridge, CB3 8RE

D. J. G. White, Department of Surgery, University of Cambridge, Addenbrooke's Hospital, Hills Road, Cambridge, CB2 2QQ

Celia Wight, Senior Transplant Coordinator, Addenbrooke's Hospital, Hills Road Cambridge CB2 2QQ and Papworth Hospital, Papworth Everard, Cambridge, CB3 8RE

T. G. Wreghitt, Clinical Microbiology and Public Health Laboratory, Addenbrooke's Hospital, Hills Road, Cambridge, CB2 2QQ

Foreword

In the late 1950s and early 1960s experimental work was begun respectively on heart and heart–lung transplantation. Developments in this field over the past 30 years have been absolutely amazing. Heart transplantation is now a routine procedure which has been elevated to therapeutic status. Transplantation of the heart and both lungs and transplantation of one lung or both lungs without the heart are now on the road to established therapy. In this book, Professor John Wallwork and his collaborators summarize beautifully the state of the art with respect to transplantation of the heart and heart–lungs. While cyclosporin has certainly contributed much to the present-day acceptance of heart and heart–lung transplantation, the oldest living heart transplant survivor, now $18\frac{1}{2}$ years after transplantation, has never received cyclosporin. The nephrotoxicity of cyclosporin has stimulated many researchers to look for better and more specific methods of immunosuppression. The concept of specific acquired tolerance may not be so great a dream after all. Its realization could pave the way for successful inter-species transplantation. The totally implantable, inexhaustible, non-heat-producing artificial heart remains an elusive but attractive goal.

The past three decades represent a wildly exciting milestone in transplantation history, and the many brilliant chapters in this book should provide ideas and inspiration for further progress in heart and heart–lung transplantation.

N. E. Shumway

Preface

In the past 10 years, heart transplantation has developed from a sporadic, esoteric activity into a widely practised routine procedure for many patients with severe cardiac disease. The number of centres undertaking cardiac transplants has proliferated from 5 in 1979 to now over 150 in the USA, more than 50 in Europe and an expanding number in other parts of the world.

For heart–lung and isolated lung transplantation, progress has been rapid in the past 7 years. Currently, however, these operations are at an early stage of development. Many of the problems have just been identified rather than solved. Results have improved considerably over the past 2–3 years and there has been a growth rate in such transplants. Advances in distant organ procurement and refinements in surgical technique, combined with a greater understanding of lung rejection, have all led to this.

Because so much is changing in the field of combined and isolated lung transplantation, the chapters in this book dealing with this subject will date soonest and will inevitably need revision in the next few years. What of progress in general related to transplantation of intrathoracic organs? Some of the major areas which will see further development in the next 5–10 years can be identified. First and most importantly are developments to maximize the availability and appropriate use of that most scarce resource—donor organs.

The debate concerning how best to improve consent for organ donation will continue. In the end it is a greater awareness among the general public of the success of cardiac transplantation that will break down barriers and prejudice to organ donation. Intra-professional jealously and rivalry, so petty and destructive, are now less strong. Inevitably the better organization of an equitable distribution of organs to maximize overall benefit is beginning to take effect.

The impact of 'required request' to improve the availability of donor organs is uncertain. On the face of it, the arguments for its introduction are strong. After initial enthusiasm in the USA and increase in transplant activity, difficulties are beginning to arise over the practical application of such schemes. How should they be implemented? Who should do the asking? How to avoid the lukewarm, half-hearted approach of those who 'comply with the rules' with disinterest or frank obstruction? Careful and considered monitoring and reappraisal of 'required request' schemes should help to avoid these obvious pitfalls. It is important that the professional personnel responsible for the direct contact with bereaved relatives should be appropriately trained and supportive.

Tragically, even when consent is obtained for organ donation, many organs, particularly hearts and lungs, are damaged or lost because of inadequate or inappropriate care of the donor. Attention has been focused on this area. A better understanding is emerging not just of the simple haemodynamic aspects of donor care, but of complex biochemical and endocrine changes that occur after brain death. Hopefully, this will lead to an overall improvement in the number and quality of donor organs available.

Even if, however, all possible donor organs were made available for transplantation and used, the demand would continue to rise beyond supply. Indeed, in parallel with developments in transplant medicine we all hope that fewer people will die prematurely from accidents and trauma and thus truly reduce the potential donor pool.

In an era of organ shortages it seems perverse to generate more recipients, for instance by resuscitation of the moribund or by the use of mechanical 'bridges to transplantation'. The ethical issues are complex. Should we reduce overall the survival say from 100 donor organs by transplanting patients with a less favourable outcome? Should we in the interest of cost benefit and efficiency maximize outcome by denying individual patients access to a chance of transplantation? Should we, however, increase the use of mechanical assist devices, particularly the total artificial heart, which may lead to improvements that will enable a permanently implantable device to be available to relieve the pressure on allograft transplantation?

We have all already made choices. The most obvious is the imposition of age limits for the acceptance of recipients which by their very arbitrary nature have changed with time. Some would say they rise as the transplant surgeons themselves age!

These dilemmas are heightened in transplantation above other restrictive forms of medical care because of the finite resource of available allograft organs. No amount of investment in buildings, equipment or personnel can do more than approach these finite limits.

One way to help solve these problems is to divide transplantation into development and service activities. For instance, neonatal heart transplantation, use of the artificial heart and clinical experiments in other support devices are developmental. These activities should be properly supported in centres with special interests and expertise and evaluated.

Heart transplantation is a service commitment for the most part. How best to apply this therapy depends on regular audit of results and resource use and adaptation on a national and local scale to the conclusions of such monitoring. Heart–lung transplantation is at the half-way house between development and service commitment which all medical advances must pass through.

An equitable distribution of donor organs for the benefit of the largest number of patients awaiting transplantation seems an obvious goal. With a proliferation of transplant centres in most countries with established programmes it has become more difficult. How do you avoid the larger units taking all the best donors and perhaps not necessarily using them to best benefit by transplanting the moribund at the expense of a smaller unit who cannot then transplant an 'elective' patient with a better prognosis? Spectacular saves do not necessarily reflect sound medical science.

We have attempted to overcome this difficulty in the UK through the United Kingdom Transplant Service by abandoning the registration of patients for cardiac transplantation in 'emergency' or 'urgent' categories. Organ distribution works on a strict rotation of offers, so that small and large units alike have equal access to organs. However efficient we become in procuring, harvesting and storing organs for transplantation, there remains the basic imbalance between demand and supply. For heart–lung transplantation this can only be solved by the development of reliable, permanent and implantable mechanical organs or by the exciting possibility of the widespread successful use of xenografts.

Turning now from the problem of donor organs, the operative and early survival results are now uniformly good in established centres with a one-year survival of 80% or more. The major development for the continued success of heart transplantation in the mid- and long term must be the prevention of coronary occlusive disease in the transplanted heart. The ultimate fate of most transplanted hearts will be a failure as a result of coronary occlusive disease which occurs in 40% of hearts at 5 years, as seen on angiograms. This disease is progressive at a variable rate. Similar problems with lung transplantation will need to be overcome in order to make this a long-term viable proposition.

The pathology and risk factors are not yet fully understood; further research in the field of molecular biology related to cardiology and immunology will be needed to mirror the surgical clinical progress made in the last decade—perhaps not as spectacular and obviously newsworthy as the heart transplant operation itself but surely of greater importance!

To help answer this and other problems in heart and heart–lung transplantation, accurate documentation of large numbers of patients need to be analysed. Only then can the importance of risk factors for coronary occlusive disease, the impact of improved immunosuppressive regimens, or the potential for HLA and DR matching be validated statistically.

Registration of patients in the international register held by Dr M. Kaye on behalf of the International Heart Transplant Society provides essential demographic data. It is, however, only valuable if the input is complete and updated. Making registration in the USA mandatory is a welcome but unfortunate necessity and I would urge all units worldwide to complete their annual returns accurately. Only then can potentially embarrassing and erroneous conclusions based on inadequate data be avoided.

Other registers should be supported, such as the one held in Heidelberg by Dr G. Opelz which demontrates the effects of HLA and DR matching on the outcome of heart transplantation. Although little practically can be done today, advances in organ preservation and storage may subsequently enable us to take advantage of any benefits that may be shown to arise as a result of better matching.

This book, I hope, has documented the progress of heart and heart–lung transplantation to the present day. There are omissions, but I hope few commissions. The authors are drawn worldwide for their expertise and have produced excellent comprehensive chapters. I thank them all for their contributions. I thank also my secretary Pam Norman, and above all my retired colleague Ben Milstein whose editing assistance has been truly invaluable.

John Wallwork
Papworth Everard, 1988

Contents

Part I

Heart Transplantation

Steven L. Lansman, M. Arisan Ergin
and Randall B. Griepp

1

History of Cardiac Transplantation

INTRODUCTION

Cardiac transplantation, once characterized as 'a fantastic speculation for the future' (Marcus *et al.*, 1951), is now widely accepted by the medical and lay communities as an effective therapeutic procedure. Although there was a 60-year history of sporadic experimentation, in 1964 there still remained 'some problems which require solution before the golden moment in tissue transplantation is upon us' (Shumway and Lower, 1964). These 'key problems' can be categorized into five areas: (1) technique; (2) recipient protection and graft preservation during transfer; (3) physiology of the transplanted heart; (4) immunology; (5) legal/logistic. This chapter reviews some of the major experimental and clinical efforts in heart transplantation and their contributions toward solving these problems.

Contributions have been divided into clinical and experimental work, and the latter into three historically overlapping types — those involving heterotopic non-auxiliary models, heterotopic auxiliary models, and orthotopic models. These models are schematized in Fig. 1.1.

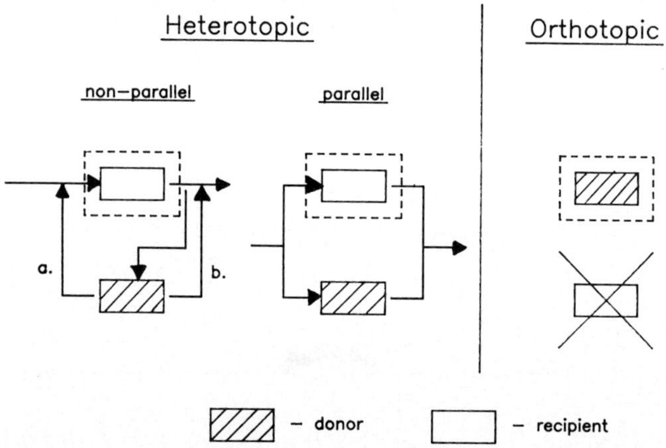

Fig. 1.1. *Schematization of experimental heart transplant models (graft outflow: a, Carrel model; b, Mann model).*

EXPERIMENTAL HEART TRANSPLANTATION

Heterotopic non-auxiliary heart transplantation

The first cardiac transplant was performed by Alexis Carrel and C. C. Guthrie at the University of Chicago in 1905 (Carrel and Guthrie, 1905). In seeking to establish techniques of vascular anastomoses, 'the replantation of a limb, the transplantation of the heart and kidney, and the replantation of the thyroid gland were performed'. The full description of their heart transplant experiment is as follows (Carrel and Guthrie, 1905):

> The heart of a small dog was extirpated and transplanted into the neck of a larger one by anastomosing the cut ends of the jugular vein and the carotid artery to the aorta, the pulmonary artery, one of the venae cavae and a pulmonary vein. The circulation was reestablished through the heart, about an hour and 15 minutes after the cessation of the beat; 20 minutes after the reestablishment of the circulation, the blood was actively circulating through the coronary system. A small opening being made through the wall of a small branch of the coronary vein, an abundant dark hemorrhage was produced. Then strong fibrillar contractions were seen. Afterward contractions of the auricles appeared, and about an hour after the operation, effective contractions of the ventricles began. The transplanted heart beat at the rate of 88 per minute, while the rate of the normal heart was 100 per minute. A little later tracings were taken. Owing to the fact that the operation was made without aseptic technique, coagulation occurred in the cavities of the heart after about two hours, and the experiment was interrupted.

Although the exact details of their experiment are not known, the most likely arrangement of anastomoses is depicted in Fig. 1.2. Perhaps one of the difficulties with this model was that atrial inflow under arterial pressure

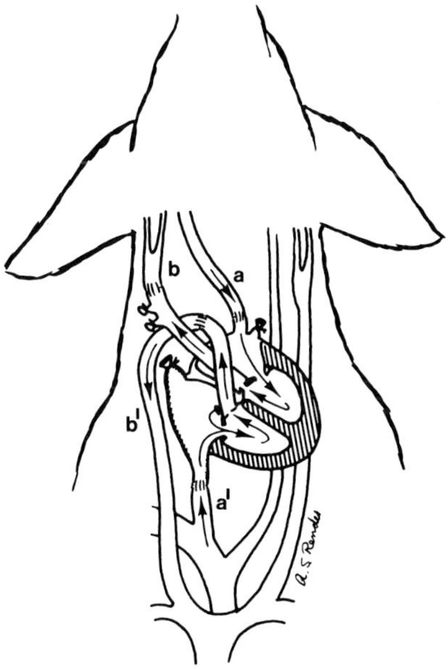

Fig. 1.2. *Possible anastomotic arrangement used by Carrel and Guthrie in 1905 (a, distal carotid artery; a′, proximal carotid artery; b, distal jugular vein; b′, proximal jugular vein). (From Najarian, J. S. and Simmons, R. L. (Eds) (1972).* Transplantation, *p. 532. Lea and Febiger, Philadelphia. Reproduced by permission.)*

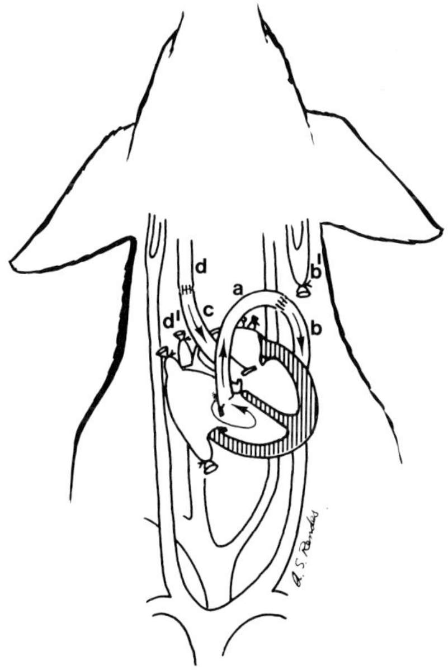

Fig. 1.3. *Anastomotic arrangement used by Mann and co-workers in 1933 (a, pulmonary artery; b, proximal jugular vein; b′, distal jugular vein, ligated; c, aorta; d, distal carotid artery; d′, proximal carotid artery, ligated). (From Najarian, J. S. and Simmons, R. L. (Eds) (1972).* Transplantation, *p. 532. Lea and Febiger, Philadelphia. Reproduced by permission.)*

combined with aortic outflow under venous pressure provided poor coronary perfusion during most of the cardiac cycle.

Despite these problems, this experiment addressed several of the key problems discussed above. In terms of technique, it demonstrated that cardiac transplantation was possible, and provided a model wherein all four chambers had pumping function. Perhaps more important, the demonstration that the heart could be separated from its blood supply and sutured into the circulation of a second animal, and yet recover organized contractions, brought into focus the issue of 'myocardial preservation' during the ischaemic transfer period. Lastly, rudimentary physiological observations were made on the transplanted heart.

The next reference to transplantation of the mammalian heart was in 1933 by Mann, Priestley, Markowitz and Yater, working at the Mayo Clinic and Georgetown University (Mann *et al.*, 1933). Seeking a denervated heart model, these authors systematically studied technical aspects of transplanting the canine heart into the carotid–jugular circulation. Their most successful model, shown in Fig. 1.3, was simple, with only the right ventricle functioning as a pump, yet the problem of coronary perfusion inherent in Carrel's model was solved. The aorta was anastomosed to either the proximal or distal cut end of the carotid artery, establishing arterial inflow to the coronary circulation, while the pulmonary artery was anastomosed to the recipient jugular vein, establishing venous outflow via the coronary sinus. Mann made contributions toward several of the 'key problems' with this model. In terms of technique, the model was reliably successful. The longest survival was 8 days and the mean survival 4 days.

Regarding myocardial preservation, the authors advised avoiding ventricular distension prior to establishing contractions, and avoiding coronary air embolism. In addition, well-documented observations on 'the general behavior of the transplanted heart' were made. The heart rate was found to be 'surprisingly constant' at 100–130 beats/min and the ECG was 'surprisingly normal'. Observing that both donor and recipient heart rates increased with exercise, whereas thyroxine increased only the donor rate, the authors concluded that thyroxine directly induced tachycardia, but that central nervous inhibition maintained a constant recipient rate. Lastly, the authors made the first observations on the phenomenon of cardiac allograft rejection, noting 'histologically the heart was completely infiltrated with lymphocytes, large mononuclears and polymorphonuclears'. They concluded (Mann *et al.*, 1933):

> It is readily seen that the failure of the homotransplanted heart to survive is not due to the technique of transplantation but to some biologic factor which is probably identical to that which prevents survival of other homotransplanted tissues and organs.

Interest in cardiac transplantation waned until 1951 when Marcus, Wong and Luisada (1951), working at the Chicago Medical School, reported their experience with a slightly modified Mann preparation (Marcus I technique). These authors were interested in cardiac transplantation *per se*:

> The problem which we are attempting to explore can then be stated as follows: Can a combination of highly specialized tissues . . . the heart be grafted in a mammalian animal? Can such a graft live in an homologous environment? Can such a graft actually function by receiving and delivering blood? Whether it might so function as to replace its counterpart in the host is a matter of fantastic speculation for the future.

Marcus focused on the problem of donor organ preservation and decided that improved survival might be obtained in two ways. Concerned that autonomic stimulation during graft excision might induce arrhythmias and ventricular distension, the authors performed bilateral cervical vagotomy in the donor dogs and injected cocaine into the pericardium prior to harvesting. In addition, it was felt that any period of ischaemia was harmful and an elaborate system of 'interim parabiotic perfusion' was developed whereby the graft was cannulated and perfused by a third animal during transfer. The results, however, were disappointing; only 10 of 22 experiments were successful and maximum survival was 48 h, demonstrating that more complicated procedures are not necessarily better ones. The authors noted that 'perhaps the greatest deterrent to long survival of the transplanted heart is the biologic problem of tissue specificity' and commented (Marcus, Wong and Luisada, 1951):

> . . . a transplanted heart or heart–lung preparation might be used for replacement of a diseased organ. The latter must be considered, at present, a fantastic dream, and does not fall within the scope of present considerations.

In 1953, Marcus, Wong and Luisada again modified the Mann preparation, so that the donor left ventricle would act as a pump (Marcus, Wong and Luisada, 1953). The proximal end of the divided recipient common carotid artery was anastomosed to the donor left atrium and the recipient distal common carotid to the donor innominate artery, so that the donor left ventricle supplied blood to its own coronary arteries and to the recipient cerebral circulation. Maximum survival with this technique was still 48 h.

The Mann preparation remained a valuable tool for evaluating the transplanted heart (Hairston, 1965; Cooper, 1968). In 1953, Downie, working at the Ontario Veterinary College, reported excellent results with the original Mann technique: 23 of 30 experiments were successful. Ischaemic times ranged from 30 to 45 min, and the maximum survival time was 10 days. Downie demonstrated that with simple techniques successful heterotopic transplantation was routinely possible and he attributed his improved results to the use of penicillin and the availability of convenient commercial suture material. Commenting upon possible clinical application, Downie (1953) stated:

> In the present state of knowledge it is not likely that homotransplantation of the usual tissues afflicted by disease will achieve great prominence clinically . . . homotransplantation of tissues has a melancholy record of failure in surgery. . . . The attempt to transplant tissues successfully from one subject to another is probably lacking in certain fundamental pieces of knowledge, much as is the case with our knowledge of carcinogenesis. In the one case we do not know why a cell continues to proliferate when it should not. In our case we do not know why a cell invites destruction when it ought to survive.

In 1962, Demikhov published a volume documenting, among other experiments, his work with heterotopic cardiac transplantation (Demikhov, 1962). He states that in 1940 he transplanted a dog heart into the inguinal region of a second animal and in 1946 he performed intrathoracic heterotopic cardiac transplants. Twenty-four anatomical variants were tried and in 1956 an intrathoracic heterotopic graft continued to beat for 32 days. The

TABLE 1.1
Maximum Survival in Experimental Heterotopic Non-Auxiliary Heart Transplantation

Reference	*Survival*
Carrel and Guthrie (1905)	2 h
Mann *et al.* (1933)	8 days
Marcus, Wong and Luisada (1951)	2 days
Downie (1953)	10 days
Demikhov (1962)*	32 days

* Operation took place in 1956.

long survival of this animal strengthened Demikhov's fervent belief that failures of all transplanted organs were due to technical rather than immunological factors (Demikhov, 1962):

On the basis of physiological, clinical and macroscopic observations, it can be stated that the period of function of the transplanted heart in a foreign organism objectively established for 32 days is not in agreement with current immunological views regarding reactions of incompatibility to a homotransplant.

Maximal survival times of heterotopic, non-functioning cardiac transplants are reviewed in Table 1.1.

Heterotopic auxiliary heart transplantation

Intrathoracic heterotopic cardiac transplantation, performed without interrupting the recipient's circulation, raised the possibility that a cardiac allograft might assume some or all of the circulatory load.

Demikhov performed 22 canine intrathoracic auxiliary heart transplants between 1951 and 1955 (Demikhov, 1962). With the donor heart fully resuscitated, the recipient heart was excluded from the circulation by ligating its great vessels and mitral annulus. In 1955, one such animal awoke from anaesthesia, stood up and drank, but died suddenly after 15 h of auxiliary heart function. Death was attributed to superior vena caval thrombosis. This animal was the first in which the circulation was completely supported for a significant period of time by a transplanted heart. Reemtsma, also studying canine intrathoracic auxiliary heart transplants, reported improved graft survival using amethopterin or azathioprine immunosuppression, but initially donor heart circulatory function was not measured (Reemtsma, 1964). However, in a subsequent series (McGough, Brewer and Reemtsma, 1966) the recipient heart was fibrillated, transferring total circulatory function to the donor heart. In one such experiment, the donor heart maintained the circulation for 4 h.

TABLE 1.2
Maximum Survival in Experimental Heterotopic Auxiliary Heart Transplantation

Reference	*Survival*
Demikhov (1962)*	15 h
McGough, Brewer and Reemstma (1966)	4 h
Johansson, Soderlund and William-Olsson (1967)	1 h

* Operation took place in 1955.

Later, Johansson, Soderlund and William-Olsson (1967), at the Karolinska Institute in Stockholm, reported a technique of intrathoracic heterotopic transplantation in which the graft functioned as an auxiliary left heart bypass pump. The donor venae cavae were ligated and coronary venous return was vented via a tube connecting the donor pulmonary artery and recipient right atrium. Parallel systemic circulation was established via tubes connecting the recipient and donor left atria and aortae. In this model, total left heart bypass was demonstrated by clamping the recipient aorta. In particular, during induced recipient heart fibrillation, the donor heart functioned as a left heart bypass pump, yet adequate cardiac output was maintained for periods of up to 1 h. The pulmonary circulation was maintained passively by the elevated central venous pressure.

These experiments with heterotopic auxiliary cardiac transplantation are listed in Table 1.2.

Orthotopic cardiac transplantation

By the early 1950s the technical feasibility of cardiac transplantation was well established and transplanted heart physiology was being studied. However, development in the third, 'orthotopic', phase of experimental cardiac transplantation awaited solutions to problems involving the critical 'transfer period', during which the recipient heart is excised and the donor heart is excised and implanted. Specifically, the problems concerned the means of maintaining the recipient and preserving the graft during this transfer period, and the development of a simplified surgical technique to minimize its length.

In 1953, Neptune and colleagues addressed all of these problems in their published report, entitled 'Complete homologous heart transplantation' (Neptune *et al.*, 1953). Clearly interested in orthotopic heart transplantation *per se*, the authors attempted to simplify the procedure by transplanting an entire heart–lung block, thus avoiding the multiple pulmonary venous anastomoses. The problem of donor myocardial protection and recipient preservation were simultaneously solved as both animals were 'placed in an ordinary beverage cooler for the production of hypothermia' (Neptune *et al.*, 1953):

> By the use of hypothermia we have been able to completely stop all circulation for periods up to 30 minutes without subsequent morbidity or mortality. It occurred to us that such a period of time would be more than ample to perform a complete transplantation of the heart — removal of the recipient animal's heart and the substitution by a donor heart.

The authors reported successful heart–lung transplantation in 3 dogs with survival of up to 6 h with these techniques. Although subsequent technical developments obviated the need to transplant the entire heart–lung block, hypothermia has remained indispensable during cardiopulmonary bypass for recipient protection and during the ischaemic period for donor graft preservation.

In 1957, Webb and Howard reported on, 'Restoration of function of the refrigerated heart' (Webb and Howard, 1957), and demonstrated that canine hearts, heparinized and flushed with potassium citrate, can survive for prolonged periods at low temperatures (4°C) yet return to adequate function when transplanted heterotopically (Marcus II technique). Perhaps anticipating current long-distance procurement procedures, Webb and Howard (1957) commented:

> Demonstration that the heart can be maintained viable and functional for periods of at least 8 hours by refrigeration in a nutrient medium has been of great value to us in experimental work in cardiac and cardiopulmonary transplants. When the problems of immunology are solved and transplantation becomes a clinical possibility, it will presumably require several hours for obtaining the heart, preparation of the recipient and total reimplantation. The practices outlined would seem to make cardiac transplantation completely feasible so far as this time element is concerned.

In 1958, Goldberg, Berman and Akman, at the University of Maryland, reported the first three experimental orthotopic cardiac transplants (Goldberg, Berman and Akman, 1958). In terms of technique, the authors comment: 'The chief innovation was transection of the left auricle to circumvent the anastomoses of the several pulmonary veins.' In other words, the recipient heart was excised so as to leave a posterior 'cuff' of left atrium containing the openings of the multiple pulmonary veins, thus requiring one large, relatively simple left atrial anastomosis rather than multiple small pulmonary venous anastomoses. The cavae were reconnected with methylmethacrylate tubes and the aorta and pulmonary arteries were re-anastomosed. The recipient circulation was maintained with cardiopulmonary bypass during the transfer and the donor heart was arrested with potassium citrate prior to excision, but hypothermia was not employed for either. Interestingly, the authors comment: 'further study of the conditions which make for the least injury to the myocardium in transport is indicated.' Ischaemic times ranged from 25 to 33 min and the longest support of the circulation by the allograft was approximately 20 min.

Webb, Howard and Neely, in 1959, using their previously described method of 'refrigeration' (Webb and Howard, 1957) to preserve the donor heart, and the pump-oxygenator to maintain the recipient, accomplished 12 successful orthotopic transplants (Webb, Howard and Neely, 1959). The aortic and pulmonary anastomoses were sutured, whereas the individual pulmonary veins were joined using vascular couplers. Interestingly, the authors noted that these latter anastomoses could be facilitated by leaving a left atrial cuff on all four recipient pulmonary veins. Donor heart ischaemic times ranged from 2 to 4 h. Two dogs succumbed within minutes of surgery, but the remaining 10 survived for periods ranging from 30 to 450 min.

In 1959, Cass and Brock, working at Guy's Hospital in London, reported six methods of cardiac excision and replacement (Cass and Brock, 1959). The first five were autotransplants, but the sixth was an orthotopic transplant, significant because the authors describe a method in which the native heart was 'separated from the venae cavae and pulmonary veins by dividing through the walls of the atria', thus forming both right and left atrial 'cuffs'. This is the first description of the now standard practice of combining the multiple pulmonary venous and vena caval anastomoses into two atrial anastomoses. Suture line bleeding limited the experiment's success, although the graft did maintain the circulation for 1 h.

In 1960, Lower and Shumway published a cardinal paper in orthotopic transplantation (Lower and Shumway, 1960) in which previously described advances in technique, recipient support and donor preservation were integrated into a single approach. Recipient protection during the transfer period was provided by cardiopulmonary bypass under conditions of moderate hypothermia (30°C), induced by surface cooling. Hypothermia was also employed for donor heart preservation by rapidly immersing the excised heart in iced saline (4°C) for 5 min. The heart was implanted using suture anastomoses and the ischaemic time, averaging 1 h, was minimized by combining the pulmonary venous and vena caval anastomoses into two atrial 'cuff' anastomoses (Fig. 1.4).

Five of 8 consecutive transplant recipients survived 6–21 days, eating and exercising normally in the postoperative period. This was the first description of a simple, routinely successful technique for mammalian orthotopic cardiac transplantation whereby recipients returned to normal activity, their circulation supported by a transplanted heart.

No immunosuppression was given to these animals and death was apparently due to rapid myocardial failure associated with massive infiltration of

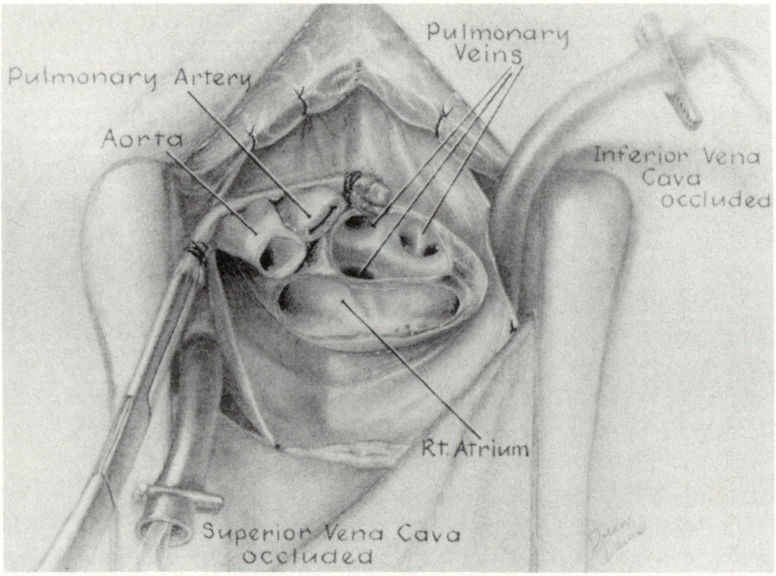

Fig. 1.4. *Essentials of the surgical technique used by Lower and Shumway in 1960 in the first successful series of orthotopic canine cardiac transplants. Recipient pericardial cavity after removal of the recipient heart. Note the long stumps of the aorta and pulmonary artery and the combination of venous anastomoses into the atrial cuffs. (From Lower, R. R., Stofer, R. C. and Shumway, N. E. (1961). Homovital transplantation of the heart.* J. Thorac. Cardiovasc. Surg. **41**, *196–204. Reproduced by permission.)*

round cells and interstitial haemorrhage. Lower and Shumway (1960) concluded:

> Observations on these animals suggest that, if the immunologic mechanisms of the host were prevented from destroying the graft, in all likelihood it would continue to function adequately for the normal life span of the animal.

Kondo and colleagues, in 1965, working at the Maimonides Hospital in Brooklyn, New York, used the technique of Lower and Shumway but reported a different approach to recipient protection (Kondo *et al.*, 1965). In this series, rapid donor heart excision and immersion in iced saline were preceded by donor surface cooling to 27°C. Recipients, surface cooled to 16°C, underwent cardiac replacement during a 60 min period of hypothermic circulatory arrest followed by surface rewarming. In 37 experiments, 18 animals survived more than 1 week, 12 more than 2 weeks, and 1 animal survived for 213 days. These experiments, performed on puppies, were conducted without immunosuppression and the authors attributed the long survivals to the relative immunological incompetence of very young animals.

Following the initial report by Lower and Shumway, a number of reports

pulseless and comatose. Management included vasopressors, tracheostomy, mechanical ventilation, femoral embolectomy and below-knee amputation. Elsewhere in the hospital a young patient was dying of irreversible brain damage, but the team was faced with the same legal/logistic problems (Hardy *et al.*, 1964):

> . . . experience with the previous case had underscored the fact that, for a homotransplant to succeed, the donor and the recipient must 'die' at almost the same time; although this might occur, the chances that both prospective donor and prospective recipient would enter fatal collapse simultaneously were very slim . . . the prospective recipient went into terminal shock . . . and it was obvious that if heart transplantation were to be performed it must be done at once. Meanwhile, the condition of the prospective donor was not such that death appeared to be immediately imminent. At this time a tranquilizing drug was given to the larger of the two chimpanzees.

Eventually, events forced a difficult decision, as 'the patient was on cardiopulmonary bypass and the prospective human donor lingered on in the recovery ward. The larger chimpanzee had already been anaesthetized in an adjacent operating room'. It was decided to proceed using the primate heart. The suture technique of Lower and Shumway (1960) was employed, but donor graft preservation was provided by retrograde coronary sinus perfusion with chilled, oxygenated blood. The transplant, technically satisfactory, was unable to maintain the circulatory load and approximately 1 h after cardiopulmonary bypass attempts at circulatory support were abandoned.

Interestingly, in 1966, a mirror image experiment was performed at the Medical College of Virginia by Lower (Griepp, 1984). Studies were performed on the resuscitation of human cadaver hearts after kidney donor harvesting. In one such experiment, the resuscitated heart was successfully transplanted into a baboon. The large donor heart precluded closing the animal's chest, but satisfactory circulatory support was maintained for several hours until the experiment was electively terminated.

Although never reported in the medical literature, this experience was well known to several surgeons interested in cardiac transplantation. It confirmed for human donor hearts the laboratory observations that the heart could be stopped, removed, resuscitated, and successfully transplanted.

On 3 December 1967, the first successful clinical cardiac transplant was performed by Barnard at the Groote Schuur Hospital in Cape Town, South Africa (Barnard, 1967). The historical context in which the procedure took place was described (Barnard, 1967):

> This achievement did not come as a surprise to the medical world. Steady progress towards this goal has been made by immunologists, biochemists, surgeons and specialists in other branches of medical science all over the world during the past decades to ensure that this, the ultimate in cardiac surgery, would be a success.

In the following paragraph, a somewhat broader perspective on transplantation was offered:

> The dream of the ancients from time immemorial has been the junction of portions of different individuals, not only to counteract disease, but also to combine the potentials of different species. This desire inspired the birth of many mythical creatures which were purported to have capabilities normally beyond the power of a single species. The modern world has inherited these dreams in the form of the sphinx, the mermaid and the chimerical forms of many heraldic beasts.

A 54-year-old man dying of end-stage ischaemic heart disease received the heart of a young man with severe brain injury, who was certified dead 5 min after the absence of ECG activity, spontaneous respirations and reflexes. At that time, the donor chest was opened and cardiopulmonary bypass was initiated to resuscitate the heart. The donor was cooled to 26°C, and the heart, cooled to 16°C, was vented via the left ventricular apex, removed, and immersed in iced saline. The aortic cannula provided coronary perfusion during implantation. The recipient recovered, but succumbed to pseudomonas pneumonia after 18 days.

Three days after this first cardiac transplant, Adrian Kantrowitz, in Brooklyn, New York, transplanted the heart of an anencephalic infant into an 18-day-old child with Ebstein's anomaly using deep hypothermia (Kantrowitz *et al.*, 1968). Although the procedure was technically satisfactory, the recipient developed unremitting acidosis and lived only $6\frac{1}{2}$ h.

In these early cases, failure to come to grips with the concept of brain death created difficult logistic situations. Similar considerations prompted Shumway to comment (Shumway, Dong and Stinson, 1969):

> It should be underlined that no one can transplant a dead heart. The hearts which have been transplanted by surgeons all over the world could have been resuscitated in the donors, and the chests could have been closed, leaving these hopelessly brain-injured persons to the fate of infection or peripheral vascular collapse. Death of the donor is a diagnosis which must be made by the neurological and neurosurgical team.

No other cardiac transplants were done in 1967, but by the end of 1968, 102 had been performed in 17 countries. Early results were discouraging, however, and by 1970 all but several institutions had abandoned the procedure. During the 1970s, clinical investigations, principally at Stanford University, California, steadily established the key elements necessary for success in cardiac transplantation. One-year survival increased from 22% in 1968 to 65% in 1978 (Griepp, 1979), with rehabilitation to normal function in 90% (Christopherson *et al.*, 1976). Early clinical results (Stinson *et al.*, 1970), infectious complications (Stinson, 1971), and the haemodynamics of the transplanted heart were reported (Griepp *et al.*, 1971a; Stinson *et al.*, 1972), indications and contraindications for the procedure were defined (Griepp *et al.*, 1971b), and donor management described (Griepp *et al.*,

1971c). The diagnosis of cardiac allograft rejection was greatly advanced by Philip Caves, who developed a bioptome for obtaining repeated transvenous endomyocardial biopsies, and by Margaret Billingham, who described a histological system for grading rejection in these specimens (Caves *et al.*, 1974). The treatment of rejection was greatly enhanced by the use of rabbit antithymocyte globulin (Griepp *et al.*, 1972; Bieber *et al.*, 1976; Baumgartner *et al.*, 1978), and survival was prolonged by the control of graft arteriosclerosis (Griepp *et al.*, 1977) and the advent of cardiac re-transplantation (Copeland *et al.*, 1977). In addition, donor organ availability increased as the concept of 'brain death' became accepted (Report Ad Hoc Committee Harvard, 1968; Black, 1978) and methods of long-distance procurement were developed (Watson *et al.*, 1979; Thomas *et al.*, 1978).

The 1980s have witnessed a worldwide wave of enthusiasm for cardiac transplantation, spurred on by promising results with cyclosporin immunosuppression at Stanford University (Oyer *et al.*, 1983). In terms of logistics, national computerized procurement networks have arisen to help satisfy the growing demand for donors.

Thus, the current success of cardiac transplantation is grounded in a long progression of experimental and clinical advances. Beginning with an isolated heart transplant performed as a technical exercise in 1905, slowly, accumulated experimental efforts yielded solutions to problems involving technique, recipient and graft protection, post-transplant function and immunology, and provided a foundation for subsequent clinical human heart transplantation. Recent work has concentrated on refining these solutions and on addressing the legal and logistic issues involved in human cardiac transplantation.

REFERENCES

Barnard, C. N. (1967). A human cardiac transplant: an interim report of a successful operation performed at Groote Schuur Hospital, Capetown. *S. Afr. Med. J.* **41**, 1271–1274.

Baumgartner, W. A., Reitz, B. A., Bieber, C. P., Oyer, P. E., Shumway, N. E. and Stinson, E. B. (1978). Current expectations in cardiac transplantation. *J. Thorac. Cardiovasc. Surg.* **75**(4), 525–530.

Bieber, C. P., Griepp, R. B., Oyer, P. E., Wong, J. and Stinson, E. B. (1976). Use of rabbit antithymocyte globulin in cardiac transplantation. *Transplantation* **22**(5), 478–488.

Black, P. M. (1978). Brain death. *New Engl. J. Med.* **299**(7), 338–344.

Carrel, A. and Guthrie, C. C. (1905). The transplantation of veins and organs. *Am. Med.* **10**, 1101–1102.

Cass, M. H. and Brock, Sir R. (1959). Heart excision and replacement. *Guy's Hosp. Reps.* **108**, 285–290.

Caves, P. K., Billingham, M. E., Stinson, E. B. and Shumway, N. E. (1974). Serial transvenous biopsy of the transplanted human heart. Improved management of acute rejection episodes. *Lancet* **1**, 821–826.

Christopherson, L. K., Griepp, R. B. and Stinson, E. B. (1976). Rehabilitation after cardiac transplantation. *J. Am. Med. Ass.* **236**(18), 2082–2084.

Cooper, D. K. C. (1968). Experimental development of cardiac transplantation. *Br. Med. J.* **4**, 174–181.

Copeland, J. G., Griepp, R. B., Bieber, C. P., Billingham, M., Schroeder, J. S., Hunt, S., Mason, J., Stinson, E. B. and Shumway, N. E. (1977). Successful retransplantation of the human heart. *J. Thorac. Cardiovasc. Surg.* **73**(2), 242–247.

Demikhov, V. P. (1962). *Experimental Transplantation of Vital Organs* (B. Haigh, Trans.). Consultants' Bureau, New York.

Downie, H. G. (1953). Homotransplantation of the dog heart. *Am. Med. Ass. Arch. Surg.* **66**, 624–636.

Goldberg, M., Berman, E. F. and Akman, L. C. (1958). Homologous transplantation of the canine heart. *J. Int. Coll. Surgeons* **30**(5), 575–586.

Griepp, R. B. (1979). A decade of human heart transplantation. *Transplant. Proc.* **11**(1), 285–292.

Griepp, R. B. (1984). The history of experimental heart transplantation. *Heart Transplant.* **3**(2), 145–151.

Griepp, R. B., Stinson, E. B., Bieber, C. P., Reitz, B. A., Copeland, J. G., Oyer, P. E. and Shumway, N. E. (1977). Control of graft arteriosclerosis in human heart transplant recipients. *Surgery* **81**, 262–269.

Griepp, R. B., Stinson, E. B., Clark, D. A., Dong, E. Jr. and Shumway, N. E. (1971c). Cardiac transplantation in man. IX. The cardiac donor. *Surg. Gyn. Obstet.* **133**, 792–798.

Griepp, R. B., Stinson, E. B., Dong, E. Jr., Clark, D. A. and Shumway, N. E. (1971a). Hemodynamic performance of the transplanted human heart. *Surgery* **70**, 88–95.

Griepp, R. B., Stinson, E. B., Dong, E. Jr., Clark, D. A. and Shumway, N. E. (1971b). Determinants of operative risk in human heart transplantation. *Am. J. Surg.* **122**, 192–197.

Griepp, R. B., Stinson, E. B., Dong, E. Jr., Phillips, R. C., Morrell, R. M. and Shumway, N. E. (1972). The use of antithymocyte globulin in human heart transplantation. *Circulation* **45–46**(Suppl. I), 147–153.

Hairston, P. (1965). Heart transplantation: past, present and future. *J. Thorac. Cardiovasc. Surg.* **50**(1), 1–8.

Hardy, J. D., Chavez, C. M., Kurrus, F. D., Neely, W. A., Eraslan, S., Turner, D., Fabian, L. W. and Labecki, T. D. (1964). Heart transplantation in man. *J. Am. Med. Ass.* **188**(13), 114–122

Johansson, L., Soderlund, S. and William-Olsson, G. (1967). Left heart bypass by means of a transplanted heart. *Scand. J. Thor. Cardiovasc. Surg.* **1**, 23–26.

Kantrowitz, A., Huller, J. D., Joos, H., Cerroti, M. M. and Carstensen, H. E. (1968). Transplantation of the heart in an infant and an adult. *Am. J. Cardiol.* **22**, 782–790.

Kondo, Y., Grundel, F. O., Chaptal, P. A., Meier, W., Cottle, H. E. and Kantrowitz, A. (1965). Immediate and delayed orthotopic homotransplantation of the heart. *J. Thorac. Cardiovasc. Surg.* **50**(6), 781–791.

Lower, R. R., Dong, E. Jr. and Shumway, N. E. (1965). Long-term survival of cardiac homografts. *Surgery* **58**(1), 110–119.

Lower, R. R. and Shumway, N. E. (1960). Studies in orthotopic homotransplantation of the canine heart. *Surg. Forum* **11**, 18–19.

Lower, R. R., Stofer, R. C. and Shumway, N. E. (1961). Homovital transplantation of the heart. *J. Thorac. Cardiovasc. Surg.* **41**(2), 196–204.

Mann, F. C., Priestley, J. T., Markowitz, J. & Yater, W. M. (1933). Transplantation of the intact mammalian heart. *Arch. Surg.* **26**, 219–224.

Marcus, E., Wong, S. N. T. and Luisada, A. A. (1951). Homologous heart grafts: transplantation of the heart in dogs. *Surg. Forum* **2**, 212–217.

Marcus, E., Wong, S. N. T. and Luisada, A. A. (1953). Technique of interim parabiotic perfusion. II. Transplantation in dogs. *Archives of Surgery* **66**, 179–191.

McGough, E. C., Brewer, P. L. and Reemtsma, K. (1966). The parallel heart: studies of intrathoracic auxiliary cardiac transplants. *Surgery* **60**(1), 153–158.

Neptune, W. B., Cookson, B. A., Bailey, C. P., Appler, R. and Rajkowski, F. (1953). Complete homologous heart transplantation. *Am. Med. Ass. Arch. Surg.* **66**, 174–178.

Oyer, P. E., Stinson, E. B., Jamieson, S. A., Hunt, S. A., Billingham, M., Scott, W., Bieber, C. P., Reitz, B. A. and Shumway, N. E. (1983). Cyclosporin A in cardiac allografting: a preliminary experience. *Transplant Proc.* **15**, 1247–1252.

Reemtsma, K. (1964). The heart as a test organ in transplantation studies. *Ann. N. Y. Acad. Sci.* **120**, 778–785.

Report of the Ad Hoc Committee of the Harvard Medical School to Examine the Definition of Brain Death (1968). A definition of irreversible coma. *J. Am. Med. Ass.* **205**(6), 85–88.

Shumway, N. E., Dong, E. and Stinson, B. (1969). Surgical aspects of cardiac transplantation in man. *Bull. N.Y. Acad. Med.* **45**(5), 387–393.

Shumway, N. E. and Lower, R. R. (1964). Special problems in transplantation of the heart. *Ann. N.Y. Acad. Sci.* **120**, 773–777.

Stinson, E. B., Griepp, R. B., Clark, D. A., Dong, E. Jr. and Shumway, N. E. (1970). Cardiac transplantation in man. VIII. Survival and function. *J. Thorac. Cardiovasc. Surg.* **60**, 303–321.

Stinson, E. B., Griepp, R. B., Schroeder, J. S., Dong, E. Jr. and Shumway, N. E. (1972). Hemodynamic observations one and two years after cardiac transplantation in man. *Circulation* **45**, 1183–1193.

Thomas, F. T., Szentpetery, S. S., Mammana, R. E., Wolfgang, T. C. and Lower, R. R. (1978). Long-distance transportation of human hearts for transplantation. *Ann. Thorac. Surg.* **26**(4), 344–350.

Watson, D. C., Reitz, B. A., Baumgartner, W. A., Raney, A. A., Oyer, P. E., Stinson, E. B. and Shumway, N. E. (1979). Distant heart procurement for transplantation. *Surgery* **86**(1), 56–59.

Webb, W. R. and Howard, H. S. (1957). Restoration of function of the refrigerated heart. *Surg. Forum* **8**, 302–306.

Webb, W. R., Howard, H. S. and Neely, W. A. (1959). Practical methods of homologous cardiac transplantation. *J. Thorac. Surg.* **37**(3), 361–366.

Margaret J. Dallman
and Peter J. Morris

2

The Rejection Reaction

INTRODUCTION

The transplantation of many organs, including heart and heart–lung (as evidenced in this volume), kidney, liver and pancreas is now quite successful. Despite more effective immunosuppression in recent years, the rejection of the transplanted organ by the recipient remains a continuing problem in all cases. The immunological nature of tissue rejection was firmly established over 40 years ago when Gibson and Medawar (1943) and Medawar (1944, 1945) found that skin grafts between genetically disparate humans and rabbits underwent rapid necrotic changes and were sloughed off. The rejection process displays marked specificity and memory for donor tissue and is accompanied by infiltration with leucocytes.

Since that time, our knowledge of the immune system has increased greatly and has been applied to the study of transplantation responses. We believe that the immune system responds to a foreign tissue in the main, as shown in Fig. 2.1. As may be seen, the events resulting in the destruction of the graft may be divided into two general parts: the afferent phase, when the immune system is alerted to the presence of the foreign tissue, and the efferent phase, when tissue destruction is effected. However, as will become evident in the subsequent sections in this chapter, we still remain very unsure of the exact mechanisms involved in both these phases of the immune response to a foreign tissue graft (see Table 2.1 for terminology). In this short review of the subject we can only highlight some of the current concepts and controversies in this extremely complex area, which is so central to the practice of transplantation.

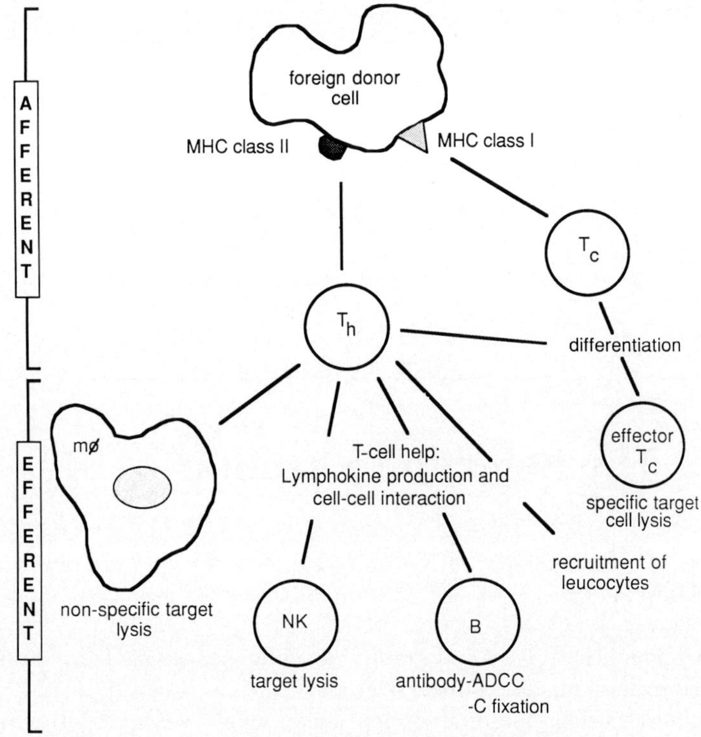

Fig. 2.1. *Immune response to an allograft. MHC classes I and II antigens are presented to the T lymphocytes of the recipient. Once triggered, the T helper cell produces a number of soluble lymphokines which are required for the proliferation, differentiation and recruitment of other leucocytes of the immune system. A variety of effector mechanisms may be involved in the efferent or destructive phase of the immune response. (MHC, major histocompatibility complex; T_h, T helper cell; T_c, T cytotoxic cell; mφ, macrophage; NK, natural killer; ADDC, antibody-dependent cellular cytotoxicity; C, complement).*

AFFERENT PHASE

Antigens

It is the foreign antigens (or glycoproteins) present on the cells of transplanted tissue that provoke graft rejection. The most important of these antigens in transplantation responses are those glycoproteins encoded by genes within the major histocompatibility complex (MHC). Differences in these cell surface antigens between donor and recipient were shown by Snell (1953) to cause more rapid rejection of both skin and tumour grafts than

TABLE 2.1
Terminology of Grafts

AUTOGRAFT	Transplantation of an individual's own tissue to another site, e.g. skin grafting in burn patients, a coronary artery bypass graft with saphenous vein
SYNGENEIC GRAFT (ISOGRAFT)	Transplantation of tissues between genetically identical members of the same species, e.g. kidney grafting between monozygotic twins
ALLOGRAFT	Transplantation of tissues between genetically disparate individuals of the same species, e.g. cadaveric heart or kidney transplantation
XENOGRAFT	Transplantation of tissues between individuals of different species, e.g. baboon heart to a human

antigenic differences coded for by other genetic loci. Although the MHC is the main genetic region controlling the rejection of heart, kidney and skin grafts (Bildsoe *et al.*, 1970; Bildsoe, 1972), primary grafts, identical with the recipient at the MHC, may be rejected under the influence of the so-called minor histocompatibility antigens (Goulmy, 1985; Peugh *et al.*, 1986). The structure and distribution of minor histocompatibility antigens has been difficult to assess. This is due mainly to our inability to raise antisera directed at minor histocompatibility antigens, which makes analysis of the presence of these molecules on certain cell types and of their biochemical nature extremely difficult.

One of the most notable aspects of the MHC (and one of the most frustrating for the transplantation surgeon) is the very high degree of polymorphism in the antigens it encodes. The biological significance of this polymorphism is not clearly defined, although the intimate involvement of the MHC in cellular interactions of the immune response suggests that the extensive polymorphism has evolved as a by-product of immune defence mechanisms against infection. However, it means that in transplantation it is possible to graft completely MHC identical material only between monozygotic twins. Thus, in the great majority of organ transplants, tissue rejection is a major problem, either as an acute reaction or as a more chronic process.

It may be seen from Fig. 2.2 that the MHC (called in the human the human leucocyte antigen or HLA region) encodes two types of antigens that induce transplantation rejection. The class I molecules are glycoproteins comprised of two chains, the heavy chain (mol. wt 45 kD), which is polymorphic, and a non-variable light chain, B_2 microglobulin (mol. wt 12 kD).

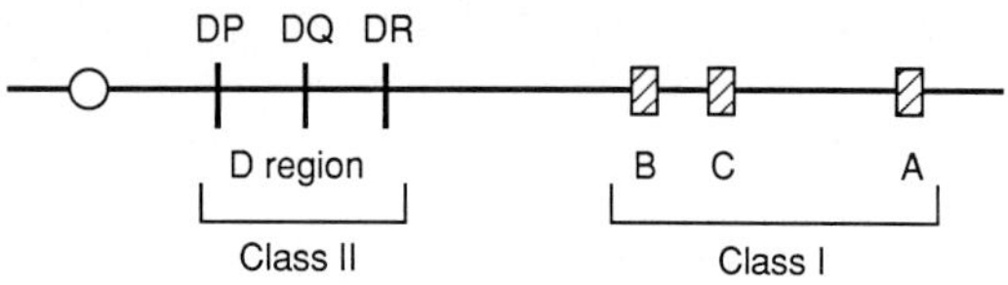

Fig. 2.2. *Simplified version of the genetic map of the MHC (or HLA region) of man. Solid bars indicate the position of loci encoding for class II antigens and hatched bars those encoding for class I molecules. Position in relation to the centromere (○) is shown.*

Such molecules are expressed on virtually all nucleated cells and are, in general, responsible for activating T cells of the CD8 phenotype (see Fig. 2.1). The class II molecules are also glycoproteins but comprised of two chains of similar molecular weight (alpha chain, mol. wt 35 kD; beta chain mol. wt 28 kD) and stimulate T cells mainly of the CD4 phenotype (see Fig. 2.1). The tissue distribution of class II antigens is far more restricted than that of class I molecules, being expressed only by B lymphocytes, dendritic cells and some endothelial cells. However, during the course of an immune response, most other cell types, with a few exceptions, may be induced to express class II molecules (Lampert, Suitters and Chisholm, 1981; Mason, Dallman and Barclay, 1981; Fellous *et al.*, 1982; de Waal *et al.*, 1983; Dallman and Mason, 1984; Wong *et al.*, 1984).

Incompatibility for either class I or class II antigens alone between donor and recipient may result in graft rejection. This has been demonstrated both in clinical transplantation and unequivocally in experimental transplantation using inbred animals differing only at well-defined regions of the MHC (Klein, 1977).

Stimulation of the recipient immune response

Although it is clear that MHC antigens stimulate graft rejection, the manner in which they are presented to the recipient is not so clearly understood. It is thought that bone marrow derived cells within the transplant, the so-called passenger leucocytes, play an important role in host sensitization. Of such cells, the dendritic cell seems to be a particularly potent stimulus of immune responses, at least in *in vitro* assay systems (Steinman and Witmer, 1978; Klinkert *et al.*, 1980; Mason, Pugh and Webb, 1981). These cells express particularly high levels of MHC class II antigens as well as MHC class I antigens and, as such, may be able to stimulate directly recipient T cells to initiate the rejection response (see Fig. 2.1). Passenger leucocytes with the characteristics of dendritic cells are found in a wide variety of organs (Hart and Fabre, 1981a; Daar *et al.*, 1983) and a number of experimental transplantation systems has been used to dissect the role of the dendritic cell in graft rejection.

Such experiments have been essentially of two types. First, grafts have been depleted of their own passenger leucocytes either by such means as irradiation or tissue culture of the graft, or by exchange with dendritic cells of recipient type (Guttman, Lindquist and Ockner, 1969; Steinmuller and Hart, 1971; Stuart *et al.*, 1971; Lafferty *et al.*, 1976; Emma and Jacobs, 1981). This latter situation is achieved by placing grafts in immunosuppressed animals of recipient origin and allowing the replacement of passenger leucocytes by cells of recipient type to result from the natural turnover of bone marrow derived cells. Secondly, induction of a rejection episode in long-term surviving grafts has been attempted using leucocytes of tissue donor origin (Lechler and Batchelor, 1982). In these types of experiments, the presence or origin of the passenger leucocyte may influence graft survival, but really clear data implicating the dendritic cell as the primary or only stimulus of graft rejection in *all* donor–recipient pairs are lacking. Further, one must interpret these experimental data with some caution when considering clinical transplantation rejection, since in rodents often the only cell within the graft to express MHC class II antigens is the passenger leucocyte, and thus this cell may be very important in recipient sensitization (Frelinger *et al.*, 1979; Katz, Tamaki and Sachs, 1979; Hart and Fabre, 1981b). However, in man (Fuggle *et al.*, 1983) vascular endothelial cells constitutively express these molecules and as such may also stimulate the rejection reaction.

The site of sensitization of the host is also of some debate since initiation of the immune response may occur either within the graft or within the draining lymphoid tissue (Billingham, Brent and Medawar, 1954; Mitchison, 1954; Strober and Gowans, 1965). The prolonged survival of grafts in anatomical positions lacking lymphatic drainage such as the brain (Medawar, 1948) or hamster cheek pouch (Billingham and Silvers, 1964) or when surgically deprived of lymphatic drainage (Barker and Billingham, 1968; Tilney and Gowans, 1971) suggests that sensitization may occur in the graft draining lymph nodes. However, it is also likely, particularly in fully vascularized organ grafts, that lymphocytes from the blood enter the transplant and become sensitized *in situ* (Pedersen and Morris, 1970, 1974).

Cellular events

Before discussing the cellular events involved in graft rejection, it is useful to give a brief outline of the cellular interactions which we believe to occur within the immune system (see Fig. 2.1). It is quite clear that, for the majority of antigens, including MHC antigens, T helper lymphocytes are required to interact with B lymphocytes which produce antibody, cytotoxic precursor lymphocytes which differentiate into effector cytotoxic cells, and macrophages which develop into cytocidal effector cells. Further, the T helper cell has an important role in attracting other leucocytes to the site of an immune reaction and also in increasing the activity of other cells such as the natural killer (NK) cell. This interaction may require direct cell–cell contact or be mediated via soluble molecules called lymphokines (Lafferty, Andrus and Prowse, 1980; Robb, 1984; Garland, 1986; Oppenheim *et al.*, 1986). The majority of T helper cells have the CD4 phenotype and interact with class II antigens (Cantor and Boyse, 1975a,b; Klein, Chiang and Hauptfeld, 1977). However, there seems to be a minority population of lymphocytes with the CD8 phenotype which may react with class I antigens to provide T cell help (Okada and Henney, 1980; Meuer *et al.*, 1982).

It has been clear for many years that T lymphocytes play an essential role in graft rejection, since both congenitally athymic nude mice (Rygaard, 1974), and T cell deprived animals (Rolstad and Ford, 1974; Hall, Dorsch and Roser, 1978), fail to reject either xenografts or allografts. Further, experiments both in the mouse (Loveland *et al.*, 1981) and rat (Dallman, Mason and Webb, 1982) have defined the central role of the T helper cell in skin graft rejection. These studies have shown that adoptive transfer of cells of the CD4 phenotype, but not of the CD8 phenotype, restores skin graft rejection in T cell deprived animals. More recently, such adoptive transfer studies have been extended by other workers to examine the cellular requirements for experimental heart and kidney allograft rejection (Gurley, Lowry and Clarke-Forbes, 1983; Hall, DeSaxe and Dorsch, 1983; Lowry, Gurley and Clarke-Forbes, 1983). Similar results have been obtained by these workers, although it has sometimes been found that, while cells of the CD4 phenotype are able to restore rejection alone, $CD8^+$ cells are required to restore the kinetics of the response to that of first set rejection in normal animals (Tilney *et al.*, 1984). These findings are somewhat confounded by the recent demonstration that in certain mutant mouse strains which differ only by a few amino acids in their class I molecules, only the $CD8^+$ cell is required to restore graft rejection (Sprent *et al.*, 1986). This may well be a reflection of the fact that it is possible, in a limited number of situations, to generate class I directed, $CD8^+$ helper cells. Recent data suggest that this is indeed the case (Rosenberg *et al.*, 1986; Rosenberg, Mizuochi and Singer, 1987). Such studies, however, give little information about the effector mechanisms of graft rejection and this area will be discussed later.

It has traditionally been thought that alloantigens on the surface of, for example, donor dendritic cells within the grafted organ, are able directly to stimulate T cells of the recipient that react with either class I or class II antigens. However, during an immune response to other non-MHC molecules (e.g. viral antigens) processing of the antigen by accessory cells (e.g. the dendritic cell or macrophage) of host origin occurs to allow presentation of antigen in association with self-MHC molecules (MHC restriction). Recent work suggests that processing and presentation in association with self-MHC molecules may also occur for alloantigens (Sherwood, Brent and Rayfield, 1986). In these experiments, host strain peritoneal cells, sensitized by donor alloantigen, could transfer an accelerated rejection response of donor strain skin to naive host strain mice. This was not due simply to transfer of sensitized T cells, since T cell depleted adherent cells transferred the effect. It was suggested that dendritic cells or other accessory cells carrying processed antigen were stimulating host T cells. In summary, it seems possible that host T cells may be stimulated by direct interaction with cells of donor origin and, in addition, with processed antigen in a self-MHC restricted fashion.

Stimulation of B lymphocytes is a much simpler process, since it is known that B lymphocytes may be activated by direct interaction with antigens via their surface immunoglobulin receptors. Following an interaction with T helper cells or lymphokines derived from T helper cells, they are able to differentiate and proliferate into antibody-secreting plasma cells.

EFFERENT PHASE

The efferent or effector phase of graft rejection still arouses much controversy and stimulates much experimental research. There is a variety of immune-mediated effector mechanisms all of which may result in tissue destruction. The specific cytotoxic T cell, activated macrophages and delayed type hypersensitivity reactions (DTH), natural killer (NK) cells, antibody-dependent cell mediated cytotoxicity (ADCC) and complement-dependent antibody mediated cytotoxicity may all, in principle, result in graft rejection. The relative roles of each of these effector mechanisms in graft rejection is not clearly defined — indeed it may be that each or all of these mechanisms are important, depending on the immune status of the recipient.

Specificity of rejection

The actual nature of tissue destruction during rejection may itself be informative; that is, graft destruction shows specificity for cells carrying donor alloantigens. Indeed, the elegant experimental system of Mintz and Silvers (1967, 1970) demonstrated an exquisite specificity of donor cell lysis. These workers bred allophenic mice to use as tissue donors. Such allophenic, or tetraparental, mice are bred by fusing the embryos from mice of two different genetic origins. The tissues of the resulting mosaic offspring are made up of patches of cells from each parental type. The experiments were performed using mice with different coat colours. When skin was grafted to mice of either parental origin the cells of non-identical type were rejected, leaving only cells of recipient type intact and capable of hair growth (Fig. 2.3). It is

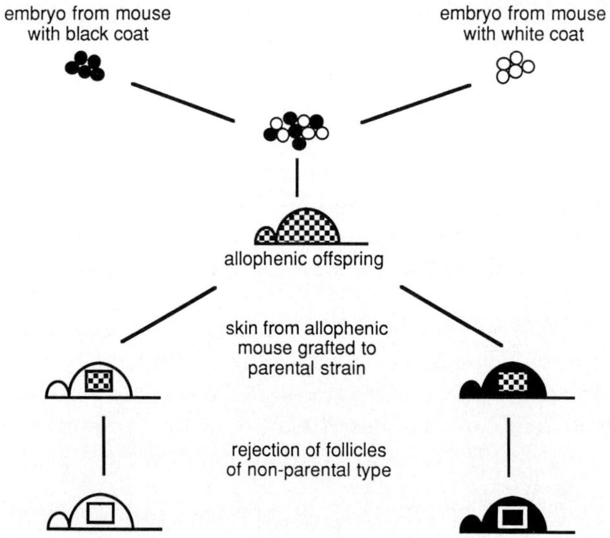

Fig. 2.3. *Use of allophenic mice to demonstrate the specificity of skin graft rejection.*

very difficult to imagine how an essentially non-specific effector mechanism such as that involved in DTH lesions could have been operating to mediate graft rejection in these experiments.

Antibody in graft destruction

Preformed antibodies directed at MHC antigens resulting from previous exposure to HLA incompatible tissue (e.g. in the form of a previous transplant or pregnancy) may undoubtedly be the cause of hyperacute rejection in man, where the organ fails immediately following revascularization (Kissmeyer-Nielsen *et al.*, 1966; Morris and Ting, 1982). Rejection is accompanied by deposition of antibody and complement within the graft and infiltration by polymorphonuclear leucocytes (Williams *et al.*, 1968; Patel and Terasaki, 1969). The presence of such antibodies directed at donor alloantigens in a recipient is now routinely assessed before transplantation in the crossmatch test. Until recently it was thought that a positive crossmatch indicated the presence of HLA-directed cytotoxic antibodies and thus represented a contraindication to transplantation. However, autoantibodies directed at non-HLA antigens which are harmless to a graft may also result in a positive crossmatch (Ting and Morris, 1977, 1981), and in recent years much effort has been expended to discriminate such autoantibodies from HLA antibodies (Ting and Morris, 1978; Chapman *et al.*, 1986).

The role of antibody in acute or chronic rejection is not well understood. Many of the changes seen in acute rejection such as arteriolar thrombosis, interstitial haemorrhage and fibrinoid necrosis of the arteriolar walls have been considered to be due predominantly to antibody (Dunnill, 1984). This is also true of the intimal fibrosis seen in organs undergoing chronic rejection. However, although antibodies, both donor-specific and non-specific, may appear in recipients, their appearance does not necessarily precede rejection, and indeed their presence may be compatible with unimpaired graft function.

Antibody may also cause tissue damage via the K cell, which is yet another type of leucocyte, in antibody-dependent cellular cytotoxicity (ADCC). Antibody may act as a bridge between donor tissue, to which it is bound specifically, and the K cell, to which it is bound via a receptor for the Fc portion of immunoglobulin. This interaction results in the activation of the lytic mechanism of the K cell and tissue damage. The specificity of K cells is identical to that of the antibody involved (Perlmann and Holm, 1969) and no bystander lysis of nearby cells is seen (Perlmann and Perlmann, 1970; Moller and Svehag, 1972). ADCC activity may be recovered from graft infiltrating cells (Tilney *et al.*, 1975) but their role, if any, in graft rejection has not been defined *in vivo*.

The specific cytotoxic T cell

In *in vitro* systems, MHC mismatched lymphocytes will proliferate in response to one another, resulting in the generation of T lymphocytes that will lyse, specifically, target cells of the MHC mismatched type (Häyry and Defendi, 1970; Hodes and Svedmyr, 1970). It has been suggested (Häyry and Defendi, 1970) that this represents a complete *in vitro* model for allograft rejection, the proliferation phase representing expansion of reactive cells following recognition of alloantigens, and the cytotoxic cells representing the effector cells of graft destruction. This is certainly a very attractive view and one which has held widespread belief for many years. Indeed, cells with specific cytotoxic effector activity may be recovered from rejected grafts (Tilney *et al.*, 1975). However, clear evidence implicating this cell as the unique effector mechanism of cell-mediated allograft rejection is lacking. As described in the previous section, skin allograft rejection may be restored in T cell deprived animals of the CD4 type alone (Loveland *et al.*, 1981; Dallman, Mason and Webb, 1982). As the latter authors have pointed out, however, these studies do not exclude a role for the cytotoxic effector cell in graft rejection for two reasons. First, although both the T cell deprived animals used in these experiments, and congenitally athymic animals, are unable to reject allografts unless restored with normal lymphocytes, such animals may generate a good cytotoxic T cell response mediated by $CD8^+$ cells when provided only with cells of the CD4 phenotype (i.e. T cell help) (Gillis *et al.*, 1979; Hale, 1980; Hunig and Bevan, 1980; Wagner *et al.*, 1980;

Mason *et al.*, 1984). Secondly, it has been clearly demonstrated that while the majority of cytotoxic cells are $CD8^+$ and directed at class I antigens, there is a minority, but significant, population of $CD4^+$ cytotoxic cells reactive with class II antigens (Swain *et al.*, 1981; Krensky *et al.*, 1982).

Probably the clearest demonstration that such cells may effect tissue damage has been gained from experiments in which cloned populations of donor-specific cytotoxic T cells have been used to mediate both tumour (Engers, Glasebrook and Sorenson, 1982) and skin (Tyler *et al.*, 1984) destruction. These experiments must, however, be interpreted with a certain degree of caution since cloned cells represent a highly selected, *in vitro* maintained population, whose functional capacity may be different from that of *in vivo* activated cells.

Further evidence comes from studies where the contribution of cell subpopulations in the destruction phase has been at least partially eliminated either in T cell deprived animals or by the use of monoclonal antibodies. In the former experiments, restoration of heart graft rejection to a normal first set tempo either across an MHC class I (Lowry *et al.*, 1985) or, in some cases, a full MHC disparity (Tilney *et al.*, 1984) in immunocompromised animals occurs only if the cells of both the CD4 and CD8 phenotype are injected, implicating the CD8 cytotoxic cell in rejection. In the latter experiments, monoclonal antibodies reacting with cells of either the CD4 or CD8 subtype in the mouse have been used to deplete cell populations *in vivo*. As may be expected from previous work, antibodies depleting the CD4 subset prolonged skin allograft survival. Further, antibodies depleting the CD8 subset lead to some prolongation of survival, again suggesting that the CD8 cytotoxic T cell is important in rejection (Cobbold *et al.*, 1984).

Other experiments favouring the role of the cytotoxic cell in graft rejection come in part from our own laboratories. In these studies, rats in certain strain combinations were treated with cyclosporin A to prevent renal allograft rejection. While the cells recovered from these grafts demonstrated high levels of non-specific or NK-like activity, donor-specific cytotoxicity was absent (Bradley, Mason and Morris, 1985).

There is, however, some evidence that graft destruction may occur in the apparent absence of specific cytotoxic T cells and conversely that the presence of such cells within a graft may not always lead to graft destruction.

The male specific H-Y antigen (an example of a minor histocompatibility antigen) was first detected by the rejection of male skin grafts by female mice of the same strain. Using a variety of mouse strains, it was found that although female mice could often reject male skin, they did not always mount a detectable cytotoxic T cell response. Further, it became clear that in some strains of mice the females were able to generate H-Y specific cytotoxic cells but did not reject skin grafts (Hurme *et al.*, 1977, 1978a,b). This evidence, showing a lack of correlation between rejection and cytotoxic cell response, suggested that, for destruction of minor histo-incompatible skin grafts at least, the cytotoxic T cell was neither sufficient nor required.

Some very recent experiments from our own laboratories have demonstrated the presence of cytotoxic effector cells within a graft that is not rejected (Dallman, Wood and Morris, 1987). In this work, rats are given a donor-specific preoperative blood transfusion which prolongs survival of a subsequent renal allograft indefinitely. However, the cells extracted from such grafts show a high and persistent degree of donor-specific T cell mediated cytotoxicity. At face value, these results may be taken to suggest that the cytotoxic T cell is not sufficient for graft rejection under these circumstances. It is, however, difficult to draw such a conclusion at this time since it is possible that the action of such cells may be blocked *in situ* by, for instance, an enhancing antibody. This does, however, remain an intriguing observation and is the first report of the presence of cytotoxic *effector* cells within an organ graft that is not ultimately rejected.

Delayed type hypersensitivity reaction

The main problem with implicating DTH reactions in allograft rejection is that, although it is clear that the $CD4^+$ T cell is involved (Loveland and McKenzie, 1982), the effector mechanisms mediating tissue damage are not clearly defined. This lesion, however, does imply a specific lymphocyte–antigen interaction followed by an essentially non-specific effector phase (as described by Koch in 1891 in the tuberculin skin reaction — see Florey and Jennings, 1970), characterized by an infiltrate of lymphocytes and cells of the monocyte–macrophage lineage. It is notable that the tissue necrosis that accompanies DTH reactions varies greatly in different species, being extremely severe in guinea-pigs but mild in rats or mice. In contrast, all of these species reject allografts with comparable facility.

Further support for the role of DTH reactions in graft rejection comes from the studies on rejection of H-Y disparate grafts. Although cytotoxic cell responses do not correlate well with graft rejection, the presence of DTH reactions to H-Y antigens follows closely the ability of female mice to reject male skin (Liew and Simpson, 1980).

Lowry, Gurley and Clarke-Forbes (1983) found that irradiated animals reconstituted with CD4 cells reject their grafts, yet do not develop a detectable specific cytotoxic cell response even within the grafted tissue. The absence of specific cytotoxicity was taken to suggest that such activity is not required for graft rejection in this model.

As may be seen from the preceding two sections, there is much evidence for and against the involvement of both the specific cytotoxic effector and DTH effector mechanisms in graft rejection. It seems likely that neither mechanism is unique in its ability to cause graft rejection and that, in the absence of one mechanism, another may become involved.

Natural killer cells

Unlike the effector mechanisms described above, the NK cell apparently does not need to interact with antigen in order to become lytic to target cells; NK cells may be recovered from, for instance, the blood or spleen and are immediately able to lyse a panel of NK sensitive targets (Herberman *et al.*, 1979). These targets are largely of tumour origin, but the cell surface molecule(s) allowing interaction with the NK cell is unknown. While clearly the NK cell is a potent source of cytotoxic activity, a role for it in graft rejection remains to be established. Indeed, our own work in a variety of experimental models indicates that grafts survive indefinitely in the presence of high levels of NK effector activity (Bradley, Mason and Morris, 1985; M. J. Dallman, K. J. Wood and P. J. Morris, unpublished data).

Cell-mediated effector mechanisms have largely been implicated in acute allograft rejection and certainly the experimental systems described above have largely concentrated on this type of rejection. However, it is possible that cellular events may also be involved in hyperacute rejection, as demonstrated in the miniature swine model (Kirkman *et al.*, 1979). The cellular events accompanying human allograft rejection have relied largely on a phenotypic analysis of graft infiltrates. Although this may be an extremely useful tool in the diagnosis and subsequent management of clinical graft rejection, it is difficult to use this information to increase our understanding of the effector mechanisms involved in tissue destruction, since there is only a poor correlation between phenotype and function.

Target cells of graft destruction

The precise targets in allograft rejection are not clearly defined. It seems likely, however, that damage to the vascular endothelium, which may express both class I and class II MHC antigens, would result in rapid cell necrosis and graft loss (Kauntz *et al.*, 1963; Waksman, 1963). Indeed, the predominantly vascular changes that occur during rejection of an organ graft suggest that this is the case (Porter, Calne and Zukoski, 1964; Laden and Sinclair, 1971; Dvorak *et al.*, 1979). It is also possible that parenchymal cells may be targets for tissue destruction and perhaps may be more important in chronic rejection, although once again the endothelium would appear to be a key target. This is particularly evident after cardiac transplantation, where much of the extensive atheroma-like changes in the coronary arteries of the graft after transplantation must reflect a chronic rejection reaction.

CONCLUSIONS

The mechanism of the rejection reaction remains uncertain. Nevertheless, there has been considerable progress in our understanding of the reaction compared with our rather simplistic conception of the process in the early days of transplantation immunology. At present, our attempts to prevent or decrease the severity of rejection are directed at either HLA matching of donor and recipient (not at present logistically possible in cardiac transplantation) and more potent immunosuppression. In the latter area, certainly the advent of cyclosporin has led to a decrease in the more acute rejection reactions after cardiac transplantation and better graft survival as a result. Nevertheless, immunosuppression today remains relatively non-specific, with not inconsiderable side effects as a result. Further advances in immunosuppression must depend on a better understanding of the mechanisms of the rejection reaction, which will allow the development of more specific and more effective immunosuppressive strategies than we have available at present.

REFERENCES

Barker, C. F. and Billingham, R. E. (1968). The role of afferent lymphatics in the rejection of skin homografts. *J. Exp. Med.* **128**, 197–221.

Bildsoe, P. (1972). Organ transplantation in the rat. The importance of the Ag-B (or H-1) locus. *Acta Pathol. Microbiol. Immunol. Scand.*, sec. B, *Microbiology* **80**, 221–230.

Bildsoe, P., Sorenson, S. F., Pettirossi, O. and Simonsen, M. (1970). Heart and kidney transplantation from segregating hybrid to parental rats. *Transplant. Rev.* **3**, 36–45.

Billingham, R. E., Brent, L. and Medawar, P. B. (1954). Quantitative studies on tissue transplantation immunity. II The origin, strength and duration of actively and adoptively acquired immunity. *Proc. Roy. Soc. Lond.*, ser. B, *Biol. Sci.* **143**, 58–80.

Billingham, R. E. and Silvers, W. K. (1964). Studies on homografts of foetal and infant skin and further observations on the anomalous properties of pouch skin grafts in hamsters. *Proc. Roy. Soc. Lond.*, ser. B, *Biol. Sci.* **161**, 168–190.

Bradley, J. A., Mason, D. W. and Morris, P. J. (1985). Evidence that rat renal allografts are rejected by cytotoxic T cells and not by non-specific effectors. *Transplantation* **39**, 169–175.

Cantor, H. and Boyse, E. A. (1975a). Functional subclasses of T lymphocytes bearing different Ly antigens. i. The generation of functionally distinct T cell subclasses is a differentiative process independent of antigen. *J. Exp. Med.* **141**, 1376–1389.

Cantor, H. and Boyse, E. A. (1975b). Functional subclasses of T lymphocytes bearing different Ly antigens. ii. Cooperation between subclasses of Ly+ cells in the generation of killer activity. *J. Exp. Med.* **141**, 1390–1399.

Chapman, J. R., Taylor, C. J., Ting, A. and Morris, P. J. (1986). Immunoglobulin class and specificity of antibodies causing positive T cell crossmatches: relationship with renal transplant outcome. *Transplantation* **42**, 608–613.

Cobbold, S. P., Jayasuriya, A., Nash, A., Prospero, T. D. and Waldmann, H. (1984). Therapy with monoclonal antibodies by elimination of T cell subsets *in vivo*. *Nature* **312**, 548–551.

Daar, A. S., Fuggle, S. V., Hart, D. N. J., Dalchau, R., Abdulaziz, Z., Fabre, J. W., Ting, A. and Morris, P. J. (1983). Demonstration and phenotypic characterization of HLA-DR-positive interstitial dendritic cells widely distributed in human connective tissues. *Transplant. Proc.* **XV**(1), 311–315.

Dallman, M. J. and Mason, D. W. (1984). Induction of Ia antigens on murine epidermal cells during the rejection of skin allografts. *Transplantation* **36**, 221–223.

Dallman, M. J., Mason, D. W. and Webb, M. (1982). The roles of host and donor cells in the rejection of skin allografts by T-cell-deprived rats injected with syngeneic T-cells. *Eur. J. Immunol.* **12**, 511–518.

Dallman, M. J., Wood, K. J. and Morris, P. J. (1987). Specific cytotoxic T cells are found in the non-rejected kidneys of blood transfused rats. *J. Exp. Med.* (in press).

de Waal, R. M. W., Bogman, M. J. J., Mass, C. N., Cornelissen, L. M. H., Tax, W. J. M. and Koene, R. A. P. (1983). Variable expression of Ia antigens on the vascular endothelium of mouse skin allografts. *Nature* **303**, 426–429.

Dunnill, M. S. (1984). Histopathology of rejection in renal transplantation. In *Kidney Transplantation: Principles and Practice*, 2nd edn, pp. 355–382. (P. J. Morris, Ed.). Grune and Stratton, New York.

Dvorak, H. F., Mihm, M. C. Jr., Dvorak, A. M., Barnes, B. A., Manseau, E. J. and Galli, S. J. (1979). Rejection of fresh-set skin allografts in man. The microvasculature is the critical target of the immune response. *J. Exp. Med.* **150**, 322–337.

Emma, D. A. and Jacobs, B. B. (1981). Prolongation of skin allograft survival following donor irradiation and organ culture explantation. *Transplantation* **31**, 138–139.

Engers, H. D., Glasebrook, A. L. and Sorenson, G. D. (1982). Allogeneic tumour rejection induced by the intravenous injection of Lyt-2+ cytolytic T lymphocyte clones. *J. Exp. Med.* **156**, 1280–1285.

Fellous, M., Nir, U., Wallach, D., Merlin, G., Rubenstein, M. and Revel, M. (1982). Interferon dependent induction of mRNA for the major histocompatibility antigens in human fibroblasts and lymphoblastoid cell lines. *Proc. Nat. Acad. Sci. USA* **79**, 3082–3086.

Florey, H. W. and Jennings, M. A. (1970). In *General Pathology*, 4th edn, pp. 124–174 (H. W. Florey, Ed.). Lloyd-Luke, London.

Frelinger, J. G., Hood, L., Hills, S. and Frelinger, J. A. (1979). Mouse epidermal Ia molecules have a bone marrow origin. *Nature* **282**, 321–323.

Fuggle, S. V., Errasti, P., Daar, A. S., Fabre, J. W., Ting, A. and Morris, P. J. (1983). Localization of major histocompatibility complex (HLA-ABC and DR) antigens in 46 kidneys. *Transplantation* **35**, 385–390.

Garland, J. M. (1986). Growth, receptors and Interleukin-3. *Immunol. Today* **7**, 104–105.

Gibson, T. and Medawar, P. B. (1943). The fate of skin homografts in man. *J. Anat.* **77**, 299–310.

Gillis, S., Union, N. A., Baker, P. E. and Smith, K. A. (1979). The *in vitro* generation and sustained culture of nude mouse cytolytic T lymphocytes. *J. Exp. Med.* **149**, 1460–1476.

Goulmy, E. (1985). Class I restricted human cytotoxic T lymphocytes directed against minor transplantation antigens and their possible role in organ transplantation. *Prog. Allergy* **36**, 44–72.

Gurley, K. E., Lowry, R. P. and Clarke-Forbes, R. D. (1983). Immune mechanisms in organ allograft rejection. II T helper cells, delayed-type hypersensitivity and rejection of renal allografts. *Transplantation* **36**, 401–405.

Guttman, R. D., Lindquist, R. R. and Ockner, S. A. (1969). Renal transplantation in the inbred rat IX. Hemopoietic origin of an immunogenic stimulus of rejection. *Transplantation* **8**, 472–484.

Hale, A. H. (1980). Elicitation of primary cytotoxic T lymphocytes in nude mice. *Cell. Immunol.* **55**, 236–239.

Hall, B. M., DeSaxe, I. and Dorsch, S. E. (1983). The cellular basis of allograft rejection *in vivo.* III Restoration of first set rejection of heart grafts by T helper cells in irradiated rats. *Transplantation* **36**, 700–705.

Hall, B. M., Dorsch, S. and Roser, B. (1978). The cellular basis of allograft rejection *in vivo*. i. The cellular requirements for first-set rejection of heart grafts. *J. Exp. Med.* **148**, 878–889.

Hart, D. N. J. and Fabre, J. W. (1981a). Demonstration and characterization of Ia-positive dendritic cells in the interstitial connective tissues of rat heart and other tissues, but not brain. *J. Exp. Med.* **154**, 347–361.

Hart, D. N. J. and Fabre, J. W. (1981b). Major histocompatibility complex antigens in rat kidney, ureter and bladder. *Transplantation* **31**, 318–325.

Häyry, P. and Defendi, V. (1970). Mixed lymphocyte cultures produce effector cells: model *in vitro* for allograft rejection. *Science* **160**, 133–135.

Herberman, R. B., Djeu, J. Y., Kay, H. D., Ortaldo, J. R., Riccardi, C., Bonnard, G. D., Holden, H. T., Fagnani, R., Santoni, A. and Puccetti, P. (1979). Natural killer cells: characteristics and regulation of activity. *Immunol. Rev.* **44**, 43–70.

Hodes, R. J. and Svedmyr, E. A. J. (1970). Specific cytotoxicity of H-2 incompatible mouse lymphocytes following mixed culture *in vitro*. *Transplantation* **9**, 470–477.

Hünig, T. and Bevan, M. J. (1980). Specificity of cytotoxic T cells from athymic mice. *J. Exp. Med.* **152**, 688–702.

Hurme, M., Chandler, P. R., Hetherington, C. M. and Simpson, E. (1978b). Cytotoxic T-cell responses to H-Y: correlation with the rejection of syngeneic male skin grafts. *J. Exp. Med.* **147**, 768–775.

Hurme, M., Hetherington, C. M., Chandler, P. R., Gordon, R. D. and Simpson, E. (1977). Cytotoxic T cell responses to H-Y: Ir genes and associative antigens map in H-2. *Immunogenetics* **5**, 453–459.

Hurme, M., Hetherington, C. M., Chandler, P. R. and Simpson, E. (1978a). Cytotoxic T-cell responses to H-Y: mapping of the Ir genes. *J. Exp. Med.* **147**, 758–767.

Katz, S. I., Tamaki, K. and Sachs, D. H. (1979). Epidermal Langerhans cells are derived from cells originating in the bone marrow. *Nature* **282**, 324–326.

Kauntz, S. L., Williams, M. A., Williams, P. L., Kapros, C. and Dempster, W. J. (1963). Mechanism of rejection of homotransplanted kidneys. *Nature* **199**, 257–260.

Kirkman, R. L., Colvin, R. B., Flye, M. W., Williams, G. M. and Sachs, D. H. (1979). Transplantation in miniature swine. VII Evidence for cellular immune mechanisms in hyperacute rejection of renal allografts. *Transplantation* **28**, 24–30.

Kissmeyer-Nielsen, F., Olsen, S., Petersen, V. P. and Fjeldborg, O. (1966). Hyperacute rejection of kidney allografts associated with pre-existing humoral antibodies against donor cells. *Lancet* **2**, 662–665.

Klein, J. (1977). Allograft reaction against H-2 region antigens. *Transplant. Proc.* **9**, 847–852.

Klein, J., Chiang, C. L. and Hauptfeld, V. (1977). Histocompatibility antigens controlled by the I region of the murine H-2 complex. II. K/D region compatibility is not required for I-region cell-mediated lymphocytotoxicity. *J. Exp. Med.* **145**, 450–454.

Klinkert, W. E. F., LaBadie, J. H., O'Brien, J. P., Beyer, C. F. and Bowers, W. E. (1980). Rat dendritic cells function as accessory cells and control the production of a soluble factor required for mitogenic responses of T lymphocytes. *Proc. Nat. Acad. Sci. USA* **77**, 5414–5418.

Krensky, A. M., Reiss, C. S., Mier, J. W., Strominger, J. L. and Burakoff, S. J. (1982). Long-term human cytolytic T-cell lines allospecific for HLA-DR6 antigen are OKT4+. *Proc. Nat. Acad. Sci. USA* **79**, 2365–2369.

Laden, A. M. K. and Sinclair, R. A. (1971). Thickening of arterial intima in rat cardiac allografts. *Am. J. Pathol.* **63**, 69–84.

Lafferty, K. J., Andrus, L. and Prowse, S. J. (1980). Role of lymphokine and antigen in the control of specific T cell responses. *Immunol. Rev.* **51**, 279–314.

Lafferty, K. J., Bootes, A., Dart, G. and Talmage, D. W. (1976). Effect of organ culture on the survival of thyroid allografts in mice. *Transplantation* **22**, 138–149.

Lampert, I. A., Suitters, A. J. and Chisholm, P. M. (1981). Expression of Ia antigen on epidermal keratinocytes in graft-versus-host disease. *Nature* **293**, 149–150.

Lechler, R. I. and Batchelor, J. R. (1982). Restoration of immunogenicity to passenger cell-depleted kidney allografts by the addition of donor strain dendritic cells. *J. Exp. Med.* **155**, 31–41.

Liew, F. Y. and Simpson, E. (1980). Delayed-type hypersensitivity responses to H-Y: characterisation and mapping of Ir genes. *Immunogenetics* **11**, 255–266.

Loveland, B. E., Hogarth, P. M., Ceredig, Rh. and McKenzie, I. F. C. (1981). Cells mediating graft rejection in the mouse. I. Lyt-1 cells mediate skin graft rejection. *J. Exp. Med.* **153**, 1044–1057.

Loveland, B. E. and McKenzie, I. F. C. (1982). Delayed-type hypersensitivity and allograft rejection in the mouse: correlation of effector cell phenotype. *Immunology* **46**, 313–320.

Lowry, R. P., Clarke-Forbes, R. D., Blackburn, J. H. and Marghesco, D. M. (1985). Immune mechanisms in organ allograft rejection. V. Pivotal role of the cytotoxic-suppressor T cell subset in the rejection of heart grafts bearing isolated class I disparities in the inbred rat. *Transplantation* **40**, 545–550.

Lowry, R. P., Gurley, K. E. and Clarke-Forbes, R. D. (1983). Immune mechanisms in organ allograft rejection. I. Delayed-type hypersensitivity and lymphocytoxicity in heart graft rejection. *Transplantation* **36**, 391–401.

Mason, D. W., Dallman, M. J., Arthur, R. P. and Morris, P. J. (1984). Mechanisms of allograft rejection — the roles of cytotoxic T-cells and delayed-type hypersensitivity. *Immunol. Rev.* **77**, 167–184.

Mason, D. W., Dallman, M. J. and Barclay, A. N. (1981). Graft-versus-host disease induces expression of Ia antigen in rat epidermal cells and gut epithelium. *Nature* **293**, 150–151.

Mason, D. W., Pugh, C. W. and Webb, M. (1981). The rat mixed lymphocyte reaction: roles of a dendritic cell in intestinal lymph and T-cell subsets defined by monoclonal antibodies. *Immunology* **44**, 75–87.

Medawar, P. B. (1944). The behaviour and fate of skin autografts and skin homografts in rabbits. *J. Anat.* **78**, 176–199.

Medawar, P. B. (1945). A second study of the behaviour and fate of skin homografts in rabbits. *J. Anat.*, **79**, 157–176.

Medawar, P. B. (1948). Immunity to homologous grafted skin; fate of skin homografts transplanted to brain, to subcutaneous tissue and to anterior chamber of eye. *Br. J. Exp. Path.* **29**, 58–69.

Meuer, S. C., Hussey, R. E., Penta, A. C., Fitzgerald, K. A., Stadler, B. M., Schlossman, S. F. and Reinherz, E. L. (1982). Cellular origin of interleukin 2 (IL2) in man: evidence for stimulus restricted IL2 production by T4+ and T8+ lymphocytes. *J. Immunol.* **129**, 1076–1079.

Mintz, B. and Silvers, W. K. (1967). 'Intrinsic' immunological tolerance in allophenic mice. *Science* **158**, 1484–1486.

Mintz, B. and Silvers, W. K. (1970). Histocompatibility antigens on melanoblasts and hair follicle cells: cell localised homograft rejection in allophenic skin grafts. *Transplantation* **9**, 497–505.

Mitchison, N. A. (1954). Passive transfer of transplantation immunity. *Proc. Roy. Soc. Lond.*, ser. B, *Biol. Sci.* **142**, 72–87.

Möller, G. and Svehag, S-E. (1972). Specificity of lymphocyte-mediated cytotoxicity induced by *in vitro* antibody-coated target cells. *Cell. Immunol.* **4**, 1–19.

Morris, P. J. and Ting, A. (1982). Studies of HLA-DR with relevance to renal transplantation. *Immunol. Rev.*, **66**, 103–131.

Okada, M. and Henney, C. S. (1980). The differentiation of cytotoxic T cells *in vitro*. II. Amplifying factor(s) produced in primary mixed lymphocyte cultures against K/D stimuli require the presence of Lyt 2+ cells but not Lyt 1+ cells. *J. Immunol.* **125**, 300–307.

Oppenheim, J. J., Kovacs, E. J., Matsushima, K. and Durum, S. K. (1986). There is more than one interleukin 1. *Immunol. Today* **7**, 45–56.

Patel, R. and Terasaki, P. I. (1969). Significance of the positive crossmatch in kidney transplantation. *New Eng. J. Med.* **280**, 735–739.

Pedersen, N. C. and Morris, B. (1970). The role of the lymphatic system in the rejection of homografts: a study of lymph from renal transplants. *J. Exp. Med.* **131**, 936–969.

Pedersen, N. C. and Morris, B. (1974). The rate of formation and the composition of lymph from primary and secondary renal allografts. *Transplantation* **17**, 48–56.

Perlmann, P. and Holm, G. (1969). Cytotoxic effects of lymphoid cells *in vitro*. *Adv. Immunol.* **11**, 117–193.

Perlmann, P. and Perlmann, H. (1970). Contactual lysis of antibody-coated chicken erythrocytes by purified lymphocytes. *Cell. Immunol.* **1**, 300–315.

Peugh, W. N., Superina, R. A., Wood, K. J. and Morris, P. J. (1986). The role of H-2 and non-H-2 antigens and genes in the rejection of murine cardiac allografts. *Immunogenetics* **23**, 30–37.

Porter, K. A., Calne, R. Y. and Zukoski, C. F. (1964). Vascular and other changes in 200 canine renal homotransplants treated with immuno-suppressive drugs. *Lab. Invest.* **13**, 810–824.

Robb, R. J. (1984). Interleukin 2: the molecule and its function. *Immunol. Today* **5**, 203–209.

Rolstad, B. and Ford, W. L. (1974). Immune responses of rats deficient in thymus-derived lymphocytes to strong transplantation antigens (Ag-B). Graft-versus-host activity, allograft rejection, and the factor of immunization. *Transplantation* **17**, 405–415.

Rosenberg, A. S., Mizuochi, T., Sharrow, S. O. and Singer, A. (1987). Phenotype specificity and function of T cell subsets and T cell interactions involved in skin allograft rejection. *J. Exp. Med.* **165**, 1296–1315.

Rosenberg, A. S., Mizuochi, T. and Singer, A. (1986). Analysis of T-cell subsets in rejection of K^b mutant skin allografts differing at class I MHC. *Nature* **322**, 829–831.

Rygaard, J. (1974). Skin grafts in nude mice. 2 Rat skin grafts in nude mice of three genetic backgrounds (BALB-c, C3H, C57-BL). The effects after preparation by thymus grafts. *Acta Pathol. Microbiol. Immunol. Scand.*, sec. A, *Pathology* **82**, 93–104.

Sherwood, R. A., Brent, L. and Rayfield, L. S. (1986). Presentation of alloantigens by host cells. *Eur. J. Immunol.* **16**, 569–574.

Snell, G. D. (1953). Genetics of transplantation. *J. Nat. Cancer Inst.* **14**, 691–704.

Sprent, J., Schaeffer, M., Lo, D. and Korngold, R. (1986). Properties of purified T cell subsets. II *In vivo* responses to class I vs class II H-2 differences. *J. Exp. Med.*, **163**, 998–1011.

Steinman, R. M. and Witmer, M. D. (1978). Lymphoid dendritic cells are potent stimulators of the primary mixed leukocyte reaction in mice. *Proc. Nat. Acad. Sci. USA* **75**, 5132–5136.

Steinmuller, D. and Hart, E. A. (1971). Passenger leukocytes and induction of allograft immunity. *Transplant. Proc.* **3**(1), 673–675.

Strober, S. and Gowans, J. C. (1965). The role of lymphocytes in the sensitization of rats to renal homografts. *J. Exp. Med.*, **122**, 347–360.

Stuart, F. P., Bastien, E., Holter, A., Fitch, F. W. and Elkins, W. L. (1971). Role of passenger leukocytes in the rejection of renal allografts. *Transplant. Proc.* **3**(1), 461–464.

Swain, S. L., Dennert, G., Wormsley, S. and Dutton, R. W. (1981). The Lyt phenotype of a long-term allospecific T-cell line. Both helper and killer activities to IA are mediated by Ly-1 cells. *Eur. J. Immunol.* **11**, 175–180.

Tilney, N. L. and Gowans, J. L. (1971). The sensitisation of rats by allografts transplanted to alymphatic pedicles of skin. *J. Exp. Med.* **133**, 951–962.

Tilney, N. L., Kupiec-Weglinksi, J. W., Heidecke, C. D., Lear, P. A. and Strom, T. B. (1984). Mechanisms of rejection and prolongation of vascularized organ allografts. *Immunol. Rev.* **77**, 185–216.

Tilney, N. L., Strom, T. B., MacPherson, S. G. and Carpenter, C. B. (1975). Surface properties and functional characteristics of infiltrating cells harvested from acutely rejecting cardiac allografts in inbred rats. *Transplantation* **20**, 323–330.

Ting, A. and Morris, P. J. (1977). Renal transplantation and B cell crossmatches with autoantibodies and alloantibodies. *Lancet* **2**, 1095–1097.

Ting, A. and Morris, P. J. (1978). Reactivity of autolymphocytotoxic antibodies from dialysis patients with lymphocytes from chronic lymphocytic leukemia (CLL) patients. *Transplantation* **25**, 31–33.

Ting, A. and Morris, P. J. (1981). Positive crossmatch transplants — safe or not? *Transplant. Proc.* **13**, 1544–1546.

Tyler, J. D., Galli, S. J., Snider, M. E., Dvorak, A. M. and Steinmuller, D. (1984). Cloned Lyt-2+ cytolytic T lymphocytes destroy allogeneic tissue *in vivo*. *J. Exp. Med.* **159**, 234–243.

Wagner, H., Hardt, C., Heeg, K., Röllinghoff, M. and Pfizenmaier, K. (1980). T-cell derived helper factor allows the *in vivo* induction of cytotoxic T cells in nu/nu mice. *Nature* **284**, 278–280.

Waksman, B. H. (1963). The pattern of rejection in rat skin homografts and its relation to the vascular network. *Lab. Invest.* **12**, 46–57.

Williams, G. M., Hume, D. M., Hudson, R. P., Morris, P. J., Kano, K. and Milgrom, F. (1968). Hyperacute renal homograft rejection in man. *New Engl. J. Med.* **279**, 611–618.

Wong, G. H. W., Clark-Lewis, I., Harris, A. W. and Schrader, J. W. (1984). Effect of cloned interferon-gamma on expression of H-2 and Ia antigens on cell lines of hemopoetic, lymphoid, epithelial, fibroblastic and neuronal origin. *Eur. J. Immunol.* **14**, 52–56.

D. Glenn Pennington

3

Circulatory Support Before Transplantation

INTRODUCTION

The recent success of cardiac transplantation in centres around the world is well documented in this book. Patients who receive cardiac transplants have an excellent chance for survival and great promise of leading active, useful lives. However, the widespread application of cardiac transplantation is still limited by several factors. The most important factor is the scarcity of donor organs, so that while awaiting a donor heart many patients die or suffer injuries to vital organs which make them no longer eligible for transplantation. Recently, dramatic advances have been made in the application of circulatory support devices to maintain organ viability until donor hearts are available. The reasons for this success can be attributed to two important factors. The first is cyclosporin therapy, which has substantially reduced the severity of infections, which are a constant threat to immunosuppressed patients who have received circulatory devices. The second has been the improvement in the efficiency of circulatory devices, including the greater understanding of problems related to host–device interfaces. This chapter chronicles the history and current status of the use of circulatory devices in patients prior to heart transplantation. Since this is such a rapidly expanding field, the experiences cited here may well represent only a fraction of those which will be accomplished by the time this book is published.

HISTORICAL REVIEW

All of the initial implantations of devices to support the circulation as a bridge to transplantation were performed at the Texas Heart Institute by Cooley *et al.* (1969), Norman *et al.* (1978) and Frazier *et al.* (1983). The dramatic implantation of the Liotta artificial heart in a 47-year-old man in April of 1969 introduced the possibility of temporary circulatory support prior to cardiac transplantation (Cooley *et al.*, 1969). The implantation of the Liotta heart, the use of an abdominal left ventricular assist device in a patient with a stone heart in 1978 (Norman *et al.*, 1978) and the subsequent implantation of the Akutsu heart in a 36-year-old man in 1981 all met with the same result: the development of infection and multiple organ failure. However, there were also difficulties with the devices. The abdominal left ventricular assist device was awkward to implant and could injure the abdominal organs. The Akutsu heart partially obstructed the pulmonary veins, resulting in moderately severe hypoxaemia requiring extracorporeal membrane oxygenation (ECMO). The efficiency of the devices has been significantly improved since then, but this chapter will consider the questions that still remain in developing appropriate devices.

Because of the complexities involved in the use of total artificial hearts and implantable assist devices, the period from 1978 to 1984 saw attempts in several centres to use less complicated devices to bridge patients to transplantation. This era was introduced by the success of Reemtsma and his associates in supporting three patients with intra-aortic balloons (IAB) prior to cardiac transplantation (Reemtsma *et al.*, 1978). All three patients survived and were able to leave the hospital. They were the first successful cases of bridging to transplantation with any type of mechanical device. Because of the success of the IAB in post-cardiotomy and myocardial infarction patients, a large experience has accumulated and great confidence in it has been gained. It is now the most commonly used initial technique for dealing with the potential transplant recipient who develops cardiogenic shock. The success of this system has been emphasized by the remarkable achievements of Hardesty, Griffith and associates at the University of Pittsburgh. In their experience, patients who were supported with IAB prior to cardiac transplantation fared as well after transplantation as those who did not require IAB support (Hardesty *et al.*, 1986). Although the worldwide results of IAB use in cardiac transplant patients have not been collated, it is clear that it is highly successful.

Another method of carrying out support prior to cardiac transplantation was the use of veno-arterial ECMO (Pennington *et al.*, 1983, 1984). This was performed by Pennington and associates at St. Louis University in 2 patients who were thought to be excellent transplant candidates. Unfortunately both patients died, one shortly after transplantation and the other 1 month later. Both deaths were related in part to complications related to the ECMO system. The use of ECMO in cardiac transplant recipients has been rather limited in comparison with other methods, but it can still be useful in initial resuscitative efforts.

On 5 September 1984, P. E. Oyer and colleagues at Stanford University (personal communication) implanted a Novacor (Novacor Medical Corporation, Oakland, CA) electrical implantable left ventricular assist system into a 51-year-old man with ischaemic cardiomyopathy. Nine days later his heart was transplanted and after a somewhat difficult course he recovered and is now doing well. This was the first successful case of bridging to transplantation with a ventricular assist device, and the first use of an implantable electrical left ventricular assist system. The following day, Hill and associates at Pacific Medical Centre in San Francisco used an external pneumatic Pierce–Donachy left ventricular assist device (Thoratec Laboratories Corporation, Berkeley, California) for 52 h to support a 47-year-old man with post-infarction cardiogenic shock prior to cardiac transplantation (Hill *et al.*, 1986). This patient also survived after a long and difficult hospital course and is doing reasonably well. This was the first successful use of an *external* ventricular assist device for bridging to transplantation and it has been followed by a moderate number of similar cases to be outlined in this chapter.

On 1 December 1982, DeVries and associates placed the first permanent total artificial heart in Dr Barney Clark in Salt Lake City (DeVries *et al.*, 1984). Three other patients had permanent total artificial hearts implanted by DeVries and his team during the period from 25 November 1984 to 4 April 1985. On 6 March 1985, Vaughn and Copeland at the University of Arizona implanted the Phoenix total artificial heart into a 33-year-man for 36 h prior to his second cardiac transplant (Vaughn *et al.*, 1986). The patient had apparently rejected the first transplant and was dying of heart failure. Unfortunately, he died of bleeding, pulmonary oedema and other complications. However, on 29 August 1985, Copeland and associates removed the heart of a 25-year-old man with severe cardiomyopathy and cardiogenic shock and replaced it with a Jarvik-7 total artificial heart (J-7 TAH). This patient was supported with the J-7 TAH for 9 days prior to successful cardiac transplantation and subsequently became the first patient to leave hospital after being 'bridged to transplantation' with an implantable, orthotopic, artificial circulatory support device (Levinson *et al.*, 1986a). Subsequent bridging procedures have employed a variety of circulatory support devices with moderate success. This therapeutic option is now a growing and important part of cardiac transplantation programmes.

DESCRIPTION OF DEVICES AND TECHNIQUES OF INSERTION

Intra-aortic balloon

The IABs introduced by Reemtsma and associates in their early experience were all placed via a femoral arteriotomy. However, in recent years percutaneous techniques have been successfully employed. Since the IAB is a standard part of the cardiac surgeon's and cardiologist's armamentarium, a description of these devices and their insertion is not necessary. Most potential cardiac transplant recipients who develop unstable haemodynamics and low cardiac output should be treated initially with intra-aortic balloon pumps, since they can often be stabilized without the need for more complicated, sophisticated and expensive systems.

Extracorporeal membrane oxygenation

Extracorporeal membrane oxygenation for circulatory support has been available since the introduction of cardiopulmonary bypass and the development of the membrane oxygenator. Considerable experience with ECMO in respiratory failure was accumulated in the early 1970s (Zapol *et al.*, 1979). However, in recent years attention has focused more on the use of ECMO to support patients with cardiac and cardiopulmonary failure (Pennington *et al.*, 1983, 1984). The system currently in use at St. Louis University (Fig. 3.1) consists of a Scimed membrane lung (Scimed, Inc., Minneapolis), a heat exchanger and a blood pump. Both the Biomedicus pump (Biomedicus, Inc., Eden Prairie, Minnesota) and a simple Debakey roller pump have been employed. The pump is connected to the patient by standard cardiopulmonary bypass cannulae. Continuous intravenous heparinization is used to maintain the activated clotting time between 150 and 200 sec. It now seems imperative to use both proximal and distal arterial and venous cannulae in order to avoid the development of leg oedema or ischaemia. An IAB may be used in the other femoral artery in order to provide a pulse, although we do not believe that pulsatile flow is essential for the success of ECMO therapy. One of the chief advantages of the ECMO perfusion system is that it can be easily transported on a small trolley to all areas of the hospital, making it rapidly available to the cardiac intensive care unit, cardiac catheterization laboratory and emergency room. A technique for fast femoral cannulation (Bard Corporation, Santa Anna, California) has been used by Phillips and associates in Des Moines, Iowa (Phillips, 1986) for rapid establishment of femorofemoral ECMO. ECMO can supply flows of up to 3–4 litres/min and can quickly establish normal haemodynamics, permitting speedy resuscitation of patients, and so giving

Current techniques for the implantation of the centrifugal pumps prior to cardiac transplantation employ a sternotomy and, if the patient is unstable, standard cardiopulmonary bypass. Simple pursestring sutures placed in the right or left atrium allow introduction of the cannulae. A standard aortic cannula is passed through a pursestring suture into the ascending aorta of the main pulmonary artery for return of flow. Some investigators have used a paediatric endotracheal tube or a similar longer tube for the aortic cannulation in an attempt to avoid embolization of the cerebral vessels (Rose *et al.*, 1985). The necessity of this technique has not been proven.

External pulsatile ventricular assist devices

The Pierce–Donachy pump is a paracorporeal pneumatic sac-type device constructed of a machined polycarbonate housing with an angle port design that contains a flexible seam-free segmented polyurethane sac (Fig. 3.2) (Donachy *et al.*, 1978). It utilizes Bjork–Shiley (Shiley, Irvine, California) inlet and outlet valves and has a stroke volume of 65 ml with a dynamic ejection fraction of approximately 0.75. Pump inlet cannulae are available for the atria or the left ventricular apex. In potential cardiac transplant recipients, a large-bore, wire-wound segmented polyurethane cannula fitted with a felt washer to permit suture fixation to the myocardium is inserted into the left ventricular apex. The 14 French Dacron graft on the polyurethane outflow cannula may be sutured to the aorta or the pulmonary artery depending on whether left or right ventricular support is required. In cases in which atrial cannulation is used, the 51 French Sarns (Ann Arbor, Michigan) venous drainage cannula coated with the segmented polyurethane Biomer (Ethicon Corporation, Summerville, New Jersey) and shaped to a right angle configuration can be easily fitted into either atrium with a simple pursestring suture around the atrial appendage. It is also possible to pass the atrial cannula through a pursestring suture into the left

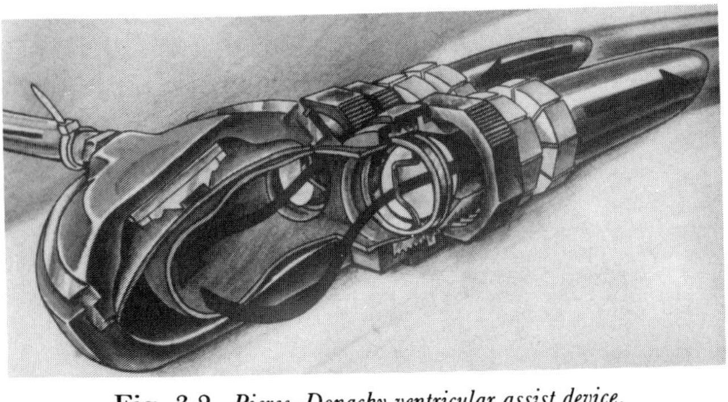

Fig. 3.2. *Pierce–Donachy ventricular assist device.*

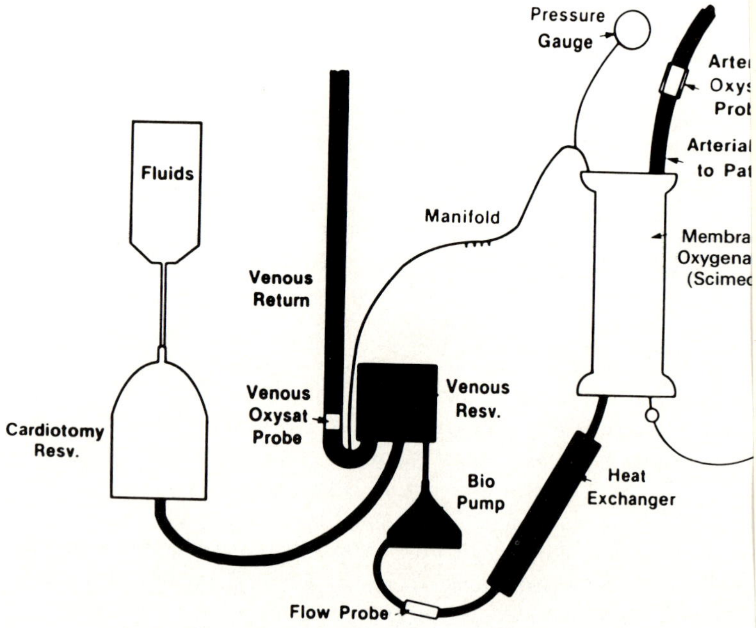

Fig. 3.1. *Extracorporeal membrane oxygenator perfusion circuit.*

time for the necessary diagnostic procedures to be carried out. There definitive method of circulatory support may be established.

Centrifugal pumps

Centrifugal circulatory assist pumps developed by Biomedicus, Inc. Prairie, Minnesota) and Centrimed Corporation (Minneapolis, Min have been used to bridge patients to transplantation. The Biomedicus (Biopump) is widely employed for the treatment of post-cardiotomy genic shock (Magovern, Sang and Maher, 1985; Zumbro *et al.*, 1985 Centrimed pump is newer and has had limited clinical use. Apparen first success with a centrifugal pump to bridge a patient to cardiac tran tation was achieved in Minneapolis by Joyce and colleagues in a 25-ye man who was supported with a Centrimed pump for 1 day prior to plantation. The centrifugal blood pumps utilize rotating cones to ge energy which is recovered in the form of pressure/flow work. While ating at a given constant speed, the pumps generate nearly constant pr over a wide range of flow rates. The pumping action is transmitted by netic coupling to the mated drive magnet. Although there are no sp cannulae designed for the Biomedicus or Centrimed pumps, most inve tors have been able to adapt standard cardiopulmonary bypass can atrium near the entrance of the right superior pulmonary vein. Although the control system is capable of functioning in a synchronized mode, synchronization is rarely used in patients who are expected to undergo cardiac transplantation. A manual, set-rate mode or a fill-to-empty mode that operates by activating a Hall effect switch when the sac is full is used. When the pump is operating in the fill-to-empty mode, the rate × stroke volume (65 ml) equals pump flow. Heparin is not necessary during normal flow periods, but it is used if the pump flow falls below 3000 ml/min.

Implanted ventricular assist devices

It has long been the goal of several pioneering research groups to develop a permanent, implantable, left ventricular assist device which would not require tubes or wires which traverse the skin. Currently the National Heart, Lung, and Blood Institute is sponsoring the development of these devices. Although the components of these systems which will make them totally implantable have not been perfected, excellent pumps have been developed. It is now feasible to use these sophisticated systems with externalized energy sources to bridge patients to transplantation. Two systems, the Novacor pump and the Thermedics pump, have been used in modified forms in humans prior to cardiac transplantation.

The Novacor model 100 left ventricular assist system (LVAS) is composed of a balanced solenoid energy converter, dual pusher plate sac-type blood pump and a microprocessor-based control and monitoring console (Portner *et al.*, 1983). The integrated energy converter and blood pump (Fig. 3.3) are connected to the patient by Dacron conduits to the left ventricular apex and the ascending aorta. A percutaneous cable is brought out from the right

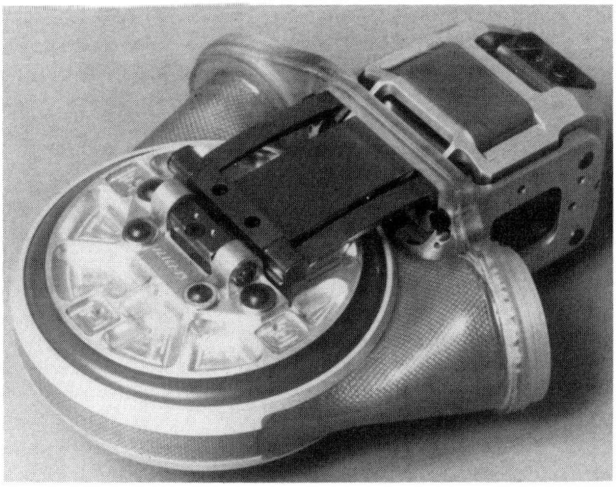

Fig. 3.3. *Novacor left ventricular assist system.*

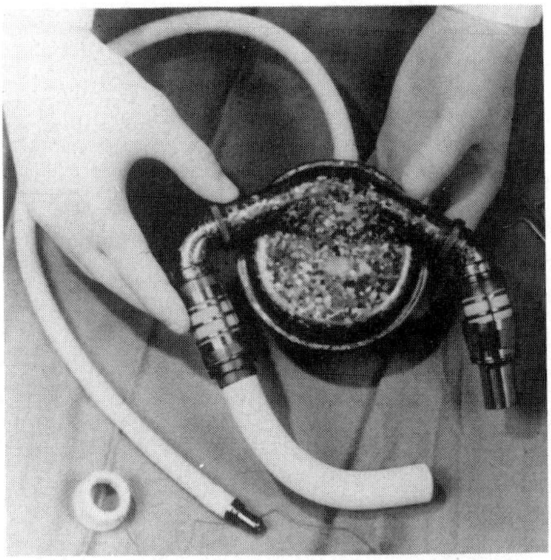

Fig. 3.4. *Thermedics ventricular assist system.*

lower quadrant of the abdomen to connect to an extracorporeal control console. The conduits contain 21 mm Carpentier–Edwards pericardial valves which allow unidirectional blood flow through the pump. Electrical energy is converted into hydraulic work which is used to eject blood from the pump. Synchronous counter-pulsation is possible by sensing pump fill and eject rates, based upon signals from displacement transducers within the energy converter. The blood sac has a highly smooth surface which is designed not to require anticoagulation, although some centres have used anticoagulants. The Novacor pump is designed for implantation in the left ventricular apex only and is not appropriate for left atrial or right atrial use.

The Thermedics model 14 VAD is a pusher plate blood pump driven by a pneumatic external console (Fig. 3.4) adapted from the permanent Thermedics electrical LVAS. The inflow and outflow conduits consist of 20 mm diameter woven Dacron grafts containing glutaraldehyde-preserved porcine xenograft valves. The prosthetic interface covering the flexible pump bladder and metal components consists of flocked polyester fibrils. When the conduits are coupled to the pump housing, the uniform blood/material surface immediately attracts and binds a thin fibrin–cellular coagulum. The control system provides either synchronized counter-pulsation or fixed-rate pumping. The metal inflow cannula is inserted into the left ventricular apex by sewing a silicone rubber ring with an attached Teflon sewing cuff to the epicardium. A circular knife is used to excise a wedge of myocardium, permitting insertion of the metal inflow tube. The Thermedics model 14 VAD in its current configuration is designed for use in the left ventricle only. Heparinization may be used during the initial implantation, but is not required while the VAD is in place.

Orthotopic biventricular replacement devices

Although the initial orthotopic replacements of the heart involved several different devices, the most commonly used device is the Jarvik-7 artificial heart. The Liotta, Akutsu, Phoenix and Berlin hearts have been used in 1 patient each and the Pennsylvania State University heart and the Unger Ellipsoid heart in 2 patients each. Although it is beyond the scope of this review to describe each of these devices in detail, a description of the Jarvik-7 heart will be given, as it is representative of this group of devices. The two J-7 TAH ventricles are made of polyurethane with polyurethane bases and Medtronic disc valves. The diaphragm is composed of three layers of Avcothane with interposed layers of Dacron mesh and graphite. The maximum stroke volume of each ventricle is 100 ml. Connections to the natural atria and great vessels are made with a 'quick-connect' system. Recent modifications of the system allowed a 40% decrease in the d*p*/d*t* of the Utah pneumatic drive system. In addition, a revision of the valve housing at the point of connection to the sac is planned for the Jarvik-8 TAH in an attempt to decrease blood clotting at that interface. The Jarvik-7-70 can be implanted in smaller people, and has been used in larger patients at higher pumping rates in order to decrease the tendency toward thrombosis. Anticoagulation regimens of continuous heparin or coumadin in conjunction with dipyridamole or aspirin have been used.

PATIENT SELECTION

Because of the scarcity of donor hearts it is imperative that appropriate selection criteria be used for patients who are to be bridged to transplantation. The ultimate outcome of heart transplant recipients requiring assist devices should be similar to that in those who did not require circulatory support. The first criterion is whether the patient has deteriorated to the point that use of a mechanical device is the only way of preventing death or impairment of vital organs.

Patients who are being considered for assist devices should have the most efficient care, including optimal drug therapy, correction of acid-base imbalance, correction of hypoxaemia and blood volume replacement. Most patients who are candidates for devices should have an IAB as the initial method of mechanical support. In some instances, patients might not be able to have an IAB because of arterial obstruction, but these cases will be rare because severe peripheral vascular disease may be considered a contraindication to cardiac transplantation.

Haemodynamic criteria

The haemodynamic criteria for circulatory assistance have been well established: cardiac output index less than 1.8 litres/m^2 per min; left and/or right atrial pressures greater than 20 mmHg, urine output in an adult less than 20 ml/h; systemic vascular resistance greater than 2100 dyn sec/cm^5; and other evidence of decreasing peripheral perfusion such as cool extremities, weak foot pulses, mental confusion or decreased sensorium. Patients who meet these criteria may be observed for a period of a few hours, but they will probably not survive if allowed to continue in that condition. Norman *et al.* (1977) have demonstrated that the mortality rate in such patients is in excess of 90%.

Cardiomyopathy

Most patients with cardiomyopathy have a history of chronic illness and gradual decompensation. However, haemodynamic deterioration can occur abruptly and the rapid downhill course may necessitate mechanical circulatory assistance in order to prevent death. Some patients who have already been selected as heart transplant recipients will deteriorate suddenly while awaiting a donor heart. If there has not been a prior evaluation, it may be necessary to attempt to establish the diagnosis after circulatory assistance has begun. Endomyocardial biopsy to determine the presence of an acute viral cardiomyopathy is appropriate, since it is possible for myocardial recovery to occur. One patient treated with a left ventricular centrifugal pump for viral myocarditis at San Antonio, Texas, recovered completely and did not require transplantation, but this is a rarity (C. Moore, 1986, personal communication). It may be anticipated that the majority of patients with cardiogenic shock resulting from viral cardiomyopathy will not recover and will require transplantation.

Post-cardiotomy

Patients with post-cardiotomy shock treated with circulatory assist devices have been studied most extensively. Well over 500 such patients have been supported with various types of devices, with recovery rates ranging from 30% to 50% (Rose *et al.*, 1985; Pennington *et al.*, 1985b; Gaines *et al.*, 1985; Park *et al.*, 1986). Evidence of myocardial recovery in our own series of post-cardiotomy patients has been as high as 50%, in spite of the fact that the overall survival rate is less (Pennington *et al.*, 1985b). We and others have made extensive efforts to determine which post-cardiotomy patients might be expected to regain myocardial function. One factor mitigating against recovery has been an acute perioperative myocardial infarction. In our recent series of 26 post-cardiotomy patients treated with the Pierce–Donachy VAD, there were 9 survivors and 17 deaths. Only one of the 9 survivors had conclusive evidence of myocardial infarction (electrocardiographic and enzymatic changes or positive biopsy). However, of the fatal cases there was evidence of acute perioperative myocardial infarction in 75%. Another important consideration is the presence of biventricular failure (Pennington *et al.*, 1985a). Right ventricular failure is a frequent accompaniment of left ventricular failure and is sometimes predominant. If biventricular support is required, the assist methods become more complicated and the probability of survival diminishes. Perioperative myocardial infarctions often involve both left and right ventricles and/or the ventricular septum. Necropsy in 14 of the fatal cases showed that 10 had visible evidence of acute perioperative infarctions. Six of these involved both ventricles or the ventricular septum. Therefore, it would seem from our series that acute perioperative infarction and biventricular failure is a combination that would strongly mitigate against myocardial recovery.

Acute myocardial infarction shock

These patients may qualify for circulatory support prior to cardiac transplantation. They present a difficult problem because they have not usually been screened for transplantation prior to the need for circulatory assistance. On the other hand, this is a group who might have a better chance for survival in that they have not usually had a progressive chronic illness which has left them severely debilitated. If the sequelae of the initial cardiogenic shock can be prevented by medical therapy or circulatory assistance, these candidates may make excellent cardiac transplant recipients. Their management is further complicated because they may present in the emergency room, intensive care unit or cardiac catheterization laboratory with an acute massive infarct and cardiogenic shock, without a previous study of the coronary arteries or cardiac function. Therefore, it may be appropriate in some instances to institute circulatory support before cardiac catheterization.

The primary concern in choosing patients for bridging to transplantation is whether the patient is truly a candidate for cardiac transplantation. Our belief is that a strong contraindication to transplantation, such as renal failure requiring dialysis, would also be a contraindication to the institution of circulatory support. As will be noted in the subsequent descriptions of clinical experience, 2 patients with circulatory support had severe renal failure requiring dialysis at the time of cardiac transplantation. However, the yield from such cases must be expected to be small and the commitment of resources and donor hearts to such patients must be strongly questioned. Some features such as sepsis, severe coagulopathy, cerebral injury or liver failure must be considered strict contraindications to both mechanical support and cardiac transplantation. It is incumbent upon all investigators in this field to apply very stringent criteria to patient selection in order to ensure the most prudent distribution of donor hearts.

MANAGEMENT TECHNIQUES

Type of support required

The determination of whether there is a left ventricular, right ventricular or biventricular failure is an important concept in circulatory assistance. Early investigators focused their attention on mechanical support of the left ventricle and depended upon inotropic drugs to treat associated right ventricular failure (Bernhard *et al.*, 1979; Holub *et al.*, 1979). However, it has become apparent that primary right ventricular failure may occur in spite of reasonable left ventricular function. In many instances, severe biventricular failure may not be recognized early in the course of circulatory support (Pennington *et al.*, 1985a). Pierce (1979) emphasized the problem of right ventricular failure in patients undergoing left ventricular bypass, and subsequently described the use of a right ventricular assist device as a primary means of support (Parr *et al.*, 1980). Biventricular devices have now been applied successfully (Turina, Bosue and Serring, 1978; Pennington *et al.*, 1985a; Park *et al.*, 1986). It may be theorized that the incidence of biventricular failure will be higher in patients with cardiomyopathy than in patients with ischaemic disease. However, in the experiences to be described in this chapter, there are clear instances of isolated and bilateral ventricular failure in patients with both ischaemic and non-ischaemic cardiomyopathy.

The aetiology of the heart failure has not been useful in determining the need for biventricular support. Haemodynamic criteria are the most useful in determining the type of support required. In general, the atrium with the higher pressure indicates the ventricle with predominant failure. However, if circulatory support is established for either the right or left side, it may 'unmask' failure of the other ventricle. It is not unusual to find that after the establishment of left ventricular bypass in a patient with apparently satisfactory right ventricular function, the right atrial pressures begin to rise, left atrial pressures fall, left pump filling is impaired and the patient develops a rapid downhill course leading to death (Pennington *et al.*, 1985a). This vicious cycle may be interrupted by the use of biventricular mechanical support. In our study of post-cardiotomy patients with biventricular failure, the survival rate was significantly higher among patients who received biventricular mechanical support than in those who received only a left ventricular assist device and increasing doses of isoproterenol to stimulate the right ventricle (Pennington *et al.*, 1985a). The determination of the type of support required is of utmost importance in determining the type of device to be used. If there is proven severe biventricular dysfunction in a patient already selected for cardiac transplantation who suddenly deteriorates, an orthotopic biventricular type device is appropriate. On the other hand, if there is satisfactory right ventricular function and left ventricular dysfunction, it is more reasonable to use a left ventricular support device. If the patient develops right ventricular failure after the insertion of a left ventricular pump, it is then necessary to employ another device to support the right ventricle. Since the Novacor and Thermedics devices are not designed for right ventricular support, another type of device must be used. It is important that the type of failure and the type of support needed are assessed carefully in all patients being considered for circulatory support prior to cardiac transplantation.

Operation for insertion

Site

The more sophisticated systems require insertion in the operating room with full cardiopulmonary bypass and the usual cardiac surgical environment. However, patients who suddenly deteriorate in the intensive care unit, the emergency room or the cardiac catheterization laboratory can be placed on circulatory support systems rapidly without the need for a sternotomy. A system for rapid placement of femoral cannulae has been employed by Phillips (1986) with success. A kit for initiation of femorofemoral circulatory assistance has been designed by Bard Corporation. Wallwork and associates maintained a patient on femorofemoral bypass for several days prior to successful cardiac retransplantation. Apparently flows as high as 4 litres/min can be obtained with these methods. At St. Louis University, 2 patients were placed on femorofemoral bypass in the intensive care unit and maintained for 3 and 5 days prior to cardiac transplantation. D. M. Rose and associates of New York (personal communication) have placed a transeptal left atrial cannula for patients who deteriorate in the cardiac catheterization laboratory. Using left atrial–femoral artery bypass, flows in the range of 3–4 litres/min were obtained in 6 patients with cardiogenic shock following myocardial infarction. Regardless of whether emergency support is established by peripheral cannulation or transeptal techniques, it is doubtful that such systems can be maintained over the period required to obtain a donor heart. Unless a donor heart is known to be available, these patients should have a definitive system inserted while they await transplantation.

Incision

The incision depends upon the type of device to be inserted. The ECMO system and the systems for rapid support described above require percutaneous techniques or cutdown. The more complex systems require sternotomy and cardiopulmonary bypass. In some circumstances, perfusion may have to be initiated with femorofemoral cannulation, particularly when the patient has undergone a previous cardiotomy or is in profound shock. In the first case described by Hill and associates they implanted a Pierce–Donachy left ventricular assist device through a left thoracotomy, whereas the subsequent cardiac transplant was performed through a median sternotomy (Hill *et al.*, 1986). Although the lateral thoracotomy approach seemed to have the advantage of leaving the sternum undisturbed for later transplantation, it proved to be a cumbersome and difficult technique which they have abandoned. The need for a second sternotomy does not present an inordinately high risk of infection or wound complications.

Cannulation and pump placement

At present, the centrifugal pumps are used in conjunction with standard cardiopulmonary bypass cannulae which can be passed into the great vessels or cardiac chambers through simple pursestring sutures. The Pierce–Donachy, Novacor and Thermedics pumps all require that grafts be sutured to the outflow vessel. Difficulty may arise if the patient has had previous coronary bypass grafts. Occasionally, the pump outflow graft must be sutured to the innominate artery or to an unusual site on the ascending aorta. The Pierce–Donachy pump and the centrifugal pumps can be used in the left atrium or ventricle. If it is apparent that the patient's heart is not going to recover and that transplantation will indeed be required, it is usually preferable to cannulate the left ventricle. The pulsatile pumps seem to fill better from a left ventricle which contracts to fill the pump chamber actively rather than when it is filled passively from the atrium. We have found that low levels of vacuum (−5 to −10 mmHg) may be required with ventricular cannulation, whereas −15 to −25 mmHg is often required with left atrial cannulation. One of the frequent problems of left ventricular cannulation in post-cardiotomy patients is a small left ventricle or a hypertrophied ventricle which compromises the internal volume. This is rarely a problem with cardiac transplant recipients since most of them have dilated left ventricles.

It is extremely important during the implantation of the devices that the positions of the cannulae and the pump be carefully considered. If the device can be positioned in such a way that the patient is able to be mobile, this will greatly facilitate recovery. The Pierce–Donachy (Thoratec) ventricular apex cannula is available in varying lengths to facilitate placement of the pump on the abdominal wall. For placement of the Novacor pump, we have used a single incision extending through the sternum and beyond the umbilicus. We incise the rectus sheath on both sides of the linea alba and dissect the rectus muscle anterior to the posterior rectus sheath, creating a large pocket for the pump. This incision has the advantage of providing a muscle layer to cover the pump and avoids the difficulties involved in placement inside the peritoneal cavity. In one patient at Stanford University, in whom the Novacor pump was placed inside the peritoneal cavity, there was erosion of the colon requiring a separate operation. However, there may be some patients with a small muscular abdomen in whom our bilateral incision may not be feasible, necessitating placement of the device inside the peritoneal cavity. The positioning of the Jarvik-7 artificial heart has been an important consideration in permanent recipients as well as candidates for cardiac transplantation. The Jarvik-7 (100 ml) pump can present considerable problems for smaller patients or those with a small anteroposterior thoracic diameter. The development of the Jarvik-7-70 (70 ml) heart has greatly facilitated the placement of this device, particularly in smaller men and women. In a recent study, Jarvik *et al.* (1986) suggest that the J-7 or J-7-70 device may be used in virtually all adult potential cardiac recipients.

Control of bleeding

Bleeding was a complication in more than 50% of patients receiving ventricular assist devices for post-cardiotomy heart failure. However, we have gradually begun to reduce the frequency of bleeding by several techniques, including meticulous attention to control of bleeding; reversal of the heparin used for cardiopulmonary bypass; and generous applications of Avitene, Surgicel, fibrin glue and topical thrombin spray for local control of bleeding. Often the bleeding is diffuse and apparently related to coagulopathy, necessitating the administration of large amounts of fresh frozen plasma and platelets. The pulsatile devices produce a large d*p*/d*t* which creates stress at the suture lines used to place the outflow grafts. These sites often require reinforcement with pledgeted mattress sutures in order to prevent bleeding.

Wound closure

Closure of the wound is a controversial issue in circulatory device techniques perhaps as there are separate considerations in cardiac transplant recipients as compared to post-cardiotomy patients. It has been our policy to leave the sternum open in post-cardiotomy patients and simply close the skin, or to use a plastic or rubber covering for the skin incision. This method avoids compression of the heart and allows easy accessibility if cardiac tamponade is suspected. However, closure of the sternum with wire has the advantages of allowing mobilization during the period awaiting transplantation and of limiting the bleeding from the sternal edges. At present, we attempt to close the sternum in all transplant candidates. If there is obvious haemodynamic compromise, it may be necessary to remove the sternal wires and simply close the skin and subcutaneous tissue.

Anticoagulation

The need for anticoagulants with circulatory assist devices complicates the patient's course as well as the subsequent transplantation. The simpler systems such as ECMO and the percutaneous femorofemoral techniques obviously require continuous heparinization. The centrifugal pumps placed through sternotomy incisions have been used without anticoagulants by Magovern, Sang and Maher (1985). However, most investigators who use the various centrifugal devices have identified fibrin in the pump heads in some patients, although thrombo-embolism has not been a common problem. At present, we believe that patients with Biomedicus or Centrimed pumps should be anticoagulated with heparin as soon as the initial bleeding from the operation has subsided. On the other hand, the Pierce–Donachy pump can be used without heparin as long as the flow is maintained above 3 litres/min. Using anticoagulation during the weaning period only in more than 25 patients with the Pierce–Donachy pump, we have had only three instances of pump thrombus and no instance of embolization. In those three instances we made the mistake of intermittently clamping the cannulae in order to test for cardiac recovery, thus precipitating sac thrombus by interrupting flow. When clamping methods were not employed, thrombus did not develop in the sacs.

Patients receiving the Novacor device prior to transplantation have almost all had some type of anticoagulation, usually continuous heparin. Since this device employs bovine pericardial valves, it may be that anticoagulation with heparin is not necessary. However, the current procedure is to give heparin as soon as the initial bleeding has stopped after implantation of the device (usually after 24 h). In one patient maintained at our hospital with the Novacor device for 91 days, we were able to change to a regimen of oral Coumadin and Persantin, during which time he had no evidence to suggest thrombo-embolic events. He received heparin intermittently, when the prothrombin time rose above 30%.

The anticoagulation regimen required with the Jarvik device is still not clearly defined, nor is it entirely established for any of these devices. In the initial experiences with the Jarvik-7, DeVries employed a generous heparinization schedule along with aspirin and Persantin. This often resulted in bleeding which led to several complications. At present, most investigators using the Jarvik device use continuous heparinization and Persantin. Aspirin is not given because of the danger of bleeding at the time of transplantation. Thrombo-embolism has been a problem in several patients with the Jarvik-7, but measures are being taken to prevent thrombo-emboli by more intensive anticoagulation and by design modifications. Unfortunately, none of the systems described in this chapter can be relied upon to function safely over more than a few weeks without the threat of thrombo-embolism, unless some type of anticoagulation is employed.

Drive parameters

The initial goal of assistance is to establish high flows as soon as possible in order to reverse ischaemic changes in the vital organs. The minimum value of 2 litres/m^2 per min of systemic flow is absolutely imperative for a successful outcome, but it is desirable to maintain higher flows. The actual drive parameters vary, depending upon the device employed. The non-pulsatile centrifugal pumps are driven at rates which produce optimal flow without regard to the patient's intrinsic cardiac rate. However, if the patient's own heart is contributing a significant percentage of the cardiac output, it may be possible to use flows in the range of 2500–3000 ml/min, particularly with the centrifugal devices. The Pierce–Donachy device can function in several different modes, including a set-rate manual mode, a fill-to-empty mode in which the pump only empties when it is filled, or an ECG synchronized mode in which the pump can be made to counterpulsate. Much of the experience with the Pierce–Donachy pump in postoperative patients has been with the fill-to-empty mode, without synchronization. More recently, we have employed synchronization of the VAD in order to have it function in a counterpulsating mode in patients in whom the heart might recover.

The Novacor LVAS has the advantage of being able to function during any portion of the left ventricular cycle. It is possible gradually to increase or decrease the portion of blood pumped by the native left ventricle according to its recovery. While these synchronizing techniques may facilitate ventricular recovery, the patients with whom we are concerned will not have myocardial recovery, and therefore weaning techniques are not of great importance. In order to provide optimal assistance, the effects of the Novacor LVAS on intrinsic left ventricular function can be assessed by a left ventricular Millar transducer-tipped catheter. A computer within the console provides on-line beat-to-beat readout of pumping parameters. In general, when using left atrial cannulation in order to obtain adequate left VAD filling, left atrial pressure is maintained in the range of 10–15 mmHg. When apex cannulation is employed, left atrial pressures in the range of 5–10 mmHg will provide excellent left pump filling. Although it was at first feared that biventricular assist devices would present difficult problems of synchronization of the left and right pumps, this has not been an important clinical problem. It is usually anticipated that left ventricular flow will exceed right ventricular flow by 500–1000 ml/min because of the return of bronchial flow to the left ventricle. Centrifugal pumps are run to provide the highest flow possible, without regard to the cardiac cycle.

When using the Pierce–Donachy pump, the right and left pumps are usually run in the fill-to-empty mode. Alternatively, we have driven the left VAD on the ECG-synchronized mode with the right VAD in the fill-to-empty mode. Curiously, in some patients with biventricular Pierce–Donachy VADs functioning in the fill-to-empty mode, a natural synchronization of the pumps occurs and the flows in both become similar. Regardless of which drive parameters are employed, synchronization of the pumps is not necessary. The Jarvik TAH does not have the problem of working in synchrony with a natural heart since the ventricles have been removed. Both the right and left ventricular pumps' degree of filling and emptying can be measured from the pneumatic exhaust, using a pneumotachygraph and a computerized system (COMDU™).

Operation for removal and transplantation

The patient is transported to the operating room using the portable energy sources provided by the various devices. Cardiopulmonary bypass is initiated through the groin or chest. It is highly desirable to remove all prosthetic graft material from the great arteries in order to avoid leaving a nidus for infection. Occasionally, it has been considered more of a risk to try to accomplish complete removal than to leave a small rim of graft in place, but this has been rare. Standard cardiac transplantation techniques are employed. The atria are divided near the AV groove and the aorta and pulmonary artery are divided near the valves. Patients with Jarvik-7 TAH may have slightly smaller atrial cuffs after removal of the device, but this has not created difficulty. The large pocket in the abdominal wall created for the Novacor LVAS must be inspected carefully for haemostasis, and be well drained.

One patient in our series with Novacor LVAS in place for 91 days had a clean abdominal wall space without fluid or blood collection, which healed without complication. This was particularly important since there had been cellulitis surrounding the driveline leading from the abdominal pocket. After removal of the LVAS, the driveline tract was debrided and packed open. The rather large tracts created by the placement of the Pierce–Donachy cannulae must also be packed open, gently debrided from time to time and allowed to heal without suture closure. While these tracts have not healed as fast in the immunosuppressed patients as in our other patients, they have all healed without infection or residual problems.

CLINICAL EXPERIENCE

After the historic cases outlined earlier in this chapter, a virtual explosion of interest occurred in the field of bridging patients to cardiac transplantation. While experience had previously been limited to only a few centres with very sophisticated devices, the development of less expensive systems and the greater availability of devices has allowed the technique to become widespread. The data presented in this chapter are derived from various sources, mostly by direct communication with the various investigators. The data are incomplete in some instances, but are a reasonable indication of the current status of the use of various systems to bridge patients to transplantation.

Results

The results of the use of the various devices according to the type are presented in Tables 3.1–3.5.

Extracorporeal membrane oxygenation

In Table 3.1A (see also Table 3.1B), the non-thoracotomy approach to bridging is shown, beginning with the 2 patients previously mentioned from St. Louis University who were bridged to transplantation with a femorofemoral ECMO system. Although neither of these patients ultimately survived, both were stabilized haemodynamically with temporary systems until hearts became available. Unfortunately, complications related to the ECMO system developed in each: an iliac vein thrombosis with subsequent pulmonary embolus in one, and a groin wound infection leading to sepsis in the other, who lived a month after transplantation. However, Gifford and his colleagues of Cambridge, England, supported a patient with a percutaneous femorofemoral system for several days and then performed a successful transplantation (Gifford *et al.*, 1986). Bolman and his colleagues at Washington University supported a patient with an ECMO system for 48 h after an acute rejection episode, and the patient underwent successful retransplantation (Bolman *et al.*, 1987).

The obvious limitation of the ECMO system is the length of time it can be safely relied upon. Both survivors were maintained for less than 72 h. The problems of anticoagulation, immobilization, bleeding and sepsis limit the usefulness of this technique for prolonged maintenance. However, ECMO can be extremely useful in the immediate resuscitation of a patient, regardless of whether it is inserted in the emergency room, the operating room, the intensive care unit or the cardiac catheterization laboratory. Our current use of the femorofemoral ECMO system is to provide emergency resuscitation for periods of 24–48 h. If a decision has been made to pursue transplantation and if irreparable organ damage has not occurred, a more sophisticated system such as a Pierce–Donachy, Novacor or Jarvik-7 device can be implanted.

Centrifugal pumps

In Table 3.2A (see also Table 3.2B), the rather impressive results with centrifugal pumps are tabulated. The first patient who was supported at the Minnesota Heart Institute with a Centrimed pump is doing extremely well. All the other patients were supported with the Biomedicus device which was described earlier. The encouraging part of this experience is that 10 of the 15

TABLE 3.1A
*Bridge to Transplantation With ECMO**

Age	*Sex*	*Date*	*Institution*	*Diagnosis*	*Device*	*Pumping Duration (days)*	*Complications*	*Outcome*
52	M	3-2-83	SLU†	Cardiogenic shock	ECMO	3	Sepsis Renal failure	Died 1 month after transplant Sepsis
25	M	31-5-83	Papworth Hosp., England	Chronic rejection of donor heart	ECMO	4.2	None	?
25	M	16-7-83	SLU	Myocarditis	ECMO	5	Sepsis Pulmonary infarcts	Died 1 day after transplant Pulmonary infarcts Sepsis
32	M	7-9-86	Washington Univ.	Acute rejection post-transplant	ECMO	2.0	Neurological deficit (recovered)	Retransplanted (doing well)

* Extracorporeal membrane oxygenation.
† St. Louis University, Missouri.

TABLE 3.1B
Patient Not Transplanted From ECMO

Age	*Sex*	*Date*	*Institution*	*Diagnosis*	*Device*	*Pumping Duration (days)*	*Reason Not Transplanted*	*Outcome*
38	M	27-11-82	SLU	Viral cardiomyopathy	ECMO	2	Renal failure Bleeding	Died

patients (67%) who underwent transplantation were discharged from the hospital. The mean time of device support was 3.4 days, emphasizing the importance of obtaining donor hearts early in the course of circulatory support. The limitation of the centrifugal pumps has been the relatively high incidence of fibrin formation and occasional thrombus in the pump heads. For this reason, we believe that anticoagulation with heparin is essential as soon as the initial bleeding has stopped. These systems may be appropriate for periods of up to 1 week, but it is doubtful whether pumping beyond that time will lead to a successful outcome.

External pulsatile ventricular assist device

Table 3.3A (see also Table 3.3B) demonstrates the outstanding success experienced with the use of the Pierce–Donachy external VAD. Half of this group of patients required biventricular assistance, made possible by the versatility of the Pierce–Donachy pump. The length of time required to obtain a donor heart in this group was 7.6 days. A young woman at Pennsylvania State University was maintained for 22 days prior to transplantation, during which period she suffered no ill effects from the pump, and she went on to have a highly successful transplant. For two of our own patients treated at St. Louis University we were able to obtain donor hearts within a very short period. These patients had completely uneventful courses and were discharged from the hospital after a shorter recuperative period than our average transplant patients. Recently, the data for the Pierce–Donachy VAD patients has been nicely summarized and reported by Farrar *et al.* (1986). One of the potential problems with this device is that it is an external pump which must be carried on the patient's abdominal wall, making it subject to kinking of the cannulae and other difficulties during mobilization. However, one of the patients in this series was able to get out of bed and have some activity in spite of the need for continuous pumping. It is not known whether this pump is suitable for periods of support extending beyond 3 weeks. However, there is concern that the large cannulae required to traverse the abdominal wall might be subject to tract infection, bleeding and mechanical kinking. The excellent blood contact surface of this pump is a definite advantage which makes it a desirable system for intermediate (less than 1 month) use.

Implanted ventricular assist devices

As shown in Table 3.4A (see also Table 3.4B), 8 patients underwent cardiac transplantation after support with implantable paracorporeal left ventricular assist systems (LVAS). The first successful case was a patient at Stanford who received the Novacor left ventricular assist device. The longest time that this device was implanted was 91 days in a patient at St. Louis University.

TABLE 3.2A

Bridge to Transplantation With Centrifugal Pumps

Age	*Sex*	*Date*	*Institution*	*Diagnosis*	*Device*	*Cannulation*	*Duration (days)*	*Complications*	*Outcome*
32	M	7-84	Univ. Hosp., Augusta, GA	Failed allograft	Biomedicus BVADs	LA-Ao RA-PA	0.5	Mediastinal sepsis	Died 2 weeks after 2nd cardiac Tx.
42	M	9-85	Univ. Hosp., Augusta, GA	Failed allograft	Biomedicus BVADs	LV-Ao RA-PA	0.5	Sepsis, multiple organ failure	Died 5 days after 2nd cardiac Tx.
25	M	15-1-86	Minneapolis Heart Inst.	Unknown	Centrimed LVAD	LV-Ao	0.5	None	Alive, at home
58	M	2-86	Texas Heart Inst.	Ischaemic cardiomyopathy	Biomedicus LVAD	LV-Ao	0.5	None	Died 2 weeks post-op. of sepsis
46	F	2-86	Washington Univ.	Ischaemic cardiomyopathy	Biomedicus LVAD	LV-Ao	2.0	None	Doing well
Unk.	M	23-5-86	Humana Hosp., San Antonio, CA	Ischaemic/post-cardiotomy	Biomedicus LVAD	LA-Ao	3.0	Multiple organ failure, dialysis, jaundice, unconscious	Full recovery Working full time

44	M	26-6-86	Univ. Hosp., Augusta, GA	Ischaemic cardiomyopathy Vent. aneurysm	Biomedicus LVAD	Pulm. vein-Ao	4.0	Hospitalized 5 weeks Leg wound problems Enterobact. from chest tube	Survived, doing well
17	Unk.	17-7-86	Mercy Hosp., Des Moines, Iowa	Unknown	Biomedicus RVAD	RA-PA	2.0	None	Doing well
57	M	7-86	Washington Univ.	Ischaemic post-cardiotomy	Biomedicus LVAD	LV-Ao	2.0	Renal failure, liver failure, neuro. Sepsis	Complete recovery Working full time
48	M	9-86	Washington Univ.	CAD/acute MI	Biomedicus LVAD	LV-Ao	0.5	None	Complete recovery
37	M	10-86	Washington Univ.	Reiter's synd. AVR	Biomedicus LVAD	LV-Ao	2.0	None	Working full time
56	F	7-10-86	Cleveland Clinic, Ohio	Mitral stenosis (rheumatic)	Biomedicus LVAD	LA-Ao	3.4	None	Alive, at home
50	M	12-11-86	Cleveland Clinic, Ohio	Cardiomyopathy	Biomedicus LVAD	LA-Ao	2.5	Bleeding	Alive, at home
55	M	11-86	UCLA*	AVR/MVR Post-cardiotomy	Biomedicus BVADs	LA-Ao RA-PA	Unk.	Fungal sepsis Renal failure	Died
43	M	11-86	UCLA	Post-cardiotomy Cardiac arrest	Biomedicus BVADs	LA-Ao RA-PA	5.0	Renal failure Sepsis	Died

* University of California at Los Angeles.

TABLE 3.2B

Patients Not Transplanted From Centrifugal Pumps

Age	*Sex*	*Date*	*Institution*	*Diagnosis*	*Device*	*Cannulation*	*Duration (days)*	*Complications*	*Outcome*
35	M	3-8-85	Cleveland Clinic, Ohio	Acute MI	Biomedicus LVAD	LA-Ao	5.0	Bleeding	Died
52	M	1-86	Humana Hosp., San Antonio, CA	Flu., cardiogenic shock	Biomedicus LVAD	Unk.	5.0	Dialysis (6 wks) Pseudomonas, septicaemia, gangrene	Recovered, weaned and not transplanted
62	M	7-86	Univ. Hosp., Augusta, GA	MI/CABG	Biomedicus LVAD	LV-Ao	7.0	Sepsis	Patient extubated
30	M	22-8-86	Cleveland Clinic, Ohio	Cardiomyopathy	Biomedicus BVAD	RA-PA LA-Ao	3.0	Bleeding	Died
42	M	1-12-86	Cleveland Clinic, Ohio	Idiopathic cardiomyopathy	Biomedicus LVAD	LA-Ao	15.4	Bleeding Ventricular thrombus	Died

The prolonged period of support was necessitated by the development of antibodies which made it difficult to find a suitable donor. Fortunately, the antibody level fell from a PRA of 85% to a PRA of 0% over a 2½-month period, allowing successful transplantation. The average length of time prior to transplantation in these patients was 28 days, indicating the capability of these devices to serve as longer term devices. The current limitation to permanent implantation of these systems is the need for an externalized drive line to provide electrical power, and to vent air in the absence of a compliance chamber. In the patient who was sustained for 91 days, cellulitis occurred in the drive line tract and necessitated antibiotic therapy. Had the patient continued longer, it is possible that this infection would have led to complications, preventing transplantation. Fortunately, after transplantation the opened tract healed well in spite of immunosuppression.

Orthotopic biventricular replacement devices

The experience with orthotopic biventricular cardiac replacement (TAH) is shown in Table 3.5A. To date, the only survivors of transplantation after this type of circulatory support have been patients who received the Jarvik device manufactured by Symbion Corporation, Salt Lake City, Utah (Copeland, 1986; Joyce *et al.*, 1986a, b; Griffith *et al.*, 1986; Levinson *et al.*, 1986). Forty patients have received 42 devices. The Jarvik-7 (100 ml) was used in 14 instances and the Jarvik-7-70 (70 ml) in 26. Of the 40 patients, 32 underwent orthotopic transplantation, 21 of whom were living in mid-March 1987. Five patients still had the Jarvik-7 device in place. The length of time on the Jarvik-7 prior to transplantation ranged from 1 to 243 days, with an average time of 18 days and a median time of 9 days. In general, the devices have worked well without major complications. In almost every case, the patients who died prior to transplantation developed complications related to events occurring prior to placement of the Jarvik-7 such as renal failure, liver failure and pulmonary disease.

Seven patients died after receiving transplants. A 40-year-old Minnesota woman who was supported for 45 days (Joyce *et al.*, 1986b) died 9 months after transplantation of multiple complications, including renal failure requiring dialysis, driveline infection and mediastinitis. A 40-year-old woman from the University of Arizona died of acute rejection of her second donor heart after living for 243 days with her second Jarvik-7. This fascinating case was complicated by high antibody levels (PRA of 90%), resulting in a positive crossmatch against 90 potential donors. Eventually, after extensive immunosuppressive therapy and irradiation, she had a second transplant but died of acute rejection shortly after. It appears that the length of time of implantation of the Jarvik-7 was not a factor in determining sur-

TABLE 3.3A

Bridge to Transplantation With External Pulsatile Ventricular Assist Device

Age	*Sex*	*Date*	*Institution*	*Diagnosis*	*Device*	*Pumping Duration (days)*	*Complications*	*Outcome*
47	M	6-9-84	PMC*	Acute MI	Pierce–Donachy LVAD	2.2	Amputated leg due to IABP Acute renal failure	Doing well
16	M	24-3-85	Univ. Louisville, Kent.	Viral cardiomyopathy	Pierce–Donachy BVADs	5	Acute renal failure	Alive, doing well
54	M	14-5-85	SLU†	Acute MI	Pierce–Donachy LVAD	1.5	None	Alive, doing well
24	F	21-7-85	Penn. State Univ.	Cardiomyopathy	Pierce–Donachy LVAD	22	Respiratory failure Infection	Alive, doing well
42	F	22-10-85	SLU	Cardiomyopathy	Pierce–Donachy LVAD	0.4	Bleeding	Doing well
33	M	25-10-85	PMC	Cardiomyopathy	Pierce–Donachy BVADs	3.5	None	Alive, doing well
53	M	9-1-86	Harley Street Clinic, London	CABG Re-do	Pierce–Donachy LVAD Roller pump RVAD	0.5	Initial biventricular failure	Alive, doing well
35	M	1-86	Medical Coll., Wisconsin	Idiopathic cardiomyopathy	Pierce–Donachy BVADs	3	None	Doing well
42	M	14-2-86	Cardiovascular Research Inst., Sion, Switzerland	Cardiomyopathy	Pierce–Donachy BVADs	4.1	None	Doing well
20	M	22-3-86	Penn. State Univ.	Cardiomyopathy	Pierce–Donachy LVAD	7	Infection	Died 4 weeks post-transplant
29	M	3-5-86	Univ. Louisville, Kent.	Idiopathic cardiomyopathy	Pierce–Donachy LVAD	21	Respiratory failure	Doing well

52	M	6-5-86	Univ. Hosp., Augusta, GA	Acute MI shock	Pierce–Donachy LVAD	0.8	None	Alive, at home
40	M	29-5-86	Cardiovascular Research Inst., Sion, Switzerland	Dilated cardiomyopathy	Pierce–Donachy BVADs	4.0	None	Alive, at home
41	M	17-6-86	PMC	Acute MI	Pierce–Donachy BVADs	1.6	None	Alive, at home
25	M	19-12-86	Penn. State Univ.	Cardiomyopathy	Pierce–Donachy LVAD	31	Fungal infection	Recovering, doing well
34	M	31-12-86	SLU	Idiopathic cardiomyopathy	Pierce–Donachy LVAD	24	Minor CVA	At home, recovered
25	M	24-1-87	Penn. State Univ.	Cardiomyopathy	Pierce–Donachy LVAD	3	None	Alive, at home
41	M	13-2-87	SLU	Cardiomyopathy	Pierce–Donachy BVAD	3	Infection	Recovering
53	M	28-2-87	PMC	AMI	BVAD	1.5	None	Doing well
51	M	20-3-87	PMC	AMI	BVAD	3	None	Doing well
30	F	24-3-87	Ohio State Univ.	Viral cardiomyopathy	BVAD	22	None	Doing well
20	F	7-4-87	Univ. Louisville, Kent.	Post-partum cardiomyopathy	LVAD	1	None	Doing well
34	M	9-4-87	SLU	Cardiomyopathy	Pierce–Donachy BVADs	75	Antibodies developed	Doing well
38	M	23-4-87	Ohio State Univ.	Cardiomyopathy	BVAD	13	None	Doing well
41	M	13-5-87	Univ. Hosp., Augusta, GA	Cardiomyopathy	BVAD	40	Multiple organ failure	Died
46	M	30-6-87	Univ. Louisville, Kent.	Acute MI	BVAD	2	None	Doing well
50	M	2-7-87	PMC	Acute MI	BVAD	10	Cardiac tamponade	Doing well
32	M	13-7-87	PMC	Cardiomyopathy	BVAD	2	None	Doing well

* Pacific Medical Centre.

† St. Louis University, Missouri.

TABLE 3.3B

*Patients Not Transplanted From External Pulsatile Ventricular Assist Device**

Age	Sex	Date	Institution	Diagnosis	Device	Pumping Duration (days)	Reason Not Transplanted	Outcome
27	F	16-4-82	SLU†	Cardiomyopathy	Pierce–Donachy LVAD	4.5	Bleeding Renal failure	Died
					Medtronic RVAD	4.0		
32	M	27-9-82	SLU	Cardiomyopathy	Pierce–Donachy LVAD	5	Renal failure	Died
50	M	12-6-85	SLU	Post-CPB shock	Pierce–Donachy LVAD	22	Sepsis	Died
					Biomedicus RVAD	6		
48	M	30-7-85	SLU	Acute MI	Pierce–Donachy LVAD	3	Renal failure	Died
					Biomedicus RVAD	3		
48	M	1-8-85	Penn. State Univ.	Acute MI	Pierce–Donachy BVADs	13	Respiratory failure Renal failure Sepsis	Died
52	M	11-10-85	PMC	Acute MI	Pierce–Donachy BVADs	0.1	Aspiration	Died
27	F	30-10-85	Univ. Louisville, Kent.	Cardiomyopathy	Pierce–Donachy BVADs	0.8	Renal failure Pulmonary hypertension	Died
45	M	8-12-85	Univ. Hosp., Augusta, GA	Cardiomyopathy	Pierce–Donachy BVADs	2.6	Bleeding	Died
22	F	22-5-86	Cardiovascular Research Inst., Sion, Switzerland	Cardiomyopathy	Pierce–Donachy LVAD	1	Bleeding	Died
55	M	22-6-86	Univ. Louisville, Kent.	Acute MI	Pierce–Donachy LVAD	0.2	Bleeding PAH	Died
25	M	9-9-86	Univ. Louisville, Kent.	Cardiomyopathy	Pierce–Donachy BVADs	2.6	Bleeding Coagulopathy	Died

* Since unsuccessful bridge-to-transplant procedures are not always documented, this table is not comprehensive.

† St. Louis University, Missouri.

TABLE 3.4A

Bridge to Transplantation With Internal Pulsatile Ventricular Assist Device

Age	*Sex*	*Date*	*Institution*	*Diagnosis*	*Device*	*Pumping Duration (days)*	*Complications*	*Outcome*
21	M	9-2-78	THI*	P.O. shock	ALVAD #7	5	ATN Sepsis	Died 15 days post-transplant
51	M	5-9-84	Stanford Univ., CA	Ischaemic cardiomyopathy	Novacor	9	Tamponade	At home, doing well
47	M	19-1-86	THI	Cardiomyopathy	Thermedics	41	Sepsis Multiple organ failure	Died 49 days post-heterotopic transplant
53	M	20-5-86	THI	Cardiomyopathy	Thermedics	19	Sepsis Multiple organ failure	Died 41 days post-transplant
47	M	5-6-86	Stanford Univ., CA	Acute MI	Novacor	3.2	None	At home, doing well
46	M	10-9-86	SLU†	Ischaemic cardiomyopathy	Novacor	91	None	At home, doing well
30	F	11-9-86	Stanford Univ., CA	Cardiomyopathy	Novacor	2.4	Tamponade	Died post-transplant
37	M	2-12-86	THI	Cardiomyopathy	Thermedics	25	Acute rejection	Died in OR during heterotopic transplant

* Texas Heart Institute.

† St. Louis University, Missouri.

TABLE 3.4B

Patients Not Transplanted From Internal Pulsatile Ventricular Assist Device

Age	*Sex*	*Date*	*Institution*	*Diagnosis*	*Device*	*Pumping Duration (days)*	*Complications*	*Outcome*
39	M	4-4-85	Stanford Univ., CA	Ischaemic cardiomyopathy	Novacor	16	Renal failure Fungal pneumonia	Died
28	M	13-2-86	SLU*	Cardiomyopathy	Novacor	29	Multiple organ failure Sepsis	Died
55	M	30-4-86	THI†	Cardiomyopathy	Thermedics	5	Multiple organ failure	Died
38	M	26-12-86	Johns Hopkins Univ.	Acute MI	Novacor	65	Renal failure Bleeding	Died
28	F	13-2-87	Stanford Univ. CA	Acute rejection, 2nd transplant	Novacor	0.1	Rejection of 2nd transplant	Died
38	F	18-4-87	Detroit Henry Ford Hospital	Viral cardiomyopathy	Novacor	0.25	Unknown	Died
58	M	3-7-87	Univ. Pittsburgh, PA	Cardiomyopathy	Novacor	0.5	Severe blood reaction	Died

* St. Louis University, Missouri.

† Texas Heart Institute.

vival, since 4 of the 7 deaths occurred in patients who had the Jarvik device in place for less than 1 week.

The overall survival rate at the time of writing, among recipients of Jarvik-7 devices who ultimately had transplants is 73%. The current survival rates can be attributed to several factors, including the alteration of the Utah drive system to decrease the d*p*/d*t* and therefore decrease the incidence of haemolysis (DeVries *et al.*, 1986), and the introduction of J7-70 to allow for better fitting in smaller patients (Jarvik *et al.*, 1986).

An interesting aspect of this study is the evaluation of those patients who did not receive transplants (Table 3.5B). It is to be expected that some patients receiving devices as proposed bridges to transplantation will never receive transplants, since a certain percentage of patients will develop complications which prohibit transplantation. In this entire experience, we have identified 31 such patients. The reasons included the development of renal failure, liver failure, cerebral injury or infections such as mediastinitis, pneumonia or in the driveline. The investigative team must prepare the patient and the family prior to device implantation for the possibility that complications may preclude transplantation. In such instances, the patient may simply die of a complication or become dependent upon the assist device for a prolonged period. Long-term pump dependence is most likely in patients with increased levels of antibodies, which preclude transplantation, but do not result in the death of the patient. A man at Pennsylvania State University had been supported with the Pennsylvania State total artificial heart for nearly a year. In order to ensure the most efficient use of donor organs, it is necessary for the 'bridging experience' to be a screening mechanism. If criteria for transplantation are strictly maintained, it is reasonable to expect a rejection rate of about 30% and a survival rate in transplanted patients greater than 70%.

Management of complications

Bleeding

In spite of the surgeon's best efforts, bleeding may continue and lead to cardiac tamponade and hypotension. Recently, we have discontinued the reinfusion of shed whole blood because it appears to aggravate the coagulopathy. We have continued to collect the shed blood, and wash the red cells for reinfusion. Our approach is to use large amounts of fresh frozen plasma, platelets and washed red blood cells for volume replacement. The development of cardiac tamponade can be very insidious, since the mechanical device will continue to function in most instances in spite of moderately severe tamponade. The usual pattern in patients with left ventricular assist devices is an increase in right and left atrial pressures, accompanied by decreased left ventricular pump filling which does not improve with volume

TABLE 3.5A

*Bridge to Transplantation With a TAH**

Age	*Sex*	*Date*	*Institution*	*Diagnosis*	*Device (TAH)*	*Pumping Duration (days)*	*Complications*	*Outcome*
47	M	4-4-69	THI†	Ischaemic cardiomyopathy Postoperative shock	Liotta	2.5	Anatomical fit	Died 1 day post-transplant
36	M	23-7-81	THI	Coronary artery disease Postoperative shock	Akutsu	2.3	Hypoxaemia–ECMO Anatomical fit	Died of heart rejection 8 days post-transplant
33	M	6-3-85	Univ. Arizona	Ischaemic cardiomyopathy Post-transplant cardiogenic shock	Phoenix	0.5	Bleeding, pulmonary oedema, pneumonia, sepsis, pulmonary hypertension	Died 36 h after 2nd transplant
25	M	29-8-85	Univ. Arizona	Viral cardiomyopathy	Jarvik-7	9.0	Embolic strokes	Tx. on 9th day, did well Alive, at home
44	M	18-10-85	Penn. State Univ.	Acute congestive cardiomyopathy	Penn. State Pneumatic	11.0	Post-transplant renal failure Fungal sepsis Pancreatitis	Died 17 days post-transplant
47	M	24-10-85	Univ. Pittsburgh, PA	Cardiomyopathy Cardiogenic shock	Jarvik-7	4.0	None	Alive
40	F	18.12.85	Minneapolis Heart Inst., Minn.	Cardiomyopathy	Jarvik-7-70	45.0	Renal failure, bleeding, respiratory failure, ischaemic leg–IABP, superficial driveline infection	Died 9 months post-transplant
39	M	3-2-86	Univ. Pittsburgh, PA	Acute myocardial infarction Shock	Jarvik-7	12.0	Respiratory failure Bleeding	Alive
40	F	3-2-86	Univ. Arizona	Viral myocarditis	Jarvik-7-70	246 (total 2 TAH)	Transplanted heart failed, second TAH required	Died of acute rejection of 2nd donor heart

41	M	3-2-86	THI	Cardiomyopathy	Jarvik-7	32.0	None	Alive and well
26	F	6-3-86	Herzchirurgie, Salzburg	Cardiomyopathy	Ellipsoid heart, Unger	1	Bleeding	Rejection of donor heart Died 10 days post-op
39	Unk.	7-3-86	Free Univ., Berlin	Cardiomyopathy	Berlin	4	Renal failure Respiratory failure	Died 2 days post-transplant
42	M	1-5-86	Univ. Pittsburgh, PA	Cardiomyopathy	Jarvik-7	2	Infection	Died of acute onset delayed rejection 2 months post-transplant
41	M	1-5-86	Ottawa Heart Inst.	Cardiomyopathy	Jarvik-7-70	7	None	Alive, at home
53	M	6-5-86	Karolinska Inst., Stockholm	Ischaemic cardiomyopathy	Jarvik-7-70	10	None	Alive, at home Working part-time
47	Unk.	13-5-86	Univ. Vienna	Cardiomyopathy	Ellipsoid heart, Unger	9	Unknown	Died at transplant
22	M	14-5-86	Hospital La Pitié, Paris	Acute viral myocarditis	Jarvik-7	13	None	Alive, at home, working
32	M	13-6-86	Univ. Pittsburgh, PA	Cardiomyopathy	Jarvick-7-70	8	Unknown	Alive, at home, working
40	M	18-6-86	Hospital La Pitié, Paris	Idiopathic cardiomyopathy	Jarvik-7	15	None	Alive, at home
34	M	26-6-86	Hospital La Pitié, Paris	Idiopathic cardiomyopathy	Jarvik-7	14	Infection	Alive, at home, working
40	M	30-7-86	Univ. Pittsburgh, PA	Hyperacute rejection of 1st transplant	Jarvik-7-70	12	Unknown	Alive, at home, working
32	F	4-8-86	Hospital La Pitié, Paris	Post-partum cardiomyopathy	Jarvik-7-70	1	None	Alive, at home, working
42	M	14-9-86	Hospital La Pitié, Paris	Ischaemic cardiomyopathy	Jarvik-7-70	1	Neurological and resp. complications post-transplant	Died 15 days post-transplant
58	F	7-10-86	Univ. Pittsburgh, PA	Viral cardiomyopathy	Jarvik-7-70	2	Rejection	Died at transplant
Unk.	Unk.	8-10-86	Unknown	Cardiomyopathy	Ellipsoid heart, Unger	10	Unknown	Died 6 weeks post-transplant
44	M	12-10-86	Univ. Pittsburgh, PA	Cardiomyopathy	Jarvik-7-70	8	Unknown	Alive, at home
35	M	17-10-86	Hospital La Pitié, Paris	Cardiomyopathy	Jarvik-7	16	None	Alive, at home, working
20	M	17-10-86	Hospital La Pitié, Paris	Terminal cardiomyopathy	Jarvik-7	24	None	Alive, at home

TABLE 3.5A—continued

Age	*Sex*	*Date*	*Institution*	*Diagnosis*	*Device (TAH)*	*Pumping Duration (days)*	*Complications*	*Outcome*
54	M	22-10-86	Univ. Pittsburg, PA	Idiopathic cardiomyopathy	Jarvik-7-70	5	Unknown	Alive, good condition
37	M	30-10-86	Ottawa Heart Inst.	Coronary artery disease	Jarvik-7-70	1	Cardiac arrest post-transplant	Died 4 weeks post-transplant
40	M	2-11-86	Papworth Everard Hospital, Cambridge, UK	End-stage ischaemic cardiomyopathy	Jarvik-7	2	Unknown	Alive, good condition
Unk.	Unk.	4-11-86	Unknown	Cardiomyopathy	Ellipsoid heart, Unger	22	Unknown	Died at transplant
28	F	11-11-86	Minneapolis Heart Inst.	Giant cell myocarditis Cardiomyopathy	Jarvik-7-70	4	Unknown	Alive, good condition, at home
38	M	21-11-86	Midwest Heart Surgical Inst., Milwaukee	Cardiomyopathy	Jarvik-7-70	4	Unknown	Alive, good condition at home
43	M	8-12-86	Hospital La Pitié, Paris-	Ischaemic cardiomyopathy	Jarvik-7	21	Hepatitis	Died 17 days post-transplant
26	M	20-12-86	Univ. Pittsburgh, PA	Viral cardiomyopathy	Jarvik-7-70	4	Unknown	At home, good condition
55	M	7-1-87	Univ. Pittsburg, PA	Ischaemic cardiomyopathy	Jarvik-7-70	5	Sepsis	Died 32 days post-transplant
48	M	8-1-87	Midwest Heart Surgical Inst.	Ischaemic cardiomyopathy	Jarvik-7-70	15	Unknown	Died 1 day post-transplant
43	M	13-1-87	Hospital La Pitié, Paris	Non-obstructive cardiomyopathy	Jarvik-7	21	Unknown	Died at transplant
38	M	14-1-87	Univ. Pittsburgh, PA	Idiopathic cardiomyopathy	Jarvik-7-70	34	Sepsis	Died 1 day post-transplant
56	M	17-1-87	Univ. Florida	Ischaemic cardiomyopathy	Jarvik-7-70	9	Fungal infection	Died 7 weeks post-transplant

35	M	28-1-87	Henri-Mondor, Paris	Acute rejection	Jarvik-7-70	5	Fungal infection	Died 36 days post-transplant
47	M	2-2-87	Ottawa Heart Inst.	Post-cardiotomy	Jarvik-7-70	6	Unknown	Stable condition
47	M	3-2-87	Hospital La Pitié, Paris	Ischaemic cardiomyopathy	Jarvik-7	7	Unknown	Died at transplant
56	M	26-2-87	Hospital La Pitié, Paris	Acute myocardial infarction	Jarvik-7	12	Unknown	Good condition
57	M	27-2-87	Univ. Pittsburg, PA	Acute myocardial infarction	Jarvik-7-70	14	Unknown	Died 2 months post-transplant
15	M	8-4-87	Minneapolis Heart Inst.	Idiopathic cardiomyopathy	Jarvik-7-70	25	Unknown	Doing well
39	M	21-4-87	Univ. Pittsburgh, PA	Idiopathic cardiomyopathy	Jarvik-7-70	6	Unknown	Doing well
39	M	22-4-87	Univ. Arizona	Acute rejection of 1st transplant	Jarvik-7-70	12	Unknown	Doing well
37	M	1-5-87	Hospital La Pitié, Paris	Ischaemic cardiomyopathy	Jarvik-7	31	Unknown	Recovering
39	M	5-5-87	Univ. Arizona	Viral cardiomyopathy	Jarvik-7-70	31	Unknown	Recovering
50	M	13-5-87	Minneapolis Heart Inst.	CABG redo	Jarvik-7-70	18	Unknown	Recovering
24	M	19-5-87	Ottawa Heart Inst.	Congenital heart disease	Jarvik-7-70 Jarvik-7	6 2	Rejected first transplant; 2nd TAH used	Recovering
40	M	28-5-87	DesMoines Mercy Medical Center	CABG redo	Jarvik-7	1	Unknown	Died 2 weeks post-transplant
47	M	3-6-87	Univ. Pittsburgh, PA	Acute rejection of 1st transplant	Jarvik-7-70	7	Unknown	Recovering
35	M	17-6-87	San Diego Sharp Memorial Hospital	Failed donor heart	Jarvik-7-70	11	Unknown	Recovering
47	M	25-6-87	St. Luke's Hospital, Milwaukee	CABG redo	Jarvik-7-70	3	Unknown	Recovering

* Biventricular replacement device.
† Texas Heart Institute.

TABLE 3.5B

*Patients Not Transplanted From TAH**

Age	*Sex*	*Date*	*Institution*	*Diagnosis*	*Device (TAH)*	*Pumping Duration (days)*	*Reason Not Transplanted*	*Outcome*
48	M	17-3-86	Penn. State Univ.	Unknown	Penn. State Pneumatic	396	Unknown	Died
43	M	22-3-86	Univ. Pittsburgh, PA	Ischaemic cardiomyopathy	Jarvik-7-70	18	Multi-organ failure	Died
26	M	13-4-86	Hospital La Pitié, Paris	Valvular disease, CHF	Jarvik-7-70	10	Pulmonary infection	Died
55	M	10-5-86	Hospital La Pitié, Paris	Cardiomyopathy	Jarvik-7-70	14	Multi-organ failure	Died
18	M	14-7-86	Hospital La Pitié, Paris	Acute rejection of 1st donor heart	Jarvik-7-70	1	Unknown	Died
48	F	30-9-86	Karolinska Inst., Stockholm	Congenital tricuspid valve anomaly; calcif. right ventricle	Jarvik-7-70	190 days (2 TAH)	Rejected 1st donor heart; 2nd J-7-70 implanted	Died

48	M	13-10-86	THI†	Cardiomyopathy	Jarvik-7-70	4	Multi-organ failure	Died
47	M	11-11-86	Hospital La Pitié, Paris	Ischaemic cardiomyopathy	Jarvik-7	16	Unknown	Died
27	F	17-11-86	Hospital La Pitié, Paris	Post-partum cardiomyopathy	Jarvik-7-70	6	Renal failure Respiratory failure	Died
40	F	25-11-86	Univ. Arizona	Ebstein's anomaly	Jarvik-7-70	9	Multi-organ failure	Died
30	F	26-12-86	Hospital La Pitié, Paris	Acute rejection of 1st transplant	Jarvik-7-70	6	Unknown	Died
47	M	31-12-86	Hospital La Pitié, Paris	Non-obstructive cardiomyopathy	Jarvik-7	9	Unknown	Died
Unk.	Unk.	9-1-87	Free Univ. Berlin	Ischaemic cardiomyopathy	Berlin	4	Unknown	Died
Unk.	Unk.	23-1-87	Free Univ. Berlin	Ischaemic cardiomyopathy	Berlin	Ongoing	Unknown	Unknown
55	M	22-2-87	Hospital La Pitié Paris	Acute myocardial infarction	Jarvik-7	8	Sepsis	Died
29	M	23-5-87	Hospital La Pitié, Paris	Acute rejection of 1st transplant	Jarvik-7-70	15	Unknown	Died

* Biventricular replacement device.
† Texas Heart Institute.

replacement or increasing vacuum. In such circumstances, immediate re-exploration is required. Cardiac tamponade has complicated the course of patients with virtually all the devices described in this chapter. We have had to re-explore patients with assist devices as many as 3 times during the first 48 h after operation. The need for blood or blood product transfusions markedly increases the likelihood of the development of antibodies, and may strikingly limit the transplant possibilities. Therefore, it is highly desirable to use washed red blood cells and type-specific platelets for volume replacement. The need for multiple transfusions also increases the risk of cytomegalovirus (CMV) infection unless CMV negative blood is used.

Arrhythmias

One of the advantages of orthotopic ventricular replacement is the absence of ventricular arrhythmias. Actually, ventricular arrhythmias are of no immediate consequence in patients with biventricular assist devices. However, persistent ventricular fibrillation may result in myocardial injury (Rich *et al.*, 1982) and should be interrupted whenever possible. It is possible to support a patient with ventricular fibrillation with a left ventricular assist device only (Norman *et al.*, 1981). However, recurrent ventricular arrhythmias, in patients with left ventricular assist only, may be an indication for insertion of a right ventricular assist device.

Thrombo-embolism

Thrombo-embolism remains a potential threat for all types of ventricular assist systems. While the incidence of embolization is rare in this series, the incidence of thrombus in the pumps or cannulae is not uncommon. One patient with the ECMO system had a thrombus in an iliac vein, leading to pulmonary embolus which contributed to his death. Several patients sustained neurological deficits, but there were no recorded instances of systemic embolization in patients supported with centrifugal pumps, the Pierce–Donachy pulsatile pump or the Novacor left ventricular assist device. Insufficient data were available from the Thermedics patients, but no known instances of embolization occurred. The first patient to have a successful transplant after support with the Jarvik orthotopic ventricles was a 25-year-old man from Tucson, who had an episode of cerebral embolism when his anticoagulation regimen was not optimal (Levinson *et al.*, 1986). Fortunately, his cerebral symptoms resolved and he recovered completely. The incidence of thrombo-embolism in the various patients in this chapter cannot be related to the pump employed, since the time on the device varied greatly. However, it is clear that all the devices can cause thrombo-embolism, and therefore anticoagulation is advised for all cases who require assistance for more than a few days.

Renal failure

In spite of high perfusion flows after placement of the assist devices, renal failure frequently progressed. In our experience, using various types of ventricular assist devices in more than 100 patients at St. Louis University over the past 9 years, we have never had a patient survive who required haemodialysis for renal failure. However, several patients from other institutions required dialysis and survived cardiac transplantation (Farrar *et al.*, 1986; Joyce *et al.*, 1986b; L. Gray, 1986, personal communication). Notable among these was a 16-year-old boy at the University of Louisville who required biventricular assistance and who was dialysed for several weeks before eventual renal recovery (Gray, 1986). The centrifugal pumps and the ECMO systems lend themselves very well to on-line ultrafiltration or dialysis. Haemodialysis is less complicated in patients with assist devices because satisfactory cardiac output can usually be maintained by the device. In spite of these advantages, which make dialysis more feasible in assist device patients, complete renal failure remains a very important factor in the failure of many patients to survive and ultimately to receive a cardiac transplant.

Infection

Infection was one of the more frequent causes of death in patients who did not survive transplantation, and was a common reason for patients not receiving a transplant after being supported with an artificial device. However, driveline infections did not occur in any of the patients who were supported for 1–18 days with total artificial hearts, but never transplanted. The Pennsylvania State University patient who was maintained with biventricular orthotopic support (Penn State TAH) for 11 days died of fungal mediastinitis. The other Penn State TAH patient who has been supported for nearly a year on a total artificial heart apparently had a driveline infection which was successfully treated (Magovern *et al.*, 1986). The 40-year-old woman from Minnesota previously discussed also developed a driveline infection (Joyce *et al.*, 1986b). There is still controversy over how best to handle the threat of infection in patients who require prolonged support. For example, some believe that patients should have continuous antibiotic treatment during their entire period of perfusion. However, this has not been shown to prevent infections, and may create the problem of superinfection. Driveline infections may best be handled by opening the driveline tract and treating it with surgical debridement, a procedure used in at least two patients with Jarvik-7 devices. In the 91-day patient with the Novacor device at St. Louis University, two different episodes of cellulitis around the driveline were treated with antibiotics and resolved. However, just prior to transplantation, infection recurred. At present, our policy is to withdraw antibiotics in patients who are stable and whose drainage tubes have been removed. We believe that the devices are less likely to become infected if the patients are haemodynamically stable and have a reasonable nutritional status. An important consideration in the development of infection in these patients may be the fact that immunosuppression occurs early in their course. Ward *et al.* (1986) have reported a selective effect of cardiopulmonary bypass on immunological parameters, and Stelzer *et al.* (1987) have demonstrated T-cell depression and complement activation in long-term Jarvik-7 recipients. A recent study of T-cell lymphocytes in patients with assist devices at St. Louis University revealed marked depression of the total lymphocyte count and of the T-cell lymphocytes during the early days of perfusion (McBride *et al.*, 1987). However, once the patient had stabilized and the haemodynamics had improved, the immunosuppression diminished. We are only just beginning to learn about the fascinating relationship between circulatory assist devices and the patient's immune mechanisms.

ECONOMIC CONSIDERATIONS

The approximate costs of the various devices described in this chapter are given in Table 3.6. The costs may change with increased production, but the more sophisticated devices are moderately expensive. With the exception of the Jarvik-7, the cost increases if biventricular assistance is required. Although the costs of the devices are important, they are not the most important in determining the feasibility of this technology. The major costs are those related to the intensive care and prolonged hospital stay of patients in whom transplants cannot be done within a short period of device implementation, or in patients who develop major complications. Since it was anticipated that all patients described in this chapter would have died without mechanical support, it is obvious that the most economic choice would have been to withhold support. Although such a course is morally unacceptable, physicians are obliged to consider not only the patient's welfare but the fiscal burden of allocating resources in the most responsible

TABLE 3.6
Cost of Bridging Devices

Device	*Console ($)*	*Pump ($)*
ECMO	10 000	1 200
Biomedicus	12 000	450
Pierce–Donachy	32 000	10 400
Novacor LVAS	55 069	19 597
Jarvik-7	59 700	18 600

manner. Patients without a reasonable probability of successful transplantation and long-term survival must be denied current mechanical support devices, since none of the devices is considered suitable for permanent use. Furthermore, private and government agencies who determine eligibility for third-party payment must recognize that the results described in this chapter approximate those in patients who did not require mechanical support. Such extensive and successful experience must now be regarded as acceptable clinical practice, rather than experimental investigation. Most of the costs of the devices described in this chapter were paid by government contracts or grants, hospitals or individuals. However, it is apparent that these sources of funding are inadequate for the appropriate distribution of mechanical support technology.

EPIDEMIOLOGICAL CONSIDERATIONS

The use of the Jarvik artificial heart for permanent implantation has been criticized as a technique which provides little benefit to patients, and presents the threat of allocation of large amounts of money which would be better spent on other aspects of health care (Preston, 1985; Jonsen, 1986). In spite of these concerns, the development and application of circulatory support systems, including ventricular assist devices, was given a sound endorsement by the working group on mechanical circulatory support of the National Heart, Lung and Blood Institute (1985). The recommendations of this group included an appeal for cost-effectiveness, and the need to present a balanced view of these devices to the public, so that problems and failures, as well as successes, can be anticipated. Others argue that the use of mechanical circulatory support devices to bridge patients to transplantation leads to a misallocation of donor organs. Annas (1985) particularly challenged the use of temporary artificial hearts, while Relman (1986) generally supported their use as bridges to cardiac transplantation. Some would argue that critically ill patients should not be given preferential consideration for organs which would then be denied to fitter patients who might have a better chance of a successful result. However, it is not clear that there is a substantial difference in mortality in favour of patients who do not require mechanical support. Furthermore, 25 patients who received circulatory support devices were denied transplantation because they developed contra-indications. This screening process ensured that the precious supply of donor hearts was not wasted on patients who did not have a reasonable chance of survival. It is possible for patients to improve during the waiting period, from better nutrition, loss of oedema, improved pulmonary function and increased motor strength. Such improvement might be critical in patients with long-standing cardiac disability, but improvement can only be expected if the assist devices allow for patient mobility. Bedridden patients are likely to develop oedema, muscle wasting and pulmonary complications.

Another frequently voiced concern about the use of mechanical devices as bridges for transplantation is the possibility that hospitals will be inundated with large numbers of patients with assist devices for whom donor hearts will never become available. It is clear that there is a severe limitation of donor organs. There are approximately 15 000 potential heart transplant recipients per year in the USA, but only 2000 potential donor hearts (Evans *et al.*, 1986). However, of the patients accepted for transplantation in the various programmes, about 20% per year die before an organ becomes available (Copeland *et al.*, 1985). If all these patients had been candidates for assist devices in 1985, the number would be only about 180. Since about half the patients who die while waiting have acute episodes out of the hospital, it is unlikely that they would ever become candidates for circulatory support. Therefore, a realistic number of patients who might receive assist devices as 'bridges' would probably be less than 100 per year. Of course, if these patients were maintained indefinitely, they would become a much larger fraction of recipients every year. Unfortunately, with the current mechanical devices which require some type of driveline traversing the body wall, the incidence of infection can be expected to be high and this will limit the potential for patients to survive more than a year.

Current laboratory models of permanently implantable left ventricular assist systems (Program and Abstracts, 1986) and orthotopic ventricles (Pierce, 1986) will not require transcutaneous tether, and will offer potential for much longer survival. When these devices become available for clinical use, patients, families and physicians may be faced with the choice of maintaining permanent assist devices or pursuing transplantation. However, the number of recipients will probably always exceed the number of available human donor hearts, making it necessary for a substantial number of patients to be totally dependent upon mechanical devices. Depending upon the success of these permanent mechanical devices, the role of cardiac transplantation will have to be reassessed. The problems of blood compatibility, mechanical failure and threat of infection inherent in mechanical systems will have to be compared with the long-term risks of immunosuppression, infection and accelerated atherosclerosis associated with heart transplantation.

REFERENCES

Annas, G. J. (1985). No cheers for temporary artificial hearts. *Hastings Center Rep.* **15**, 27–28.

National Heart, Lung and Blood Institute (1985). *Artificial Heart and Assist Devices:*

Directions, Needs, Costs, Societal and Ethical Issues. Working Group on Mechanical Circulatory Support of the HLBI, Bethesda, MD.

Bernhard, W. F., Berger, R. L., Stetz, J. P., Carr, J. G., Colo, N., McCormick, J. R. and Fishbein, M. C. (1979). Temporary left ventricular bypass: factors affecting patient survival. *Circulation*, Suppl. I, **60**(2), 131–141.

Bolman, R. M., Spray, T. L., Cance, C., Saffitz, J., Genton, R. E. and Eisen, H. (1987). Heart transplantation in patients requiring preoperative mechanical support. *J. Heart Transplant.* **5**(5), 374 (Abstract).

Cooley, D. A., Liotta, D., Hallman, G. L., Bloodwell, R. D., Leachman, R. D. and Milam, J. D. (1969). Orthotopic cardiac prosthesis for two-staged cardiac replacement. *Am. J. Cardiol.* **24**, 723–730.

Copeland, J. G. (1986). Early human experiences with the pneumatic orthotopic biventricular externally driven blood pump (total artificial heart). *J. Heart Transplant.* **5**(3), 183.

Copeland, J. G., Emery, R. W., Levinson, M. M., Copeland, J., McAleer, J. M. and Riley, J. E. (1985). The role of mechanical support and transplantation in treatment of patients with end stage cardiomyopathy. *Cardiovasc. Surg. Suppl. to Circulation* **72**, II-7–12.

DeVries, W. C., Anderson, J. L., Joyce, L. D., Anderson, F. L., Hammond, E. H., Jarvik, R. K. and Kolff, W. J. (1984). Clinical use of the total artificial heart. *New Engl. J. Med.* **310**, 273–278.

DeVries, W., Mays, B., Hasting, S. L., Johnson, S. and Oser, A. (1986). Effect of drive system modification on hematologic profiles of two permanent total artificial heart recipients. *Am. Soc. Artif. Intern. Org.* (Abstract).

Donachy, J. N., Landis, D. L., Rosenberg, G. *et al.* (1978). Design and evaluation of a left ventricular assist device: the angle port pump. In *Assisted Circulation*, pp. 344–352 (F. Unger, Ed.). Academic Press, New York.

Evans, R. W., Mannion, D. L., Garrison, L. P. Jr and Maier, A. M. (1986). Donor availability as the primary determinant of the future of heart transplantation. *J. Am. Med. Ass.* **255**, 1892–1898.

Farrar, D. J., Hill, D. J., Gray, L. A., Pennington, D. G., McBride, L. R., Ross, D., Glenville, B., Galbraith, T. A. and Carpentier, A. (1986). Bridge to cardiac transplantation in eight patients at six institutions using prosthetic left and right ventricles. *Circulation* **74**, (Abstract 879), II-220.

Frazier, O. H., Painvin, G. A., Urrutia, C. O., Igo, S. R. and Cooley, D. A. (1983). Mechanical circulatory support: clinical experience at the Texas Heart Institute. *Heart Transplant.* **2**, 299–306.

Gaines, W. E., Pierce, W. S., Donachy, J. H., Rosenberg, G., Candis, D. L., Richenbacher, W. E. and Waldhansen, J. A. (1985). The Pennsylvania State University paracorporeal ventricular assist pump. Optimal methods of use. *World J. Surg.* **9**, 47–53.

Gifford, D., Wheeldon, D., Wallwork, J. and Spratt, P. (1986). Balloon counterpulsation together with Bio-Medicus pump closed circuit membrane oxygenation for left ventricular assist: a case report. *J. Extracorp. Technol.* **18**, 29–33.

Griffith, B. P., Kormas, R. L., Wei, L. M., Borovetz, H. S., Trento, A. and Hardesty, R. L. (1986). Use of the total artificial heart as an interim device: initial experience in Pittsburgh with four patients. *J. Heart Transplant.* **5**(3), 210.

Hardesty, R. L., Griffith, B. P., Trento, A., Thompson, M. E., Ferson, P. F. and Bahnson, H. T. (1986). Mortally ill patients and excellent survival following cardiac transplantation. *Ann. Thorac. Surg.* **41**, 126–129.

Hill, J. D., Farrar, D. J., Hirshon, J. J., Compton, P. G., Avery, G. J. and Brent, B. N. (1986). Use of a prosthetic ventricle as a bridge to cardiac transplantation for postinfarction cardiogenic shock. *New Engl. J. Med.* **314**, 626–628.

Holub, D. A., Hibbs, C. W., Sturm, J. T., Edmonds, C. H., McGee, M. G., Fuhrman, T. M., Trono, R., Igo, S. R. and Norman, J. C. (1979). Clinical trials of an abdominal left ventricular assist device (ALVAD): progress report. *Trans. Am. Soc. Artif. Intern. Org.* **25**, 197.

Jarvik, R. K., DeVries, W. C., Semb, K. H. B., Koul, B., Copeland, J. G., Levinson, M. L., Griffith, B. P., Joyce, L., Cooley, D. A., Frazier, O. H., Cabrol, C. and Keon, W. J. (1986). Surgical position of the Jarvik-7 total artificial heart. *J. Heart Transplant.* **5**(3), 184.

Jonsen, A. R. (1986). The artificial heart's threat to others. *Hastings Center Rep.* 9–11.

Joyce, L. D., Johnson, K. E., Pierce, W. S., DeVries, W. C., Semb, B. K. H., Copeland, J. G., Griffith, B. P., Cooley, D. A., Frazier, O. H., Cabrol, C., Keon, W. J., Unger, F., Bucherl, E. S. and Wolner, E. (1986a). Summary of the world experience with clinical use of total artificial hearts as heart support devices. *J. Heart Transplant.* **5**(3), 229.

Joyce, L. D., Pritzker, M. R., Kiser, J. C., Nicoloff, D. M., Kersten, T. E., VonRueden, T. J., Eales, F., Johnson, K. E., Jorgensen, C. R., Goebel, F. L. and VanTassel, R. A. (1986b). Use of the mini Jarvik-7 total artificial heart as a bridge to transplantation. *J. Heart Transplant.* **5**(3), 203.

Levinson, M. M., Smith, R. G., Cork, R., Gallo, J., Icenogle, T., Emery, R., Ott, R. and Copeland, J. G. (1986). Three recent cases of the total artificial heart before transplantation. *J. Heart Transplant.* **5**(3), 215–228.

Magovern, J. A., Pennock, J. L., Campbell, D. B., Pae, W. E. Jr, Pierce, W. S. and Waldhausen, J. A. (1986). Bridge to heart transplantation: the Penn State experience. *J. Heart Transplant.* **5**(3), 196.

Magovern, G. J., Sang, B. P. and Maher, T. D. (1985). Use of a centrifugal pump without anticoagulants for postoperative left ventricular assist. *World J. Surg.* **9**, 25–36.

McBride, L. R., Pennington, D. G., Tsai, C. C., Kanter, K. R., Miller, L. W., Naunheim, K. S. and Rusevich, S. A. (1987). Influence of ventricular assist devices on lymphocytes. *J. Heart Transplant.* **5**(5), 379 (Abstract).

Norman, J. C., Cooley, D. A., Igo, S. R., Hibb, C. W., Johnson, M. D., Bennett, J. G., Fugna, R. M., Trono, R. and Edmunds, C. H. (1977). Prognostic indices for survival during postcardiotomy intraaortic balloon pumping. *J. Thorac. Cardiovasc. Surg.* **74**, 709.

Norman, J. C., Cooley, D. A., Kahan, B. D., Keats, A. S., Massin, E. K., Solis, R. T., Luper, W. E., Brook, M. I., Klino, T., Frazier, O. H., Hacker, J., Duncan, J. M., Dasco, C. C., Winston, D. S. and Ruel, G. J. (1978). Total support of the circulation of a patient with a postcardiotomy stone-heart syndrome by a partial artificial heart (ALVAD) for 5 days followed by heart and kidney transplantation. *Lancet* **1**, 1125.

Norman, J. C., Duncan, J. H., Frazier, O. H., Hauman, G. L., Ott, D. A., Reul, G.

J. and Cooley, D. A. (1981). Intracorporeal (abdominal) left ventricular assist devices or partial artificial hearts. *Arch. Surg.*, **116**, 1441–1445.

Park, S. B., Liebler, G. A., Burkholder, J. A., Maher, T. D., Benckart, O. H., Magovern, G. J. Jr, Christlieb, I. Y., Kao, R. L. and Magovern, G. J. Sr (1986). Mechanical support of the failing heart. *Ann. Thorac. Surg.* **42**, 627–632.

Parr, G. V. S., Pierce, W. S., Rosenberg, G. and Waldhausen, J. A. (1980). Right ventricular failure after repair of left ventricular aneurysm. *J. Thorac. Cardiovasc. Surg.* **80**, 79.

Pennington, D. G., Codd, J. E., Merjavy, J. P., Swartz, M. T., Kaiser, G. C., Barner, H. B. and Willman, V. L. (1983). The expanded use of ventricular bypass system for severe cardiac failure and as a bridge to cardiac transplantation. *Heart Transplant.* **3**, 38–46.

Pennington, D. G., Merjavy, J. P., Codd, J. E., Swartz, M. T., Miller, L. L. and Williams, G. A. (1984). Extracorporeal membrane oxygenation for patients with cardiogenic shock. *Circulation* **70**, Suppl I, 130–137.

Pennington, D. G., Merjavy, J. P., Swartz, M. T., Codd, J. E., Barner, H. B., Laganoff, D., Bashiti, H., Kaiser, G. C. and Willman, V. L. (1985a). The importance of biventricular failure in patients with postoperative cardiogenic shock. *Ann. Thorac. Surg.* **39**, 16–26.

Pennington, D. G., Samuels, S. O., Williams, G., Palmer, D., Swartz, M. T., Codd, J. E., Merjavy, J. P., Lagunoff, D. and Joist, J. H. (1985b). Experience with the Pierce–Donachy ventricular assist device in postcardiotomy patient with cardiogenic shock. *World J. Surg.* **9**, 37–46.

Phillips, S. J. (1986). Percutaneous cardiopulmonary bypass and innovations in clinical counterpulsation. In *Critical Care Clinics*, Vol. 2, No. 2, pp. 297–318. Saunders, Philadelphia.

Pierce, W. S. (1979). Clinical left ventricular bypass problems of pump inflow obstruction and right ventricular failure. *Am. Soc. Artif. Intern. Org. J.* **2**, 1.

Pierce, W. S. (1986). The artificial heart — 1986. Partial fulfillment of a promise. *Am. Soc. Artif. Intern. Org. Trans.* **32**, 5.

Portner, P. M., Oyer, P. E., Jassawalla, J. S., Miller, P. J., Chen, H., LaForge, D. H., Green, G., Ream, A. K. and Shumway, N. (1983). An alternative in end-stage heart disease: long term ventricular assistance. *Heart Transplant.* **3**, 47–57.

Presten, T. A. (1985). Who benefits from the artificial heart? *Hastings Center Rep.* **15** (1), 5–7.

Program and Abstracts (1986). Devices and Technology Branch Contractors Meeting, pp. 29–35.

Reemtsma, K., Krusin, R., Edie, R., Bregman, D., Dobelle, W. and Hardy, M. (1978). Cardiac transplantation in patients requiring mechanical circulatory support. *N. Engl. J. Med.* **298**, 670–671.

Relman, A. S. (1986). Artificial hearts — permanent and temporary. *New Engl. J. Med.* **314**, 644–645.

Rich, G. F., Smith, K. W., Gendorf, J., Murashita, J. and Peters, J. R. (1982). Recovery with biventricular bypass after induced massive infarction. *Trans. Am. Soc. Artif. Intern. Org.* **28**, 547.

Rose, D. M., Laschinger, J., Grossi, E., Krieger, K. H., Cunningham, J. N. and

Spencer, F. C. (1985). Experimental and clinical results with a simplified left heart assist device for treatment of profound left ventricular dysfunction. *World J. Surg.* **9**, 11–17.

Stelzer, G. T., Ward, R. A., Wellhausen, S. R., McLeish, K. R., Johnson, G. S. and DeVries, W. C. (1987). Alterations in select immunologic parameters following total artificial heart implantation. *Artif. Org.* **11**, 52.

Turina, M. T., Bosue, R. and Serring, A. (1978). Paracorporeal artificial heart in postoperative heart failure. *Artif. Org.* **2**, 273.

Vaughn, C. C., Copeland, J. G., Cheng, K., Austin, J., Levinson, M. and Emery, R. W. (1986). Interim cardiac replacement with a mechanical heart: staged cardiac transplantation. *Texas Heart Inst. J.* **13**, 45–52.

Ward, R., Stelzer, G., Wellhausen, S. and DeVries, W. (1986). Effect of cardiopulmonary bypass (CPB) on select immunologic parameters. *Am. Soc. Artif. Intern. Org.* (Abstract).

Zapol, W. M., Snider, M. T., Hill, J. D., Fallat, R. J., Bartlett, R. H., Edmunds, L. H., Morris, A. H., Pierce, E. C. II, Thomas, A. N., Proctor, H. G., Drinker, P. A., Pratt, P. C., Bagniewski, A. and Miller, R. G. (1979). Extracorporeal membrane oxygenation in severe respiratory failure. *J. Am. Med. Ass.* **242**, 2193.

Zumbro, G. L., Shearer, G., Kitchens, W. R. and Galloway, R. F. (1985). Mechanical assistance for biventricular failure following coronary bypass operation and heart transplantation. *Heart Transplant.* **4**(3), 348–352.

Mark E. Thompson

4

Recipient Selection and Assessment: Indications For Transplantation*

INTRODUCTION

Cardiac transplantation has met with increasing success over the past 20 years. This procedure can restore almost unrestricted physical activity, in contrast to the severe physical limitations imposed by end-stage heart failure. Most candidates for cardiac transplantation are in New York Heart Association (NYHA) Class IV prior to operation as a result of (1) idiopathic cardiomyopathy (45%); (2) ischaemic cardiomyopathy (50%); and (3) miscellaneous causes (5%), such as end-stage valvular heart disease. They require a thorough cardiac assessment, usually including complete cardiac catheterization, in order to identify those who might benefit from alternative modes of treatment (Baumgartner *et al.*, 1979; Thompson, 1986) as well as those who require transplantation.

Alternative forms of conventional treatment and promising experimental therapy must be considered before a decision is made to undertake cardiac transplantation. Recent advances in coronary artery bypass grafting in patients with depressed left ventricular function, and the treatment of refractory cardiac arrhythmias using electrophysiological testing to identify effective drug therapy, or the use of subendocardial myocardial resection along

* Adapted from 'Selection of candidates for cardiac transplantation', *Journal of Heart Transplantation* **3**(1), 65, 1983; and from 'Candidate selection for cardiac transplantation', published in *Corde* (Argentina), 1986.

with aneurysmectomy, may be appropriate therapy in some circumstances (Horowitz *et al.*, 1959; Josephson, Harken and Horowitz, 1979; Manley *et al.*, 1979; Akins and Austen, 1981). Patients with active myocarditis may be identified by endomyocardial biopsy and can be treated with a trial of azathioprine and prednisone (Mason, Billingham and Ricci, 1980; Fowles and Mason, 1982). Caution must be exercised in considering the use of immunosuppressive therapy in this circumstance, however, as its complications may preclude consideration of transplantation in the future, especially if severe infection is encountered. There is some evidence to suggest that improvement in patients with myocarditis is independent of therapy (Dec *et al.*, 1985). Patients with severe congestive heart failure may show temporary improvement with unloading therapy or newer inotropic agents (Chatterjee and Parmley, 1983; Cohn, 1986; Colucci, Wright and Braunwald, 1986). Those with hypertrophic cardiomyopathy may benefit from the use of beta-blockade, or calcium channel blocking agents, while beta-blockade alone has been reported to be beneficial in some patients with idiopathic cardiomyopathy (Hubner *et al.*, 1973; Swedberg *et al.*, 1979; Rosing *et al.*, 1981). Although it is not possible to state with certainty what proportion of patients otherwise acceptable for cardiac transplantation may be suitable for alternative treatment, this figure was approximately 20% in the early experience at Stanford and at the University of Arizona (Baumgartner *et al.*, 1979; Carrier *et al.*, 1986). It must be remembered, however, that employment of one of the treatment alternatives will in most cases be simply a temporizing measure, and that transplantation may ultimately be required. Thus, the total number of patients awaiting transplantation should not be expected to decline significantly, except as a result of intervening death.

PRE-TRANSPLANTATION ASSESSMENT

A thorough review of the history, physical examination and routine laboratory data is essential for all potential recipients. These preliminary studies are to identify the patients most likely to benefit from cardiac transplantation, and to identify any systemic illness which may limit the patient's ability to recover. Cardiac catheterization will establish the aetiology of the heart failure, and will determine whether any conventional treatment would be of benefit.

In individuals with a severely depressed ejection fraction (<15–20%) and an elevated wedge pressure (>25–30 mmHg) while on optimal therapy, and with echocardiographically demonstrated normal cardiac valves, complete left heart catheterization with angiography may be unnecessary and unwise because of the potential complications. In any case, it is doubtful if patients with such significantly impaired left ventricular function would respond favourably to conventional operative intervention. Irreversible changes in the central nervous system and hepatic and renal function as a result of long-standing congestive heart failure must be excluded. Good dental hygiene should be restored to remove a potential source of postoperative infection, and the patient should be screened for previous exposure to the Epstein–Barr virus (EBV), toxoplasmosis, cytomegalovirus, tuberculosis and fungal diseases. This information is important, as immunosuppression may reactivate latent infection, and infection may be transmitted from the donor to the recipient (Hakim *et al.*, 1985).

IMMUNOLOGICAL SCREENING FOR RECIPIENT AND DONOR MATCHING

Immunological studies are carried out to identify a suitable match between donor and recipient. This matching is based mainly on ABO blood type. The limited time between donor identification and the transplant operation, as well as the limited number of donors, makes routine use of HLA typing between donor and recipient impractical. Also, there have been few studies indicating that HLA matching is important in the long-term survival of cardiac transplant recipients (Stinson *et al.*, 1981). Mismatch at the HLA_2 locus has been associated with more rapid development of graft coronary atherosclerosis in those treated with azathioprine, but not in those treated with CyA (Zusman *et al.*, 1985).

Potential recipients are screened for preformed antibodies using a broad panel of HLA antigens. In those patients in whom no pre-existing antibodies are identified, the donor-specific lymphocyte cytotoxicity test is not routinely performed, as the chance of a positive crossmatch is remote. An increase in preformed antibodies in a potential recipient makes it more difficult to identify compatible donors. In these patients, a donor-specific lymphocyte crossmatch is recommended prior to transplantation. The time required to conduct such a test, and the limited number of facilities available distant from the transplant centre, limit the potential number of donors available for any given recipient. In critically ill patients with a high percentage of preformed antibodies, cardiac transplantation is sometimes done without awaiting the result of the donor-specific lymphocyte crossmatch. In this circumstance, acute accelerated rejection may not occur, but indolent rejection may develop which is more difficult to control (Rabin, 1983). Thus the pretransplant donor-specific lymphocyte cytotoxicity crossmatch has a less well-defined role than it had in the early years of cardiac transplantation. Many of the original immunological guidelines used for cardiac transplantation were based on the principles established for renal transplantation. The extent to which these may need to be modified for cardiac transplantation remains to be investigated. Nevertheless, some credence must be accorded to the donor-specific lymphocyte cytotoxicity crossmatch in circumstances where it is practical to use it.

There have been some instances of acute rejection after cardiac transplantation in which an immunological response between recipient and donor endothelial antigen systems has been identified, as opposed to preformed antibodies against the HLA system. At present, pre-transplant matching between donor and recipient endothelial antigen systems is not carried out. Such testing might be recommended in the future, if the importance of this interaction in acute rejection is demonstrated (Rabin, 1983).

Psychosocial evaluation

Potential recipients must exhibit psychosocial stability and an ability to co-operate with a rigorous medical treatment programme. One can then be reasonably certain that the patient will be able to tolerate the psychological stress of transplantation and to co-operate with the extended care required during the follow-up for the remainder of the patient's lifetime. Patients benefit from strong emotional support provided by family and friends. In addition, there must be adequate financial resources to cover the cost of the operation and the period of follow-up.

LIFE EXPECTANCY PRIOR TO TRANSPLANTATION AND DONOR AVAILABILITY

Potential recipients with severe heart failure have an average life expectancy of approximately 30–60 days (Baumgartner *et al.*, 1979), although prediction of 1-year survival for patients being considered for cardiac transplantation is an uncertain exercise (Stevenson *et al.*, 1986). Rough guidelines have been suggested to supplement the physician's judgement. The level of circulating catecholamines has been shown to correlate with the severity of heart failure, and may be of prognostic significance (Levine *et al.*, 1982). In patients with dilated cardiomyopathy, multivariant analysis taking into consideration the presence of left intraventricular conduction delay, the mean right and left atrial pressures, and the presence or absence of ventricular arrhythmias may be used to predict 1-year mortality (Unverferth *et al.*, 1984; Daly *et al.*, 1986). In patients with ischaemic heart disease, the prognosis is best predicted by the extent of left ventricular dysfunction and the presence of complex cardiac arrhythmias (Frishman, Furberg and Friedewald, 1984). These guidelines can be used to identify those patients who need urgent assessment.

In the USA, it is estimated that approximately 15 000 patients die from heart disease annually; these might be considered for cardiac transplantation

(Evans *et al.*, 1986). Using strict criteria designed to identify patients with a high probability of survival and rehabilitation following transplantation, Stanford University accepted only 11.3% of 1125 potential candidates referred between 1977 and 1981 (Pennock *et al.*, 1982). Similarly, at the University of Arizona, approximately 30% of patients under age 50 referred for cardiac transplantation were accepted, and about 20% of these ultimately underwent transplantation (Carrier *et al.*, 1986). Only 20% of patients over age 50 were accepted, and 10% of these ultimately underwent the procedure (Carrier *et al.*, 1986). We deduce that in the USA 2000–5000 patients per year might benefit from cardiac transplantation (Pennock *et al.*, 1982). If one extends the upper age limit to 60 years, the figure becomes 25 200, and reaches 41 000 if the upper age limit is extended to 65 years (Evans *et al.*, 1984).

Widening of the criteria for selection of cardiac transplantation candidates will lead to greater numbers of individuals on the waiting list without a corresponding increase in the number of donors, and this must depend on demonstrating favourable long-term postoperative survival. Otherwise, there will be an increasing number of deaths among potential candidates for cardiac transplantation awaiting suitable donors. At present, the exact number of patients who die awaiting cardiac transplantation is not known, but in the University of Arizona experience during 1975–85 this number approached 20% (Carrier *et al.*, 1986). In the National Heart Transplantation Study, approximately 60% of suitable recipients underwent cardiac transplantation, while the remaining 40% either died or remained on the waiting list (Evans *et al.*, 1984). At present, approximately 1100 suitable hearts are available for transplantation each year (Evans *et al.*, 1986). Thus, the major limitation on cardiac transplantation programmes is the lack of donors. These statistics emphasize the importance of choosing candidates most likely to benefit from the procedure, and explain why a large number of patients die awaiting transplantation.

RECIPIENT SELECTION

Table 4.1 lists the pre-transplantation screening tests for cardiac transplantation candidates and Table 4.2 the primary criteria for recipient selection. Cardiac transplantation candidates should be in NYHA Class IV as a result of refractory heart failure, and have an estimated life expectancy of less than 6–12 months. An upper age limit of 50–55 years for recipients is based on early experience at Stanford University, because older patients have a less favourable long-term survival after transplantation (Baumgartner *et al.*, 1979). At the University of Pittsburgh and the University of Arizona, patients between ages 50 and 55 years have similar mean survival times to

TABLE 4.1

Pre-transplantation Screening Tests

Complete history and physical examination	Complete blood count
BUN/creatinine/glucose	Urinalysis
ECG	Electrolytes
Chest radiograph	Liver function tests
Pulmonary function tests	Pulmonary vascular resistance
Cardiac catheterization	Anergy panel
Epstein–Barr viral titres	Cytomegalic viral titres
Toxoplasmosis serology	
Immunology Testing	
Donor/recipient compatibility	
ABO blood typing	
Reactive antibodies	

TABLE 4.2

Primary Criteria for Recipient Selection

Terminal heart disease with an estimated life expectancy of <6–12 months
Age less than 50–55 years
Normal or reversible renal and hepatic function
Absence of active infection
Absence of pulmonary infarction in the preceding 8 weeks
Absence of insulin-dependent diabetes mellitus or hyperglycaemia requiring treatment with insulin or oral hypoglycaemic agents
Psychosocial stability and a supportive social milieu

Contraindications

A pulmonary vascular resistance in excess of 6 Wood units (orthotopic transplantation)
Crossmatch incompatibility between recipient and donor
Significant peripheral vascular or cerebrovascular disease
Active peptic ulceration
Drug addiction
Alcoholic cardiomyopathy and continued alcohol abuse
Co-existing systemic illness which may limit life expectancy or compromise recovery from cardiac transplantation
Pre-existing malignant disease
Chronic bronchitis and chronic obstructive lung disease

younger ones (Thompson, 1986; Carrier *et al.*, 1986). The lower limit for cardiac transplantation depends upon identification of a young individual who is prepared to co-operate fully in the extended recovery phase and in the long-term follow-up. Between 1968 and 1984, 105 operations in patients under age 20 were reported in the International Heart Transplantation Registry (Kaye, 1984). The average age of recipients was 14 $\pm$ 4.4 years (range <1 year to 19 years). The 1- to 3-year actuarial survival rate in this group is approximately 55%. Although transplanting patients under age 10 does not diminish the donor pool for older patients, the issue of transplantation in infants and children does raise ethical and socio-economic questions.

Patients should not have active infection at the time of transplantation, and there should not have been a pulmonary infarction within the preceding 8 weeks. In some patients with severe heart failure, it may take more than 8 weeks for a pulmonary infarct to resolve. Patients with pulmonary infarction close to the time of transplantation may develop cavitation and postoperative infection, especially after initiation of the immunosuppressive regimen (Young *et al.*, 1985).

Insulin-dependent diabetes mellitus is a relative contraindication to cardiac transplantation. High-dose steroid therapy, which is part of the immunosuppressive regimen, complicates the control of diabetes mellitus. Diabetes mellitus is associated with a higher incidence of peripheral vascular disease, renal disease and peripheral neuropathy. These complications may develop at an accelerated rate following transplantation. For this reason, restraint must be exercised when cardiac transplantation is considered in such patients.

A pulmonary vascular resistance in excess of 6–8 Wood units is an absolute contraindication to orthotopic cardiac transplantation, and so at the time of catheterization this measurement is essential. A fixed pulmonary vascular resistance in excess of 6 Wood units frequently leads to acute right ventricular failure after cardiac transplantation, and may account for a postoperative mortality of approximately 5% (Griepp *et al.*, 1971; Baumgartner *et al.*, 1979). A fixed pulmonary vascular resistance is defined as one which does not decrease when the oxygen saturation rises, or one which cannot be altered by the use of vasodilating or inotropic agents (Schroeder, 1979). It has been possible to use a larger donor heart in patients with a pulmonary vascular resistance of 5–6 Wood units, and the pulmonary vascular resistance has gradually fallen in the first weeks after transplantation. Even so, the immediate postoperative period may be characterized by a decreased cardiac output, elevated pulmonary artery pressures and the need for longer than usual administration of inotropic support and pulmonary vasodilators.

The demonstration of preformed antibodies in the recipient's serum to the donor's lymphocytes is a relative contraindication to cardiac transplantation (Weil *et al.*, 1981; Pennock *et al.*, 1982). In this case there is greater difficulty in controlling postoperative rejection, even when an acute rejection response does not occur (Rabin, 1983). For this reason, the long-term prognosis of this group of patients is less favourable. While this guideline is followed less strictly at present, it is still a factor worth considering.

Peripheral vascular and cerebrovascular disease may lead to an increased incidence of postoperative complications and are relative contraindications to cardiac transplantation. An active bleeding ulcer at the time of transplantation may be aggravated by the steroids and the stress of operation. The use of H2-blocking drugs (i.e. ranitidine HCl) to reduce the level of gastric acid secretion has been a great step forward in the past 5 years, making peptic ulcer disease a less frequent contraindication or complication of the procedure.

Drug addiction and chronic alcoholism are two behavioural traits which identify candidates as less suitable for transplantation because of the potential inability to co-operate or tolerate the rigorous long-term follow-up. These patients may also be unable to tolerate the emotional stress associated with the procedure.

Co-existing illnesses which limit life expectancy, such as previous malignant disease and chronic obstructive pulmonary disease, also make patients less than ideal candidates for cardiac transplantation.

Emphysema and chronic bronchitis, as the major components of chronic obstructive lung disease, may represent a contraindication to cardiac transplantation if the degree of airway obstruction is severe (FEV_1/FVC ratio $<45\%$ of predicted). Bronchiectasis, characterized by chronic cough and sputum production, represents a further contraindication to cardic transplantation because it will be more difficult to treat once immunosuppression starts. Asthma, alone or in association with any of the above conditions, is a relative contraindication because it may be reversible with bronchodilator therapy. Patients become less suitable for transplantation as the degree of airway obstruction increases. Those with severe airway obstruction (FEV_1/FVC ratio $<45\%$ of predicted), despite optimum medical therapy, or requiring systemic corticosteroids for control of bronchospasm, would not be suitable transplant candidates. Interstitial lung disease, regardless of the aetiology, is also a contraindication to transplantation when the degree of restriction is severe (FEV $<50\%$ of predicted). Patients with severe lung disease often fail to improve after cardiac transplantation.

It is frequently difficult to separate signs and symptoms of obstructive or restrictive lung disease from those of congestive heart failure. Furthermore, the distinction is not easily made by pulmonary function studies, since congestive heart failure can result in pulmonary function abnormalities. Congestive heart failure can result in a restrictive defect as seen in interstitial lung disease, or in an obstructive defect as seen in emphysema or chronic bronchitis. In patients being considered for transplantation, it may not be possible to improve the cardiac failure sufficiently to allow pulmonary function tests to be done. Therefore, previous pulmonary function studies (performed when the patient was not in congestive heart failure) should be reviewed to determine the patient's current pulmonary function.

Cardiac transplantation in patients requiring inotropic and/or mechanical circulatory assistance

The critically ill patient is an urgent problem for those involved in cardiac transplantation. These patients require intravenous administration of inotropic agents such as dobutamine, dopamine and amrinone, or a combination of these drugs, to maintain adequate blood pressure, cardiac output and cerebral and renal perfusion. This intensive treatment of heart failure is used to prevent deterioration of organ systems which would otherwise preclude cardiac transplantation. At the University of Pittsburgh, approximately one-third of patients undergoing cardiac transplantation require inotropic support. An additional 10% of patients need intra-aortic counter-pulsation in addition to inotropic support (Hardesty *et al.*, 1986).

As cardiac transplantation becomes an increasingly accepted form of treatment, the number of donor hearts available for any one transplantation centre declines dramatically. Consequently, the waiting time between identification of a critically ill recipient and transplantation has increased. In the first years of our experience, a satisfactory donor could usually be identified within 6 days. Two years ago, the average waiting time for identification of a donor was approximately 2 weeks; at present, this waiting period may extend to 3 or 4 weeks (Hardesty *et al.*, 1986). As a result of the longer waiting period, fewer patients survive long enough to allow donor identification. This increased time delay has prompted the use of a totally implantable circulatory assist device — the Jarvik-7 mechanical heart — in 5 patients at the University of Pittsburgh. Three of these 5 patients underwent successful orthotopic transplantation; one experienced complications which precluded cardiac transplantation while being maintained on the Jarvik-7 heart, and the other died of mediastinitis following transplantation.

In spite of the severe illness exhibited by the moribund patients who require extensive preoperative inotropic and mechanical support prior to cardiac transplantation, the survival rate in this group is comparable to those who are less ill, provided vital organ function is maintained and infection does not supervene (Hardesty *et al.*, 1986). For this reason, strict attention is given to the use of aseptic techniques when intravascular monitoring catheters are used. When at all possible, indwelling intravascular lines and urinary bladder catheters are avoided.

It is therefore reasonable to consider transplantation in this group, although it must be recognized that enormous personnel time and institutional resources are required. Inevitably, the waiting time for the less severely ill candidates is extended. For this reason, if a decision is made to support critically ill patients vigorously, the effort should be limited to those who are excellent candidates for transplantation.

The survival rate of 80% in both groups — the electively transplanted patients and those who are critically ill — provides ample justification for considering cardiac transplantation in patients who can be adequately maintained with maximal medical support (Hardesty *et al.*, 1986).

SELECTION CRITERIA FOR REPEAT CARDIAC RE-TRANSPLANTATION

A second or third cardiac transplantation may be required in patients who develop acute irreversible rejection shortly after the initial procedure, or in those who develop ventricular dysfunction as a result of chronic rejection and/or accelerated graft atherosclerosis (Weil *et al.*, 1981). The guidelines for selecting patients requiring cardiac re-transplantation are the same as those for the initial procedure. The survival in these patients is approximately 30% at two years (Copeland *et al.*, 1977). The number of re-transplantation operations will remain limited because of the increasing demand for donors and because few recipients are suitable for a second or third operation.

HETEROTOPIC CARDIAC TRANSPLANTATION

The selection criteria for patients receiving a heterotopic cardiac transplant are similar to those for orthotopic transplantation, except that heterotopic cardiac transplantation (Cooper and Lanza, 1984) may be considered for patients with an elevated pulmonary vascular resistance (approximately 6 Wood units), since the recipient's right ventricle remains functional and has previously adapted to the pressure overload in the pulmonary circuit. With time, there may be a decline in pulmonary vascular resistance and the transplanted right ventricle may undergo sufficient hypertrophy to contribute to forward pulmonary flow. A patient being considered for heterotopic cardiac transplantation should not have significant tricuspid insufficiency, as a competent native right ventricle is initially necessary to propel blood through the pulmonary circuit.

The major advantage of heterotopic cardiac transplantation is that the recipient's own heart, under some circumstances, may remain sufficiently functional during periods of acute graft rejection or periods of arrhythmia to support the patient's circulation in circumstances which would otherwise be fatal (Losman and Barnard, 1982). The disadvantages of heterotopic transplantation include the development of systemic or pulmonary emboli as a result of clot formation in the dilated and poorly functioning ventricles of the native heart. Mural thrombi in the native heart may become infected. The native heart should not contain prosthetic valves which could prove to be a nidus for infection. Heterotopic transplantation can be considered a reasonable alternative to orthotopic transplantation in selected circumstances (Losman and Bernard, 1982).

PERSPECTIVE

Improved survival statistics over the past 18 years have resulted in a renewed world-wide interest in cardiac transplantation. With the increasing number of centres, there has been a rapid increase in the number of cardiac transplantations performed each year. Proper selection of recipients continues to be an important consideration for any transplantation programme. The introduction of newer immunosuppressive techniques raised the hope that the selection criteria for cardiac transplantation recipients could be widened. However, experience to date indicates that these criteria should remain relatively unchanged from those developed at Stanford in the early 1970s. They should not be looked upon as exclusionary, but rather as guides to identification of a patient most likely to benefit from cardiac transplantation.

This is an important precept, since logistical considerations preclude transplantation of all potential donors. Likewise, a patient and his family should not be asked to undergo the rigours of transplantation unless there is a reasonable chance of benefit.

CONCLUSIONS

Cardiac transplantation is entering an era where it is no longer considered as experimental therapy for patients with intractable heart failure. The number of patients undergoing cardiac transplantation remains limited, however, because of the relative lack of donors. Advances in the use of mechanical assist devices have permitted the development of a staged cardiac transplantation procedure in which seriously ill patients may be supported for a short period of time prior to definitive orthotopic cardiac transplantation. At present, the mechanical assist device is reserved for younger patients with no other contraindications to cardiac transplantation, and who are faced with imminent death because of heart failure unresponsive to all other means of support. This form of interim support does not, however, solve the problem posed by the relative lack of suitable donors. For this reason, efforts to develop a permanently implantable mechanical heart will persist. While the mechanical heart does not represent a viable alternative to cardiac transplantation as it is now practised, further improvements may make this possibility a reality. Many of the same standards for patient selection will remain, regardless of the treatment used.

ACKNOWLEDGEMENT

The author wishes to thank Irvin Paradis, MD, Assistant Professor of Medicine and the Director of Bronchoscopy Service, Pulmonary Medicine Division, University of Pittsburgh, for his comments regarding obstructive lung disease.

REFERENCES

Akins, C. W. and Austen, W. G. (1981). Revascularization of the myocardium. *Curr. Prob. Surg.* **18**, 4.

Baumgartner, W. A., Reitz, B. A., Oyer, P. E. *et al.* (1979). Cardiac homotransplantation. *Curr. Prob. Surg.* **16**, 1.

Carrier, M., Emery, R. W., Riley, J. E. *et al.* (1986). Cardiac transplantation in patients over 50 years of age. *J. Am. Coll. Cardiol.* **8**, 285.

Chatterjee, K. and Parmley, W. W. (1983). Vasodilator therapy for acute myocardial infarction and chronic congestive heart failure. *J. Am. Coll. Cardiol.* **1**, 133.

Cohn, J. N., Archibald, D. G., Ziesche, S., Franciosa, J. A. *et al.* (1986). Effect of vasodilator therapy on mortality in chronic congestive heart failure. *New Engl. J. Med.* **314**, 1547.

Colucci, W. S., Wright, R. F. and Braunwald, E. (1986). New positive inotropic agents in the treatment of congestive heart failure: mechanisms of action and recent clinical developments. *New Engl. J. Med.* **314**, 349.

Cooper, D. K. C. and Lanza, R. P. (Eds) (1984). *Heart Transplantation.* MTP Press, Hingham, Mass.

Copeland, J. G., Griepp, R. B., Bieber, C. P. *et al.* (1977). Successful retransplantation of the human heart. *J. Thorac. Cardiovasc. Surg.* **73**, 242.

Daly, P. A., Viquerat, C., Simonston, C. *et al.* (1986). Predictors of early death in young transplantable dilated cardiomyopathy. *J. Am. Coll. Cardiol.* **7**, 44A (Abstract).

Dec, F. W. Jr, Palacois, I. F., Fallon, J. T. *et al.* (1985). Active myocarditis in the spectrum of acute dilated cardiomyopathies: clinical features, histologic correlates, and clinical outcome. *New Engl. J. Med.* **312**, 885.

Evans, R. W., Manninen, D. L., Garrison, L. P. and Maier, A. M. (1986). Donor availability as the primary determinant of the future of heart transplantation. *J. Am. Med. Ass.* **255**, 1892.

Evans, R. W., Manninen, D. L., Overcast, T. D. *et al.* (1984). *The National Heart Transplantation Study: Final Report*, vols 1–5. Batelle Human Affairs Research Centers, Seattle.

Fowles, R. E. and Mason, J. W. (1982). Endomyocardial biopsy. *Ann. Int. Med.* **97**, 887.

Frishman, A. M., Furberg, C. D. and Friedewald, W. T. (1984). Beta-adrenergic blockade for survivors of acute MI. *New Engl. J. Med.* **310**, 430.

Griepp, R. B., Stinson, E. B., Dong, E. *et al.* (1971). Determinants of operative risk in human heart transplantation. *Am. J. Surg.* **122**, 192.

Hakim, M., Wreghitt, T., Cory-Pearce, R. *et al.* (1985). Significance of donor-transmitted disease in cardiac transplantation. *Heart Transplant* **4**, 120.

Hardesty, R. L., Griffith, B. P., Trento, A. *et al.* (1986). Mortally ill patients and excellent survival following cardiac transplantation. *Ann. Thorac. Surg.* **41**, 126.

Horowitz, L. N., Josephson, M. E., Farshidi, A. *et al.* (1959). Recurrent sustained ventricular tachycardia. III. Role of the electrophysiologic studies in selection of antiarrhythmic regimens. *Circulation*, **58**, 987.

Hubner, P. J., Ziady, G. M., Oakley, C. M. *et al.* (1973). Double blind trial study of propranolol and practolol in hypertrophic cardiomyopathy. *Br. Heart J.* **35**, 1116.

Josephson, M. E., Harken, A. H. and Horowitz, L. N. (1979). Endocardial excision: a new surgical technique for treatment of recurrent ventricular tachycardia. *Circulation* **10**, 1430.

Kaye, M. P. (1984). The International Heart Transplantation Registry. First official report — May 1984. *Heart Transplant* **3**, 278.

Levine, T. B., Francis, G. S., Goldsmith, S. R. *et al.* (1982). Activity of the sympathetic nervous system and renin–angiotensin system assessed by plasma hormone levels and their relationship to hemodynamic abnormalities in congestive heart failure. *Am. J. Cardiol.* **49**, 1659.

Losman, J. G. and Barnard, C. N. (1982). Heterotopic heart transplantation: a valid alternative to orthotopic transplantation: results, advantages, and disadvantages. *J. Surg. Res.* **32**, 297.

Manley, J. C., King, J. F., Zeft, H. J. *et al.* (1979). The 'bad' left ventricle. Results of coronary surgery and effect on late survival. *J. Thorac. Cardiovasc. Surg.* **72**, 841.

Mason, J. W., Billingham, M. E. and Ricci, D. R. (1980). Treatment of acute inflammatory myocarditis assisted by endomyocardial biopsy. *Am. J. Cardiol.* **45**, 1037.

Pennock, J. L., Oyer, P. E., Reitz, B. A., Jamieson, S. W. *et al.* (1982). Cardiac transplantation in perspective for the future. Survival, complications, rehabilitation, and cost. *J. Thorac. Cardiovasc. Surg.* **83**, 168.

Rabin, B. S. (1983). Immunologic aspects of human cardiac transplantation. *Heart Transplant* **2**, 188.

Rosing, D. R., Condit, J. R., Maron, B. J. *et al.* (1981). Verapamil therapy: a new approach to pharmacologic treatment of hypertrophic cardiomyopathy. *Am. J. Cardiol.* **48**, 545.

Schroeder, J. S. (1979). Current status of cardiac transplantation. *J. Am. Med. Ass.* **241**, 2069.

Stevenson, L. W., Fowler, M. B., Schroeder, J. S., Dracup, K. A. *et al.* (1986).

Patients denied cardiac transplantation for non-medical criteria: a control group. *J. Am. Coll. Cardiol* **7**, 9A (Abstract).

Stinson, E. B., Griepp, R. B., Payne, R. and Dong, E. Jr. (1981). Correlation of histocompatibility matching with graft rejection and survival after cardiac transplantation in man. *Lancet* **2**, 459.

Swedberg, K., Waagstein, F., Hjalmerson, A. *et al.* (1979). Prolongation of survival in congestive cardiomyopathy by beta receptor blockade. *Lancet* **1**, 1374.

Thompson, M. E. (1986). Transplantation review. In *Progress in Cardiology*, vol. 15 (P. Yu, Ed.). Lea and Febiger, Philadelphia (in press).

Unverferth, D. V., Magorien, R. D., Moeschberger, M. L. *et al.* (1984). Factors influencing the one-year mortality of dilated cardiomyopathy. *Am. J. Cardiol.* **54**, 147.

Weil, R., Clarke, D. R., Iwaki, Y. *et al.* (1981). Hyperacute rejection of a transplanted human heart. *Transplantation* **32**, 71.

Young, J. N., Yazbeck, J., Esposito, G. *et al.* (1985). The influence of acute preoperative pulmonary infarction on the results of cardiac transplantation. Report of the International Society for Heart Transplantation, Sixth Scientific Sessions. *Heart Transplant* **4**, 600.

Zusman, D. R., Stinson, E. B., Oyer, P. E., Baldwin, J. C. *et al.* (1985). Determinants of accelerated graft atherosclerosis (AGAS) in conventional and cyclosporine treated heart transplant recipients. *Heart Transplant* **4**, 587.

Celia Wight and Marguerite Brown

5

Organ Procurement — The Role of the Coordinator: UK, Europe, USA

INTRODUCTION

The greatest single problem facing cardiac transplant units throughout the world is the shortfall in suitable donor organs. Unlike other surgical procedures, transplantation cannot take place in isolation — it requires the cooperation of medical and nursing colleagues working in intensive care units, often many miles from a transplant centre, and the support of the general public who must have no objection to organ donation (Wight, 1986).

Following a general moratorium on heart transplantation, worldwide interest was renewed in the late 1970s. This was in response to the good results, in terms of quality and length of life, reported from the Stanford University Medical Centre, advances in the field of immunosuppression, in particular the introduction of cyclosporin which resulted in a markedly improved patient survival, and improvements in the methods of preserving the donor heart prior to transplantation.

The first heart–lung transplant operation was carried out in the Stanford University Medical Centre in 1981 (Reitz *et al.*, 1982) and the procedure is now undertaken in about a dozen of the 180 cardiac transplant units throughout the world. The major initial difficulties experienced were the shortage of referred donors having acceptable lung function and being free of infection, coupled with problems then experienced in the preservation of lung tissue. These problems necessitated the movement of ventilated brain-stem dead donors from the place of death to the transplant centre, with all the associated logistical and emotional difficulties. Better methods of lung preservation and improving donor management now allow distant procurement of these organs (Wallwork *et al.*, 1987) and could be one of the reasons for the increase in the number of patients identified as suitable heart–lung donors. Also by the late 1970s, there was a wider availability of sophisticated life-support maintenance for patients in deep coma. Although many of these patients would survive this state, some would die as a result of irreversible brain-stem injury. Having recognized this clinical state, the majority of the United States of America and many Western European countries had clarified the diagnosis of brain-stem death.

BRAIN-STEM DEATH

Brain-stem death was recognized as early as 1959 (Mollaret and Goulon, 1959) when renal transplantation was in its infancy and long before the clinical development of heart and heart–lung transplantation. It is important to emphasize this fact, as the ethical problems associated with brain-stem death would still exist even in the absence of organ transplantation. In 1974, following the report of the Ad Hoc Committee of the Harvard Medical School (1968), the Minnesota Criteria were published. These recommendations were to influence thinking and practice throughout the world. In the UK in 1976 and 1979, memoranda on brain death were issued by the Conference of Medical Royal Colleges and Their Faculties in the UK (1976, 1979), and the Department of Health and Social Security (DHSS, 1983) provided a code of practice, 'Cadaveric organs for transplantation', which also includes the diagnosis of brain-stem death.

The most recent guidelines for the recognition of brain-stem death in the USA were in a Report of the Medical Consultants to the President's Commission for the Study of Ethical Problems in Medicine, Biomedical and Behavioural Research (1981). Thirty-one States have passed brain-stem death laws and six other States have appellate court decisions which recognize the brain death standard. Many other countries throughout the world have also laid down criteria for the diagnosis of brain-stem death, although not always within a legal framework.

CONSENT

All the major religious groups support organ donation and transplantation as a good and charitable act, although some such as the Jewish Rabbinate and the Watch Tower Society for Jehovah's Witnesses state that an individual must have expressed his intent during his lifetime. In 1982, a Special Commission in Saudi Arabia declared that organ donation was permissible under Islamic Law. Refusals for organ donation are therefore more likely to be for cultural rather than religious reasons. This is particularly so among ethnic minority groups, and in some countries in Southern Europe and the Far East.

Individual countries have made efforts to increase organ donation, for example the 1961 Human Tissues Act in the UK and the 1968 Uniform Anatomical Gift Act in the USA. These and similar laws in other countries brought about the introduction of donor card schemes which are now widely available throughout the Western world. Gallup polls indicate that although the majority of Western populations are aware of transplantation, only a minority carry a donor card (DHSS, 1985; Gallup, 1986). Although distribution of donor cards may act as a publicity tool to promote discussion on organ donation, as a method of providing more organs for transplantation this 'opting in' system has been a failure.

In European countries such as Austria and Belgium, where 'opting out' systems have been introduced, it is assumed that the patient wished to be a donor unless he had stated otherwise during his lifetime. Little long-term improvement has been seen, underlining the necessity for the cooperation of the medical profession in the referral of brain-stem dead patients as potential organ donors.

The most effective method to date in gaining consent from bereaved relatives is the 'Required Request' or 'Routine Referral' system adopted in the USA. Legislation was introduced in Oregon, New York and California in 1985 and is now federal law in the majority of the States. In order to comply with the law, hospitals must formulate policies which outline a systematic and compassionate approach on the question of organ donation to the relatives of all patients who fulfil the criteria for brain-stem death. The required request laws have provided a much needed stimulus to hospitals involved in the participation of transplantation. The law also decreases the emotional burden on physicians, as they are required to ensure that the family are approached and may make that statement as part of the introduction to the subject. The law has also been well accepted by the public who should now always be given the opportunity to consider organ donation before support systems are withdrawn. Much European interest has been expressed over the legislation, but to date little, if any, progress has been made in this direction.

ORGAN PROCUREMENT SERVICES

The major organ-matching service in Western Europe is the Eurotransplant Service (ETS), which is located in the Netherlands. For the registration of patients awaiting a renal transplant and the allocation of available donor kidneys, this service is exclusive to the Netherlands, Belgium, Luxembourg, Germany and Austria. The UK Transplant Service (UKTS) similarly serves the whole of the UK, which for the purposes of transplantation includes Eire. France Transplant and the Rhone–Méditerranée Services cover France, while Scandia Transplant provides a service for Norway, Denmark and Sweden. Italy Transplant covers only Northern Italy. So far, Spain does not have a national organ-matching service, although organization in the Catalonian region of Spain is well developed (Wight, 1988). All these organizations facilitate the exchange of available donor material primarily within their own catchment area. Should there be no suitable local recipient, the kidney will be offered to another transplant service. A significant increase in multiple organ donation in Europe occurred in 1984. Prior to that time, available donor hearts were offered between the very few cardiac transplant centres on an informal basis. With an increase in transplant units and in the interest of a more equitable distribution, this practice is now discouraged and the referral of available hearts and/or lungs is made through the national organ-matching services. Each cardiac transplant unit registers its patients with its own national agency, but only if the patient's condition becomes critical will the agency, on request, register the patient with the other European services.

As with other organs, each region and country retains the right to use available hearts and lungs for its own population. Only if there is no suitable recipient will the organs be offered to another country.

As there are still relatively few cardiac transplant centres in Western Europe, patients requiring such therapy may travel to another country where the treatment is available. This is considered to be correct practice on humanitarian grounds. Under European Economic Community (EEC) agreements, patients are entitled to treatment in another member country free of charge to the patient—reimbursement being made at government level. Patients from countries outside the EEC may be treated, but will have to pay the full charges and will only receive treatment if there is no suitable entitled recipient registered at that time.

It has been recognized for some time that as the demand for suitable hearts and lungs for transplantation continues to outstrip the supply, the condition of many patients becomes critical during the waiting period. Since critically ill patients take priority over others, inequalities in the referral and distribution systems began to emerge. In 1987 in the UK, a working party consisting of transplant surgeons, coordinators, and members of the DHSS and UKTS met and decided, in order to make better use of this scarce resource and in the interests of a more equitable distribution, that for heart and heart–lung transplantation the 'urgent' category should be abandoned. Available donor organs would be offered to the heart transplant units on a strict rotational basis, and advice to transplant coordinators on the referral sequence is given by the UKTS. Should a heart or heart–lung operation take place involving organs offered on an informal basis, the transplant unit concerned is required to report prospectively to UKTS and to be placed at the bottom of the list. Success of this scheme necessitates the cooperation of regional transplant coordinators who, working at grass roots level, are responsible for the logistics of organ referral and removal. In addition, cooperation of the transplant units themselves in the notification to UKTS of intended and completed transplant operations is essential.

The recent and rapid increase in multiple organ donation has brought its own problems. There is great potential for confusion in the intensive care units, which underlines the importance of improved communications and trust not only between the donating units and transplant coordinators but also between the transplant units themselves. The organization of multiple organ donation can run more smoothly when all communication between the intensive care unit and transplant centre concerned are channelled through the local transplant coordinator (Wight, 1987). This potential for confusion now seems to have moved to the operating theatre where four separate surgical teams, possibly unknown to each other, may gather for organ removal. An initiative pioneered in Cambridge, England, in providing one single surgical team trained to remove and preserve all organs and tissue for transplantation, has met with approval from operating theatre staff and it is hoped that in time more such teams will be trained and available, thereby contributing to professional goodwill towards multiple organ donation (Wight, 1988).

In the USA the Federal Government has become increasingly involved in organ donation and transplantation. Prior to October 1987 the situation was similar to that in Europe. Approximately 110 organ procurement agencies, either affiliated to a hospital or acting independently, formed a network to match available donor organs with waiting recipient patients. Two computerized systems, 24-Alert — sponsored by the North American Transplant Coordinators Organization — and the United Network for Organ Sharing (UNOS), existed for the registration of patients awaiting an organ transplant and for the distribution, in particular, of extra-renal organs. In an effort to increase organ donation and to provide a more equitable distribution of available material, Public Law 99-509 was passed in late 1986 and became effective from 1 October 1987. UNOS was awarded a contract to set up a national network for organ procurement and transplantation. Hospitals are required to develop organ-recovery policies in order to be reimbursed by Medicare; in addition, the law requires all organ procurement organizations and transplant programmes to be UNOS members in order to be eligible for Medicare reimbursement. Whether this serious attempt to rationalize organ procurement and transplantation in the USA, combined with other initiatives from Europe, does indeed provide a system that is fair and equitable to both the professional and public communities is awaited with keen interest.

THE TRANSPLANT COORDINATOR

The transplant coordinator has become a vital member of the transplant team. Coordinators involved in procurement are responsible for determining the suitability of organs for transplant, assisting with the clinical management of the donor and ensuring that the proper legal and medical criteria have been met in declaration of death. In addition, they often take part in consultations with the next of kin on the possibility of organ donation.

As a result of the increasing recognition of the role of the transplant coordinator in the USA, there are plans to provide a national accrediting examination in order to unify standards of knowledge in this field. This examination is being organized through the North American Transplant Coordinators' Organization. Since there is a growing number of transplant centres as well as of waiting recipients, the transplant coordinator will continue to serve as a crucial link in the organ-recovery process.

REFERENCES

Ad Hoc Committee of the Harvard Medical School (1968). A definition of irreversible coma. *J. Am. Med. Ass.* **205**, 85–88.

Conference of Medical Royal Colleges and Their Faculties in the UK (1976). Diagnosis of death. *Br. Med. J.* **ii**, 1187–1188.

Conference of Medical Royal Colleges and Their Faculties in the UK (1979). Diagnosis of death. *Br. Med. J.* **i**, 3320.

DHSS (1983). Cadaveric organs for transplantation. A Code of Practice including the diagnosis of brain death. Department of Health and Social Security, London.

DHSS (1985). Public Health Service health resources and services administration. *HRS-A-OC 85-2.* Department of Health and Social Security, London.

Gallup (1986). Social Surveys for the British Kidney Patients' Association. Gallup, London.

Mollaret, P. and Goulon, M. (1959). Le cama depassé (mémoire preliminaire). *Rev. Neurol.* **101**, 3–15.

Reitz, B. A., Wallwork, J., Hunt, S. A., Pennock, J. L., Gillingham, M. E., Oyer, P. E., Stinson, E. B. and Shumway, N. E. (1982). Heart–lung transplantation: successful therapy for patients with pulmonary vascular disease. *N. Engl. J. Med.* **306**, 557–564.

Report of the Medical Consultants on the Diagnosis of Death to the President's Commission for the Study of Ethical Problems in Medical, Biochemical and Behavioral Research (1981). Guidelines for the determination of death. *J. Am. Med. Ass.* **246**, 2184–2186.

Wallwork, J., Jones, D. K., Cavarocchi, N., Hakim, M. and Higenbottam, T. (1987). Distant procurement of organs for clinical heart–lung transplantation using a single flush technique. *Transplantation* **44**(5), 654–658.

Wight, C. (1986) The role of the transplant co-ordinator (Leading Article). *Cyclosporin Qtly* **7**.

Wight, C. (1987) Organ donation. *Prof. Nurse* **3**(2), 43–44.

Wight, C. (1988) Organ procurement in Western Europe. *Transplant. Proc.* **20**, 1003–1006.

Timothy B. Icenogle, Robert W. Emery
and Jack G. Copeland

6

Donor Operation — Myocardial Protection: Current and Future Practice

INTRODUCTION

Cardiac transplantation has become an accepted form of therapy for properly selected patients with end-stage heart disease for whom no other treatment remains. The process of transplantation is a complex one. Each step is critical to the patient's survival. One of the earliest steps is the appropriate preparation and management of the cardiac donor.

After the usual careful screening and selection of a heart donor, a series of events is initiated which will lead to the transplant procedure. The donor's vital signs must be maintained in a stable condition while the logistics of harvesting are being arranged. This is particularly important in distant and multiple organ procurement. Factors included in determining the timing of donor cardiectomy are: (1) stability of the donor patient, (2) local factors in the donor hospital, (3) recipient preparation time, and (4) transport time.

MANAGEMENT OF CARDIAC DONOR

Management and physiological monitoring are key factors in the care of the organ donor and achieving stability in these patients is challenging. The physiological consequences of brain death and the care of the patient prior to the pronouncement of brain death frequently result in an unstable donor

(Griepp *et al.*, 1971; Levinson and Copeland, 1987). The brain-dead patient has usually been fluid-restricted and treated with diuretics in an attempt to lower intracranial pressures. With the pronouncement of brain death, this concern is no longer relevant and the vasomotor instability associated with brain death, diabetes insipidus and previous fluid restriction then results in a need for resuscitation with several litres of crystalloid fluids. A central venous pressure (CVP) line should be placed and an infusion of crystalloid solution administered until the patient's CVP reaches 4–8 mmHg to ensure adequate pre-load. Transfusion is appropriate if the haemoglobin is less than 12 g per cent since it is anticipated that multiple organ harvesting may result in considerable blood loss. Urine output must be monitored, and the fluid loss replaced hourly with crystalloid. Diabetes insipidus should be managed with intravenous aqueous vasopressin, titrated to maintain the urine output in the range of 100–200 ml/h.

An arterial line is absolutely necessary to monitor the blood pressure. Dopamine, at a dose of 5–10 μg/kg per min, may be used to maintain vasomotor tone. Many patients requiring dopamine infusions greater than 10 μg/kg per min are hypovolaemic and need further crystalloid infusion to reduce inotropic support. In our view, if the patient with an adequate CVP requires more than 10 μg/kg per min of dopamine, he cannot be used for cardiac donation. A donor heart with an adequate pre-load which requires massive inotropic support to maintain blood pressure may not function in the immediate post-transplant period.

A loss of temperature regulation occurs in the brain-dead patient and a temperature-sensing Foley catheter can be inserted in the bladder to monitor core temperature. Hypothermia is treated with warming blankets and by warming the intravenous solutions and the gases to the ventilator. Hyperthermia is treated with cooling blankets and ice packs and is an indication for blood culture prior to acceptance of the patient as a donor.

While the donor is being stabilized, the procurement team must obtain laboratory values and chest radiograph, and the appropriate consents. Blood, urine and tracheal aspirate cultures should be studied and prophylactic antibiotics (gentamicin and cefamandol) and high-dose steroids (methylprednisolone 1 g) should be administered immediately prior to transfer to the operating room.

In the operating room, the procurement team must help position and prepare the donor and make certain that the anaesthetist is able to monitor the CVP and arterial lines. Organ procurement procedures often take place in small hospitals unaccustomed to dealing with the unstable donor patient, and courtesy is essential to ensure future referrals and proper patient management.

Consultation with other organ procurement teams is essential for a successful organ donation procedure. It is now the rare exception for the heart alone to be harvested. A clear understanding of the techniques used by the other teams will result in a smooth operative experience (Rosenthal *et al.*, 1983; Shaw *et al.*, 1983; Starzl *et al.*, 1984) and certain technical considerations should be kept in mind. The sternal retractor should be placed in such a manner that the retractor's crossbar will not interfere with the teams harvesting organs from the abdomen, allowing maximal exposure for the liver and kidney teams. The heart procurement team should open the chest as the renal or liver team opens the abdomen. After umbilical tapes have been passed around the aorta and the superior and inferior venae cavae, and the heart has been assessed, assistance may be given to the liver or kidney teams in their dissection. During the removal of the liver and/or kidneys, a member of the cardiac procurement team should stay at the table and be prepared to remove the heart rapidly in the event that the donor becomes unstable.

Some renal procurement teams do not secure the aorta above the renal arteries and require that the aortic cross-clamp be left in place after cardiectomy in order to infuse the kidneys with cold perfusate. Renal teams using Collins' solution must coordinate the initiation of their perfusion with the heart transplant team. The high potassium content in the Collins' solution can arrest the heart before the cardiac team is ready.

DONOR CARDIECTOMY

The technique of donor cardiectomy has recently been described and will be briefly reviewed here (Copeland, 1984). A median sternotomy is performed with careful attention to haemostasis. The pericardial well is created and the aorta is circled with an umbilical tape. Both cavae are dissected circumferentially and the inferior vena cava is circled with an umbilical tape. A 2–0 Teflon-coated Dacron suture is passed around the superior vena cava with a superficial stitch through the visceral pericardium to ensure that the suture does not slip. This suture is used to ligate the superior vena cava and serves as a marker for transection, which would be approximately 1 cm cephalad to this point. This manoeuvre protects the sino-atrial node, located on the medial aspect of the superior vena caval–atrial junction.

When the other teams are ready for organ harvesting, heparin (30 000 units) is injected into the superior vena cava by the cardiac surgeon. A 14-gauge plastic cannula is inserted into the ascending aorta and connected to sterile tubing from the cardioplegic solution container. The superior vena cava is then ligated and the inferior vena cava and right inferior pulmonary vein are transected and the heart allowed to exsanguinate. This decompresses the heart and the cardioplegic solution is then started. A pressurized blood pump is used to infuse the cardioplegic solution into the aortic root. A total of 500 ml of a modified buffered Krebs' solution at 4°C with 15 mmol/

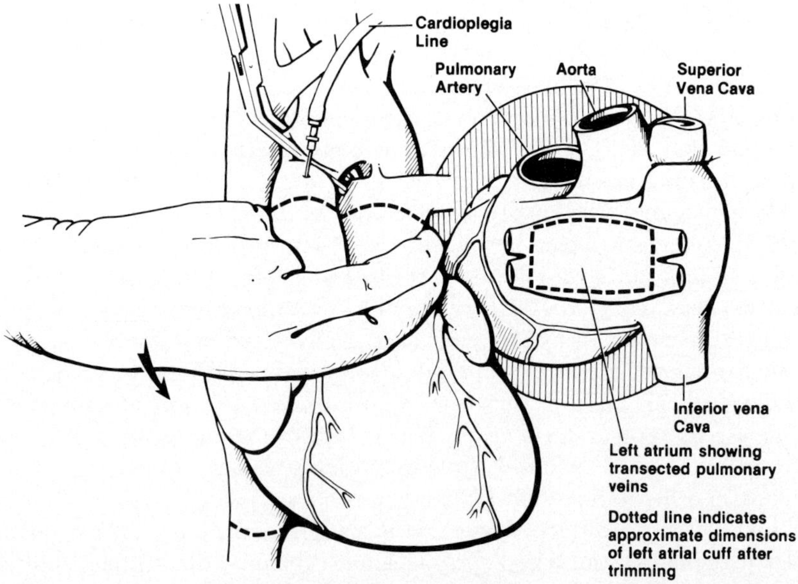

Fig. 6.1. *Lines of excision of the donor heart. (From Copeland, J. G. (1984). Heart transplantation.* Mod. Tech. Surg. Cardiothorac. Surg. **66**, *1–18. Reproduced by permission.)*

litre of potassium and 10 mmol/litre of magnesium is given. When the heart stops ejecting, the aorta is cross-clamped and the remainder of the cardioplegic solution flows in and arrests the heart. Saline at 4°C is applied topically to cool the heart during this time and two suction tip catheters are required to remove the blood and the saline effluent. The flaccid heart is elevated by the apex, the pulmonary veins are individually cut, and the left atrium dissected to the level of the transverse sinus. Only the great vessels and the superior vena cava remain attached at this point. The superior vena cava is transected approximately 1 cm cephalad to the previously placed ligature, and the surgeon places his thumb in the transverse sinus and pulls downward on the aorta and pulmonary artery to transsect the aorta distally just proximal to the take-off of the innominate artery. The left and right pulmonary arteries are then divided and thc heart is removed from the field (Fig. 6.1).

The heart is then carried by the surgeon to an adjacent table and washed in 3 basins of saline at 4°C. Care must be taken to cover the heart completely with saline and to bathe the endocardial surfaces for 10 min. The heart is cleaned of blood in the first basin and the left atrium opened with scissors by connecting the orifices of the four pulmonary veins. The scissor tips are passed from one pulmonary vein orifice to another to ensure that the orifices are indeed from the pulmonary veins. When the left atrium is

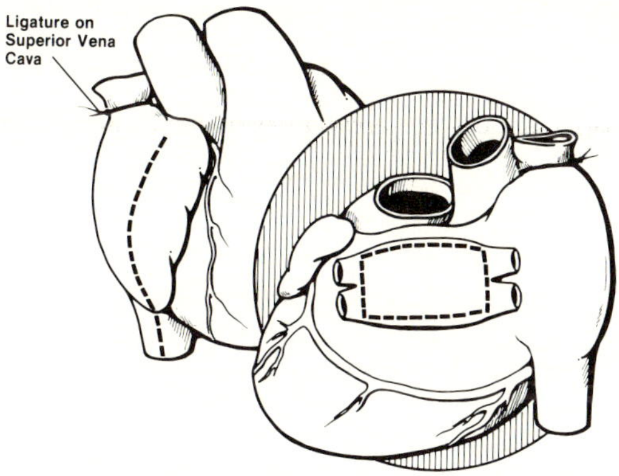

Fig. 6.2. *Incisions in the right and left atria of the donor heart. (From Copeland, J. G. (1984). Heart transplantation.* Mod. Tech. Surg. Cardiothorac. Surg. **66**, *1–18. Reproduced by permission.)*

opened, the septum is examined for a patent foramen ovale and the mitral valve inspected. Attention is then directed to the right atrium and the inferior vena caval orifice. A small incision should be made in the anterolateral margin of the right atrium from the inferior vena cava, extending superiorly towards the auricle for approximately 4–5 cm (Fig. 6.2). The final atriotomy will be made at the discretion of the transplanting surgeon at the time of the right atrial anastomosis (Fig. 6.3). The adequacy of the suture ligature in the superior vena cava should be checked at this time.

The heart should then be placed in a sterile plastic bag containing 200 ml of cold saline and air evacuated from the bag prior to sealing. The bag is then placed in a second bag with saline and, again, air evacuated. Finally,

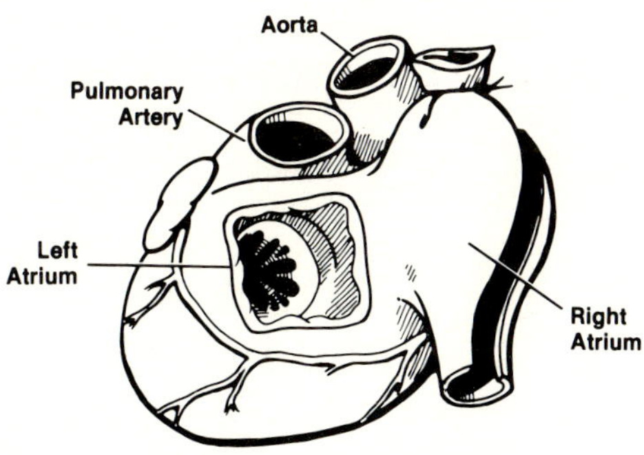

Fig. 6.3. *Final appearance of the posterior aspect of the donor heart. (From Copeland, J. G. (1984). Heart transplantation.* Mod. Tech. Surg. Cardiothorac. Surg. **66**, *1–18. Reproduced by permission.)*

the bag is placed into a sterile, 4.5 litre (1 gal.), wide-mouthed plastic jar to which saline has been added and the air evacuated. The lid is made water-tight and the jar placed into a third plastic bag, which is again sealed to make it water-tight. It is essential to evacuate air from all the bags as air is an insulator and could lead to inadequate preservation. The transport pack is placed into an ice chest and covered on all sides with crushed ice. Blood samples from the donor for serological studies as well as lymph nodes and spleen for immunological evaluation and cytotoxic crossmatching are also placed in the ice chest. The heart is then taken by the transport team for transportation.

CARDIAC PHYSIOLOGY AFTER BRAIN DEATH

Many potential donors are excluded each year because of poor cardiac performance. The aetiology of poor cardiac performance in the face of brain death deserves close scrutiny in order to determine possible methods by which more donors could be used. ECG changes following brain death were noted in donor patients early in the Stanford experience (Griepp *et al.*, 1971). The Capetown group has examined the electrocardiographic, haemodynamic and endocrine changes in experimental brain death in the Chacma baboon (Novitzky *et al.*, 1984). Brain death was initiated by inflating a Foley catheter in the subdural space to produce herniation. ECG changes were seen in all animals, and in half there were inverted T waves, ST segment elevation or an infarct pattern. Circulating catecholamines increased significantly after herniation, adrenaline rising 11-fold, noradrenaline three-fold and dopamine two-fold over baseline values. Circulating catecholamines returned to control values within 10 min and by the third hour had decreased below baseline values. Myocardial histology revealed abnormalities consisting of contraction bands, focal myocardial cell necrosis, interstitial oedema and mononuclear cell infiltration around the myocytes in 6 of 10 baboons.

Further studies using the same model indicated that interrupting the beta-adrenergic stimulation of the heart led to a reduction of tachycardia, the abolition of ventricular arrhythmias and loss of ischaemic features on the ECG (Novitzky *et al.*, 1986b). None of the animals in this group had contraction bands or coagulation necrosis on histological examination, although mononuclear cell infiltration and mild oedema were present in approximately half the animals. These results indicate that the surge of catecholamines associated with brain herniation can cause direct myocardial injury and that interruption of beta-adrenergic stimulation may prevent this damage.

Studies in a rabbit brain-death model (Walpoth *et al.*, 1985) have shown that catecholamine surge reduces the tolerance to ischaemia and reduces high-energy phosphate stores in the myocardium. Pre-medication and anaesthesia can produce a significantly lower post-brain-death catecholamine level, thus increasing high-energy phosphate levels and tolerance to ischaemia in the animal model.

After brain death in the pig, myocardial function is compromised. This is associated with depletion of myocardial high-energy phosphate and glycogen reserves whether or not there is haemodynamic support for the circulation (Wicomb *et al.*, 1986). The rate of depletion of the myocardial high-energy phosphate and glycogen reserves appears to be reduced by conversion to anaerobic glycolysis. The ability of the myocardium to undergo oxidatative phosphorylation seems to be impaired in the brain-dead animal, but the cause of this is not yet understood.

Brain-death studies in the Chacma baboon revealed that hormonal influences may also affect cardiac stability. Thyroid hormones, T3 and T4, fell sharply to 50% of control values 1 h after brain death and no circulating T3 or T4 was detectable after 16 h (Novitzky *et al.*, 1984). Cortisol levels rose in all animals within 5 min of brain death, then declined progressively to 50% of baseline at 1 h and continued to decline over the next 16 h. Insulin levels also fell in this model. Hormonal therapy has been used to reverse the deleterious effects of brain death on cardiac function (Novitzky *et al.*, 1986a). Intravenous thyroxine (T3), cortisol and insulin were infused into brain-dead pigs and the hearts excised and tested in an *ex vivo* apparatus. The hearts from the brain-dead and hormone-treated group were then compared with freshly excised hearts and hearts from untreated brain-dead pigs. The induction of brain death led to significant reductions in left ventricular pressure, stroke volume, cardiac output, and creatine phosphate and glycogen stores when compared with the freshly excised hearts. The hearts from the hormone-treated brain-dead group, however, showed no significant differences from the freshly excised hearts in stroke volume, cardiac output, creatine phosphate or glycogen stores, but did have a lower left ventricular pressure. Maintenance of intramyocardial energy stores through the preservation of oxidatative phosphorylation by hormonal modulation may salvage hearts that are currently rejected because of 'haemodynamic instability'. These results, yet to be proven in the human, offer an exciting new area for research and may have a place in the future treatment of the brain-dead patient.

A recent clinical study adds insight into the use of vasopressin in the brain-dead patient which may serve to increase haemodynamic stability (Yashioka *et al.*, 1986). Adrenaline alone versus vasopressin and low-dose adrenaline were compared for supporting haemodynamics in brain-dead patients. Vasopressin infusion at 1–2 units/h, combined with a minimal dose of adrenaline of less than 0.5 mg/h, prolonged mean survival times of brain-dead patients to 23.1 days, while the adrenaline alone group developed terminal cardiac failure within 48 h. Vasopressin enhanced the action of adrenaline and seemed to play a critical role in maintaining the pressor response to the catecholamines. Traditionally, vasopressin is not used until diabetes insipidus has developed, but it is possible that the earlier use of vasopressin may lower the requirements for catecholamine infusions, thereby making more patients acceptable organ donors. Currently, approximately 20% of organ donors may be unacceptable for cardiac donation (Novitzky *et al.*, 1984) because of haemodynamic instability. Continued research into brain-death physiology may increase the number of acceptable donors and improve the stability of those at present available.

MYOCARDIAL PRESERVATION

Myocardial preservation is of the utmost importance in the donor heart. Adequate preservation not only allows for the return of cardiac function at the end of the cross-clamp time, but also allows the heart to be transported long distances, thus increasing the donor pool. A combination of topical hypothermia and cold hyperkalaemic cardioplegia is used by most centres for preservation. The total ischaemic time accepted by most centres is approximately 4 h (Thomas *et al.*, 1978; Watson *et al.*, 1979), beginning with the interruption of the blood supply of the donor organ and ending with revascularization in the recipient. Ultrastructural studies have compared the distantly procured hearts with a mean ischaemic time of 154 min with locally procured hearts with a mean ischaemic time of 49 min (Billingham *et al.*, 1980). Post-perfusion biopsies in the on-site donors revealed myocardial changes similar to those in the transported hearts. (Ultrastructural studies done at 1 year after transplantation also revealed similarities in the myocardium.) However, endothelial changes were seen in 3 of 4 of the distantly procured hearts but in none of the on-site procured hearts, both immediately and at 1 year after transplantation. This study concluded that donor hearts could be preserved with satisfactory function for 3–4 h, with only scattered permanent endothelial damage.

Experience at the University of Arizona revealed that distant procurement of cardiac organs was associated with a decreased long-term recipient survival, and that the donor ischaemic time was the significant variable (Emery *et al.*, 1986). The 2-year survival was 85% for patients with locally procured hearts and 38% for those with a distantly procured heart. A recent reassessment of these data has determined that there is no statistically significant difference in the actuarial survivorship between those patients with locally procured hearts and distantly procured hearts. The difference between the two data probably stems from changes in immunosuppressive protocols that were not accounted for in the first study. In the USA, the number of distantly procured hearts will probably decline in the future as more heart transplant centres become active. However, the concern for the adequacy of preservation and the desire to match donor hearts more closely with recipients will provide the impetus to search for improved methods of myocardial protection.

Continuous hypothermic perfusion of the donor heart has been a research topic for many years. Copeland *et al.* (1973) proved that a canine heart could be preserved for 24–28 h using this system and then undergo successful orthotopic transplantation. Since that time, others have documented adequate function of allografts preserved by a variety of hypothermic perfusion systems in experimental animals (Cooper, 1976; Guerraty *et al.*, 1981; Tago, Subramanian and Kaye, 1983).

The St. Louis University group has shown that control of the oxidation reduction potential in the perfusion system, which serves to decrease the production of oxygen-derived free radicals, can lead to improved myocardial function (Miller *et al.*, 1985). Free radicals injure the viability of myocardial mitochondria, thus preventing oxidative phosphorylation (Otani *et al.*, 1984). These free radicals can also react with unsaturated fatty acids causing cellular damage.

Human hearts have been preserved with a similar system and successfully transplanted in the heterotopic position (Wicomb *et al.*, 1984). In 4 patients, one heart was rejected acutely, two initially had poor function which then improved, and one patient had immediate excellent donor function. Prolonged preservation of donor hearts may allow for better tissue typing, increased organ sharing through longer transports and elective scheduling of transplant procedures in the future.

Improved donor heart function may result from the reduction of oxygen-derived free radicals that are produced after preservation. The production of oxygen-derived free radicals occurs when ischaemic tissues are reperfused and oxygen combines with hypoxanthine in the presence of the enzyme xanthine oxidase. Uric acid and the superoxide radical are produced in this reaction. Treatment of the ischaemic heart preparation with superoxide dismutase or catalase enzymes which scavenge the superoxide radical and catalyse its dismutation to hydrogen peroxide and oxygen has been shown to have a protective effect during reperfusion (Shlafer *et al.*, 1982; McCord, 1985).

The beneficial effect of superoxide dismutase has been demonstrated in an orthopic heart transplant model in sheep (Stewart *et al.*, 1986). Donor hearts received cardioplegia with 30 000 units of superoxide dismutase and the recipient animals received another 60 000 units upon reperfusion. Compared with control animals, the hearts in the treated group had better left ventricular function, improved sub-endocardial blood flow, less platelet deposition and a decreased level of membrane injury products. Allopurinol, which inhibits xanthine oxidase, thereby reducing the production of free radicals, has potential use in the preservation of myocardial function. Studies in canine ischaemic myocardium demonstrated that pretreatment with allopurinol prevented the profound functional deficits seen after reperfusion when compared to control animals (Peterson *et al.*, 1985). Others (DeWall *et al.*, 1971; Manning, Coltart and Hearse, 1984; McCord, 1985) have shown a salutory effect with pretreatment of allopurinol to prevent reperfusion injury in ischaemic myocardium.

CONCLUSIONS

The successful outcome of heart transplantation is dependent upon adequate function of the donor heart. Well-established techniques for the preoperative and intraoperative care of the donor patient have been discussed. The subject of myocardial preservation, which in itself is worthy of a monograph, has been touched upon with particular reference to hypothermic perfusion and oxygen-derived free radical reperfusion injury. Perhaps the most exciting research is that being done in the area of donor physiology. By more closely understanding the effect of brain death on cardiovascular function, we may be able to achieve homeostasis in cardiac donors who would other wise be unused. This could significantly increase our pool of donor hearts and lead to a greater utilization of scarce resources.

REFERENCES

Billingham, M. E., Baumgartner, W. A., Watson, D. C., Reitz, B. A., Masek, M. A., Raney, A. A., Oyer, P. E., Stinson, E. B. and Shumway, N. E. (1980). Distant heart procurement for human transplantation. *Circulation* **62**, Suppl I, 11–19.

Cooper, D. K. C. (1976). Current research review: the donor heart, the present position with regard to resuscitation, storage, and assessment of viability. *J. Surg. Res.* **21**(5), 363–381.

Copeland, J. G. (1984). Heart transplantation. *Mod. Tech. Surg. Cardiothorac. Surg.* **66**, 1–18.

Copeland, J. G., Jones, M., Spragg, R. and Stinson, E. B. (1973). *In vitro* preservation of canine hearts for 24 to 28 hours followed by successful orthotopic transplantation. *Ann. Surg.* **178**, 687–692.

DeWall, R. A., Vasko, K. A., Stanley, E. L. and Kezdi, P. (1971). Responses of the ischemic myocardium to allopurinol. *Am. Heart J.* **82**(3), 362–370.

Emery, R. W., Cork, R. C., Levinson, M. M., Riley, J. E., Copeland, J., McAleer,

M. J. and Copeland, J. G. (1986). The cardiac donor: a six-year experience. *Ann. Thorac. Surg.* **41**(4), 356–362.

Griepp, R. B., Stinson, E. B., Clark, D. A., Dong, E. Jr. and Shumway, N. E. (1971). The cardiac donor. *Surg. Gynecol. Obstet.* **133**, 792–798.

Guerraty, A., Alivizatos, P., Warner, M., Hess, M., Allen, L. and Lower, R. R. (1981). Successful orthotopic canine heart transplantation after 24 hours of *in vitro* preservation. *J. Thorac. Cardiovasc. Surg.* **82**, 531–537.

Levinson, M. M. and Copeland, J. G. (1987). The organ donor physiology, maintenance and procurement considerations. In *Contemporary Anesthesia Practice*, vol. 10 (B. R. Brown, Ed.). F. A. Davis, Philadelphia.

Manning, A. S., Coltart, D. J. and Hearse, D. J. (1984). Ischemic and reperfusion-induced arrhythmias in the rat. *Circ. Res.* **55**(4), 545–548.

McCord, J. M. (1985). Oxygen-derived free radicals in postischemic tissue injury. *New Engl. J. Med.* **312**(3), 159–163.

Miller, L. W., Jellinek, M., Codd, J. E. and Kolata, R. J. (1985). Improved myocardial preservation by control of the oxidation-reduction potential. *Heart Transplant.* **IV**(3), 319–324.

Novitzky, D., Wicomb, W. N., Cooper, D. K. C., Rose, A. G., Fraser, R. C. and Barnard, C. N. (1984). Electrocardiographic, hemodynamic and endocrine changes occurring during experimental brain death in the chacma baboon. *J. Heart Transplant.* **IV**(1), 63–69.

Novitzky, D., Wicomb, W. N., Cooper, D. K. C. and Reichart, B. (1986a). Evidence of myocardial and renal functional recovery following hormonal treatment after brain death. *Transplant. Proc.* **XVIII**(3), 613–615.

Novitzky, D., Wicomb, W. N., Cooper, D. K. C., Rose, A. G. and Reichart, B. (1986b). Prevention of myocardial injury during brain death by total cardiac sympathectomy in the chacma baboon. *Ann. Thorac. Surg.* **41**(5), 520–524.

Otani, H., Tanaka, H., Inoue, T., Umemoto, M., Omoto, K., Tanaka, K., Sato, T., Osako, T., Masuda, A., Nonoyama, A., Kagawa, T. (1984). *In vitro* study on contribution of oxidative metabolism of isolated rabbit heart mitochondria to myocardial reperfusion injury. *Circul. Res.* **55**(2), 168–175.

Peterson, D. A., Asinger, R. W., Elsperger, K. J., Homans, D. C. and Eaton, J. W. (1985). Reactive oxygen species may cause myocardial reperfusion injury. *Biochem. Biophys. Res. Comm.* **127**(1), 87–93.

Rosenthal, J. T., Shaw, B. W. Jr, Hardesty, R. L., Griffith, B. P., Starzl, T. E. and Hakala, T. R. (1983). Principles of multiple organ procurement from cadaver donors. *Ann. Surg.* **198**(5), 617–621.

Shaw, B. W. Jr, Rosenthal, J. T., Griffith, B. P., Hardesty, R. L., Broznik, B., Hakala, T., Bahnson, H. T. and Starzl, T. E. (1983). Techniques for combined procurement of hearts and kidneys with satisfactory early function of renal allografts. *Surg. Gynecol. Obstet.* **157**, 261–264.

Shlafer, M., Kane, P. F., Wiggins, V. Y. and Kirsh, M. M. (1982). Possible role for cytotoxic oxygen metabolites in the pathogenesis of cardiac ischemic injury. *Circulation*, **66**, Suppl I, 85–92.

Starzl, T. E., Hakala, T. R., Shaw B. W. Jr, Hardesty, R. L., Rosenthal, T. J., Griffith, B. P., Iwatsuki, S. and Bahnson, H. T. (1984). A flexible procedure for multiple cadaveric organ procurement. *Surg. Gynecol. Obstet.* **158**, 223–230.

Stewart, J., Gerhardt, E. B., Wehr, C. J., Shuman, T., Merrill, W. H., Hammon, J. W. and Bender, H. W. (1986). Free radical scavengers and myocardial preservation during transplantation. *Ann. Thorac. Surg.* **42**(4), 390–393.

Tago, M., Subramanian, R. and Kaye, M. P. (1983). Light and electron microscopic evaluation of canine hearts orthotopically transplanted after 24 hours of extracorporeal preservation. *J. Thorac. Cardiovasc. Surg.* **86**(6), 912–919.

Thomas, F. T., Szentpetery, S. S., Mammana, R. E., Wolfgang, T. C. and Lower, R. R. (1978). Long-distance transportation of human hearts for transplantation. *Ann. Thorac. Surg.* **26**(4), 344–350.

Walpoth, B., Barbalat, F., Vitus, L., Fathi, N., Faidutti, B., Jardetzky, N. and Jamieson, S. (1985). Detrimental effect of endogenous and/or exogenous catecholamine stimulation on ischemic myocardial tolerance and energetics. *Heart Transplant.* **IV**(6), 606.

Watson, D. C., Reitz, B. A., Baumgartner, W. A., Raney, A. A., Oyer, P. E., Stinson, E. B. and Shumway, N. E. (1979). Distant heart procurement for transplantation. *Surgery* **86**(1), 56–59.

Wicomb, W. N., Cooper, D. K. C., Lanza, R. P., Novitzky, D. and Isaacs, S. (1986). The effects of brain death and 24 hours' storage by hypothermic perfusion on donor heart function in the pig. *J. Thorac. Cardiovasc. Surg.* **91**(6), 896–909.

Wicomb, W., Cooper, D. K. C., Novitzky, D. and Barnard, C. N. (1984). Cardiac transplantation following storage of the donor heart by a portable hypothermic perfusion system. *Ann. Thorac. Surg.* **37**(3), 243–248.

Yoshioka, T., Sugimoto, H., Uenishi, M., Sakamoto, T., Sadamitsu, D., Sakano, T. and Sugimoto, T. (1986). Prolonged hemodynamic maintenance by the combined administration of vasopressin and epinephrine in brain death: a clinical study. *Neurosurgery* **18**(5), 565–567.

C. Cabrol, I. Gandjbakhch,
A. Pavie, V. Bors, P. Dalous,
F. Baud and E. Solis

7

Surgical Procedure

INTRODUCTION

There are two main surgical procedures — orthotopic transplantation and heterotopic transplantation.

In orthotopic transplantation, the recipient's heart is excised and replaced by the donor's heart. In heterotopic transplantation, the recipient's heart is not excised and the donor's heart is anastomosed side to side to the corresponding atria and great vessels of the recipient's heart in order to give complete or partial assistance.

Orthotopic transplantation is the procedure used in most cases and will be described first.

ORTHOTOPIC TRANSPLANTATION

In order to reduce the ischaemic time of the donor's heart during a distant procurement, we have modified slightly the technique of Lower and Shumway (1960), the pioneers of the method. The procedure for harvesting the donor heart is described in Chapter 6.

Timing of donor's and recipient's operations

To minimize the ischaemic time to which the donor's heart is subjected, a precise timing is mandatory between the heart procurement and the preparation of the recipient. Usually, the recipient is not waiting in the hospital but is either at home or in another hospital located generally within three hours' travel. As soon as the possibility of obtaining a heart is mentioned, two compatible recipients are called urgently to our hospital. After a review in our unit, one is selected and prepared for transplantation. It usually takes one hour before the recipient can be placed on the operating table and another hour is necessary before the cardiopulmonary bypass can be started.

If the donor is in the adjacent operating theatre, it is easy to adjust the time between the two operations. The excision of the donor's heart may take place after the dissection of the kidneys and liver. This generally takes $2\frac{1}{2}$ h, so the recipient's operation is started $1\frac{1}{2}$ h after the beginning of the multiple organ procurement in the donor, unless pericardial adhesions (e.g. in the case of reoperation) are expected in the recipient.

In a distant procurement, after the first telephone call from the donor's hospital and when the suitability of the heart procurement (haemodynamic condition, ABO group, weight, etc.) is settled, the companies which organize the transport (air and/or road) are warned. The harvesting surgeon is sent to the donor's hospital at the beginning of the multiple organ procurement in order to assess more precisely the haemodynamic condition of the donor. He then informs the transplanting team of the expected hour of heart excision. The recipient is prepared in time and placed on the operating table approximately $1\frac{1}{2}$ h before the expected time of the donor's heart arrival in the operating room. When the harvesting surgeon clamps the aorta, he records the time when the cardiac ischaemia starts. Other telephone calls are made when the surgeon leaves the donor's hospital, when he reaches the arrival airport and finally when he is entering the transplantation hospital.

These telephone communications imply that, in our unit, an operator remains in contact with the operating theatre of the donor's hospital, the different companies which organize the transport of the donor's heart and the porter's lodge of our hospital.

Preparation of recipient

Usually, two recipients are called to come to our unit. They are carefully examined to rule out any temporary contraindications (skin or another infection, recent transfusion, pulmonary infarction, etc.).

Then the chosen recipient is prepared, beginning by a thorough shaving, washing and disinfection of the skin. In our protocol (Cabrol *et al.*, 1984), several steps are performed before the patient is transported into the operating room:

(1) Placement of a central venous pressure (CVP) catheter through the right internal jugular vein.
(2) Drawing of venous samples for ABO group, serum electrolytes, Ca^+,

phosphorus, irregular agglutinins, coagulation tests, virology, toxoplasma, etc.

(3) Infusion of 240 mg i.v. methylprednisolone in a single dose.

(4) Oral administration of 3 mg/kg azathioprine and 30 ml antacids.

(5) The patient is premedicated with 25 mg/kg i.m. cefatoxine sodium and 6.6 mg morphine, 0.22 mg scopolamine bromhydrate and 22 mg sparteine sulphate.

Then the patient is transported to the operating room where another CVP catheter, a peripheral i.v. line and an arterial catheter are placed.

Anaesthesia is induced with 0.2 mg/kg diazepam and 5–10 μg/kg fentanyl. Curarization is obtained with 0.1 mg/kg pancuronium.

After orotracheal intubation, ventilation is supported with a volume respirator with an FiO_2 of 60%. Anaesthesia is maintained with multiple injections of diazepam, fentanyl and pancuronium as needed.

A Foley catheter is placed to quantitate urinary output. Continuous electrocardiographic and arterial pressure monitoring is maintained throughout the transplant procedure. Serum electrolytes and blood gases are obtained every 30 min until the patient is in the intensive care unit (ICU).

Cardiopulmonary bypass (CPB) is established in a routine fashion and, prior to the orthotopic transplantation, pressures in the right atrium, right ventricle, pulmonary artery and left atrium are obtained.

Crossmatching between the donor and the recipient is an important point. Usually every recipient is investigated in order to detect HLA antibodies, testing his serum against a panel of potential donors' lymphocytes. If there are no antibodies, the transplantation can be done with any donor of the same ABO group. A direct donor recipient crossmatch is always made after the transplant is performed. If there are some antibodies, a direct crossmatch between the donor and the recipient must be done before the transplantation, and usually imposes an on-site procurement.

La Pitié technique

A median sternotomy and vertical pericardiotomy are made. Care is taken not to open the pleural or peritoneal cavities. Meticulous haemostasis is secured at this time. The aorta is dissected from the pulmonary artery. When the donor's heart arrives in the hospital, CPB is established with two right-angle caval cannulae for venous drainage inserted through the right atrium, as posteriorly as possible, and an arterial inflow line is inserted into the ascending aorta. The priming of the CPB circuit is done according to the fluid status of the patient. In that respect, it is often useful to interpose an ultra-filtration device in the circuit. When the donor's heart arrives in the operating room, the heart of the recipient is electrically fibrillated and the

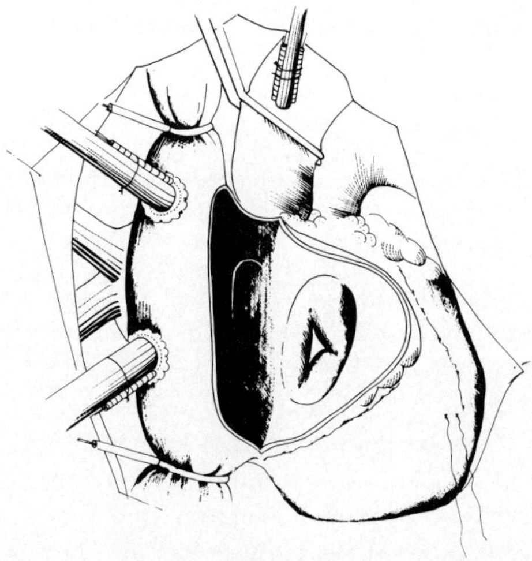

Fig. 7.1. *Electric fibrillation of the recipient's heart, aortic cross-clamp, and heart excision through the right atrial roof. The atrial incision curves down to the right anteriorly toward the atrioventricular groove. To the left it is directed toward the aortic root.*

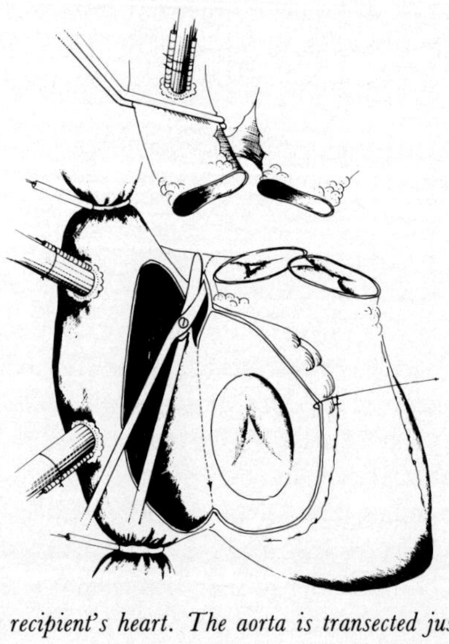

Fig. 7.2. *Removal of the recipient's heart. The aorta is transected just above the coronary ostia and the pulmonary artery is transected over the semilunar valve's commissures. The roof of the left atrium is exposed and opened posteriorly to the base of the left atrial appendage.*

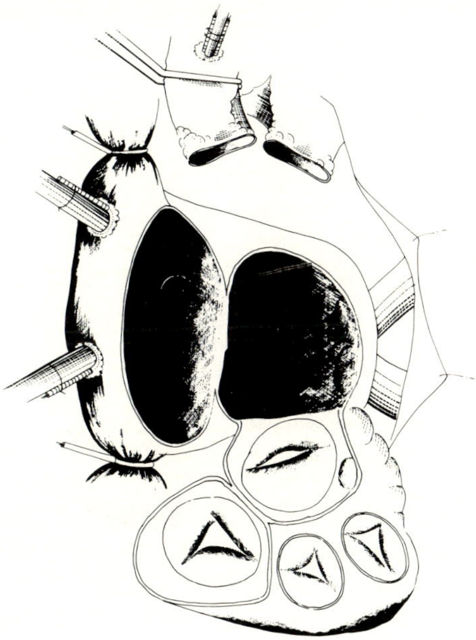

Fig. 7.3. *Transection of the atrial septum and union of the lateral and inferior incisions in the right and left atrial walls.*

aorta is cross-clamped to prevent embolization of thrombi that are often present in the dilated diseased heart. The CPB is then initiated, the caval tapes are tightened and the body temperature is lowered to 27°C.

The recipient's heart is removed by transecting the right atrial roof proximal to its appendage (Fig. 7.1). The incision curves down to the right, anteriorly toward the atrioventricular groove. To the left, it is directed toward the aortic root. The aorta is transected just above the coronary ostia and the pulmonary artery is transected over the semilunar valve commissures. The roof of the left atrium is exposed and opened posteriorly to the base of the left atrial appendage, then curving down anteriorly toward the left atrioventricular groove, usually through the coronary sinus (Fig. 7.2). The atrial septum is transected at the end, close to the mitral orifice, rejoining the lateral and inferior incisions in the right and left atrial walls (Fig. 7.3). After excision of the heart, the aorta and pulmonary artery are separated from each other by 1 or 2 cm to facilitate the anastomoses.

During that time, the plastic bags and box containing the donor's heart are opened in a sterile manner and the cooled heart placed first in a bowl containing 4°C saline, then in the pericardial cavity on the left side of the left atrial remnant. The left atrial anastomosis is performed first. Before

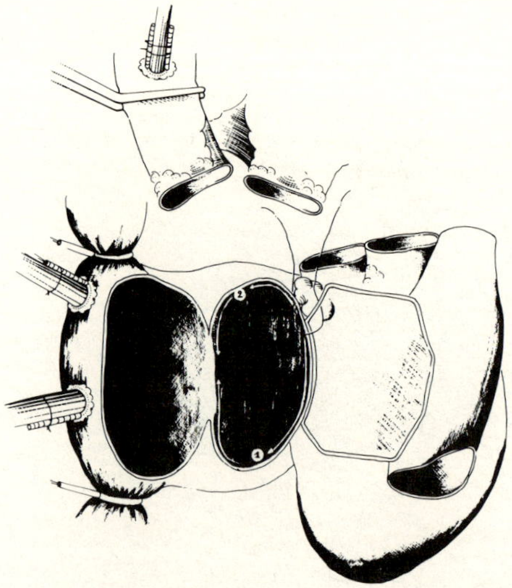

Fig. 7.4. *Placement of the 3–0 monofilament suture at the entrance of the recipient's left superior pulmonary vein and the base of the donor's left atrial appendage. The anastomosis is performed starting with the lateral and inferior sides, followed by the superior aspect and the septum.*

starting the implantation, to prevent anatomical distortion the position of the graft is assured by placing 3–0 monofilament sutures at both the entrance of the recipient's left superior pulmonary vein and the base of the donor's left atrial appendage. The anastomosis is done with 3–0 sutures,

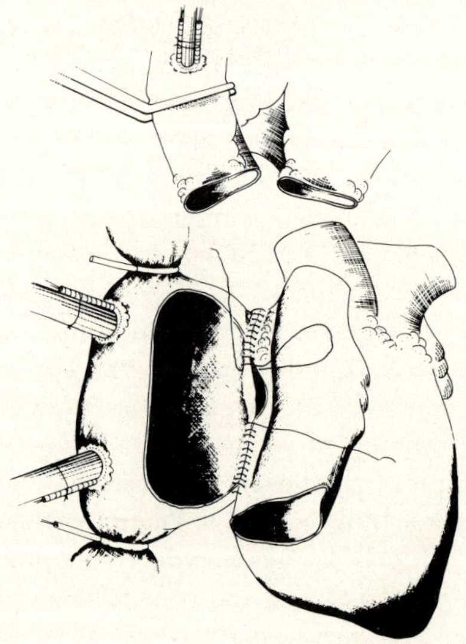

Fig. 7.5. *Final closure of the left atrium down the atrial septum.*

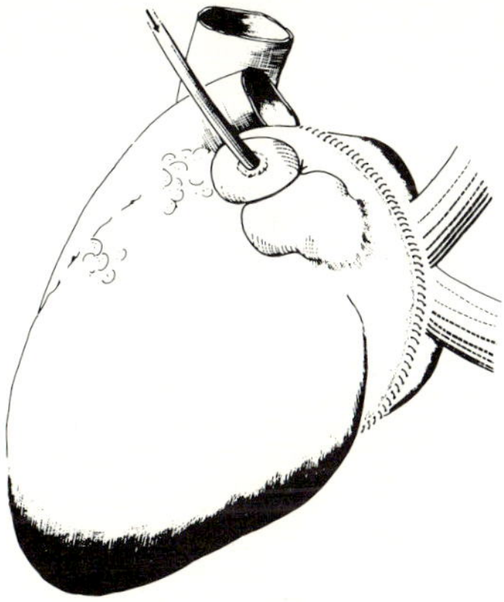

Fig. 7.6. *Placement of the left atrial perfusion catheter.*

starting with the lateral and inferior sides, followed by the superior aspect and the septum (Fig. 7.4). The whole thickness of the lateral and inferior walls is anastomosed in a single layer from the inside. The suture is brought outside at the inferior junction of the wall and interatrial septum. Another 3–0 suture is then placed and run superiorly across the roof of the left atrium and down the atrial septum. At that level, the suture incorporates the margins of the donor's left atrial edge and the recipient's entire atrial septum edge. The two 3–0 sutures, the inferior and the superior ones, are tied together (Fig. 7.5).

At this time, cold lactated Ringer's solution is infused into the left atrium through a small cannula inserted into the left atrial appendage (Fig. 7.6); this will protect the heart by maintaining a low sub-endocardial temperature and will evacuate all air, not only from the left cardiac chambers but from the pulmonary vascular bed. This manoeuvre, proposed by the Stanford group, has totally eliminated the occurrence of air emboli in our series. The aortic anastomosis is then started using a 5–0 monofilament suture. The first suture begins at the junction of the left inferior edges of both the donor's and the recipient's aorta (Fig. 7.7). The donor's aorta must sometimes be cut obliquely to fit a dilated recipient's aorta. Prior to completion of this suture line, all residual air is evacuated by allowing the Ringer's lactate infusion to fill the ascending aorta. An aspirating needle is placed in the ascending aorta and the aortic clamp is removed. Two electrodes are inserted in the right ventricular anterior wall and the heart is electrically fibrillated to prevent premature contractions that could eject some residual air. At this point, the cold infusion is stopped and a left ventricular vent is placed via the recipient's superior right pulmonary vein. This vent is left open to the pericardial

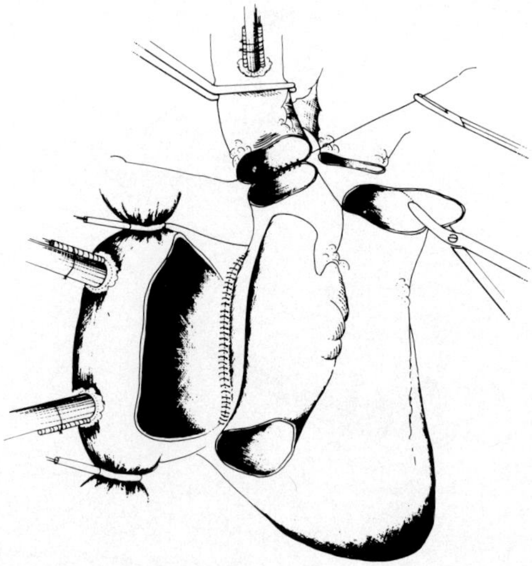

Fig. 7.7. *Initiation of the aortic anastomosis. The donor's aorta sometimes must be cut obliquely to fit a dilated recipient's aorta. All air from the left cardiac chambers is evacuated prior to the completion of this suture.*

cavity to avoid any distension of the left ventricle (Fig. 7.8). The patient is progressively rewarmed to 34°C.

The donor heart's pulmonary artery is trimmed in order to fit the recipient's pulmonary artery orifice. Then the pulmonary artery continuity is reestablished by an end-to-end anastomosis using a continuous 5–0 polypropylene suture. The anastomosis begins on the left side, suturing the inferior edges from the inside and then the superior edges from the outside. The pulmonary artery anastomosis is not completed at that time and a small gap is left anteriorly to avoid distension of the right ventricle during the right atrial anastomosis (Fig. 7.9). Before initiating the right suture line, the right atrium is opened from the inferior vena caval orifice up to the base of the right atrial appendage. In this way, the sinus node and its vascularization is preserved. The superior vena caval stump is closed with a 5–0 polypropylene double running suture. A right ventricular endomyocardial biopsy is taken through the tricuspid orifice and serves as a baseline specimen. Another biopsy is taken for bacteriological testing.

The right atrial anastomosis is then started using two 5–0 polypropylene sutures (Fig. 7.9). The first suture includes the posterior edge of the donor's right atrial aperture and the entire thickness of the left atrial wall on the septum at its mid-portion. This suture runs inside across the inferior part of the septum and the inferior right atrial wall. Another 3–0 suture is placed at the middle part of the atrial septum and joins the superior part of the poste-

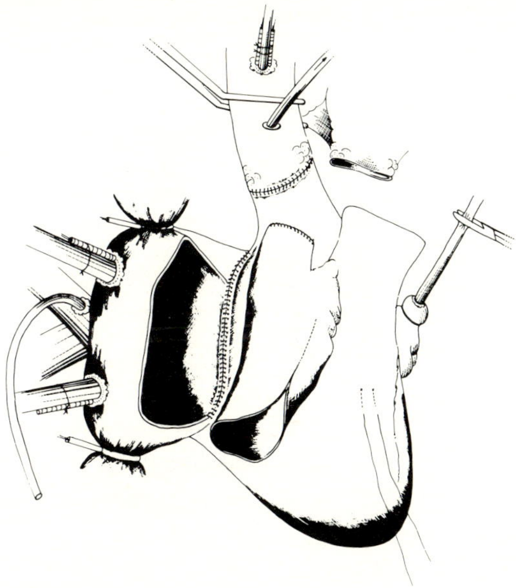

Fig. 7.8. *An aspirating needle is placed in the ascending aorta and the aortic clamp is removed. Two electrodes are inserted in the anterior wall of the right ventricle and the heart is electrically fibrillated, the cold infusion is stopped and a left ventricular vent is placed via the recipient's superior right pulmonary vein and left open to avoid distension of the left ventricle. The superior vena cava stump is closed. The right atrium is largely opened.*

rior right atrial wall of the donor's heart to the atrial septum of the recipient's heart. Subsequently, it joins the superior and anterior walls of both right atrial walls and finally is tied to the first suture.

After the right atrial anastomosis, the pulmonary artery anastomosis is completed, allowing the coronary sinus blood to expel all the air from the right cardiac chambers. All residual air from the left cardiac chambers is evacuated with precise manoeuvres. First, the caval tapes are released and, if necessary, the superior vena cava cannula is cross-clamped. Next, the lungs are reinflated. These manoeuvres increase the blood flow through the right cardiac chambers, the pulmonary vascular bed and the left cardiac chambers. The left ventricular vent is connected to the oxygenator via a gravity drainage line which is cross-clamped. Additional removal of air that may remain entrapped in the heart is done by needle aspiration of the right superior pulmonary vein, of the roof of the left atrium, and of the left ventricle through its apex (Fig. 7.10).

The left atrial appendage line is removed and the appendage carefully tied. Blood is allowed to partially fill the pericardial cavity. The clamp on

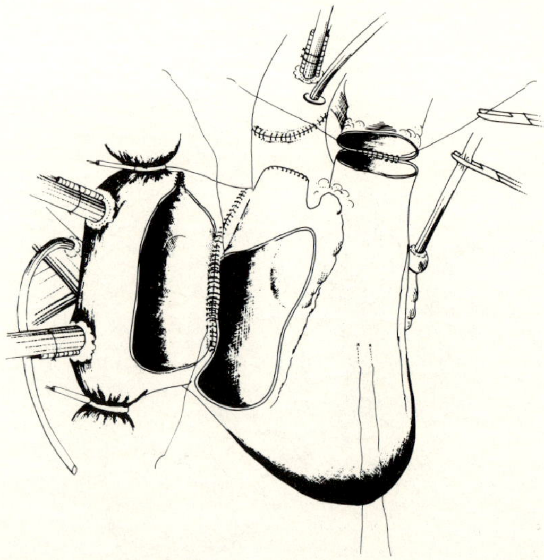

Fig. 7.9. *The pulmonary artery continuity is re-established by suturing the inferior edges from the inside and the superior edges from the outside. The anastomosis is not completed at this time to avoid distension of the right ventricle during the right atrial anastomosis. The right atrial anastomosis is started.*

the left ventricular vent is removed, allowing a smooth and efficient underwater drainage of the left cardiac chambers. These chambers are then gently massaged to evacuate residual air bubbles through the left drainage line and to prevent any air emboli to the coronary artery branches of the anterior right ventricular wall (Fig. 7.11). If such air emboli occur, the coronary arteries are carefully punctured to evacuate any air which will impair the function of the right ventricle. The heart is then electrically defibrillated if it does not start beating spontaneously. Cardiopulmonary bypass is continued for 20–30 min in order to allow myocardial recovery and rewarming of the patient to a core temperature of at least 34°C. An intravenous infusion of isoprenaline is started after the release of the aortic clamp and usually allows rapid and vigorous heart beats with a normal ECG tracing. If not, circulatory assistance is maintained and inotropic drugs are sometimes needed. When cardiac function is satisfactory, the left ventricular vent is cross-clamped and removed. The pericardial blood is aspirated and all the suture lines are carefully inspected for haemostasis. Special attention is given to the lateral part of the left atrial anastomosis, which is not easily and safely accessible when the heart is in place and CPB is stopped.

CPB is discontinued, haemostasis is completed carefully and 4 metallic markers are sutured to the cardiac borders to delineate the heart on post-

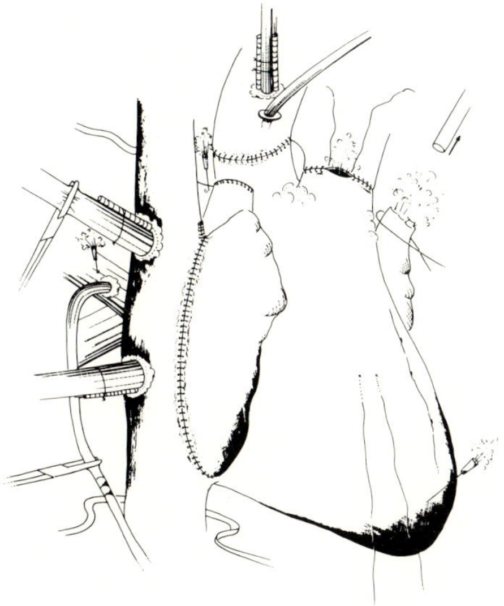

Fig. 7.10. *Completion of the pulmonary artery anastomosis after the right atrial anastomosis has been finished. All residual air is evacuated by release of the caval tapes, reinflation of the lungs, and needle aspiration of the right superior pulmonary vein, roof of the left atrium and left ventricular apex.*

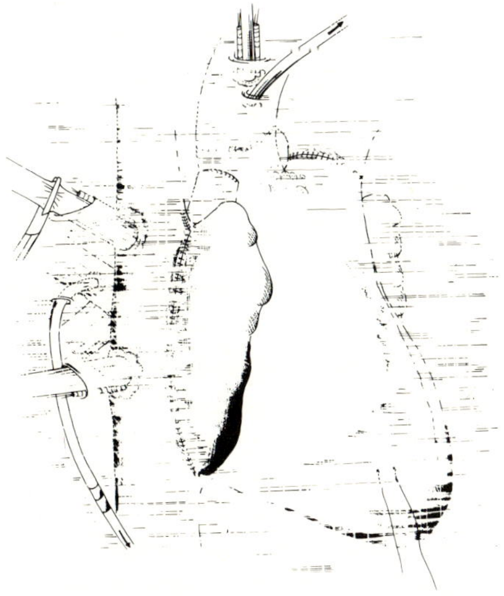

Fig. 7.11. *Underwater drainage of the left cardiac chambers with the left ventricular vent for an adequate extraction of all the residual air.*

operative chest radiographs. Two additional markers are fixed to the right border of the right ventricle as landmarks for future endomyocardial biopsies. Cardiopulmonary bypass cannulae are removed and the chest is closed as usual. The pericardium is left open to prevent any cardiac compression or tamponade.

Technical variants

In some groups the different steps are done in the following order: left atrial anastomosis, left atrial infusion with 4°C Ringer's lactate or saline, right atrial anastomosis and aortic anastomosis. After the completion of the aortic anastomosis, an aspirating vent is inserted into the ascending aorta. The aortic clamp is removed. The left atrial infusion is stopped. A left ventricular vent is placed through the right superior pulmonary vein and the mitral valve. The pulmonary artery anastomosis is performed and the de-airing manoeuvres are done as in the previously described technique. The heart is electrically defibrillated, the isoprenaline infusion is started and the patient rewarmed to 34°C.

Another operative variant is to leave the aortic anastomosis to last. Before unclamping the aorta, an aspirating needle is inserted in the ascending aorta and another in the pulmonary artery. The left atrial infusion is stopped, the left ventricular vent is placed and the usual de-airing manoeuvres are successively performed as usual.

Operative and postoperative management

It is important to mention at this point some observations on operative and immediate postoperative care.

In our experience, while the patient is in the operating room, a normal cardiac function is never established without the use of isoprenaline. Therefore, an i.v. infusion, at a dose of 0.3–0.4 mg/kg per min, is started before the aortic cross-clamp is released. The infusion is adjusted as needed, depending on the appearance and function of the heart to obtain an arterial pressure around 100 mmHg and a rate of 120 beats/min.

The electrocardiographic monitoring is particularly important. If the complexes are small and fast in sinus rhythm, the cardiac function is adequately preserved. However, if the complexes are big and arrhythmias such as complete AV blocks appear, severe haemodynamic problems will follow. Likewise, the appearance and function of the heart is significant. If the heart is without dilatation, with good contractility and in sinus rhythm, the i.v. infusion of isoprenaline is maintained, CPB is discontinued, the incision is closed and the patient is sent to the ICU. On the other hand, if dilatation of the right cavities and left ventricular insufficiency appear, more vigorous treatment is started with dopamine or adrenaline. If the cardiac function remains mediocre, the CPB is maintained until an adequate temperature around 34°C is obtained. If the heart function does not improve with these manoeuvres, the haemodynamic failure may lead to low cardiac output and death, unless a univentricular or biventricular assist device or an artificial heart is available before a second heart transplant.

Once the patient is in the ICU, *haemodynamic performance* is monitored continuously for 3–4 days in the normal cases. The isoprenaline dose is reduced progressively. During the first 5 or 6 days, the transplanted heart is dependent on the isoprenaline infusion. Therefore it is extremely important that the administration of the drug is not discontinued while the syringes and pumps are being changed, as this could lead to excessive bradycardia or complete cardiac arrest. In general, in about 7–8 days the isoprenaline is gradually discontinued, and at this time the graft is in perfect function and well adapted, in spite of a complete denervation, to maintain a normal life. Atrial pacing can, of course, also be used to maintain an adequate heart rate.

After the transplantation, the patient should be kept in strict *isolation* for at least 12 days. The minimum personnel should be in contact with him and before entering the patient's room all must wash their hands and wear cap, mask, boots and sterile gown. Also it is important to avoid bringing machines (X-ray, ECG) and any unnecessary object into the room. In 'La Pitié' (Cabrol *et al.*, 1985), the ECG electrodes that are connected to the patient have an access outside the room. Furthermore, the doors are made of glass, which permits placement of the bed in front of the door to obtain radiographs, thus avoiding the necessity for the X-ray machine to enter the room.

A nurse or a doctor is always with the patient, who is routinely examined every 6 h to confirm the absence of infection as well as hepatic, cardiac and renal dysfunction. Furthermore, an ECG and haemocultures are obtained every 8 h, chest radiographs every 12 h, serum electrolytes, CBC and blood gases every 6 h and renal function every day.

During the third week of postoperative care, the patient is transferred to *an ordinary room*. He is examined twice daily and the laboratory tests are performed twice a week while the patient is in hospital.

In the absence of complications, the patient is allowed to leave hospital in the fourth week. He will return to hospital for routine examination which consists of: physical examination, ECG, chest radiographs, serum electrolytes, CBC, renal function, hepatic function, cyclosporin levels, bacteriological tests and endomyocardial biopsy. These surveys are done every week for 3 months, then every 2 weeks until 6 months have elapsed and afterwards every month. If there is a suspicion of rejection or complications, the patient is readmitted.

With experience over the years, there is a trend to reduce the intensity of care at all stages following transplantation.

Associated treatment

The patient is extubated 12–24 h after the operation, if respiratory function is adequate. Physiotherapy is given twice a day.

The oral intake of food is established as soon as possible.

Diuretics are used to maintain a diuresis greater than 100 ml/h during the early postoperative care.

Treatment against infection

Bacteriological tests in conjunction with a rigorous physical examination are excellent tools for early identification of an infection. Throughout the patient's stay in the hospital, attention should be directed to identifying the symptoms of infection (pain, fever, fatigue, cough, abnormalities in urinary or nervous systems).

Prophylactic administration of antibiotics should be directed against the staphylococcal infections and should start early in the postoperative care and continue until the mediastinal drains are withdrawn.

Bacteriological examinations of the i.v. catheters, urinary cultures and blood cultures, as well as testing of all the natural orifices (nose, throat, anus) of the body, are routine each day for the first 2 days and then twice a week. After the 14th postoperative day, all the tests are carried out once a week.

If an infection is identified, antibiotics should start as early as possible and be modified according to cultures and antibiotic sensitivities. It is important to note that some aminoglycosides can potentiate the nephrotoxicity of cyclosporin.

Immunological surveillance

E-rosettes are obtained twice a week during the first 15 days. Serum levels of cyclosporin are measured daily during the first week and then twice a week for the first month.

Anatomopathological examination

The diagnosis of rejection by clinical or electrocardiographic examination has been abandoned since treatment with cyclosporin began. Only systematic endomyocardial biopsies permit an early diagnosis and have become the gold standard for the diagnosis of rejection. Our first biopsy is performed on the 6th–7th day of postoperative care, then once a week for 3 months or in the case of change in treatment or suspicion of rejection.

Treatment against rejection

To increase the advantages and diminish the side effects found with treatment of cyclosporin we follow these two principles:

(1) *Late* administration of cyclosporin to avoid the acute side effects of early administration.
(2) *Low* doses of cyclosporin.

'La Pitié' protocol

(a) Preoperative dose:
 – methylprenisolone 240 mg i.v.
 – oral azathioprine 5 mg/kg.
(b) Operative dose:
 – methylprednisolone 120 mg i.v. after the induction of anaesthesia and 120 mg i.v. after cardiopulmonary bypass has been discontinued.
(c) Postoperative dose:
 – methylprednisolone 300 mg i.v. in 6 doses during the first 24 h, then 240 mg on the second day, 160 mg on the third day and 120 mg on the fourth day.
 – oral azathioprine 2.5 mg/kg per day.
 – ATG 6 mg/kg per day for 3 days.

Once the patient is haemodynamically stable and when renal and hepatic function have improved (2nd–3rd day) the cyclosporin is administered by mouth (p.o.). The initial dose is 3–5 mg/kg per day in 2 doses; the dose is adjusted to a plasma level of 150–200 ng/ml. The azathioprine administration is stopped with the first dose of cyclosporin.

Corticosteroids are administered p.o. in an initial dose of 1 mg/kg per day and are gradually reduced to reach in the 6th week a dose of 0.2 mg/kg per day.

Treatment of a rejection episode

(a) Moderate rejection:
 – corticosteroid dose is increased to 100 mg of prednisone daily for 5 days.
(b) Severe rejection:
 – methylprednisolone 1000 mg/day for 3 days, ATG 6 mg/kg per day for 3 days.
 – cyclosporin treatment is unaltered.

HETEROTOPIC TRANSPLANTATION

Indications

For some groups, such as the one in Cape Town, this technique is the procedure of choice. The main advantages of this method are:

(1) It overcomes the threat of fatal donor right heart failure following orthotopic cardiac transplantation in patients with excessively high pulmonary vascular resistance.
(b) The preserved recipient heart remains functional, giving support during the initial post-ischaemic heart failure, in the case of acute rejection and when graft destruction appears induced by chronic rejection-related coronary artery disease.
(3) The reduction of the work that the diseased recipient's heart has to perform after the heterotopic transplantation could lead to an eventual improvement of this heart.

The disadvantages that other groups have found using this technique, such as a greater difficulty in the postoperative control of the ECG as well as in obtaining endomyocardial biopsies, the persistence of pre-transplant disabling symptoms (pain, arrhythmias) and the presence of thrombi in the dilated poorly contracted recipient's heart, have limited heterotopic transplantation to selected indications: (a) large patients with severe heart failure who cannot wait until a big enough graft can be found for them; (b) emergency cases when the donor's heart appears unable to support the recipient's circulation immediately; (c) patients with borderline pulmonary hypertension in whom age or technical factors (adhesions) preclude the use of the more uncertain heart–lung transplantation.

Surgical technique

We will outline the procedure described by Novitzky, Cooper and Barnard (1983), modified by Dor *et al.* (1986).

Donor heart excision

The same technique to retrieve a heart for orthotopic transplantation is used, cxcept that in the beginning of the dissection the superior vena cava is mobilized as far from the heart as possible, cranial to the azygos vein which is tied distally.

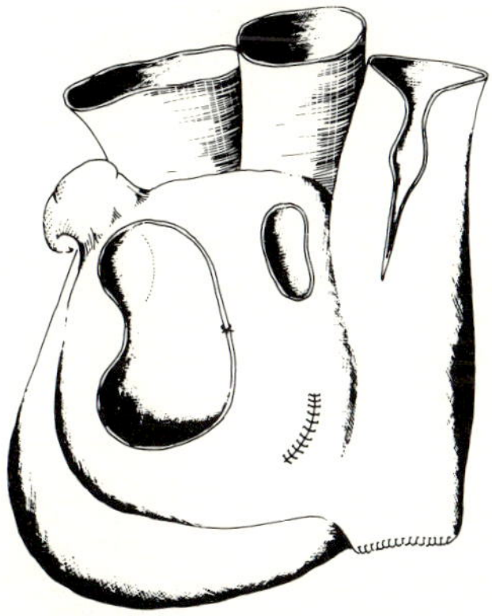

Fig. 7.12. *Preparation of the donor's heart. The orifices of the right inferior pulmonary vein and inferior vena cava are closed with a double running suture. The orifice of the right superior pulmonary vein is temporarily left open. The left atrium is opened between the two left pulmonary veins to obtain an orifice of about 4 cm in diameter. A suture placed in the midpoint of the right wall of this opening is used as a marker for the subsequent implantation.*

Once the heart is removed, it is placed in a bowl containing saline at 4°C and it is prepared for implantation in the recipient. The orifices of the right inferior pulmonary vein and of the inferior vena cava are closed with a double running suture of 5–0 polypropylene (Fig. 7.12). The orifice of the right superior pulmonary vein is temporarily left open. The left atrium is opened between the two left pulmonary veins to obtain an orifice of about 4 cm in diameter. Novitzky, Cooper and Barnard (1983) utilize a suture placed in the midpoint of the right wall of this opening as a marker to be used in the subsequent implantation. The orifice of the superior vena cava is left open and from there the posterior wall of the vein is incised longitudinally for 4 cm, passing through the orifice of the azygos vein.

Transport, timing and preparation of the recipient are the same as for orthotopic transplantation.

Recipient operation

A midline sternotomy is performed and the pericardium is opened longitudinally. A right side pleuropericardial flap is created first, by dividing the right mediastinal pleura immediately posterior to the sternum and then by extending this incision medially over the diaphragm to a point 2 cm away from the right phrenic nerve (Fig. 7.13). In this way, a triangular flap is created that comprises the parietal pericardium and the mediastinal pleura. Haemostasis of the edges of this flap must be carried out carefully, because it would be difficult to do so after the anastomosis of the allograft. The flap is allowed to fall back into the right pleural cavity, enlarging the right side of

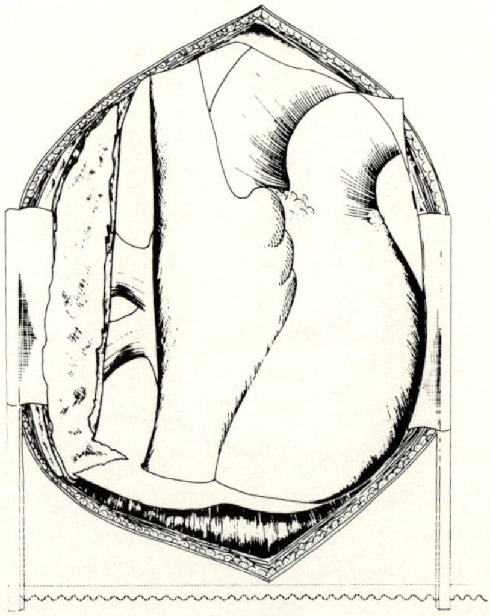

Fig. 7.13. *A right-sided pleuropericardial flap is created by dividing the right mediastinal pleura immediately posterior to the sternum and then by extending this incision medially over the diaphragm to a point 2 cm away from the right phrenic nerve. Haemostasis of the edges of this flap must be carried out carefully.*

the pericardial cavity. Thirty minutes before the expected time of the graft arrival, the patient is fully heparinized and cardiopulmonary bypass is established between the right atrium (a large double lumen cannula is introduced in the right atrial appendage and pushed down into the terminal part of the inferior vena cava) and the distal ascending aorta.

Cardiopulmonary bypass is initiated at normal temperature, keeping the heart beating (Fig. 7.14). This cardiac assistance allows one partially to clamp the anterior aspect of the main pulmonary artery and to make a longitudinal incision 3 cm long for the suture of an end-to-side 22–24 mm diameter preclotted woven Dacron graft with a 5–0 polypropylene running suture. The side biting clamp on the pulmonary artery is released, allowing the blood to fill the graft which is cross-clamped. The cardiopulmonary bypass is stopped until the donor heart arrives on the operating table. Cardiopulmonary bypass is then resumed, lowering the temperature of the recipient to 28°C. The aorta is cross-clamped and 1 litre of St. Thomas's cardioplegic solution (Plegisol) is injected into the root of the aorta. The left ventricle is decompressed with the aid of a vent, introduced by an incision in the left atrium in front of the superior right pulmonary vein.

Myocardial protection is achieved by either pouring cold saline solution (4°C) or placing iced slush over both hearts throughout the procedure.

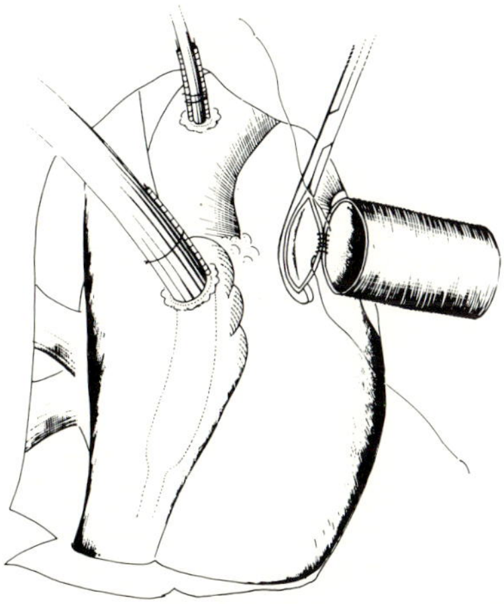

Fig. 7.14. *With the aid of a normothermic cardiopulmonary bypass, the anterior aspect of the main pulmonary artery (PA) is partially clamped. A longitudinal incision 3 cm long is made in the PA. An end-to-side anastomosis is done with a 22–24 mm diameter preclotted woven Dacron graft with a 5–0 polypropylene running suture.*

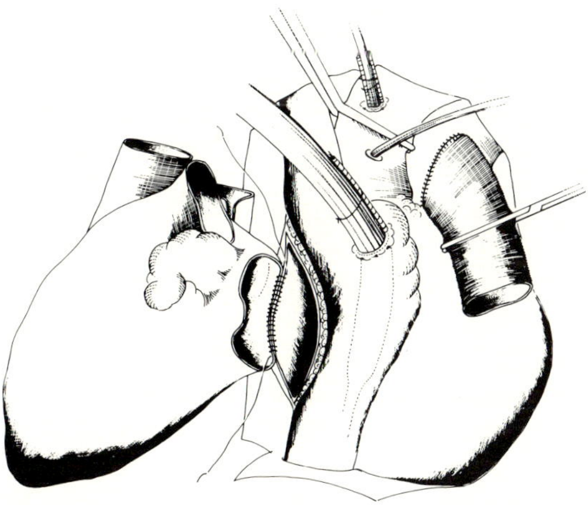

Fig. 7.15. *Left atrial anastomosis. A left atrial incision is made posterior to the inter-atrial groove from the superior to the inferior extremes of the groove. The donor heart is placed alongside the recipient heart. The midpoint of the posterior lip of the incision in the recipient's left atrium is sutured using a 5–0 polypropylene suture to the midpoint of the posterior lip of the donor's left atrium. The two atria are anastomosed by a continuous suture.*

Left atrial anastomosis

With the heart arrested, the left atrial incision is completed posterior to the inter-atrial groove from the superior to the inferior extremes of the groove as for mitral valve surgery (Fig. 7.15). The next stage is as described by Novitzky, Cooper and Barnard (1983):

> The donor heart is then placed in the right thoracic cavity, anterior to the collapsed right lung and lying alongside the recipient heart. The midpoint of the posterior lip of the incision in the recipient left atrium is sutured using double-ended 4–0 polypropylene to the midpoint of the posterior lip of the donor left atrium at the site of the previously inserted marker stitch. The two atria are anastomosed by a continuous suture, first along the posterior aspect and then along the anterior aspect. The completed anastomosis will be totally inaccessible at the end of the operation, and therefore it is essential that it be haemostatic.

The vent in the left ventricle of the recipient is removed before finishing the left atrial anastomosis. This vent is placed through the donor's right superior pulmonary vein, the anastomosis and the recipient mitral valve, in order to be in the recipient's left ventricle.

Anastomosis of right atria

After completion of the left atrial anastomosis and placement of the recipient's left ventricular vent, 5 cm of the recipient vena cava is partially and longitudinally clamped and a 4 cm longitudinal incision is made in the anterior aspect of the terminal part of the vein (Fig. 7.16). An incision of a similar length is made in the donor's superior vena cava, on its posterior aspect, starting at the cephalad orifice and going down through the caval orifice of the open azygos vein. This large aperture is anastomosed end-to-side to the incision in the recipient's superior vena cava with a 5–0 polypropylene running suture. The clamp on the recipient's superior vena cava is released and the donor's superior vena cava is clamped transversely. The suture is carefully inspected for complete haemostasis.

Aortic anastomosis

The donor's aorta is transected with sufficient length to allow lifting of the donor's heart anteriorly, but not enough to permit this heart to drop back in the right pleural cavity and compress the right lung (Fig. 7.17). A longitudinal incision equal in length to the diameter of the donor's aorta is made in the anterolateral part of the recipient's ascending aorta below the aortic clamp and the cardioplegic catheter. An end-to-side anastomosis using a 5–0 polypropylene running suture is performed between the two vessels. This anastomosis must be done with special care because of the fragility of the tissues. Two electrodes are placed on each left ventricle and electrical

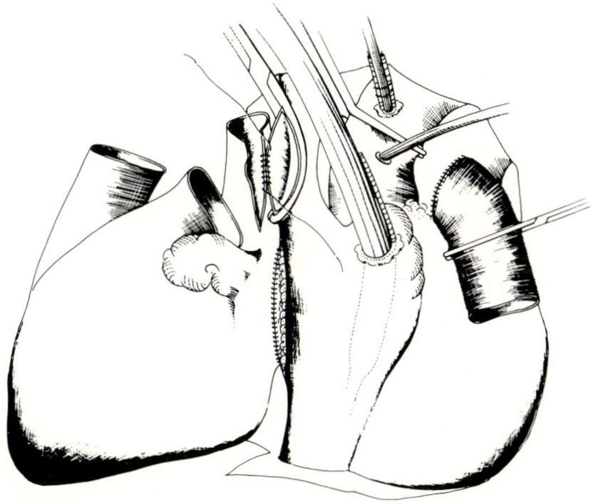

Fig. 7.16. *Anastomosis of the right atria: 5 cm of the recipient's vena cava is partially and longitudinally clamped. A 4 cm longitudinal incision is made in the anterior aspect of the terminal part of the vein. An incision of a similar length is made in the donor's superior vena cava on its posterior aspect. This large aperture is anastomosed end-to-side with a 5–0 polypropylene suture to the recipient's superior vena cava.*

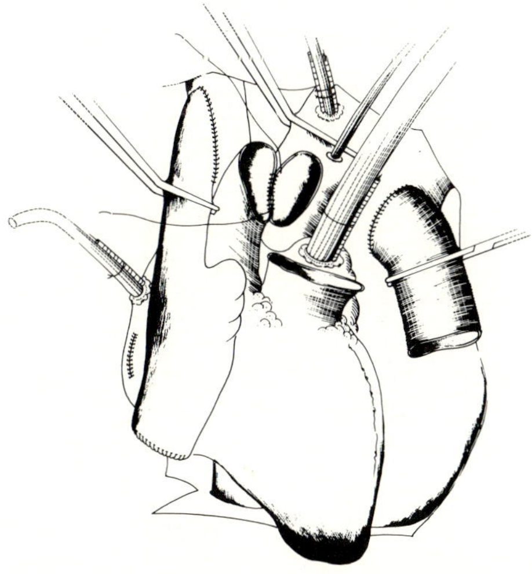

Fig. 7.17. *Aortic anastomosis. The donor's aorta is transected, long enough to lift the donor's heart anteriorly and yet avoiding this heart dropping back in the right pleural cavity. A longitudinal incision is made in the anterolateral part of the recipient's ascending aorta. An end-to-side anastomosis using a 5–0 polypropylene running suture is performed between the two vessels.*

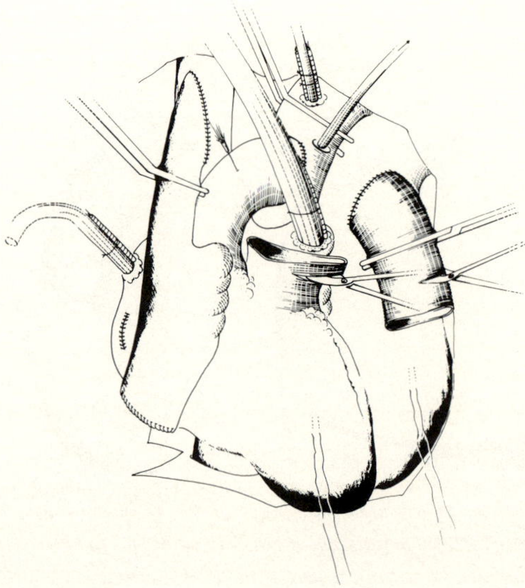

Fig. 7.18. *Two electrodes are placed on each left ventricle and electrical fibrillation is induced. The clamp on the recipient's aorta is released after the cardioplegia catheter is converted to be used as an air vent. The donor's aorta is carefully de-aired with a needle.*

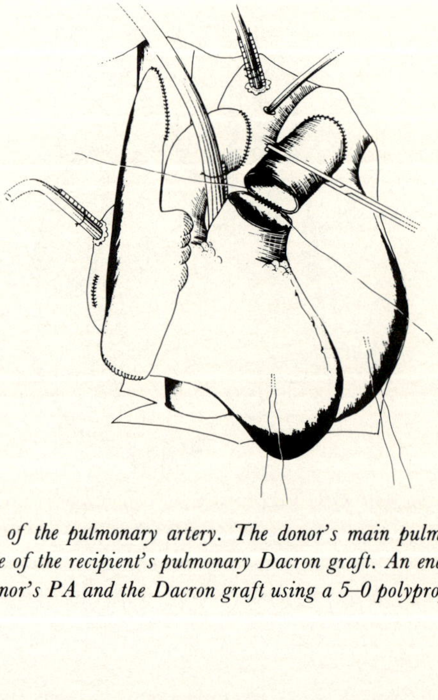

Fig. 7.19. *Anastomosis of the pulmonary artery. The donor's main pulmonary artery (PA) is trimmed to match the size of the recipient's pulmonary Dacron graft. An end-to-end anastomosis is performed between the donor's PA and the Dacron graft using a 5–0 polypropylene running suture.*

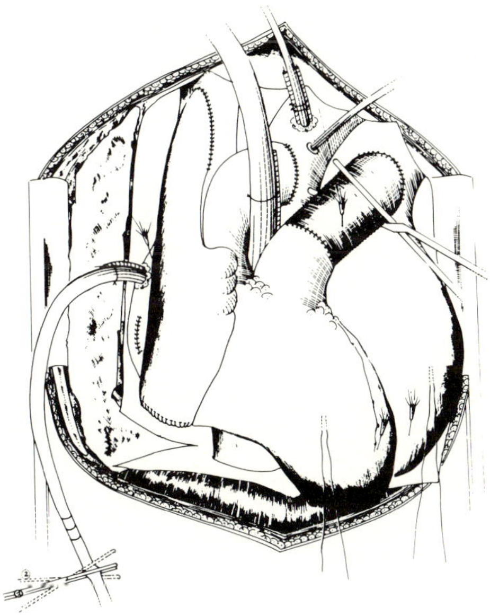

Fig. 7.20. *Both hearts are de-aired by puncturing both left atrial roofs, the two left ventricles and the recipient's pulmonary artery with a needle. The recipient's left ventricular vent is connected by a gravity line to the oxygenator and further de-airing is obtained this way.*

fibrillation is induced to avoid premature contraction before extracting all the air from both ventricles (Fig. 7.18).

The clamp on the recipient's aorta is released after the cardioplegia catheter is converted to be used as an air vent. The donor's aorta is also carefully de-aired with a needle. Both hearts are again vascularized, the clamp on the donor superior vena cava is released and the recipient's temperature is progressively raised to 34°C.

Anastomosis of pulmonary artery

The donor main pulmonary artery is trimmed to match the size of the recipient pulmonary Dacron graft, which is tailored to the correct length to bridge the gap between the two pulmonary arteries (Fig. 7.19). An end-to-end anastomosis is performed between the donor's pulmonary artery and the Dacron graft using a 5–0 polypropylene running suture. Both hearts are carefully de-aired by puncturing both left atrial roofs, the recipient's pulmonary artery and the apices of the two left ventricles with a needle (Fig. 7.20). The recipient's left ventricular vent is connected by a gravity line to the oxygenator and further de-airing is obtained in this way.

At this time, both hearts are vigorously fibrillating. Induced electrical ventricular fibrillation is stopped. The hearts may spontaneously beat or may require electrical defibrillation. A careful inspection is made of the accessible suture lines to assure haemostasis.

When the de-airing seems complete, the left ventricular vent is removed and the haemodynamic situation is estimated. In our experience, we do not rely on the donor's heart because it is recovering from an ischaemic period and the recipient's heart is doing most of the work. Therefore, all the therapeutic manoeuvres are directed to sustaining the action of the recipient's heart (vasodilators, dopamine, dobutamine, adrenaline), avoiding the use of isoprenaline which may induce life-threatening arrhythmias in this heart. So at the end of the surgical procedure (quoting again from Novitzky, Cooper and Barnard (1983)), if

> the haemodynamic status is stable, cardiopulmonary bypass is discontinued and all cannulas are removed from the patient. The heparin is neutralized with protamine sulphate. Three drains are inserted, one into the pericardial cavity posterior to the recipient heart, a second anterior to this heart, and a third in the midaxillary line at the costodiaphragmatic angle to ensure adequate drainage of the right pleural cavity.
>
> Before closure of the chest, the anaesthetist is requested to ventilate both lungs fully to ensure expansion of the right lung, particularly of the lower lobe, which has been compressed by the donor heart throughout the procedure.
>
> Some collapse of the right lower lobe is always present at the end of the operation, but with adequate physiotherapy, this lobe expands over the course of the next few days.

A few days later when the donor heart is recovering, it takes over progressively and does most of the haemodynamic work; although ejection of blood from the two hearts is asynchronous, this does not interfere substantially with the performance of either heart.

With the exception of haemodynamic care, perioperative management (anti-infectious and immunosuppressive protocols, isolation, diet, mobilization) is exactly the same as for orthotopic transplantation.

Technical variants

In the original technique described by Novitsky, Cooper and Barnard (1983) and also followed by Cooley (1984), the right atrial anastomosis is performed differently. Two caval cannulae are inserted in the recipient heart for the CPB, into the superior vena cava (SVC) through the right atrial appendage and into the inferior vena cava (IVC) through the low atrial wall. Snares are placed around the venae cavae and 'A 5 cm longitudinal incision is made into the lateral aspect of the recipient SVC and right atrium just anterior to the interatrial groove, beginning 2 to 3 cm above the junction of the vena cava and the right atrium and continuing 2 to 3 cm into the right atrium.' (Novitzky, Cooper and Barnard, 1983.)

The donor SVC, which was mobilized at the time of the donor heart excision and divided as cephalad as possible, is tied or sutured at its cephalad orifice. During the harvesting of the heart, the azygos vein was doubly ligated and divided and a longitudinal 5 cm incision was made just to the right of the inter-atrial septum in the posterior aspect of the SVC and right atrium. At least half the length of this incision must involve the right atrial wall. So, once prepared (Novitzky, Cooper and Barnard, 1983):

the donor SVC is extended alongside its counterpart. An eyelid retractor is used to retract the anterior lip of the incision in the recipient right atrium. The midpoint of the posterior lip of the incision in the recipient atrium is sutured to the most caudal point of the incision in the donor atrium, using a double-ended 5–0 polypropylene suture. The two right atria are then anastomosed by a continuous suture carried in each direction, first posteriorly and then anteriorly. At the completion of this anastomosis the ligated donor azygos vein remnant will lie at the midpoint of the anterior suture line, over which a small metal ring is tied down as a fluoroscopic reference for the passage of endomyocardial biopsy forceps into the donor heart after operation. The maneuver of suturing the midpoint of the posterior lip of the recipient atrial wall, to the most inferior aspect of the incision in the donor atrium, ensures that this anastomosis will remain wide allowing free flow of blood from one chamber to the other and permitting easy passage of the endomyocardial biopsy forceps.

The operation has been combined on occasion with other procedures in the recipient heart, such as resection of a left ventricular aneurysm, coronary artery bypass grafting, and mitral annuloplasty.

REFERENCES

Cabrol, C., Gandjbakhch, I., Pavie, A., Laskar, M. J., Cabrol, A. and Mattei, M. F. (1984). Heart and heart–lung transplantation: technique and safeguards. *Heart Transplant.* **III**, 110–114.

Cabrol, C., Gandjbakhch, I., Pavie, A., Cabrol, A., Mattei, M. F. and Leger, P. (1985). Heart transplantation in Paris, at 'La Pitié' Hospital. *Heart Transplant.* **IV**, 476–480.

Cooley, D. A. (1984). *Techniques in Cardiac Surgery*, 2nd edn, pp. 372–374. Saunders, Philadelphia.

Dor, V., Jourdan, J., Bourlon, F., Elbeze, J. P., Grinneiser, D., Isetta, C. and Montiglio, F. (1986). Evolution anatomique et hémodynamique à moyen terme du coeur assisté dans la transplantation cardiaque hétérotopique. A propos de 21 observations. *Arch. Mal. Coeur* **79**, 1037–1044.

Lower, R. R. and Shumway, N. E. (1960). Studies on orthotopic homotransplantation of the canine heart. *Surg. Forum* **11**, 18.

Novitzky, D., Cooper, C. and Barnard, C. N. (1983). The surgical technique of heterotopic heart transplantation. *Ann. Thorac. Surg.*, **36**, 476–482.

D. W. Bethune, I. Hardy, J. Kneeshaw,
R. D. Latimer and A. Oduro

8

Anaesthesia and Cardiopulmonary Bypass for Cardiac Transplantation

INTRODUCTION

It is now 20 years since the first successful transplantation of the human heart and many groups of anaesthetists have described the techniques they use for managing their patients during the recipient operation (Ozinsky, 1967; Keats *et al.*, 1969; Harrison, Bailey and Thomson, 1969; Paiment *et al.*, 1970, Fernando, Keenan and Boyan, 1978; Garman, 1981; Grebenik and Robinson, 1985; Demas *et al.*, 1986). Many different anaesthetic agents have been used successfully and it appears that each unit has based their management for these patients on the regimens that they use in patients with uncompensated cardiac failure. At Papworth Hospital, we have behaved in a similar manner and our technique for anaesthetizing patients for cardiac transplantation has evolved from the technique used for cardiac surgical patients over 17 years (Bethune *et al.*, 1981). Monitoring is established before induction, as for any critically ill patient, with percutaneous cannulation of the right internal jugular vein and an artery, preferably the radial artery on the non-dominant side. Preoperative sedation is given intravenously in the anaesthetic room, usually, using small (2 mg) aliquots of papaveretum, but both fentanyl and midazolam have been used for this purpose. Antibiotic cover is given before starting the intravenous immunosuppressive therapy.

We feel that careful monitoring is essential when starting the anti-thymocyte globulin, as in our early experience several patients had severe allergic reactions to this equine preparation. Recently, our practice has been to administer the antithymocyte globulin when the patient is on bypass. Our previous experience suggested that minimal histamine release can cause profound haemodynamic changes in the compromised patient. The patients who had marked haemodynamic changes with antithymocyte globulin before transplantation have tolerated similar doses after transplantation, with minimal symptoms. Administering the antithymocyte globulin on bypass may lead to some hypotension, but this has not been a problem.

Anaesthesia is induced with an inhalational technique using nitrous oxide and trichloroethylene. We have not been troubled with hypotension or arrhythmias related to the use of trichloroethylene as an inhalational agent; this contrasts with the observations relating to other volatile agents (Demas *et al.*, 1986). Muscle relaxation has been achieved with a variety of relaxants, including pancuronium, alcuronium and vecuronium, and anaesthesia is maintained with nitrous oxide and trichloroethylene and supplemented with intravenous papaveretum. The nitrous oxide is discontinued when the patient is heparinized prior to cannulation for cardiopulmonary bypass, to reduce any third gas effects (Bethune, 1976).

In order to minimize the possibility of infection, it is essential to use only sterilized equipment for the transplant recipient, although in many units this will be the norm for all cardiac patients. The anaesthetist should wear sterilized gloves for any procedures involving close patient contact. The airway should be protected from airborne infection and we believe that the simplest and most effective method is to use a single Pall BB50T bacterial filter between the machine circuit and the patient's catheter mount. In this position, the filter replaces the heating and humidifying properties of the upper airways (Bethune and Shelly, 1985) and provides an absolute barrier to the passage of bacteria in the respired gases. The Pall BB50T compares well as a heat and moisture exchanger with others which do not possess its bacterial filtering action (Shelly, Bethune and Latimer, 1986).

Suprapubic catheterization has been recommended to avoid the need for a urethral catheter, although in common with several other units we have not found this to be a problem and routinely use a urethral catheter which is removed on the second postoperative day.

MONITORING

Monitoring in our unit is simple — arterial and central venous pressure are displayed prior to induction, together with the ECG. Nasopharyngeal temperature is monitored, particularly in relation to the bypass period. Pulmonary artery catheters are not used in these patients, since the risk of arrhythmias and the need to remove them before the heart is excised make their benefit questionable. Skin colour and perfusion are observed, but once the chest is open the finest monitor is to watch the heart itself. Following transplantation, while the chest is open, an electromagnetic flow probe can be used on the aorta to measure the cardiac output and a surgically placed left atrial line monitors the filling pressure of the left ventricle.

CARDIOPULMONARY BYPASS MANAGEMENT

The management of cardiopulmonary bypass depends on the patient's preoperative condition. There is often a large oxygen debt and metabolic acidosis at the start of bypass, and it is helpful to maintain higher flows even though moderate hypothermia (30°C) is used routinely (Wheeldon, Bethune and Gill, 1986). The majority of the patients have a greatly expanded blood volume, and haemofiltration during bypass can be used to remove several litres of fluid. In patients who have a significant degree of pre-renal failure, haemodialysis is used during bypass to optimize the patient's condition (Hakim *et al.*, 1985). Unusual sensitivity of the transplanted heart to the serum potassium concentration has been reported (Grebenik and Robinson, 1985), although we have not observed this and have found that those patients who suffered with a chronic low cardiac output state preoperatively have an increased potassium requirement during bypass and postoperatively. It is our normal practice to give potassium supplements before discontinuing bypass to keep the serum concentration above 4.5 mmol/litre. This appears to reduce the incidence of junctional and ventricular dysrhythmias.

The haemodynamic management of the transplant recipient prior to transplantation is critical. Many of the patients are just compensated in the sitting position. Anaesthesia can, and should, be induced in such patients in the sitting position, but positioning for surgery will involve levelling the operating table. Under these circumstances the inevitable shift of blood from the periphery will result in an increase in the ventricular filling pressures. In the decompensated patient, the resulting ventricular distension will result in a fall in the cardiac output. Our technique for managing the patient at this time involves a combination of venesection of 500–1000 ml of blood, 5–10 degrees of head-up tilt and the use of nitroprusside to reduce the after-load and improve ventricular emptying. Figure 8.1 is an intraoperative trace from a patient with ischaemic cardiomyopathy who had functional mitral regurgitation preoperatively, following venesection (500 ml) and nitroprusside (0.33 ml/min with 50 mg in 250 ml). The mitral valve was competent and briefly discontinuing the nitroprusside resulted in a marked rise in the left atrial pressure which was corrected when the nitroprusside was restarted.

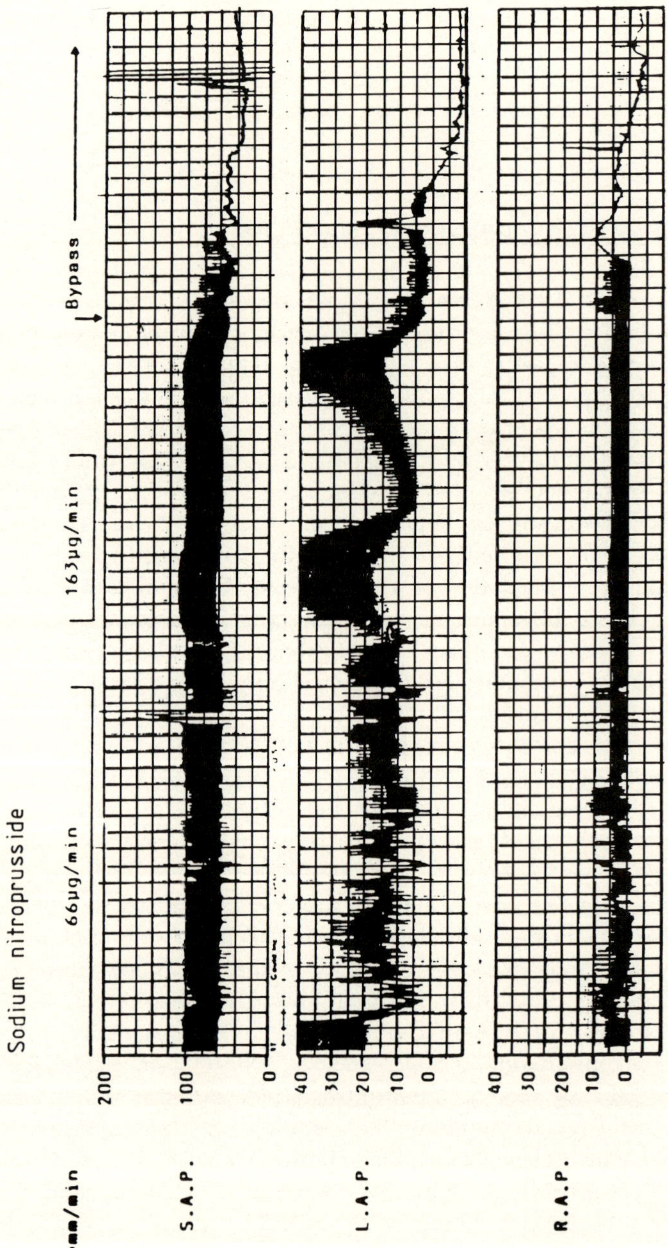

Fig. 8.1. *Effect of sodium nitroprusside on functional mitral incompetence*

The reduction in end-diastolic volume and resultant improvement in ventricular performance will, in some patients, result in a paradoxical response to nitroprusside, with a rise in systemic blood pressure. High doses of nitroprusside can be given to patients who are on the crest, or beyond, of the Frank–Starling curve without producing a hypotensive response and with a marked improvement in the cardiac output and the appearance of the heart. Figure 8.2 is the pre-bypass record of a patient with cardiomyopathy who had both low systolic and pulse pressure prior to and following induction of anaesthesia. There was no improvement with venesection and posture, but nitroprusside produced an improvement in the arterial pressures. Even at a high dose of nitroprusside (1 ml/min of 50 mg in 250 ml to a 72 kg patient) no hypotensive effect was seen. The sustained improvement in ventricular function when the nitroprusside was discontinued is not always seen, but it must reflect the improvement in ventricular contractility resulting from the reduced end-diastolic volume. Inotropes alone are not useful in these decompensated patients, with the possible exception of a bolus of calcium chloride which can be useful to counteract the occasional fall in pressure following neuromuscular blockade or positioning of the patient. The finding that inotropes are not useful without vasodilator therapy is not surprising when the pathophysiology of heart failure is considered (Braunwald, 1981), and consideration is given to the beneficial effects of vasodilator therapy in medical patients with heart failure (Forrester and Waters, 1978; Zelis *et al.*, 1979).

In the selection of patients for cardiac transplantation, a grossly raised pulmonary vascular resistance is considered a contraindication. Unfortunately, however, it is not always possible, in the intact patient, to determine the exact state of the pulmonary vasculature. Due to the nature of their disease most patients have elevated mean pulmonary artery and left atrial pressures, with near normal calculated pulmonary vascular resistances. The lowering of left atrial pressure which accompanies successful transplantation is not always accompanied by an immediate fall in the pulmonary artery pressure. In most cases the right ventricle can cope with this abnormal load, but in a few patients pulmonary hypertension after transplantation has given considerable problems, and in 2 patients bypass could only be discontinued with the help of prostacyclin to dilate the pulmonary vascular bed. Prostacyclin in these circumstances is the treatment of last resort, as it inevitably causes an increase in bleeding from every part of the operative site. The most striking finding in those patients who have given problems at the end of bypass with pulmonary hypertension is the rapidity with which the pulmonary resistance falls to normal in the immediate postoperative period.

Preoperative organ dysfunction is common in this group of patients, due to the chronic heart failure which precedes transplantation and interferes with all organ systems. Despite the severity of the organ dysfunction, it is remarkable how rapidly function will return to normal following successful

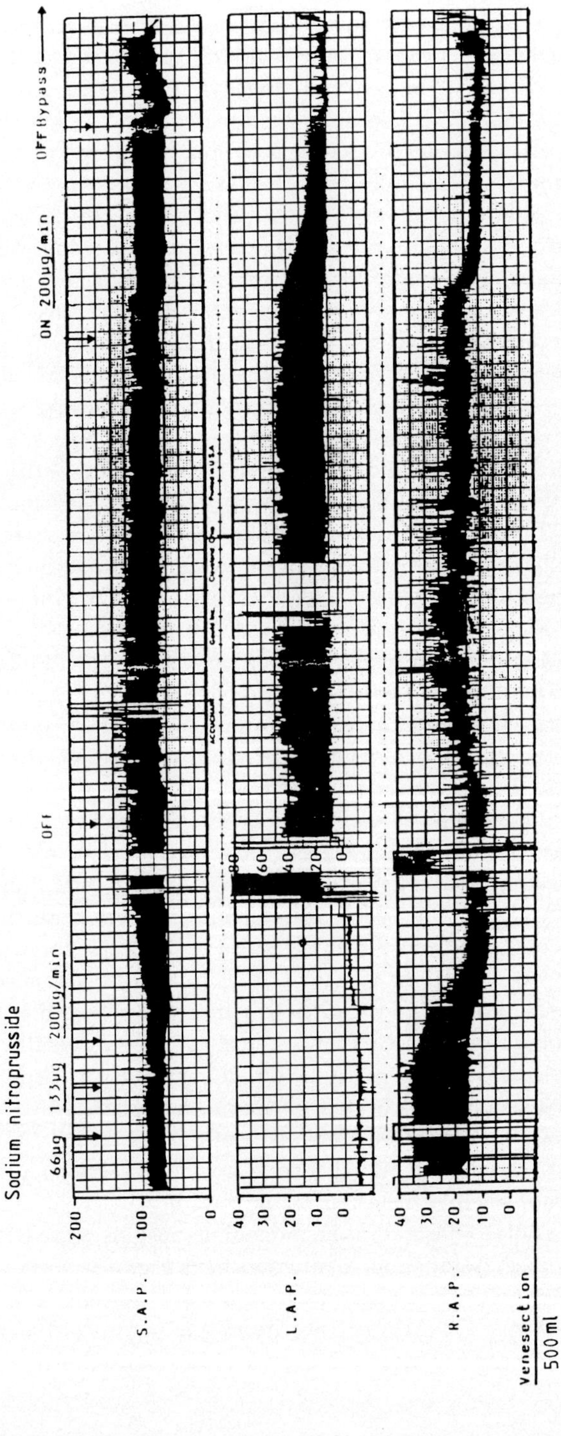

Fig. 8.2. *Paradoxical effect of sodium nitroprusside on systemic pressure and the continued effect when infusion is discontinued*

cardiac transplantation. Disturbances of liver function and the expanded blood volume would be expected to give problems with heparinization and its reversal. In practice, with careful monitoring of the activated clotting time this has not been a problem. In patients with known coagulation defects resulting from preoperative anticoagulant therapy or liver congestion, single donor plasma or fresh frozen plasma should be available at the end of the bypass period.

Postoperatively, the patients are transferred to a single cubicle in the intensive care unit. Artificial lung ventilation is continued until the patient is haemodynamically stable, awake and has no residual neuromuscular block. Extubation normally takes place 4–12 h after return to the intensive care unit. Since we adopted the Pall BB50T bacterial filter as our heat and moisture exchanger, we have been less concerned about the duration of postoperative intubation and ventilation.

Following successful transplantation, the patients are restored to a normal life and may present with surgical problems unrelated to their transplanted organs. A wide variety of general and regional anaesthetic techniques have been used in patients who have had heart and heart–lung transplants (Kanter and Samuel, 1977; Bricker and Sugden, 1985; Grebenick and Robinson, 1985, 1986; Samuels and Wyner, 1986; McKeown and Armstrong, 1986), with little evidence of superiority for a particular technique. There are theoretical advantages in the use of regional techniques whenever possible. They avoid any problems with intubation and possible infection by the tracheal route, and in the heart–lung transplants ensure that the patient can be given chest physiotherapy immediately following the operation. A purely theoretical advantage of regional anaesthesia is that it will not further depress the patient's immune system as occurs with all general anaesthetic techniques (Moudgil, 1986). Preoperative assessment should include contact with the patient's transplant centre to determine the results of the most recent follow-up assessment. This is important for several reasons, but the main interest will be in the possibility of graft atherosclerosis having been detected at follow-up coronary arteriography, as these patients cannot suffer the pain of angina with their denervated hearts. The possibility of active rejection should be considered if the patient appears unwell.

In patients with a transplanted lung there is no cough reflex, and it is important to ensure that the patient is able to co-operate with the physiotherapist and cough to command as soon as the endotracheal tube is removed. When an endotracheal tube is used following a lung transplant, care should be taken to ensure that the minimum length of tube is inserted into the trachea; with such precautions the cuff should be well above the tracheal anastomosis.

The response of the denervated heart to changes in intravascular volume and vasodilatation are abnormal in that hypovolaemia and hypotension will not cause a reflex tachycardia. Attention should be directed to the avoidance of hypovolaemia, particularly prior to regional blocks. Suitable direct-acting drugs should be available: isoprenaline for its chronotropic action, dopamine or dobutamine for inotropic effect, and a direct-acting vasoconstrictor.

Appropriate routine monitoring for most procedures would include indirect blood pressure, pulse rate and oxygen saturation from a pulse oximeter and ECG monitoring. Invasive monitoring should only be used if the surgical procedure or the patient's condition warrants it. Any suspicion of active rejection would be an indication for direct pressure monitoring.

Bacterial protection of the patient's airway is important and can most effectively be achieved by using a suitable bacterial filter, connected to the endotracheal tube or catheter mount, as a heat and moisture exchanger.

CONCLUSIONS

Anaesthesia for cardiac transplantation is an esoteric branch of our speciality, but in our department we feel that many of the lessons we have learned regarding the management of the decompensated cardiac patient have a wide application in the management of such patients who present for routine cardiac surgery and for other surgical procedures.

REFERENCES

Bethune, D. W. (1976). Organ damage after open heart surgery. *Lancet* **2**, 1410.

Bethune, D. W., Collis, J. M., Latimer, R. D. and Hardy, I. (1981). Anaesthesia for coronary artery surgery. In *Towards Safer Cardiac Surgery* (D. Longmore, Ed.), pp. 267–279. MPT, Lancaster, UK.

Bethune, D. W. and Shelly, M. P. (1985). Hydrophobic versus hygroscopic heat and moisture exchangers. *Anaesthesia* **40**, 210–211.

Braunwald, E. (1981). Heart failure: pathophysiology and treatment. *Am. Heart J.* **3**, 486–490.

Bricker, S. R. W. and Sugden, J. C. (1985). Anaesthesia for surgery in a patient with a transplanted heart. *Br. J. Anaesth.* **57**, 634–637.

Demas, K., Wyner, J., Mihm, F. G. and Samuels, S. (1986). Anaesthesia for heart transplantation. *Br. J. Anaesth.* **58**, 1357–1364.

Fernando, N. A., Keenan, R. L. and Boyan, C. P. (1978). Anaesthetic experience with cardiac transplantation. *J. Thorac. Cardiovasc. Surg.* **75**, 531–535.

Forrester, J. S. and Waters, D. D. (1978). Hospital treatment of congestive heart failure. *Am. J. Med.* **65**, 173–180.

Garman, J. K. (1981). Anesthesia for cardiac transplantation. *Cleveland Clin. Q.* **48**, 442–446.

Grebenik, C. R. and Robinson, P. N. (1985). Cardiac transplantation at Harefield. *Anaesthesia* **40**, 131–140.

Grebenik, C. R. and Robinson, P. N. (1986). Anaesthesia for surgery in a patient with a transplanted heart. *Br. J. Anaesth.* **58**, 1199–1200.

Hakim, M., Wheeldon, D., Bethune, D. W., Milstein, B. B., English, T. A. H. and Wallwork, J. (1985). Haemodialysis and haemofiltration on cardiopulmonary bypass. *Thorax* **40**, 101–106.

Harrison, G. A., Bailey, R. J. and Thomson, P. G. (1969). A heart transplantation: 4. Anaesthesia and cardio-pulmonary bypass. *Med. J. Austral.* **I**, 670–672.

Kanter, S. F. and Samuel, S. I. (1977). Anesthesia for major operations on patients who have transplanted hearts. A review of 29 cases. *Anesthesiology* **46**, 65–68.

Keats, A. S., Strong, J. M., Girigis, K. Z. and Goldstein, A. (1969). Observations during anesthesia for cardiac homotransplantation in ten patients. *Anesthesiology* **30**, 192–198.

McKeown, D. W. and Armstrong, I. R. (1986). Anaesthesia for surgery in a patient with a transplanted heart. *Br. J. Anaesth.* **58**, 1200.

Moudgil, G. C. (1986). Update on anaesthesia and the immune response. *Can. Anaesth. Soc. J.* **33**, S54–S60.

Ozinsky, J. (1967). Cardiac transplantation. The anaesthetist view: a case report. *S. Afr. Med. J.* **41**, 1268–1270.

Paiment, B., Wielhorski, W. A., Grondin, P., Lepage, G. and Dytda, I. (1970). Anaesthetic management in nine heart transplantations. *Laval. Med.* **41**, 186–190.

Samuels, S. I. and Wyner, J. (1986). Anaesthesia for surgery in a patient with a transplanted heart. *Br. J. Anaesth.* **58**, 1199.

Shelly, M. P., Bethune, D. W. and Latimer, R. D. (1986). A comparison of five heat and moisture exchangers. *Anaesthesia* **41**, 527–532.

Wheeldon, D. R., Bethune, D. W. and Gill, R. D. (1986). Perfusion for cardiac transplantation. *Perfusion* **1**, 57–61.

Zelis, R., Flaim, S. F., Moskowitz, R. M. and Nellis, S. H. (1979). How much can we expect from vasodilator therapy in congestive heart failure? *Circulation* **59**, 1092–1097.

D. J. G. White

9

Immunosuppression for Cardiac Transplantation

INTRODUCTION

Orthotopic heart transplantation and liver transplantation suffer from a major disadvantage compared with kidney or pancreas transplantation. Failure of the graft equates with the death of the patient. Furthermore, a heart graft can deteriorate at a speed which is rarely seen in liver transplantation and this can occur with little advance clinical indication, thus restricting the option to rescue the patient by re-grafting. Although the artificial heart may provide a mechanism for short-term cardiac support for such patients, in general terms the treatment of the heart transplant recipient is based on the premise that the prevention of graft rejection and its aggressive treatment is a priority which must be accommodated within every other therapeutic consideration. This priority poses a particular conflict of interests where both infection and rejection coexist. Such a scenario will often lead to a contradiction in therapeutic approaches which cannot be satisfactorily resolved. Thus, the emphasis of any immunosuppressive programme for the cardiac transplant recipient must be directed towards avoiding the horns of this particular dilemma.

HISTORY

The developments which took place in cardiothoracic surgery and its attendant technologies during the sixth and seventh decades of this century provided the necessary skills to make orthotopic heart transplantation a technically feasible procedure. The first human-to-human heart transplant was carried out in Cape Town in 1967 (Barnard, 1967). During the following year 101 cardiac transplants were performed by 64 teams and 22 countries around the world. This display of enthusiasm for an unproven clinical procedure, especially in centres with little previous experience in clinical transplantation or without significant experimental backgrounds resulted, as might be predicted, in a very poor survival rate and the cessation of heart transplant programmes by almost every centre.

With one or two notable exceptions these programmes all foundered on the inability of the clinicians to control rejection of the heart graft without exposing the recipients to fatal overwhelming infections. Thus the essential conundrum of immunosuppression in cardiac transplantation was defined — prevent rejection and risk losing the patient from infection; avoid over-immunosuppression and risk losing the patient from graft rejection. So difficult was the balancing act between these two fatal options that almost all of those transplant centres which had entered the field with such enthusiasm withdrew from the unequal contest.

One of the very few centres which was able to achieve this balance in immunosuppression was the cardiothoracic centre at Stanford University, California, USA. It was this group who, over the ensuing decade, founded the baseline principles on which heart transplant recipients are now managed.

Lower and Shumway first started to study the problems of clinical cardiac transplantation in the late 1950s with a series of experimental studies in dogs (Lower and Shumway, 1960). In 1968 these studies culminated in the inception of the clinical cardiac transplant programme at Stanford. For the next decade this one centre performed more than half of the total number of cardiac transplants worldwide. During this period several important principles were established in the control of graft rejection. These were: (a) the use of rabbit antithymocyte globulin (Bieber *et al.*, 1977); (b) the development and introduction of endomyocardial biopsy for the diagnosis of rejection (Caves *et al.*, 1973); (c) the introduction of laboratory methods for monitoring the immune status of the recipient (Bieber *et al.*, 1976); (d) the introduction of cyclosporin into clinical cardiac transplant practice (Oyer *et al.*, 1982a, b).

AZATHIOPRINE AND STEROID IMMUNOSUPPRESSION

Prior to the advent of cyclosporin, immunosuppressive protocols for cardiac transplantation had been based on the regimens developed for the recipients of kidney transplants. To the basic therapy of azathioprine and steroids was added a prolonged course of rabbit antithymocyte globulin.

The protocol in use in Stanford was as follows: azathioprine (2 mg/kg i.v.) administered immediately prior to surgery, followed by oral treatment starting on the first postoperative day and maintained at a level between 1 and 2 mg/kg dependent on avoiding leucopenia or thrombocytopenia. Immediately following surgery, 500 mg methylprednisolone was administered intravenously, followed by 125 mg/day until oral intake could be resumed. Prednisone was then started at a dose of 1.5 mg/kg per day, reducing to a maintenance level of 1 mg/kg at about 2 months postoperatively. Further gradual reduction of the daily dose was continued until a level of approximately 0.25 mg/kg per day was achieved, usually at about 1 year post-transplant. These tapering regimens depended largely upon the degree to which an individual suffered rejection episodes or the severity of the steroid side effects.

The details of this form of immunosuppression are provided largely for historical interest, since most immunosuppressive protocols of heart transplantation are now based upon cyclosporin. However, there is one component of this regimen that still plays an important role in the management of the cardiac transplant recipient — antithymocyte globulin.

ANTITHYMOCYTE GLOBULIN AND MONOCLONAL ANTIBODIES

The immunosuppressive potential of heterologous antibodies against lymphocytes was first demonstrated by Woodruff and Anderson (1963). The use of antilymphocyte serum (ALS) was soon superseded by the use of the globulin fraction containing the active antibodies (antilymphocyte globulin, ALG). Such preparations were first used clinically by Starzl (Starzl, Porter and Iwasaki, 1967), although the value of these agents has remained a matter of debate. Original preparations of ALG used lymphocytes from spleen or peripheral blood as their antigen source. These immunizations produced agents which were heavily contaminated with anti-red cell and anti-platelet antibodies, requiring extensive absorption before they could be used. This problem of contamination was resolved by the use of human thymocytes as the antigen source to produce antithymocyte globulin (ATG).

The value of ATG in the prevention or treatment of graft rejection in kidney transplant recipients has been extensively studied over the past 15 years. The multi-centre trial reported by Wechter *et al.* (1979) illustrates well the difficulties in assessing the value of such agents. The results from this study showed that 14 days of ATG (Atgam, Upjohn) delayed the onset of rejection episodes in renal transplant recipients by 2 weeks. Overall, however, only one of the four batches of ATG used produced a significant improvement in long-term graft survival compared with controls.

Why such batch variations should occur is not known, although this is a problem which has always beset commercial production of ATG. The value of ATG in heart transplantation has never been formally proved by clinical trial. However, the success of the heart transplant programme in Stanford has been ascribed in part to the use of ATG (Bieber *et al.*, 1977). This 'home-produced' rabbit anti-human thymocyte globulin (RATG) was injected intramuscularly at a dose of 2.5 mg/kg. Antithymocyte globulin was given daily for the first 3 days and then every other day at doses determined by individual patient monitoring. The aim was to reduce the T-cell number in peripheral blood samples to less than 5% of the circulating lymphocytes (it is normally over 60%) and to maintain it at this low level for at least the first 3 weeks. To ensure the continued effectiveness of the RATG, patients must be monitored to establish the number of circulating T lymphocytes by E-rosetting on a daily basis. With this information the dose can be adjusted so as to depress the T-cell numbers to the desired level.

Where prolonged courses of ATG are being used, patients also need to be monitored for the production of antibodies against the species globulin of the ATG. The production of significant titres of such anti-globulin by the patient results in the ATG being cleared from the circulation before it can bind to its target circulating T cell. When such a state of immunity is found to exist, the species in which the ATG is produced needs to be changed (i.e. from rabbit to goat).

MONOCLONAL ANTIBODIES

The availability of monoclonal antibodies following the development of hybridoma technology by Kohler and Milstein (1975) has, in principle, enabled a resolution of the problem of batch variation since this technique provides an infinite supply of antibody of constant specificity. However, the advent of this technology does pose the problems of choice of specificity, isotype and valency. Now that problems of contaminating antibodies can be avoided, a whole series of unanswered questions needs to be resolved before these antibodies can be introduced routinely as part of an immunosuppressive strategy for heart transplant recipients.

For example, is it more immunosuppressive to use anti-T-cell antibodies or would an anti-lymphocyte glubulin prove more efficient? Should the monoclonal used be lytic? If the monoclonal antibody modulates its target antigen off the surface of the lymphocyte, will the denuded lymphocyte still function? In the treatment of a rejection crisis would monoclonals against activation antigens on lymphocytes be more specific? Should the graft be pre-treated with monoclonal antibodies to remove donor antigen presenting cells? Will mixtures of different specificities be more immunosuppressive than an individual monoclonal antibody? Is it safe to give more than one course of treatment with monoclonal antibody?

All these questions are currently under investigation in different laboratories and as the answers become clear it seems probable that the use of monoclonal antibodies as part of the immunosuppressive regimen for heart transplantation will become more widespread.

CYCLOSPORIN

The introduction of this drug has had a major impact on the survival rates of all organ transplants. This is particularly the case with heart grafts, where it has significantly reduced the duration of hospital stay. The use of cyclosporin in cardiac transplantation has coincided with a substantial increase in successful clinical cardiac transplantation throughout the world.

History of cyclosporin

Cyclosporin A was first isolated from two fungal strains, *Cylindrocarpon lucidium* and *Trichoderma polysporum* (now named *Tolyplocardium inflatum*) in 1970 (Dreyfuss *et al.*, 1976). From these fungal isolates crude metabolite mixtures were prepared which were found to possess a narrow spectrum of anti-fungal properties. In 1973, Borel demonstrated the immunosuppressive properties of this mixture of metabolites and by 1975 the structure of cyclosporin A was elucidated using both chemical degradation and X-ray crystallographic techniques. The first publication of the immunosuppressive properties of cyclosporin A was by Borel (1976). Kostakis, White and Calne (1977) and Calne and White (1977) demonstrated the ability of cyclosporin A to prevent graft rejection in animal organ transplantation. These studies led to the first clinical trials of cyclosporin A both on organ transplant recipients and in the treatment of graft versus host disease in bone marrow transplantation. Since that time, worldwide interest in the drug has increased and its immunosuppressive potential has been confirmed.

Use of cyclosporin A in clinical heart transplantation

The studies which first demonstrated that cyclosporin A was of use in preventing organ graft rejection (Kostakis, White and Calne, 1977) used a heterotopic heart graft in the rat as the test system. Subsequently, Calne, White and Rolles (1978) showed the efficacy of cyclosporin A for preventing the rejection of orthotopic heart grafts in the pig.

The first clinical use of cyclosporin was in the Cardiothoracic Department of Stanford University (Oyer *et al.*, 1982a, b). In the initial protocol, cyclosporin was substituted in the conventional regimen for the azathioprine, at the same time using a lower dose of steroids and substantially curtailing the RATG used to between 2 and 4 injections (Table 9.1).

The success of this initial protocol has meant that it became the basis for all other immunosuppressive regimens for heart transplant patients which used cyclosporin. It was during these initial studies at Stanford that the concept of monitoring cyclosporin serum levels to establish the correct oral dose for any given individual patient was first reported.

Considerations in the use of cyclosporin therapy in heart transplant patients

The introduction of cyclosporin into heart transplant immunosuppression has caused a major re-evaluation of the techniques used for monitoring the patients. Cyclosporin immunosuppression by itself does not substantially decrease the number of rejection episodes; what it does do, however, is to significantly reduce their intensity and the associated morbidity (Merion, White and Calne, 1983). Thus the treatment of these rejection episodes is significantly reduced, in need, duration, and degree of potency. Indeed, one of the major problems encountered with the introduction of cyclosporin is the difficulty of diagnosing rejection episodes. The monitoring of E-rosette numbers is now of no value since T-cell numbers are normal in cyclosporin-immunosuppressed patients. With azathioprine and steroid immunosuppression, heart graft rejection could be diagnosed in the first instance by serial ECG voltage drops. Such measurements appear not to be relevant where cyclosporin is used. The diagnosis of rejection in cyclosporin patients now hinges on the histological examination of allograft tissue. Hence access to the facilities for regular endomyocardial biopsies is of major importance to the management of the cyclosporin-immunosuppressed heart transplant recipient. The diagnosis of rejection on the basis of histopathology is dealt with in detail in Chapter 15.

Another consideration in the use of cyclosporin is the best combination of other immunosuppressive drugs to use with it or indeed whether it alone is sufficient. Experimental studies have concentrated on the use of cyclosporin alone and some kidney transplant programmes have been successfully run using cyclosporin as the sole immunosuppressive, thus gaining all the benefits of avoiding the use of long-term steroid therapy (Beveridge *et al.*, 1983). However, the nephrotoxic side effects of cyclosporin make the very high doses used in cyclosporin-alone therapies undesirable, particularly in the early post-transplant phase. The advantage of using 'combination therapy'

TABLE 9.1
Immunosuppressive Regimens at Stanford University, California, USA

Initial cyclosporin regimen (28 patients, December 1980–January 1982)	
Cyclosporin	18 mg/kg per day, initial dose 10 mg/kg per day, 2 months
Prednisone	1 mg/kg per day, initial dose 0.2 mg/kg per day, 2 months
Rabbit ATG	2–4 days initial course
Modified cyclosporin regimen (74 patients, January 1982–May 1984)	
Cyclosporin	18 mg/kg per day, initial dose; thereafter dosage adjusted to maintain trough serum level, 100–300 ng/ml (radioimmunoassay)
Prednisone	1 mg/kg per day, initial dose 0.5 mg/kg per day, 1 month 0.2 mg/kg per day, 2 months
Prophylactic ATG	Discontinued
Current cyclosporin regimen (May 1984 onwards)	
Cyclosporin	16–18 mg/kg, loading dose; thereafter dosage adjusted to maintain trough serum level, 100–300 ng/ml, 1 month 50–150 ng/ml after 1 month
Azathioprine	4 mg/kg, loading dose 1–3 mg/kg per day to maintain WBC 4000–6000 mm^3
Equine ATG	7-day course 10 mg/kg per day according to T-cell rosette count
Prednisone	Randomized: (1) 0.2 mg/kg per day; (2) no corticosteroids

is that lower doses of cyclosporin can be used during this initial phase, thus reducing nephrotoxicity. The disadvantage of such combination therapy is that it increases the likelihood of infections and of the induction of EBV-induced monoclonal B-cell lymphomas.

The protocols (Table 9.1) that were successively developed by the Stanford group illustrate well the problems involved in establishing an optimal immunosuppressive regimen for heart transplantation. Initially, cyclosporin was administered at a standard dose, as part of a complex immunosuppressive cocktail. Of 28 patients treated in this way, four developed a malignant lymphoma within the first 6 months, early renal dysfunction was noted, but other complications attributed to cyclosporin such as hepatic toxicity, hirsutism and tremor appeared unimportant. The mean number of rejection episodes in the first 60 days after transplantation was 0.89 per patient in the cyclosporin group compared with 1.22 per patient in a conventionally treated historic group. The results showed an increase in the number of patients free of all rejection during this period and there appeared to be a reduction in bacterial infections in the cyclosporin-treated patients.

In an attempt to reduce the over-immunosuppression that appeared to be occurring in this patient population, as manifest by the very high incidence of lymphoma, the protocol was modified. The use of rabbit ATG was discontinued and the cyclosporin dosage was adjusted using trough serum levels of 100–300 ng/ml. This protocol was used for the next 74 heart transplant recipients and resulted in a much lower overall dose of cyclosporin and a more rapid reduction in its dosage. Only two of these patients developed lymphoma, an incidence comparable with that previously observed in conventionally treated patients. During the follow-up of these patients it became apparent that nephrotoxicity could be such a significant problem that cyclosporin therapy had to be discontinued. Furthermore, hypertension developed in most of these patients. As a result of these problems a third low-dose cyclosporin regimen was developed. Cyclosporin levels of 100–300 ng/ml continued to be the aim for the first month, but this level was then reduced to 50–150 ng/ml. In addition to this dose adjustment of cyclosporin, a prospective randomized clinical trial was started in which some patients received no oral corticosteroids, and the remainder received 0.2 mg/kg of prednisone. To compensate for this reduction in overall immunosuppression, azathioprine was administered to all patients to maintain a white cell count of between 4000 and 6000/mm^3. The use of ATG was also reinstated for the first 7 days postoperatively, maintaining a circulating T-cell count below 5% of the total lymphoid count.

Thus, the principles of the use of cyclosporin in heart transplantation are becoming clear:

(1) Avoid using large doses of cyclosporin so as to prevent long-term renal damage.
(2) Avoid using large doses of other immunosuppressants in conjunction with cyclosporin so as to avoid the risk of over-immunosuppression leading to a high lymphoma rate.

The Papworth approach to development of immunosuppressive therapy was slightly different. The initial regimen used with the introduction of cyclosporin was to abandon the use of both azathioprine and ATG, to lower the dose of steroids and to add a high dose (18 mg/kg) of oral cyclosporin. Although the results achieved with this protocol showed significant improvement in 1-year graft survival (Fig. 9.1), two problems became apparent. The first was that there was a small number of patients (Fig. 9.2) who suffered from aggressive, acute, irreversible rejection episodes as though no immunosuppression was being used at all. The second was marked nephrotoxicity occurring in almost all patients, which required rapid downward dose adjustment of the cyclosporin.

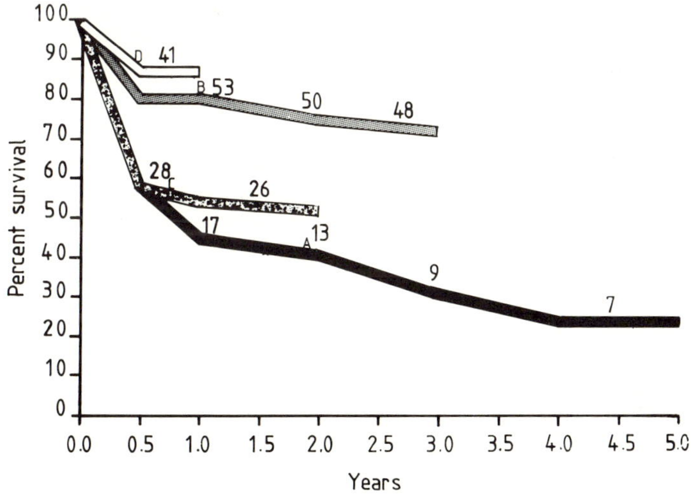

Fig. 9.1. *Survival of heart transplant recipients in Papworth divided by immunosuppressive era (A, 1979–82, n = 29; B, 1982–84, n = 66; C, 1985, n = 48, D, 1986, n = 47).*

In an attempt to overcome these problems, ATG was reintroduced for the first week post-transplant. In order to avoid increasing the risk of lymphoma, the ATG doses were adjusted by E-rosette monitoring so as to maintain T-cell numbers at approximately 10%, thus leaving some residual T-cell

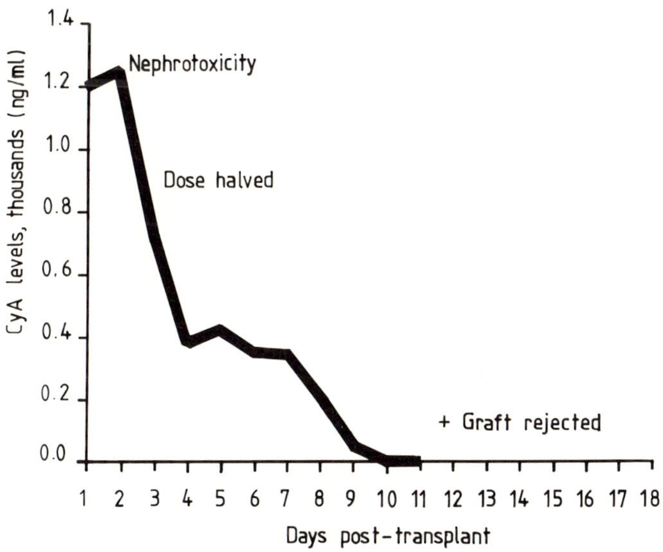

Fig. 9.2. *Result of failing to maintain cyclosporin levels in the immediate post-transplant period in the absence of ATG.*

immune competence. This schedule allowed the cyclosporin to be introduced initially at a much lower dose (2–5 mg/kg) which was adjusted on the basis of serum or whole blood cyclosporin levels. This resulted in a reduction of nephrotoxicity, although it still occurs to some extent in almost every patient treated. The incidence of acute graft rejection in the early weeks post-transplant was also reduced by this policy.

The associated hypertension remains a consistent problem in all recipients. Reports suggesting that a substitution of azathioprine for the steroids in a cyclosporin regimen reduced the hypertension led to the setting up at Papworth of a randomized prospective clinical trial of either azathioprine or steroids in conjunction with cyclosporin and ATG. The details of the immunosuppressive schedules used are given in Table 9.2. The results of this trial showed no significant difference in survival between the two groups, nor any significant difference in the number of rejection episodes per patient (pred. 0.95 re/pt, aza. 1.2 re/pt). There was no difference in renal function or dose of cyclosporin given or of diastolic hypertension between the two groups. There were, however, four deaths from infection in the steroid group. None occurred in the azathioprine group.

TREATMENT OF REJECTION EPISODES

As has already been described, the use of cyclosporin as part of an immunosuppressive protocol has made the diagnosis of rejection of the heart graft much more difficult, and this diagnosis now relies heavily on the interpretation of a biopsy. Nor can the interpretation of rejection be based purely on the evidence of mononuclear cell infiltration, as has been demonstrated by numerous studies both clinically and experimentally (Dunn *et al.*, 1979). The risks of mistreating a histopathological observation which would resolve spontaneously without biological consequences to the patient, and thus increasing the risk of infection to that patient, have to be weighed against the consequences of allowing a rejection episode to progress unchecked to irreversibility.

There are surprisingly little good research data on the treatment of rejection episodes. Clinical practice has established a regimen based on intravenous steroids as the sheet anchor of therapy. Most groups use 1 g of intravenous methyl prednisolone per day for 3 days. There is now evidence (Merion, White and Calne, 1983) that with cyclosporin treatment both the dose and duration of the steroid treatment can be reduced, although this has not yet entered into generalized clinical practice.

In severe or steroid-resistant rejection episodes, ATG provides optional therapy. Duration of ATG treatment of a rejection episode varies from

TABLE 9.2

Immunosuppressive Regimens at Papworth Hospital, Cambridge, UK

Protocol for steroid group	
Cyclosporin A	~9 mg/kg initial dose preoperatively; maintenance dose to trough levels, 200–400 ng/ml
Steroids	Perioperative i.v. methylprednisolone, 500 mg preoperatively 500 mg post-implantation 125 mg × 3 in first 24 h; maintenance, 1 mg/kg orally → 0.3 mg/kg at 14 days
Equine ATG	I.v. 10 days to maintain T cells ~10% or absolute 100 cells/ml
This is the existing protocol	
Protocol for azathioprine group	
Cyclosporin A	~9 mg/kg initial dose preoperatively; maintenance dose to trough levels, 200–400 ng/ml.
Azathioprine	2 mg/kg initial dose preoperatively i.v.; maintenance dose 1.5–2.0 mg/kg orally WBC ~5000 cells/ml
Equine ATG	I.v. 10 days to maintain T cells ~10% or absolute 100 cells/ml
Steroids	Perioperative i.v. methylprednisolone, 500 mg preoperatively 500 mg post-implantation 125 mg × 3 in first 24 h; maintenance, none

centre to centre, lasting from 3 to 10 days. Recent studies on the use of OKT3 to reverse rejection episodes in heart transplant recipients have provided good evidence that such monoclonal antibody therapy will become a more routine form of treatment (Bristow, 1987). There is now an increasing body of evidence that intravenous cyclosporin provides a useful way of reversing at least some steroid-resistant rejection episodes, but to date such treatment has not found its way into general clinical practice (Prieto *et al.*, 1986).

CHRONIC REJECTION

The slow insidious immune destruction of a graft 3–10 years post-transplant, characterized by deterioration of function and thickening of arterial walls, will undoubtedly cause more concern in the future as our ability to provide a relatively high initial 1–2 year heart graft survival becomes established. The exact immunological cause of this chronic graft rejection is not known. Anti-graft antibodies have been incriminated on the basis of very little evidence. It has also been suggested that initial inadequate immunosuppression in the first few months post-transplant leads eventually to this kind of chronic graft rejection. 'Treatment' of this condition is usually provided by increasing oral steroids. Although empirically anti-inflammatory therapy should reduce the symptoms involved in this process, there is little scientific evidence that such therapy can halt or even retard chronic rejection. In the end the only course of treatment available at present for many of these recipients is re-transplantation.

HEART–LUNG TRANSPLANTATION

The recent success of heart–lung transplantation has been directly attributed to the availability of cyclosporin immunosuppression.

The first human heart–lung transplant was carried out by Cooley in 1968 on a 2-year-old child, who died some 14 h postoperatively. Two further attempts at human heart–lung transplantation, one by Lillehei in 1969 and one by Barnard in 1971, also ended in failure when the patients died of pneumonia. One of the major reasons why heart–lung transplantation had proved so difficult at that time was the reliance upon immunosuppression with corticosteroids and azathioprine, leading to generalized leucopenia and lymphopenia, retarded wound healing and poor control of graft rejection. The failure of the tracheal anastomosis to heal properly caused particular problems in heart–lung transplantation.

The value of cyclosporin immunosuppression in heart–lung transplantation was demonstrated in monkeys in 1980 (Reitz *et al.*, 1982). These workers were impressed by the fact that cyclosporin allowed the avoidance of steroids in the early postoperative phase, thus allowing faster wound healing and particularly the healing of the tracheal anastomosis. Cyclosporin also reduced the risk of lung infection becoming a significant clinical problem. As a result of Reitz's experimental programme, the Stanford group initiated a clinical heart–lung transplant programme in the spring of 1981. To date, 26 heart–lung transplants have been performed in the Stanford series and the survival rates are 65% at 1 year and 54% at 4 years (Fig. 9.3) (McGregor, Oyer and Shumway, 1986).

One of the curiosities of heart–lung transplantation is that the *en bloc* organ transplant seems to attract less rejection than a heart transplant performed alone. Thus, in the Stanford series only 13.8% of heart biopsies from heart–lung transplant recipients showed evidence of rejection, compared

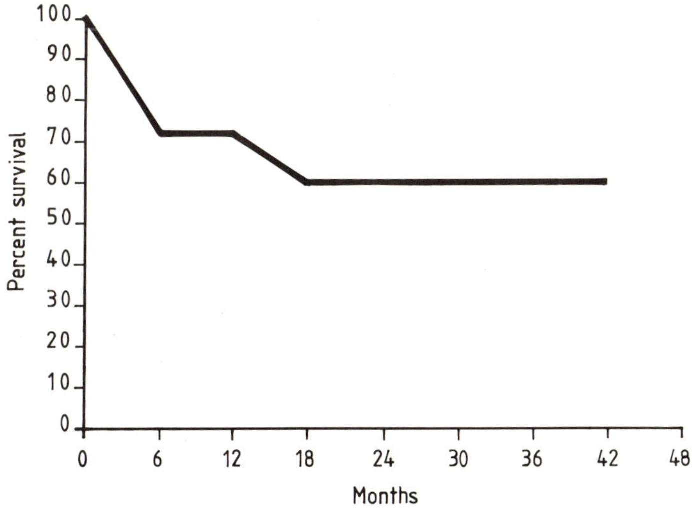

Fig. 9.3. *Actuarial survival of heart–lung transplantation at Stanford (March 1981–May 1985, n = 25)*

with 24.6% of biopsies taken from hearts transplanted alone (McGregor, Oyer and Shumway, 1986).

Experiences at Papworth echo those from Stanford (Fig. 9.4). Of 19 heart–lung transplant recipients, only 4 have died. One-year survival is 76%.

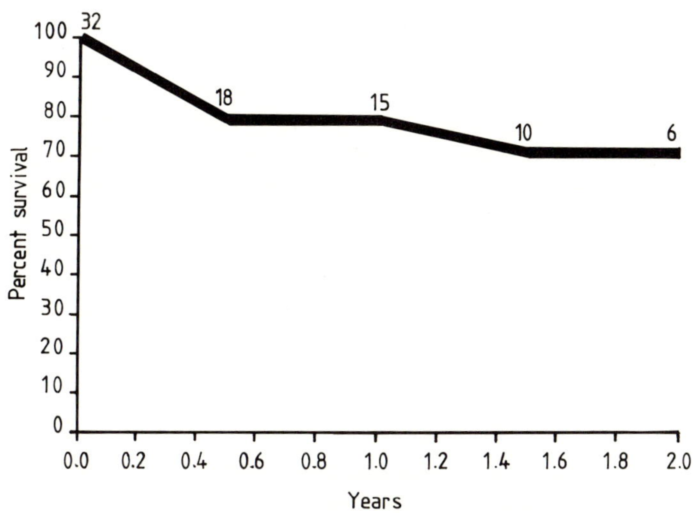

Fig. 9.4. *Actuarial survival of heart–lung transplantation at Papworth.*

MONITORING CYCLOSPORIN LEVELS

An important aid to the management of immunosuppression in heart and heart–lung transplantation is the routine (preferably daily) determination of the level of cyclosporin. This allows appropriate dose adjustment to avoid low levels precipitating a rejection crisis or high levels causing renal function to become critically impaired (see Fig. 9.2).

Cyclosporin levels depend, to a large extent, upon the ability of the individual to absorb the drug. In addition, they can be influenced by the patient's age, liver function, bile flow, other drugs and haematology. Furthermore, values returned from the laboratory will vary, dependent upon method of measurement, timing of sample and matrix measured.

Measurement of cyclosporin levels and their interpretation

Technique

There are two methods for the measurement of cyclosporin in body fluid. Each offers potential advantages and disadvantages over the other. These methods are high performance liquid chromatography (HPLC) and immunoassay. It should be stressed that neither is more 'accurate' than the other. However, they do not measure exactly the same thing. At present, the difference between these techniques concerns the specificity of the antibody used in immunoassay. The principle of this immunoassay is a competition between labelled cyclosporin tracer (currently two are available, ^{125}I and ^{3}H labelled) and cyclosporin in the patient sample for anti-cyclosporin antibody. Unfortunately all antibodies available at present bind not only cyclosporin in the patient sample but also some metabolites. The nature of immunoassays does not allow distinction between competition by metabolite or competition by whole cyclosporin. Nor at present is it known if these metabolites are immunosuppressive. Thus immunoassay-derived results give slightly higher values for 'cyclosporin' level than the true value. This excess, of the order of 10%, in most cases is not significant. However, in patients with liver dysfunction the metabolites can build up to significant levels, making immunoassay determination in these patients at best meaningless, and potentially dangerous if interpreted at face value. This difficulty can only be solved by the introduction of an antibody which does not bind the metabolites. It is anticipated that the newly developed monoclonal antibodies will resolve this problem

In its favour, however, immunoassay is relatively inexpensive, technically easy to perform, rapid, requires no pretreatment of the sample and allows almost limitless numbers of samples to be measured at one time.

The advantage that HPLC offers over immunoassay is that only whole drug is measured, which is of importance in patients with impaired hepatic function. However, compared with RIA, HPLC is relatively expensive, both

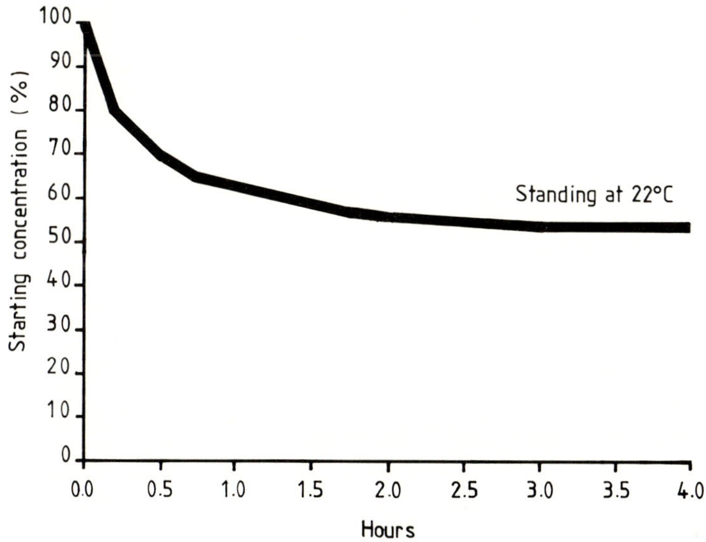

Fig 9.5 *Concentration of cyclosporin A in plasma separated at various times after being allowed to stand at 22°C (After Niederburger, personal communication).*

in terms of capital and running costs. Most HPLC methods require an initial sample extraction step. In theory, there is no limit to the number of samples that can be determined by HPLC. In practice, however, the number of columns is limited and the sample extraction process is also a rate-limiting step. Thus, centres anticipating more than 20 samples per day would find an HPLC system hard pressed to keep pace with demand.

The matrix

Initially, cyclosporin measurements were made on trough (i.e. pre-dose) serum samples. Day profile studies illustrated the value of performing the measurement as a trough level rather than attempting to take a peak sample. Peak values vary from 20 min to 4 or 5 h post-dose. The studies of Niederburger, however, questioned the wisdom of measuring cyclosporin in serum. It was demonstrated (Fig. 9.5) that, as a blood sample cooled from body temperature, cyclosporin left the plasma and entered the red cells until the serum value was diminished by 30–40% of its original value.

Thus substantial error could be introduced into cyclosporin level measurement because the value obtained was critically dependent upon the time after sampling that the serum was separated. There are three ways to overcome this problem: the sample can be left to stand at a constant temperature until equilibrium is reached (over 2 h); it can be rewarmed (forcing the cyclosporin out of the cells back into the serum); or whole blood levels can be used. Most centres have opted for this last approach.

Which level?

The therapeutic 'window' for cyclosporin immunosuppression, that is a lower level above which rejection does not occur and an upper level below which nephrotoxicity is avoided, is largely a myth. Nephrotoxicity and rejection can occur concurrently. Indeed, nephrotoxicity to some degree is an inevitable consequence of cyclosporin immunosuppression.

However, over the years a therapeutic range maximizing immunosuppressive activity while minimizing nephrotoxicity has been established in renal transplantation. This therapeutic range cannot be extrapolated in isolation, but must be used with due consideration of the other immunosuppressive agents given.

Published ranges vary somewhat, but for serum levels a range between 100 and 300 ng/ml (μg/l) is commonly accepted. In kidney transplantation this equates with a range of 200–500 ng/ml whole blood levels. Current trends in immunosuppression tend to the lower end of these scales. In heart transplantation, the tendency has been to err in favour of the top end of these therapeutic windows. Thus at Papworth, while monitoring cyclosporin *serum* levels, the mean level during the first month post-transplant was 300 ng/ml and this required an average daily dose of approximately 7 mg/kg.

The change from monitoring serum to whole blood levels however, led to disaster, with a significant increase in rejection. The whole blood range had been appropriately adjusted to 400–600 ng/ml. Was this window too low? Investigation showed that overall our average daily dosage of cyclosporin level increased to 8 mg/kg. However, those patients who had died from graft

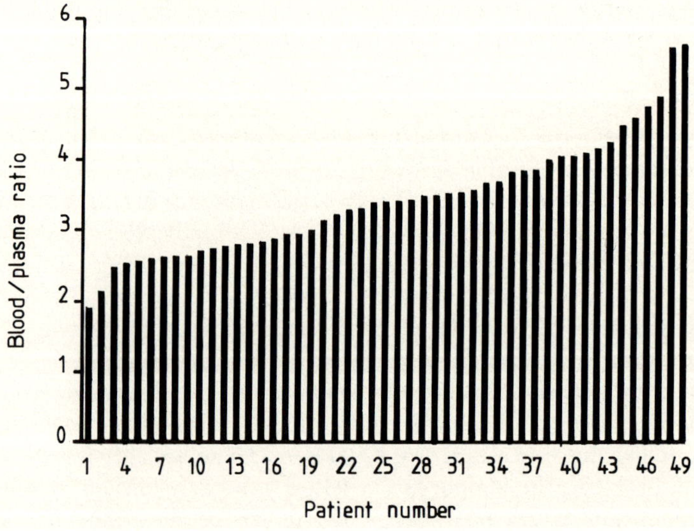

Fig. 9.6. *Variation in plasma/whole blood ratio, in 49 patients. Data displayed by rank.*

rejection were shown to have an average daily dose of only 4 mg/kg. Since this dose had been supporting whole blood levels which had proved adequate in others, why should the patients have succumbed?

Patient management policy was changed to measuring both whole blood and plasma levels. An analysis of the ratio between these two values (from the same sample) revealed the probable answer. Variation of this ratio between patients was substantial (Fig. 9.6). Analysis showed that the cause of this variation was differences in the number of red cells in the blood. Since most heart recipients have substantially greater numbers of red cells than do end-stage renal failure patients, the extrapolation of a therapeutic window from kidney to heart transplantation is not valid.

Thus the serum level measurement in heart patients probably requires a lower therapeutic level than the equivalent for a kidney recipient. Conversely, the measurement of whole blood values requires a higher therapeutic value. Measurement of cyclosporin levels for heart transplantation must be evaluated in the knowledge of the red cell content of the sample measured.

REFERENCES

Barnard, C. N. (1967). The operation. *S. Afr. Med. J.* **41**, 1271.

Beveridge, T., Wood, A. J., Calne, R. Y. and White, D. J. G. (1983). Cyclosporin in cadaveric renal transplantation: one year follow up of a multicentre trial. *Lancet* **ii**, 986.

Bieber, C. P., Griepp, R. B., Oyer, P. E., David, C. A. and Stinson E. B. (1977). Relationship of rabbit ATG clearance rate to circulating T cell level rejection and survival in cardiac transplantation. *Transplant. Proc.* **9**, 1031.

Bieber, C. P., Griepp, R. B., Oyer, P. E., Wong, J. and Stinson, E. B. (1976). Use of rabbit anti-thymocyte globulin in cardiac transplantation. Relationship of serum clearance rates to clinical outcome. Transplantation **22**, 478.

Borel, J. F. (1976). Comparative studies of *in vitro* and *in vivo* drug effects on cell mediated cytotoxicity. Immunol. **31**, 631.

Bristow, M. R. (1987). Efficiency of OKT-3 in the treatment of cardiac transplantation rejection. *Transplant. Proc.* (in press).

Calne, R. Y. and White, D. J. G. (1977). Cyclosporin A: a powerful immunosuppressant in dogs with renal allografts. *IRCS Med. Sci.* **5**, 595.

Calne, R. Y., White, D. J. G. and Rolles, K. (1978). Prolonged survival of pig orthotopic heart grafts treated with Cyclosporin A. *Lancet* **i**, 1183.

Caves, P. K., Stinson, E. B., Billingham, M. E., Rider, A. K. and Shumway, N. E. (1973). Diagnosis of human cardiac allograft rejection by serial cardiac biopsy. *J. Thorac. Cardiovasc. Surg.* **66**, 461.

Dreyfuss, M., Harri, E., Hoffmann, H., Kobel, H., Pache, W. and Tscherter, H. (1976). Cyclosporin A and C, new metabolites from *Trichoderma polysporum*. *Eur. J. Appl. Microbiol.* **3**, 125.

Dunn, D. C., White, D. J. G., Herbertson, B. M. and Wade, J. (1979). Prolongation of kidney survival during and after Cyclosporin therapy. *Transplantation* **27**, 359.

Kohler, G. and Milstein, C. (1975). Continuous cultures of fused cells secreting antibody of predefined specificity. Nature **256**, 495.

Kostakis, A. J., White, D. J. G. and Calne, R. Y. (1977). Prolongation of rat heart allograft survival by Cyclosporin A. *IRCS Med. Sci.*, **5**, 280.

Lower, R. R. and Shumway, N. E. (1960). Studies on orthotopic homotransplantation of the canine heart. *Surg. Forum* **11**, 18.

McGregor, C. G. A., Oyer, P. E. and Shumway, N. E. (1986). Heart and heart/lung transplantation. In: *Ciclosporin*, p. 346 (J. F. Borel, Ed.). Karger, Basel.

Morris, P. J. (1986). Prediction of rejection by morphometric analysis. *Transplant. Proc.* **18**, 1040.

Merion, R. M., White, D. J. G. and Calne, R. Y. (1983). Early renal rejection episodes are less aggressive with Cyclosporin A immunosuppression. *Transplant. Proc.* **15**, 2172.

Oyer, P. E., Stinson, E. B., Jamieson, S. W., Hunt, S., Reitz, B. A., Bieber, C. P., Schraeder, J. S., Billingham, M. E. and Shumway, N. E. (1982a). One year experience with Cyclosporin A in clinical heart transplantation. *Heart Transplant.* **1**, 285.

Oyer, P. E., Stinson, E. B., Reitz, B. A., Wallwork, J., Baumgartner, W. A. and Shumway, N. E. (1982b). Preliminary results with Cyclosporin A in clinical cardiac transplantation. In: *Cyclosporin A*, p. 461 (D. White, Ed.). Elsevier Biomedical Press, Amsterdam.

Prieto, C., Alcazar, J. M., Ruelope, L. M., Bello, I., Andres, A., Morales, J. M. and Rodico, J. L. (1986). Usefulness of Cyclosporine in the treatment of steroid-resistant rejection. *Transplant. Proc.* **18**, 993.

Reitz, B. A., Wallwork, J. L., Hunt, S. A., Pennock, J. L., Oyer, P. E., Stinson, E. B. and Shumway, N. E. (1982). Cyclosporin A for combined heart–lung transplantation. In: *Cyclosporin A*, p. 473 (D. White, Ed.). Elsevier Biomedical Press, Amsterdam.

Starzl, T. E., Porter, K. A. and Iwasaki, Y. (1967). Antilymphocyte serum in renal transplantation. In: *Antilymphocyte Serum.* CIBA Foundation Study Group No. 29, p. 4 (G. R. W. Wolstenhome and M. O'Connor, Eds). Little, Brown & Co., Boston.

Wechter, W. J., Brodie, J. A., Morrell, R. M., Rafi, M. and Schultz, J. R. (1979). Anti-lymphocyte globulin in renal allograft recipients. Transplantation **28**, 294.

Woodruff, M. F. and Anderson, N. A. (1963). Effect of lymphocyte depletion by thoracic duct fistula and antilymphocyte serum on the survival of skin homografts in rats. Nature **200**, 702.

P. G. I. Stovin

10

Pathology of the Excised Recipient Heart

INTRODUCTION

Although many reports of the indications for and the results of heart transplantation have appeared, there have been no reviews of the pathology encountered in the excised recipient's heart. This is because such a review would need to cover the whole range of cardiac pathology.

Although this chapter will consider selected aspects of the pathology of the recipient's heart, other aspects of the recipient's condition will be considered in so far as these features may influence the outcome of heart transplantation.

The generally accepted criteria for selection of patients for heart transplantation have been presented in Chapter 4. It can be expected that with increasing experience and improving survival the indications for heart transplantation will be widened.

It would be beyond the scope of this book to include a detailed account of the whole range of pathological lesions encountered in the excised recipient's heart, so this chapter will concentrate on a few features whose study has been facilitated by transplantation.

THE RECIPIENT HEART

End-stage heart disease

The chief criterion for acceptance of a patient for heart transplantation is that the patient should be at a late stage of the natural history of his or her

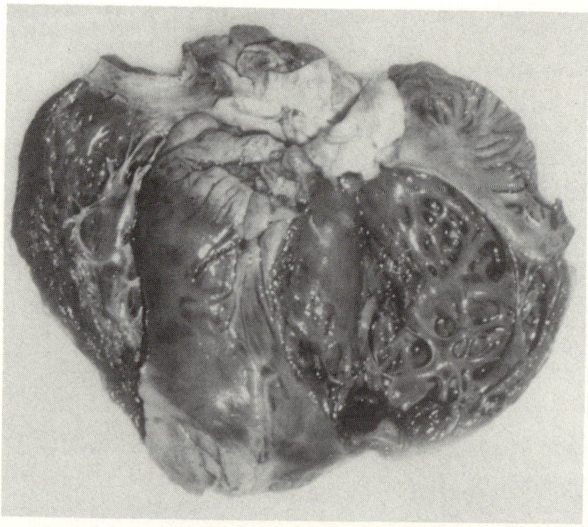

Fig. 10.1. *End-stage heart failure with endocardial thrombus in dilated right ventricle.*

heart disease. End-stage heart disease has been broadly defined by Copeland *et al.* (1985) as a prognosis of less than 1 year and is usually associated with an ejection fraction of 10% or less. At this stage the patient is having difficulty in maintaining blood pressure and there may well be some degree of liver and renal failure from inadequate perfusion of these organs. The heart itself may also be suffering from poor perfusion, which is manifest pathologically as biventricular endocardial thrombus formation and/or subendocardial recent ischaemic vacuolation or necrosis in the presence of normal coronary arteries (Fig. 10.1). In the presence of coronary artery disease it is difficult to be certain that the fresh small infarcts are due to the end-stage poor perfusion rather than to the coronary arterial narrowing.

The total artificial heart has been used to sustain or even improve such end-stage patients while waiting for a suitable donor heart to become available. This has recently been reviewed by Joyce *et al.* (1986).

Laguens, Weinschelbaum and Favaloro (1979) described elongation of the mitochondria as one of the changes seen in biopsies from patients with acute coronary insufficiency. Other changes included reduction in electron density and irregularity in the distribution of the mitochondria. At Papworth, elongation of the mitochondria (Fig. 10.2) was found in 51% of the resected recipient hearts and was not seen in the donor heart biopsies and may therefore be an indicator of end-stage heart disease.

A reduced frequency distribution of atrial granules seen on ultrastructural examination of the right atrium might also correlate with end-stage heart disease. This is a feature that I have occasionally encountered, but it is much

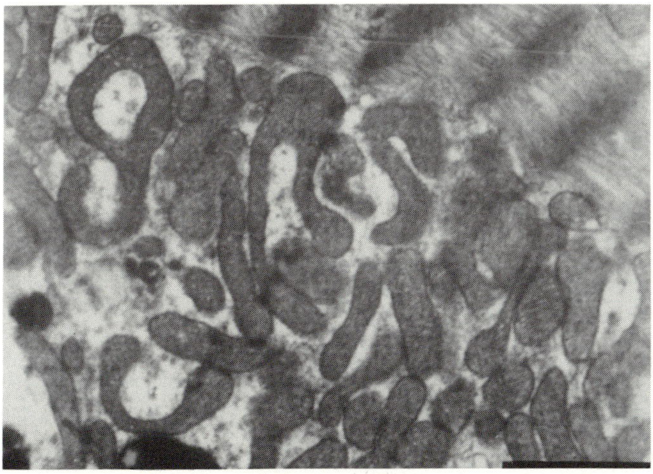

Fig. 10.2. *Elongated mitochondria seen in end-stage heart disease and in ischaemic heart disease. One mitochondrion at the top left is curled on itself to give the appearance of a ring form. Normal myocardial mitochondria are ovoid (see Fig. 10.8).* × *18 200*

less frequently seen than elongation of the mitochondria. Clinically, blood levels of atrial natriuretic hormone are increased in heart failure (Tikkanen *et al*., 1985) and following heart transplantation (Singer *et al*., 1986).

Despite its being a frequently used term, there is no very precise definition of 'end-stage' heart disease. Even though Copeland *et al.* (1985) may have given the best available clinical definition, there is bound to be the rare case that lives longer than anticipated. At the moment the pathologist is trailing behind the clinician and cannot offer any better, more reliable or distinctive histological or biochemical predictors of impending doom. Indeed, improvements in prediction are most likely to come from methods of assessing the functional reserve of the myocardium (Tan, 1986) rather than its resting function.

Because the transplant recipient is usually in a more deteriorated state than is the usual patient coming to open heart operation, and may also be more anxious, it is not surprising that ventricular dysrhythmias and even cardiac arrest occur during the induction of anaesthesia or during the operation prior to the establishment of bypass. As discussed in Chapter 8, this is a very critical time and in 1–2% of cases there may be some degree of brain damage that becomes evident postoperatively.

The next two sections will consider the commonest two groups of cardiac disease for which transplantation has been performed: ischaemic heart disease (IHD) and dilated cardiomyopathy (DCM).

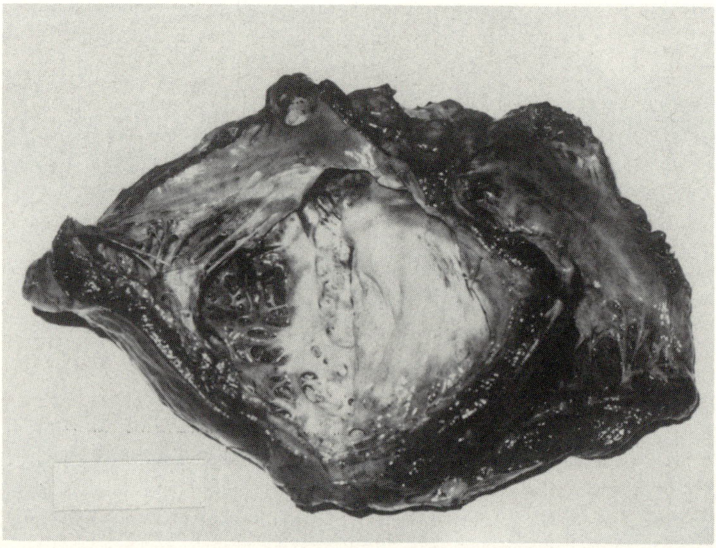

Fig. 10.3. *Myocardial infarction with previous surgical resection of a cardiac aneurysm.*

Ischaemic heart disease

This is a fairly wide range of conditions varying from extensive severe triple vessel coronary artery disease without any previous surgery to occlusive disease of one or more main arteries with or without previous bypass surgery, with or without resections of ventricular aneurysm (Fig. 10.3) and with or without previous replacement of the mitral valve because of papillary muscle infarction.

It was shown a number of years ago that previous cardiac surgery, which invariably meant previous blood transfusion, had no harmful effect on the subsequent heart transplantation (Dong *et al.*, 1973). On the contrary, previous blood transfusion appears to improve allograft survival in heart transplants (Cooper *et al.*, 1983; Szentpetery *et al.*, 1984). The effect of previous transfusion in the Papworth patients is given in Table 10.1. Of 34 patients who died after transplantation for IHD, 20 died from rejection and 6 from infection. The remaining 8 deaths were embolic events (3), malignancy (2), donor failure, recipient pulmonary vascular resistance and renal failure in 1 case each. Of the rejection deaths, only one had had a previous operation, whereas this had happened in 4 of the deaths from infection.

In most series, IHD is the diagnosis in the largest group of patients coming to heart transplantation. Ischaemic heart disease formed 59.8% of the cases described by Pomerance and Stovin (1985) from the UK. At Cape Town, 29 of 50 (58%) recipients had IHD (Cooper *et al.*, 1983), and at Stanford

TABLE 10.1
*Effect of Previous Transfusion on Deaths in IHD Transplants**

Survival		*Dead*		*Alive*
		TRANSFUSED		
	Rejection	*Infection*	*Other*	
<30 days	1	0	2	
>30 days	0	5	0	23
		NOT TRANSFUSED		
<30 days	2	1	2	
>30 days	15	4	2	26

* Patients who could have been followed up for >150 days.

48.5% of 206 cases (Jamieson *et al.*, 1981). At the other end of the scale, IHD cases formed only 14% of 180 patients considered for heart transplantation at La Pitié Hospital (Cabrol *et al.*, 1983) and 22% of 90 heart transplants in Berlin (Schuler, Warnecke and Hetzer, 1987).

In the Papworth material, only 4 out of 79 cases had severe single or double vessel disease. In 3 of these 4 patients, the occlusions at the origins of the anterior descending and circumflex branches were suggestive of an embolic episode. The vast majority had extensive triple vessel disease.

Data on blood lipids were available in 38 of the Papworth patients of whom 15 were shown to be hyperlipidaemic with serum cholesterol at 6.9 mmol/litre or higher.

The weights of the resected recipient hearts were distributed bimodally with peaks at 333 and 433 g. The total range in 82 ischaemic hearts was from 265 g to 786 g. A history of well-controlled hypertension was given in only 9 of these cases whose hearts weighed 276–648 g (mean 465.1 g). It might be that the 19 cases of the first of the bimodal groups were those unable to hypertrophy because of the lack of development of any coronary collateral circulation, whereas the heavier and larger group had developed a collateral circulation. No post-resection angiography was done on the specimens because of other investigations being undertaken. Preoperative angiography reporting varied widely between the different referring hospitals. Thus it has not been practicable to assess the degree of development of the collateral circulation in these cases. However, as one-third of the cases in each weight group had had previous operations for relief of the ischaemia, it is unlikely that the collateral circulation plays a significant part in the hypertrophy of IHD.

It is also unlikely that previous hypertension had played a significant part in the cases with an increased heart weight, since 2 of the 9 patients with treated hypertension had hearts weighing 350 g or less. Further, it is inconceivable that previously treated hypertension would have been ignored in over 80% of the case records sent by the referring cardiologists.

The degree of dilatation of the failing ischaemic left ventricle showed a normal distribution ranging from 3.5 cm diameter to 9.5 cm with a mean of 5.4 cm. These measurements were made on the fixed hearts and are therefore not comparable to the echocardiographic dimensions in either diastole or in systole. The diameter was not related to previous operations, but did show a slight correlation with the heart weight ($r = 0.43$).

The considerable ventricular dilatation to 7 cm and above, and the increased weight above 580 g in the largest 10%, raises the suspicion that there may be a dual pathology operating — a combination of ischaemia with congestive myopathy. These two conditions are the two commonest conditions for which heart transplantation is undertaken, and it would therefore be surprising if they did not occur together in some cases. This postulated dual pathology would appear to be different from the ischaemic cardiomyopathy of Dash *et al.* (1977). Histological recognition of a dual pathology is very difficult in the late extensively scarred state and must depend on an awareness of the possibility and an appreciation of a significant degree of discordance between the distribution of the scars and the distribution of the vascular stenosis and occlusions. At the time of the original examination, an accompanying cardiomyopathy was considered in 2 cases only, but was not thought to be the major lesion. In one other case, a limited focus of myocardial amyloid was present in the inferior wall of the left ventricle.

A cardiomyopathic picture defined as chronic heart failure with multiple and widespread left ventricular wall motion abnormalities, of sufficient degree to reduce significantly the left ventricular ejection fraction at rest, was studied by Dash *et al.* (1977). This ischaemic myopathy was related to the extent of the distribution of severe (>70%) stenoses of the main branches of the three chief coronary arteries. These branch vessels are the most frequent site of coronary artery narrowing (Halon *et al.*, 1983). In the study of Dash *et al.* (1977), the myopathic picture was not related to the presence or absence of a collateral circulation, nor was it related to the presence or absence of disease in the distal small coronary arteries. On ECG and angiographic criteria not all the areas of damage to the myocardium were considered to be fully transmural, although the presence of the myopathic picture correlated well with the presence of 2 or more transmural infarcts.

In a study of patients coming to necropsy with clinically unexplained heart failure, Boucher *et al.* (1979) found that in 7 of 15 patients the heart failure was due to the cardiomyopathic syndrome caused by coronary artery disease. All but two of these 7 were diabetic. Of the 8 non-ischaemic patients, 5 were myopathic and 3 had valvular disease. In the ischaemic group, the hearts weighed between 340 and 553 g and showed varying degrees of ventricular dilatation from mild to severe. The 5 cardiomyopathy hearts were heavier (483–663 g) and all were moderately or markedly dilated but had no arterial disease. Thus, this ischaemic myopathy would seem to be different from the disease in the much heavier hearts in the Papworth series with a postulated combination of IHD and DCM.

Concentric sub-endocardial necrosis or scarring is a recognized result of severe triple vessel disease (Davies, Woolf and Robertson, 1976). In the absence of coronary artery disease, similar damage is seen after open-heart surgery if myocardial preservation has been inadequate (Davies and Pomerance, 1975). Histologically, this form of ischaemic myocardial damage shows an immediately sub-endocardial zone, only a few myocytes deep, of surviving myocytes separating the damaged region from the endocardial surface.

From this brief discussion of the basic features of myocardial damage from coronary artery disease, it is difficult to pinpoint a feature that would positively identify the late result of combined past myocarditis/cardiomyopathy with coronary artery disease. The only possible indicators would be the presence of sub-epicardial scars or inflammation unrelated to partial or complete transmural infarct scars. Scattered lymphocytes can be seen in the region of incompletely organized ischaemic scars and, in the author's experience and that of others (Billingham, 1985; Yu *et al.*, 1985), are almost invariably present in some part of a resected post-infarct ventricular aneurysm. The work of Parl, Gutstein and Glasser (1980) has shown that cardiac hypertrophy itself increases the amount of myocardial fibrosis related to ischaemic damage. These authors did not assess the causes of the hypertrophy in their 86 cases.

Lastly, the study of the ischaemic hearts resected from living transplant recipients has been a very salutary personal experience for one who thought that he could give a valid cause of death from an examination of the heart at necropsy. Perhaps end-stage heart disease should be defined as the state of the heart that an experienced pathologist would accept as sufficient to be the cause of death. Twenty of the 82 hearts in the Papworth patients had fresh occlusive thrombi in the severely diseased main coronary arteries and a further 3 had recent haemorrhage into atheromatous plaques without thrombus in the lumen. The conclusion would seem to be that in most cases of cardiac death it is a dysrhythmia and not the extent or severity of the ischaemic disease that kills the patient.

Dilated cardiomyopathy

These cases form the second largest group of heart recipients: 25% in the South African series (Cooper *et al.*, 1983), 28% in the Texas series (Frazier *et al.*, 1985), 33% in Great Britain (Pomerance and Stovin, 1985) and 45% at Stanford (Jamieson *et al.*, 1981). In Paris, cardiomyopathy patients formed 77% of those on the transplant waiting list (Cabrol *et al.*, 1983), whereas in Berlin 76.7% of heart transplants were for cardiomyopathy (Schuler, Warnecke and Hetzer, 1987).

Currently, discussion centres on the extent to which myocarditis is the starting point for the subsequent development of DCM (O'Connell and Gunnar, 1982; Just and Schuster, 1983; Sekiguchi, Olsen and Goodwin, 1985). Okada and Wakafuji (1985) have estimated that about 38% of Japanese cases of DCM have an initiating myocarditis, whereas Olsen (1985b) found active myocarditis in about 25% of endomyocardial biopsies from patients with DCM. Recently, Bowles *et al.* (1986) have detected Coxsackie-B RNA sequences in 5 of 10 patients with dilated cardiomyopathy. There may be a deficiency in immunological defence mechanisms in DCM which would help explain the apparent infective origin of this condition; Anderson, Carlquist and Hammond (1982) reported reduced natural killer cell activity in half of their DCM patients.

In the Papworth series of 65 cardiomyopathy patients, only 1 had proven evidence of viral myocarditis (Lowry, Edwards and Nagle, 1982). Besides this patient, another dated the onset from an attack of chicken pox and a further 11 gave a history of a viral infection a short time before the onset of their heart failure. An additional 2 cases gave a history of worsening of the symptoms following an influenza-like illness 3 and 7 years after the initial diagnosis of cardiomyopathy. These 2 cases, coupled with the fact that the brother of the known viral infected case also underwent heart transplantation for DCM, suggest that in a number of the cases the viral infection may be incidental. Further, we have reason to believe that a proportion of normal donor hearts with normal histology and biopsy harbour toxoplasma and cytomegalovirus (Hakim *et al.*, 1985b). Thus, our experience suggests that an infective myocarditic origin for some cases of DCM is still an open question.

Besides the two brothers mentioned above, 7 other cases gave a family history of myopathy. A family history of myopathy was present in 6 of the 15 patients with mild or grossly dilated myopathy studied by Keren *et al.* (1985). On the other hand, Silver and Silver (1983) describe a positive family history as being rare in this condition.

In 3 of the Papworth patients symptoms dated from a pregnancy, in another 3 there was the possibility of an excessive alcohol intake and in 1 other there had been a past history of solvent abuse (Wiseman and Banim,

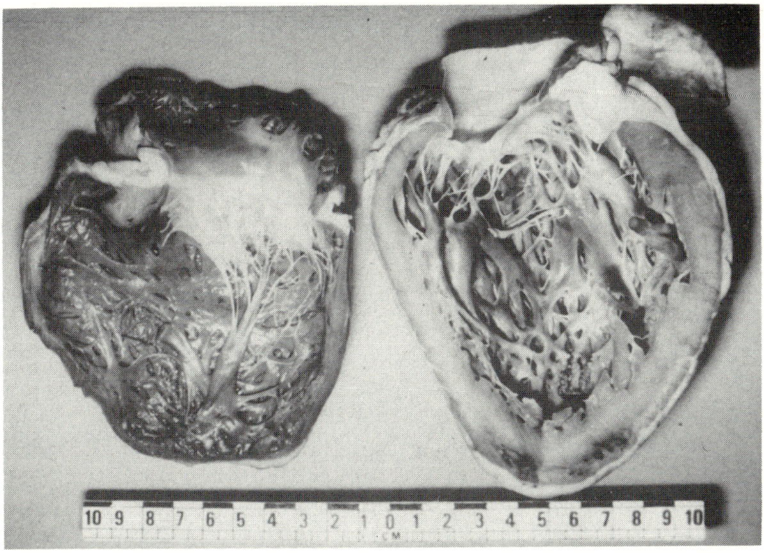

Fig. 10.4. *Dilated cardiomyopathy showing mild bilateral endocardial thickening.*

1987). For comparison, 3 of the IHD group of 82 patients had had pregnancies and there was a possibility of alcoholism in another. Although alcohol- and pregnancy-related cardiomyopathies may have a better prognosis than other forms of DCM (O'Connell and Gunnar, 1982), it is not possible to differentiate them histologically (Olsen, 1979; Fenoglio, 1982; Factor and Sonnenblick, 1985). Moreover, Sanderson, Olsen and Gatei (1986) have reported finding evidence of myocarditis in 5 of 11 East African post-partum cardiomyopathy patients. Lymphocytic infiltrates were not seen in the hearts of the 3 Papworth post-partum DCM patients.

As with the IHD group, there was a bimodal distribution of heart weights. However, in this group peaks were at 424 and 740 g. The weights ranged from 278 to 865 g, with a mean of 484.7 g. All hearts were dilated with left ventricular cavities 3.5–8.5 cm diameter (mean 5.6 cm) (Figs 10.4 and 10.5) and in 7 there were significant atheromatous narrowings of a single coronary artery. In this mixed disease group the weights ranged from 407 to 773 g, with a mean of 593.6 g. Of the 14 patients for whom data were available, 2 were hypercholesterolaemic. This compares with the 15 out of 38 IHD patients in which similar information was available. Thus, both the groups that are composed primarily of IHD and of DCM patients contain cases with dual pathology, and this may be the situation in about 10% of cases in each group.

Only 1 of the 6 DCM patients previously operated on (transfused) has died of rejection. The other 5 are well. Of the patients who had not been

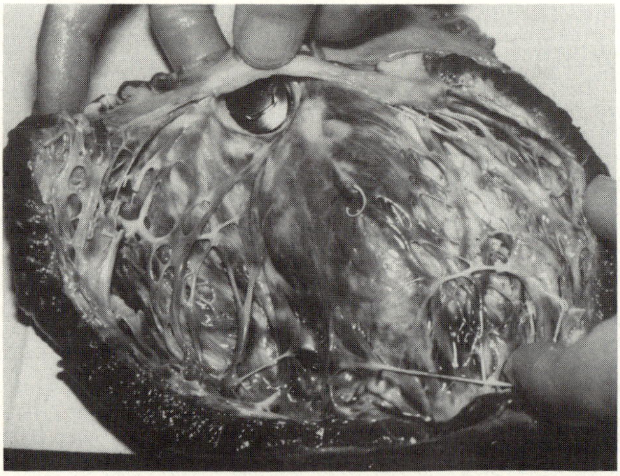

Fig. 10.5. *Dilated cardiomyopathy with previous mitral valve replacement. Note the diffuse endocardial fibrosis.*

previoulsy operated upon, 1 died from the respiratory infection present at the time of transplantation, and another from intraoperative cardiac arrest and brain damage. An inadequate heart was responsible for death in another and lung cancer in a fourth. Twelve more have died of rejection and 7 of infection.

The histology of the excised hearts showed enlargement of the myocytes and nuclear hyperchromatism, with an increase of fibrous tissue in nearly all cases. However, there was no, or only very minimal, inequality in myocyte size (anisocytosis) in half of the cases. The presence of anisocytosis (Fig. 10.6) is usually taken as a point in favour of cardiomyopathy rather than myocardial hypertrophy (Roberts, 1978; Fenoglio, 1982). Although fibrosis is regarded as a hallmark of DCM (Fenoglio, 1982; Factor and Sonnenblick, 1985), it was not present in 50% of the DCM hearts at necropsy described by Rose and Beck (1985). No fibrosis was evident in 7 (14%) of the Papworth cases, 6 of which had been symptomatic for 1 year or less. Of the cases with fibrosis, 42.5% had a similar short duration of symptoms. The fibrosis may increase with the duration of symptoms, as indicated by Rose and Beck (1985), but this can be only one of several factors operating to produce the same fibrotic end result.

The distribution of the fibrous tissue, whether it is sub-endocardial, midzonal or sub-epicardial, and whether it is perivascular, interstitial, plexiform or replacement in type, does not appear to be related to the aetiology or duration of clinical disease, and is only very poorly associated with the myocardial pathology (Anderson, Sutton and Lie, 1979; Rose and Beck, 1985). For Olson (1979) and Factor and Sonnenblick (1985) the fibrosis in DCM is

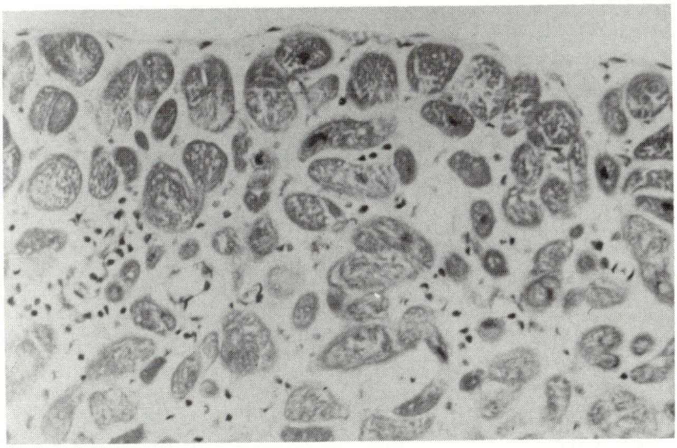

Fig. 10.6. *Dilated cardiomyopathy. Unequal-sized myocytes and interstitial fibrosis. A minimal lymphocytic infiltrate is also present. HPS × 160.*

mostly a combination of interstitial and replacement types, which can be produced by a multitude of agents. Both these authors find it impossible to distinguish alcoholic and puerperal cases histologically from other cases of DCM. The absence of distinctive histological features has also been the Papworth experience and in particular it was not possible to distinguish the histology of the solvent abuse case from other DCM cases (Wiseman and Banim, 1987). There is some evidence that the amount of interstitial fibrosis increases with the duration of the symptomatic illness (Oldershaw *et al.*, 1980; Rose and Beck, 1985).

Nuclear hypertrophy is a frequently observed feature in DCM and other forms of hypertrophy and possibly also in aging (Adler and Costabel, 1975). More recently, Unverferth *et al.* (1983) have described differences in the nucleolar structure in DCM and post-viral myocarditic patients on the one hand and normals, alcoholic and valvular heart disease on the other, with doxorubicin toxicity forming a third group. In the Papworth cases, there were 3 patients with very prominent single or double nucleoli in the hypertrophic nuclei of the myocytes. These nucleoli stained a bright pink with haematoxylin and eosin and had a well-defined border suggestive of viral inclusions (Fig. 10.7). However, on electron microscopy the structure of these bodies was that of a nucleolus.

Lymphocytic infiltrates in the myocardium in DCM were not discussed by Olsen in 1979, although later (1980) he reported finding myocarditis in 16 of 61 biopsies from patients considered to be suffering from congestive myopathy. More recently (1985a) he described focal accumulations of lymphocytes as being frequent. For Fenoglio (1982), inflammatory cells are not seen in DCM. However, Factor and Sonnenblick (1985) describe lymphocytes

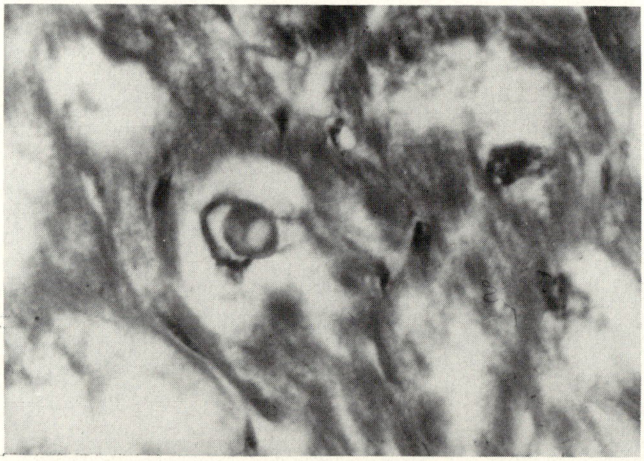

Fig. 10.7. *Prominent nucleolus in hypertrophic nucleus of DCM patient. HPS ×640.*

and histiocytes as being the most frequent cellular response. In the Papworth DCM cases, occasional scattered small lymphocytic foci were seen in 19 of 53 cases (A. Pattison, 1986, personal communication). Seven of these 19 patients gave a history of a viral illness and an eighth had suffered from Crohn's disease. Half of those patients with a history of viral-like illness had lymphocytic foci in their myocardium.

The assessment of these lymphocytic foci is not easy, partly because it is not always possible to distinguish transversely cut fibrocytes from lymphocytes in a sparsely cellular area of the section, and partly because the endothelial cells of collapsed capillaries and lymphatics may be difficult to identify. For these reasons, Edwards (1985) ignored counts of average numbers of lymphocytes less than 5 per ×400 microscopic field. However, for him any clumps of more than this number of lymphocytes represents myocarditis. Linder *et al.* (1985) have indicated that normal myocardium may contain up to 30 mononuclear cells/mm^2. Billingham (1985) has urged caution in accepting all lymphocytic infiltrates as indicating myocarditis, since these infiltrates were seen in 87% of 108 DCM cases at Stanford. Further, some normal donor hearts have also shown patchy infiltrates and only about 30% of cases considered clinically to be myocarditis showed cellular infiltrates on biopsy. These difficulties may be partly resolved if the stage of the myocarditis is taken into account (Dec *et al.*, 1985). Fenoglio *et al.* (1983) recognized acute, rapidly progressive and chronic stages and it is only this last stage that is difficult to distinguish from DCM.

In the analysis of the Papworth recipient hearts, myocarditis was recognized as areas of widespread lymphocytic infiltration, patchily distributed in the myocardium, with some myocyte damage and with some reparative

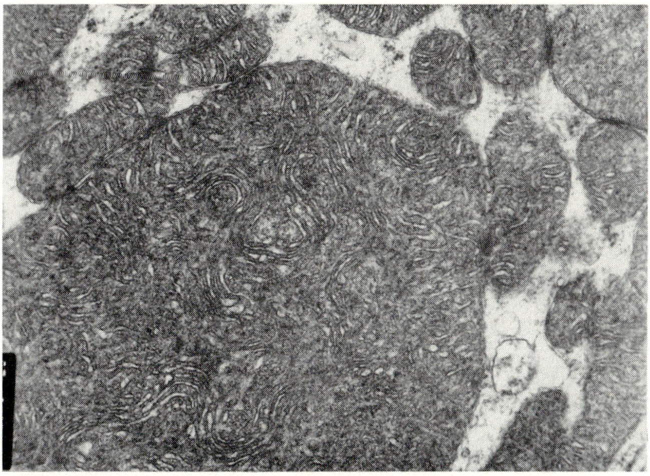

Fig. 10.8. *Giant mitochondrion. Compare the normal ovoid mitochondria on the top and right edges with the elongated ones in Fig. 10.2.* $\times 20\,800$.

fibrosis. Dilated cardiomyopathy cases had dilated ventricles with no or mild coronary artery disease, with no more than occasional small discrete foci of lymphocytes, and usually with some form of intramyocardial fibrosis. More studies are needed to clarify this important area of differential histological diagnosis.

Generally speaking, the use of electron microscopy in elucidating the nature of heart diseases and in particular DCM has been disappointing (Olsen, 1985a; Rose and Beck, 1985). This may well be due to the very small samples examined. As discussed in the chapter on detecting rejection (Chapter 15), even with 3 biopsies and using the much larger conventional sections examined with the light microscope, there is a 5% chance of missing a significant lesion (Spiegelhalter and Stovin, 1983).

Ultra-microscopical examination was made on left ventricular specimens from 53 DCM and 58 IHD hearts resected at Papworth. Mitochondriosis was seen in 8 and small mitochondria in 7 of the DCM cases, as compared to 1 and 3 IHD cases, respectively. These figures contrast with the observation of elongated mitochondria in 35 of the IHD cases and 25 of the DCM cases. Ring mitochondria (see Fig. 10.2) were seen occasionally in 5 DCM cases and in 4 of the IHD patients. Giant mitochondria (Fig. 10.8) were found in 2 IHD and in 1 DCM case. One of the DCM patients had been diagnosed on the basis of a skeletal muscle biopsy as having a mitochondrial myopathy. His ventricles showed very occasional ring and giant mitochondria — less than 0.5% of all mitochondria seen on the electron microscope grids. None

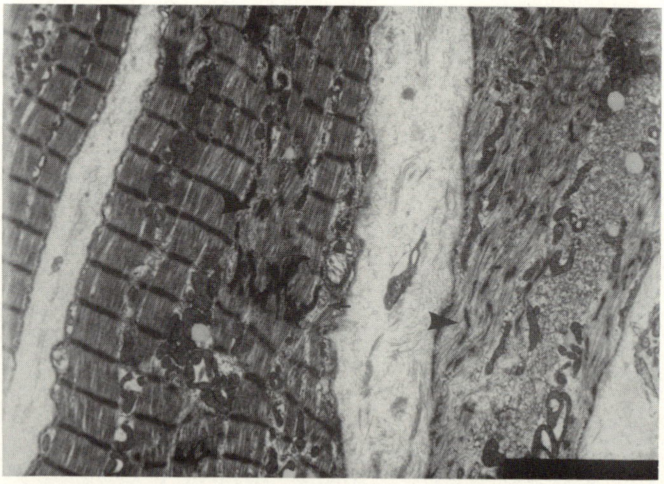

Fig. 10.9. *Degenerating myocyte to right of picture with disruption of myofibrils and distortion of and residual fragments of dark Z-band material (arrow). The irregular dark band across part of the central myocyte is a normal intercalated disc. Note the elongated mitochondria.* × *3250.*

of the cases with ring or giant mitochondria had a possible alcoholic or solvent abuse background.

The myofibrils showed a number of changes. Distorted, slurred or longitudinally running and degenerate Z-bands were seen (Fig. 10.9) more frequently in DCM cases (20) than in IHD cases (10). Attenuation of myofibrils was seen in 25 DCM but in only 8 IHD patients. In some cases the myofibrils had disappeared and their place was taken by a mass of sarcoplasmic reticulum (Fig. 10.10). This feature was encountered in 17 of the DCM cases and in 7 of the IHD cases. In other cases the myofibrils appeared to be replaced by glycogen granules or by oedema. These latter forms of replacement were seen in 6–8 cases each, in each of the two diagnostic groups. Likewise, occasional intracellular crossing-over of myofibrils was seen equally rarely in each group.

The only other feature that seemed possibly differently distributed in the two groups of cases was the position of the myocyte nucleus. In 3 of the DCM cases, nuclei were seen very close to the sarcolemma. This was not encountered in the IHD cases.

Myofibrillar attenuation, fragmentation and loss, together with proliferation of the sarcoplasmic reticulum, altered Z-bands and mitochondriosis, are generally regarded as features of hypertrophy with degeneration (Fenoglio, 1982; Rose and Beck, 1985). The ultrastructural changes in lymphocytic myocarditis have been reported by Ratcliff *et al.* (1987), who also found them to be similar to the changes in transplant rejection. Evaluation

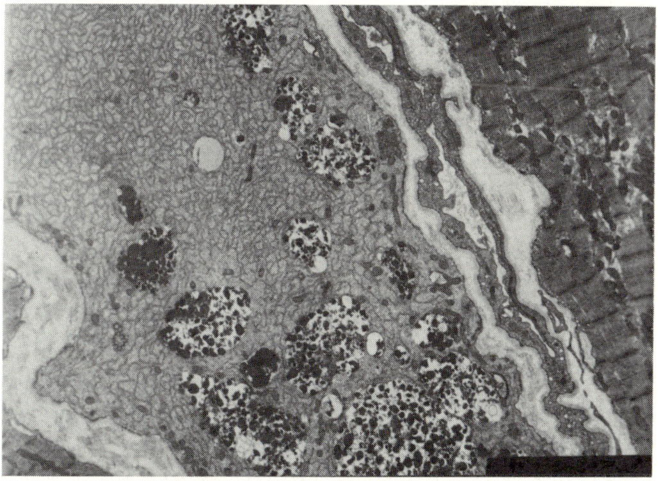

Fig. 10.10. *Mass of sarcoplasmic reticulum replacing myofibrils in degenerate myocyte. The vesicles with dark granules are lysosomal bodies.* × *2400.*

of the other features mentioned is very difficult and must await more detailed studies of individual cases.

Myocarditis

In the Papworth series, 10 patients were transplanted for myocarditis. In 5 this was rheumatic, 3 giant cell, 1 active eosinophilic endomyocarditis and 1 non-specific active myocarditis. In the Stanford series, valve disease with cardiomyopathy was the diagnosis in 5% of the recipients (Jamieson *et al.*, 1981); presumably some if not all were rheumatic. In the South African series, 12% of the recipients had rheumatic, or rheumatic with ischaemic, heart disease (Cooper *et al.*, 1983). Rheumatic disease was the reason for transplantation in 5.6% of the Texas cases (Frazier *et al.*, 1985) and valvular heart disease in 2.6% of the British cases reported by Pomerance and Stovin (1985). Three cases of sarcoid heart disease have undergone heart transplantation at Stanford and one at Harefield (H. A. Fleming, 1986, personal communication).

Of the 5 rheumatic heart disease patients in this group, 4 had had previous valve replacements. Three of these, and the fifth patient, had active rheumatic myocarditis. One of the patients with both valve replacement and active myocarditis had also had a pericardiectomy for calcified constrictive pericarditis which had been presumed, but not proved, to be tuberculous. The myocarditis in 2 of these cases contained the occasional giant cell in addition to the widespread mild lymphocytic infiltrate that was present in all

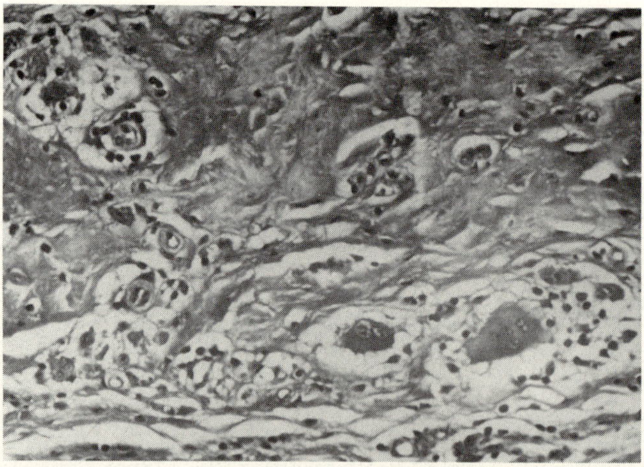

Fig. 10.11. *Active giant cell myocarditis in edge of intramyocardial scar. HPS ×200.*

4 cases. Aschoff nodules with fibrinoid degeneration of the collagen were not seen in any of the hearts. Ferrans, Rodriguez and McAllister (1985) distinguished two types of myocardial lesion in rheumatic fever: the specific granulomas and the non-specific chronic inflammatory cellular reaction. Although not typical, the giant cell granulomata in the 2 cases must be regarded as an indolent healing form of Aschoff nodule.

A rheumatic history was given by 2 other patients in the IHD group, one of whom had had an aortic valve replaced at the time of a coronary bypass graft. None of the DCM group had any evidence of rheumatic disease.

The 3 patients with giant cell myocarditis had chronic active disease which in one of them was considered to be probable sarcoid (Fig. 10.11). However, there was no evidence of any other tissue involvement to confirm this diagnosis. The importance of extracardiac involvement in the diagnosis of myocardial sarcoid has been stressed by Ferrans, Rodriguez and McAllister (1985). However, Fleming and Bailey (1981) have reported that cardiac involvement may precede evidence of other organ involvement by up to 3 years, and Roberts, McAllister and Ferrans (1977) observed that involvement of other organs in cases of myocardial sarcoidosis is often minimal.

A widespread chronic myocarditis was present in 1 of the remaining 3 patients and also in the resected donor heart removed from one of the rheumatic heart disease recipients 445 days after initial transplantation. The vast majority of the lymphocytes in this latter case were B cells on immunoperoxidase staining, and because of this continuing rejection was considered to be unlikely. There were no Aschoff nodules to indicate that this was a recurrence of the original rheumatic heart disease. Serological investigation failed to indict any virus. As not all myocarditis responds to immunosuppression (Mason, Billingham and Ricci, 1980; Fenoglio *et al.*, 1983; Daly *et al.*, 1984), it is possible that despite 445 days of immunosuppression this patient had a recurrence of his initial myocarditis.

The last case of this group was of eosinophilic myocarditis with relatively early endomyocardial fibrosis. This patient also had an aortic valve replacement and had vascularization of the pulmonary valve. He did not have any increase of circulating eosinophils nor did those present show degranulation. Degranulation, however, was present in the tissue eosinophils. Eosinophilic myocardial disorders have been recently reviewed by Spry, Take and Tai (1985) and in one case mentioned by them the mitral valve was involved.

All the cases in this group had dilated ventricles and there was none without some degree of endocardial fibrosis remote from the area of previous valve replacement. Additionally, all cases showed interstitial and replacement fibrosis consistent with healed past myocarditis. As with the DCM group, the heart weights showed a bimodal distribution: 5 below 460 g and 6 above 610 g. All 3 giant cell myocarditis cases were in the lower weight group, while 5 rheumatic cases and the eosinophilic myocarditis had the heaviest hearts.

Mild coronary artery stenoses were present in 2 cases in each of the weight groups. In the whole series the heart weights ranged from 330 to 791 g, with a mean of 570 g. These weights correlate strongly with the duration of symptoms; up to 3 years for the lighter cases, with a mean of 1.7 years compared with a mean of 20 years for the heavier cases (range 1.25–35 years). Whether the previous heart operation or the duration of symptoms was the more important factor in increasing heart weight is debatable, but all the 6 heavy hearts had had operations 1.25 or more years previously.

The heart weights of the 26 sarcoid patients of Roberts, McAllister and Ferrans (1977) ranged from 300 to 660 g, with a mean of 428 g. The relatively low weights of the 3 Papworth giant cell myocarditic cases might well be related to the 1–3 years' duration of the symptoms, but do not exclude the possibility that they are a type of myocardial sarcoid.

Endomyocardial fibrosis

There are 4 patients in this group in the Papworth series. The ages range from 6 to 44 years and the heart weights from 206 to 591 g. All had grey to white thickening of the endocardium of the right atrium and both ventricles, but this thickening was most marked in the left ventricle (Fig. 10.12), which was mildly dilated in 2 and considerably dilated in the oldest patient. This patient (aged 44) was also the only one in the group to have a plaque of thrombus in the left ventricle and a few lymphocytes in the myocardium near the thrombus. No eosinophils were seen in any of the patients. The

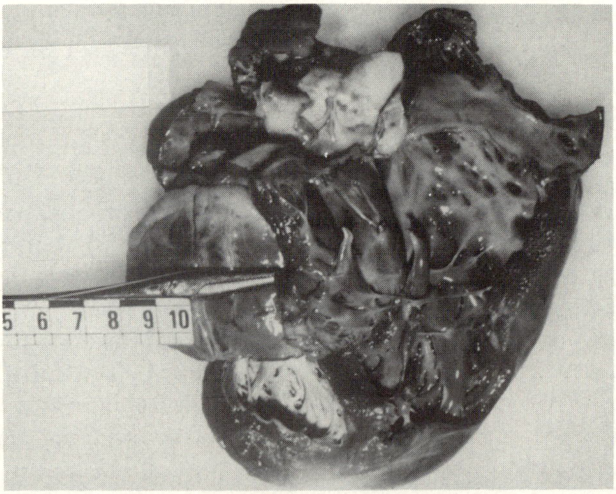

Fig. 10.12. *Endomyocardial fibrosis in both ventricles but more dense in the left which is seen through the opened right ventricle and septum.*

youngest, aged 6 years, had had a brother who had died from the same condition, while a 9-year-old girl had had a brother with a cardiomyopathy The oldest had a fairly strong family history of ischaemic heart disease. Three of the patients also gave a history of viral infection either starting or worsening their symptoms. One of the patients with a viral history was sero-negative for rheumatoid arthritis.

Histologically, the picture was of endocardial thickening by fibrous tissue with a variable increase in elastic fibrils, and with extensions of this abnormal endocardium into the myocardium. There was also a variable degree of interstitial fibrosis in the myocardium. The coronary arteries were normal.

Although Roberts and Ferrans (1975) and Olsen (1979) have both commented on the presence of eosinophils in the early active stage of this condition, the presence of these cells is not necessary for making the histological diagnosis, which rests on the involvement of several of the cardiac chambers and on the spread of the endocardial fibrosis into the myocardium. However, even in the late fibrotic stage Tai *et al.* (1987) have been able to demonstrate the presence of one or more of the different eosinophil granule proteins.

Hypertrophic cardiomyopathy

This has been the most uniform group of resected hearts, with weights ranging from 234 to 485 g (mean 366.8 g). Only the heaviest showed any dilatation of the left ventricular cavity (Fig. 10.13). The ages of the 6

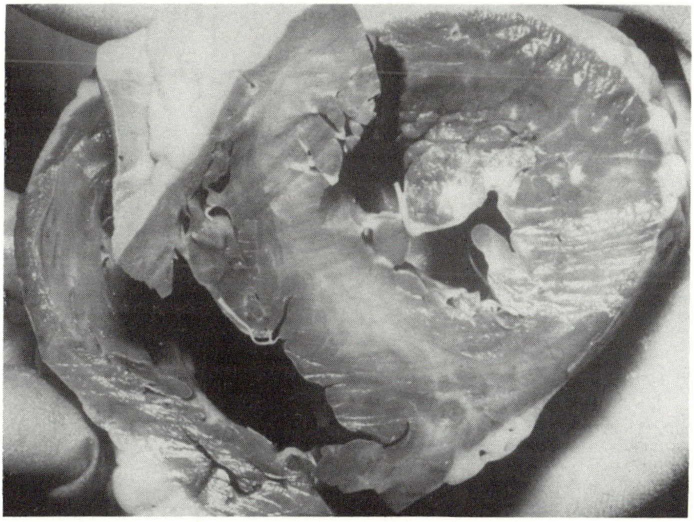

Fig. 10.13. *Hypertrophic cardiomyopathy. The left ventricular cavity is very small and there is obvious pale fibrosis in the thickened myocardium.*

patients ranged from 18 to 50 years (mean 35.2) and only one gave a family history of cardiomyopathy. Two gave a history of cerebral embolic episodes. Calcification was present in the mitral valve ring in one and in the myocardium adjacent to a pacing electrode in another. This latter also had a small focus of amyloid in the left ventricle and a patent foramen ovale. Scattered small endocardial papillomata were present in another heart. In 3 of the hearts the hypertrophy was asymmetrical, with pronounced bulging of the sub-aortic region of the septum. In all cases there were frequent multidirectional myocytes with hypertrophy and interstitial pericellular fibrosis (Fig. 10.14), and in most cases irregular intimal fibrosis of the intramyocardial arterioles.

The specificity of the pathological finding of myocyte disarray with multidirectional myofibrils within the myocytes, together with the pericellular plexiform fibrosis, has been reviewed by Wigle and Silver (1978) and by Olsen (1982). The problem is that while these features can be seen in parts of the normal or hypertrophied heart, they are seen more frequently and more widely distributed in the left ventricle in hypertrophic cardiomyopathy (HCM). The distribution of the fibrosis has been analysed by cross-sectional echocardiography by Shapiro, Kleinebenne and McKenna (1985), who found that distal ventricular hypertrophy was the most specific feature distinguishing HCM from hypertensive or athletic hypertrophy. Asymmetrical hypertrophy was seen in all three of their groups, but about 2.5 times more frequently in HCM than in either of the other two. The amount of fibrosis is

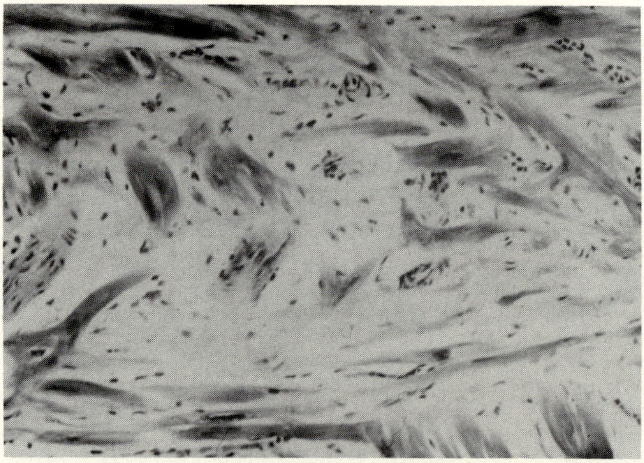

Fig. 10.14. *HCM showing the typical multidirectional myocytes with plexiform pericellular fibrosis. HPS ×70.*

also greater in HCM than in hypertension (Tanaka *et al.*, 1986). The extent of the myocyte disorganization has been quantified by Maron and Roberts (1981), who concluded that if more than 5% of a section from the interventricular septum (IVS) shows the change, then HCM is highly likely. Of

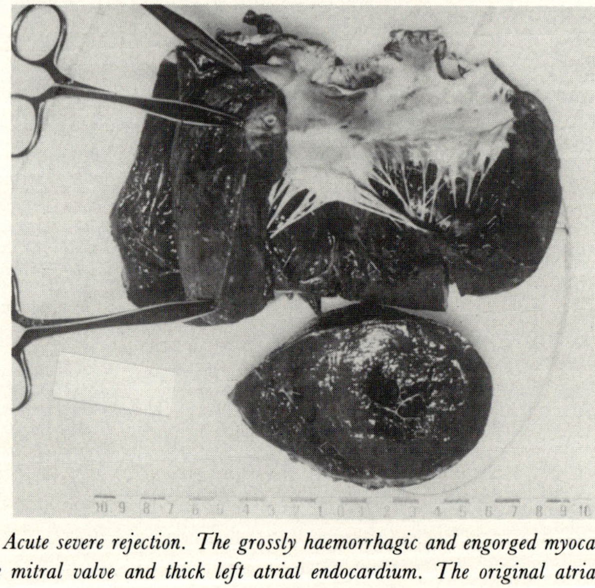

Fig. 10.15. *Acute severe rejection. The grossly haemorrhagic and engorged myocardium contrasts with the pale mitral valve and thick left atrial endocardium. The original atrial suture line is evident along the upper border.*

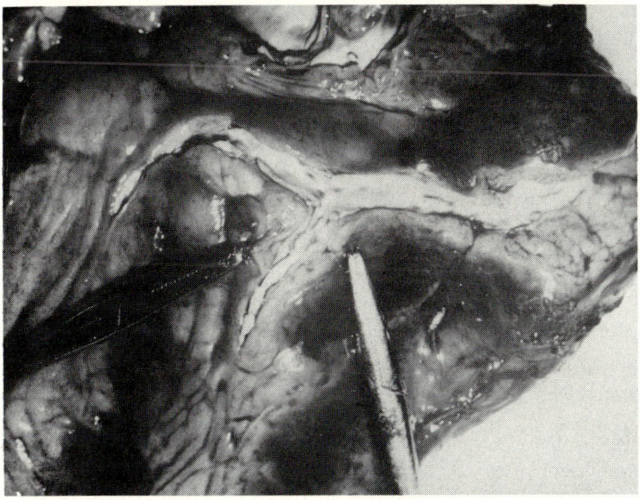

Fig. 10.16. *Chronic rejection. Right coronary artery opened to show the diffuse fairly uniform thickening of the endothelium without the focal plaques seen in atheroma.*

their 78 cases, 24% had 50% or more of the IVS affected. None of the Papworth cases showed involvement to this extent, although all had more than 5%. It may be that the Papworth cases were operated on at a relatively early stage, which might account for the relatively low heart weights and lesser degree of myocyte disorganization. The mean heart weight in the series of Tanaka *et al.* (1986) was 580 g and in the series of Maron and Roberts (1979), 535 g. In the Papworth cases, symptoms had been present for more than 10 years in 5 cases and more than 20 years in 4; the sixth patient had been symptomatic for 18 months.

Re-transplantation

This has been undertaken six times at Papworth. On three occasions this was an emergency procedure for severe acute rejection occurring at 9–41 days after transplantation (Fig. 10.15). One other emergency operation was performed because of acute-on-chronic rejection 1097 days after the original transplant operation. The remaining 2 patients were re-transplanted electively at 445 and 1168 days for recurrent myocarditis and for chronic rejection, respectively (Fig. 10.16). These 2 cases are alive 135 and 814 days after their re-transplantations, but all the emergency reoperation cases died within 13 days. The artificial heart may well be very helpful in managing acute severe irreversible rejection, to tide the recipient over until a suitable second donor heart is obtained (Joyce *et al.*, 1986).

By 1980 the Stanford group had re-transplanted 16 hearts (Watson *et al.*, 1980). The commonest indication was the accelerated coronary artery atheroma of chronic rejection, followed by unrelenting rejection. Although the survival prospect following a second transplant is less favourable than after the first, these authors found no difference in the frequency distribution of the causes of death between the first and second transplant cases. However, no mention was made of the effect of emergency compared with a more tranquil acceptance of a potential donor on the final outcome. In the South African series of 7 re-transplants after initial heterotopic transplantation, 1 was lost from early acute rejection (Lanza and Cooper, 1984). The advantage of heterotopic transplantation is that severe acute rejection of the donated heart can be tolerated by the recipient until a suitable new donor can be found, thus avoiding the possible need to accept a poor-quality donor organ in an emergency.

There is no doubt about the timing for re-transplantation in cases of severe acute rejection where increased immunosuppression has been unavailing. On the other hand, in chronic rejection the timing is more difficult to determine because the patient with a denervated transplanted heart cannot experience angina, and the main symptoms of progressive decrease in exercise tolerance, increasing weight or dyspnoea are insidiously progressive.

None of the Papworth cases of acute rejection was as acute as the case reported by Koep *et al.* (1981), in which irreversible rejection occurred on the operating table. Although a retrospective lymphocyte crossmatch showed cytotoxic antibodies in the recipient's serum, these authors give no indication of their origin. Anderson *et al.* (1979) demonstrated by an indirect immunofluorescence technique the presence of heart-reactive antibodies in 10–15% of patients coming to open-heart operation or transplantation. One of the Papworth patients initially transplanted for IHD rejected the heart at 11 days and the second heart at 6 days. His lymphocyte crossmatch showed cytotoxic antibodies on both occasions. There was mismatching at the HLA-B locus on the first and at the HLA-A locus on the second occasion. Histologically, this patient had in both the transplanted hearts an acute haemorrhagic vascular form of rejection rather than a severe cell-mediated rejection. As in the case of Lanza *et al.* (1983) there was a more vigorous rejection response to the second transplanted heart in this pre-sensitized recipient.

In another of the acutely rejecting hearts, the rejection was also of a vascular type. There were intracapillary thrombi and swelling of the vascular endothelium, with virtually no interstitial cellular infiltration. This patient was described by Hakim *et al.* (1985a). They thought that the occurrence of severe rejection and the absence of any nephrotoxicity, despite the presence of high normal blood levels, might possibly be due to an absence of cyclosporin (Cy) receptors. This patient could not be adequately sustained on cardiopulmonary bypass for the 6 h required before a replacement heart became available. Although the re-transplantation was performed, he died 12 h later. Vascular endothelial antibodies have been implicated in early acute rejection by Brasile *et al.* (1985). The major histocompatibility antigens have been demonstrated on the endothelium of the ventricles and of the small intramyocardial vessels, but not so readily on the large vessels or on the myocytes (Lautenschlager *et al.*, 1984). It may be that this vascular type of rejection is precipitated earlier than, and also is not as effectively suppressed by Cy, as the cell-mediated type of rejection.

Inadequate donor heart preservation and infection caused the deaths in the other two emergency re-transplant operations.

One of the elective re-transplantations is of interest in that his heart was originally replaced because of continuing active rheumatic carditis. For about 2 months before his re-transplantation he had been developing progressive heart failure considered to be due to chronic rejection. However, the heart showed a diffuse mild cellular infiltrate similar to that in the original heart, and which consisted almost entirely of B-cell lymphocytes. The amount of chronic arterial rejection was only mild. This appears to be a recurrence of the original pathology rather than either acute or chronic rejection.

Miscellaneous conditions

In most transplant centres the operation has been occasionally undertaken for an unusual cause of heart failure. The list includes congenital abnormalities such as ventricular septal defect with bacterial endocarditis and congenital aortic stenosis, Uhl's anomaly (Fig. 10.17), uncontrolled dysrhythmia (Watson *et al.*, 1980), post-traumatic aneurysm (Jamieson *et al.*, 1981), amyloid, myocardial storage diseases and cardiac involvement in diffuse pulmonary angiomatosis (A. Pomerance, 1986, personal communication), adriamycin cardiotoxicity, and tumours such as fibroma (M. E. Billingham, 1986, personal communication) and neurofibrosarcoma (Pomerance and Stovin, 1985). Alcoholic myopathy and puerperal cardiomyopathy cannot be separated histopathologically from DCM and have been discussed in that group. In the Papworth series it was not possible to distinguish the heart of the patient who had a history of solvent abuse from other DCM cases, and to this extent it would seem to act in a similar way to alcohol.

There is a sizable group of recipients who can be classed as failed surgical corrections of either valvular or coronary artery disease. Although their study might yield some insight into techniques for improving myocardial protection, they have been considered above under their basic cardiac disease.

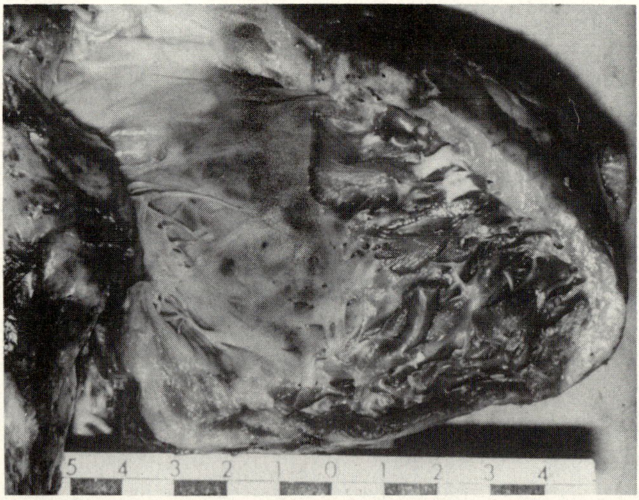

Fig. 10.17. *Uhl's anomaly. The septal half of the right ventricle viewed from the right. The cut edge of the anterior free wall of the right ventricle is pale fatty tissue and contrasts with the darker more normal cut edge of the inferior and septal walls.*

Complex transplantations

Under this heading are included heart–lung, heart–liver and heart–kidney transplants.

The pulmonary pathology of heart–lung transplants is considered in Chapter 11. The heart is not normal in these cases and shows marked right ventricular hypertrophy with dilatation of the tricuspid valve ring. Up to September 1986, 13 heart–lung transplants have been carried out at Papworth: 4 for cardiac septal defects, 2 for end-stage pulmonary fibrosis, 2 for emphysema, 2 for primary pulmonary hypertension, and 1 case each for embolic pulmonary hypertension, cystic fibrosis and eosinophilic granuloma. The heart weights of these 13 patients varied from 194 g to 696 g, with a mean of 337.9 g. Only in the heaviest heart (Eisenmenger ASD) did the grossly thickened (1.2 cm) right ventricle distort the left ventricular cavity from the usual circular cross-section into a D-shaped cross-section with a straight ventricular septum — a sort of reversed Bernheim effect. Apart from the single case of cystic fibrosis, the left ventricular cavity was not dilated and in none was there gross left ventricular hypertrophy. However, in 1 of the 2 emphysema patients there was a mild degree of left ventricular myocyte hypertrophy and in this patient the right ventricular myocytes were hypertrophied up to 60 μm diameter. The other cases showed lesser degrees of right ventricular myocyte hypertrophy, the least in 1 case of emphysema and 1 of severe pulmonary fibrosis.

There was a mild interstitial lymphocytic infiltrate mainly in the left side of the heart in both the emphysema patients, the cystic fibrosis patient, the patient with pulmonary eosinophilic granuloma and 1 of the 2 VSD patients. Both the emphysema patients showed some degree of interstitial myocardial fibrosis.

The 2 VSD hearts showed the usual billowing and thickening of the septal leaf of the tricuspid valve.

The heart–liver transplants reported by Shaw *et al.* (1985) and Figuera *et al.* (1986) were performed for severe coronary artery disease due to hypercholesterolaemia in 3 cases and for cardiomyopathy with biliary hypoplasia. The latter case is of interest because the liver transplant was undertaken 3 weeks after the heart transplantation. The 2 surviving cases have a sustained lowering of the serum cholesterol levels.

There has been one heart–kidney transplant at Papworth, on a youth of 18 who had failed to thrive from his first year of life. He had been in renal failure for some years and on continuous peritoneal dialysis for the 8 months prior to transplantation. A skeletal muscle biopsy had shown a mitochondrial myopathy. His heart weighed 278 g and showed marked myocyte hypertrophy with very prominent inclusion-like nucleoli, some interstitial fibrosis and a more marked endocardial fibrosis. Ultrastructurally, a few ring and giant mitochondria were seen in occasional myocytes. This case has been included in the DCM group above because of the mitochondrial abnormalities and the generalized 'myopathic' hypertrophy of the myocytes, even though there was little ventricular dilatation and endocardial fibrosis was present. A synchronous heterotopic renal transplant from the same donor was performed without removal or biopsy of the patient's own kidneys. A similar heart–kidney operation has been performed at Padua on an IHD patient with irreversible chronic renal failure (Galluci *et al.*, 1986). It will probably not be long before there are reports of renal transplants in heart transplant patients who have developed irreversible renal failure from their Cy treatment.

Recently, a heart–lung–liver transplant has been performed for biliary cirrhosis and primary pulmonary hypertension.

PROGNOSTIC INDICATORS

Cooper *et al.* (1983) found that the following list of factors increased patient survival after heart transplantation: age less than 40 years, rheumatic heart disease, and (if the patients survived the first 2 months) previous blood transfusion and the presence of B blood group antigen. Compatibility between donor and recipient at one or two HLA loci, and non-white donor, also increased survival. Hassell, Fowles and Stinson (1981) observed in the

Stanford transplants that congestive cardiomyopathy patients survived better than ischaemic cases, and that in both groups those under 40 did better than those over this age. In the pre-cyclosporin era, Bieber *et al.* (1981) reported that mismatches at HLA-A2 and -A3, and a serum triglyceride level above 200 mg/dl, were associated with graft atheroma. Recently, Yacoub *et al.* (1987) have reported on the factors influencing survival in the Harefield patients: age, recipient heart pathology and previous transfusion had no effect, whereas HLA-DR mismatches and donor/recipient lymphocytotoxic crossmatch did affect the prognosis. HLA-A and -B mismatches had little effect. For Keogh, Baron and Chang (1987), prior blood transfusion had a slight but not statistically significant beneficial effect.

In the Papworth experience, donor-transmitted infection with toxoplasma and CMV has been recognized as a hazard that can be determined at or very soon after operation, and effective prophylaxis is therefore possible (Hakim *et al.*, 1985b). There have also been a few instances where other donor or recipient disease present at the time of operation has led to early death, such as recipient intraoperative cardiac arrest with cerebral damage, recipient pneumonia at the time of operation, donor coronary artery disease, and excessive donor inotropic support prior to the transplant. These are cases where the risks were appreciated to be very high, but the circumstances were thought at the time to warrant completion of the operation. These potentially preventable deaths have been excluded from the following study on all the first-time heart transplants who could have survived 150 days or longer. This 150-day period was chosen because 75% of all the deaths occurred within this time. The maximum follow-up period for patients still alive is 2436 days. These considerations have allowed a study of 143 patients, of whom 49 (34.3%) have died.

Of the 71 IHD patients, 38% have died, and of the 55 DCM patients, 34.6% have died. The remaining miscellaneous group of 17 patients had a 17.7% mortality. There was no consistent difference in survival between successive decennial age groups or between the A,B or O blood groups. There was, however, a curious under-representation of group O in the IHD patients (23%) compared with the national average (45%), or to the incidence (41%) in DCM patients. Only 7 patients had rheumatic heart disease and of these 3 had died of rejection and 1 of infection, which is a higher mortality than in the group as a whole, but the numbers are very small.

Forty-five patients had received blood transfusions up to 35 years prior to the transplant operation. Of these, 13% have died of rejection and 7% of infection. Of the 98 patients not transfused, 27.6% have died of rejection and 10% of infection. There is therefore a definite beneficial effect of transfusion in reducing rejection deaths.

Whereas the donor was of the same ABO and rhesus blood group in 93 cases, there were 24 with ABO dissimilarity and 35 with rhesus dissimilarity, in 9 of which both ABO and rhesus groups were dissimilar. Deaths occurred in 31.2% of the identical group, 33.3% of the ABO non-identical group and in 41.7% of the rhesus non-identical group. However, with the small subgroup with combined dissimilarity, only 2 patients (22.2%) have died. In the rhesus mismatches the ratio of rejection to infection is 3 to 2, while in the cases without mismatch the ratio is 4 to 1, the ABO mismatches being intermediate. This might suggest that infection could be occurring because of slightly excessive immunosuppression.

HLA typing is very complex and the categorization of transplants by numbers of HLA identities is an over-simplification of the problem of assessing the effect of tissue typing. However, this does have the merit of comprehensibility and it does appear to have some value. HLA typing was available in 140 donor–recipient pairs for A and B groups and for DR in 88 pairs. Deaths from infection were distributed in an inverse frequency to that of rejection for any tissue type or combination of tissue types. Considering each of the 3 tissue types singly, with no identities 25.3% of 79 A cases, 29.8% of 94 B cases and 20.4% of 49 DR cases died of rejection. If there was one identity, then 19.3% of 57 A cases, 13.6% of 44 B cases and 16.2% of 37 DR cases died of rejection. There were only between 2 and 4 cases with 2 identities within each of the tissue types (Table 10.2). If now A + B are considered together, then the deaths from rejection are lowered only when there is identity in 1 of each group (9.1% of 22 patients) compared with 28.6% and 39.4% of 56 and 33 cases where there is none or one identity only. Numbers are even smaller if all three tissue types are considered together, but there have been no deaths from rejection or infection in the 6 cases with 1 identity in all three of the groups. The groups with 0, 1 or 2 identities were of nearly equal size (23, 30 and 26 patients) and had nearly equal incidences of death from rejection (21.7%, 20% and 19.2%, respectively). It therefore seems that it is the spread of identities rather than the number which matters. Further, the inverse frequency of rejection and of infection deaths suggests that the infections might be related to over-immunosuppression following rejection.

There was no difference between the 42 patients with identity at the HLA-A2 and -A3 loci and the 98 with dissimilarity, in respect of the incidence of death from chronic or acute rejection or infection.

Other factors which were examined were the presence of hypercholesterolaemia, history of hypertension and family history of heart disease. The only factor which might be of influence is hypertension, but the numbers are small. Of 13 hypertensives, 23% have died compared with 36.4% of 132 non-hypertensives. Deaths have occurred in 41% of the hypercholesterolaemic (>6.8 mmol/litre) and in 36% of the non-hypercholesterolaemic patients and in 35% of the patients with and 38% of the patients without a family history. On theoretical grounds it is likely that

TABLE 10.2
Effect of HLA Matching on Death From Rejection and Infection

HLA Type		*Total No. of matches*	*Rejection No.*	*Rejection %*	*Infection No.*	*Infection %*	*Other No.*
A	0	79	20	25.3	6	7.6	1
	1	57	10	17.5	5	8.8	1
	2	4	3	75	0	0	
B	0	94	28	29.8	6	6.4	1
	1	44	5	11.4	5	11.4	1
	2	2	0		0		0
A + B	0	56	16	28.6	5	8.7	1
	1	33	13	39.4	2	6.1	0
	1 + 1	22	1	11.6	4	18.2	1
	2 + 0	5	3	60	0		0
	3	1	0		0		0
DR	0	49	10	20.4	4	8.2	0
	1	37	6	16.2	1	2.7	1
	2	2	1		0		0
AB + DR	0	23	5	21.7	2	8.7	0
	1	30	6	20	1	3.3	1
	1 + 1	26	4	15.4	3	11.5	0
	2 + 0	2	2		0		0
	1 + 1 + 1	6	0		0		1
	2 + 1	1	0		0		0
	4	1	0		0		0

the follow-up on these patients is not long enough for the effect of hypercholesterolaemia to become manifest in the coronary arteries.

The effect of intraoperative blood transfusion on survival has been discussed by Shelby *et al.* (1985) and demonstrated in mice. It is difficult to assess this in the human situation, as all the operations are performed with transfusion. The experience of re-transplantation indicates that donor- and recipient-related factors are more powerful, and are not compensated for by the transfusion or the previous operation.

The most important factors promoting a satisfactory outcome of the transplant operation are the avoidance of a toxoplasma and CMV mismatch (positive donor into a negative recipient), previous transfusion in the recipient, the avoidance of rhesus mismatching between donor and recipient, a spread of identities across as many HLA groups as possible, and no infection or intraoperative cardiac arrest in the recipient.

RESEARCH AND CONCLUSIONS

The freshly excised recipient heart is a unique source of both normal and pathological tissue in relatively large bulk that can be used for a wide range of research purposes. This section will mention a number of investigations known to the author, but as heart transplantation does not appear in the title of these publications it is not possible to make any systematic check on the extent to which use is actually being made of this recipient material.

It is helpful to group the studies under anatomical, biochemical, pathological and physiological headings.

Anatomical studies of recipient hearts are typified by the ultrastructural description of the human conduction tissue by Vassall-Adams (1983). This type of study is only possible using the freshly excised recipient heart because the preservation of virtually all post-mortem tissue is not good enough for ultrastructural studies. For the purist, the fixation of human heart tissue for electron microscopical examination can never be quite as good as in the experimental animal where perfusion-fixation gives superb results. In the human case, there are the effects of the anaesthetic, the cardiac arrest, the surgical handling and the time from arrest to completion of the excision, all of which can produce artefacts. Nevertheless, this material is the best source of human heart tissue.

The distribution of neuropeptide-Y in the human heart has been studied by Kerwin *et al.* (1985), who confirmed that in the fresh state it was the same as had been seen in necropsy material.

The biochemical group includes a wide range of possible studies. Myosin variants in normal and pathological hearts have been studied by Leger *et al.* (1984). Henney, Parker and Davies (1982) have studied collagen biosynthesis in heart valves. Henney has proceeded to study with other collaborators the degradation of collagen in heart valves (Henney, Dingle and Decker, 1984; Henney and Decker, 1987).

Adomian, Laks and Billingham (1978) have used the donor heart biopsies to study the incidence of contraction bands. These authors came to the important conclusion that contraction bands are produced by the biopsy procedure and do not indicate a pathological state, as they do if seen in necropsy material.

The heart from a DCM recipient was used as one of the sources of antigen production in a study on cellular immunity in congestive cardiomyopathy by Lowry, Thompson and Littler (1985).

Pharmacological studies have assessed the inotropic effectiveness of a number of substances on congestive and ischaemic myocardium (Cameron *et al.*, 1985; English *et al.*, 1986). B-adrenergic–receptor density was shown by Bristow *et al.* (1982) to be decreased in failing human hearts.

In conclusion, therefore, heart transplantation has made it possible to get better insights into the anatomy, pathology, physiology and biochemistry of the human heart in disease and indirectly in health.

REFERENCES

Adler, C.-P. and Costabel, U. (1975). Cell number in human heart in atrophy, hypertrophy, and under the influence of cytostatics. In *Recent Advances in Studies on Cardiac Structure and Metabolism*, Vol. 6. (A. Fleckenstein and G. Rona, Eds), pp. 343–355. University Park Press, Baltimore.

Adomian, G. E., Laks, M. M. and Billingham, M. E. (1978). The incidence and significance of contraction bands in endomyocardial biopsies from normal human hearts. *Am. Heart J.*, **95**, 348–351.

Anderson, J. L., Carlquist, J. F. and Hammond, E. H. (1982). Deficient natural killer cell activity in patients with idiopathic dilated cardiomyopathy. *Lancet* **2**, 1124–1127.

Anderson, J. L., Fowles, R. E., Stinson, E. B., Yuge, C., Bieber, C. P. and Harrison, D. C. (1979). Occurrence of circulating heart-reactive antibodies in a population of cardiac transplant recipients. Correlation with cardiac rejection and subsequent course. *Circulation* **60**, 629–637.

Anderson, K. R., Sutton, M. G. St. J. and Lie, J. T. (1979). Histopathological types of cardiac fibrosis in myocardial disease. *J. Pathol.*, **128**, 79–85.

Bieber, C. P., Hunt, S. A., Schwinn, D. A., Jamieson, S. A., Reitz, B. A., Oyer, P. E., Shumway, N. E. and Stinson, E. B. (1981). Complications in long-term survivors of cardiac transplantation. *Transplant. Proc.* **13**, 207–211.

Billingham, M. E. (1985). The diagnostic criteria of myocarditis by endomyocardial biopsy. *Heart Vess.* **1**, Suppl. 1, 133–137.

Boucher, C. A., Fallon, J. T., Johnson, R. A. and Yurchak, P. M. (1979). Cardiomyopathic syndrome caused by coronary artery disease. III: Prospective clinicopathological study of its prevalence among patients with clinically unexplained chronic heart failure. *Br. Heart J.* **41**, 613–620.

Bowles, N. E., Richardson, P. J., Olsen, E. G. J. and Archard, L. C. (1986). Detection of coxsackie-B-virus-specific RNA sequences in myocardial biopsy samples from patients with myocarditis and dilated cardiomyopathy. *Lancet* **1**, 1120–1123.

Brasile, L., Zerbe, T., Rabin, B., Clarke, J., Abrams, A. and Cerilli, J. (1985). Identification of the antibody to vascular endothelial cells in patients undergoing cardiac transplantation. *Transplantation* **40**, 672–675.

Bristow, M. R., Ginsberg, R., Minobe, W., Cubicciotti, R. S., Scott-Sageman, W., Lurie, K., Billingham, M. E., Harrison, D. C. and Stinson, E. B. (1982). Decreased catecholamine sensitivity and B-adrenergic-receptor density in failing human hearts. *New Engl. J. Med.* **307**, 205–211.

Cabrol, C., Gandjbakhch, I., Pavie, A., Cabrol, A., Mattei, M. F., Lienhart, A., Gluckman, J. C. and Rottembourg, J. (1983). Transplantation cardiaque. Etat actuel a l'hôpital de La Pitié. *Presse Med.* **12**, 2521–2526.

Cameron, D., English, T. A. H., Gristwood, R. W., Morl, C. J., Owen, D. A. A. and Wallwork, J. (1985). Positive inotropic actions of SK&F 94120 on human isolated ventricular myocardium. *Br. J. Pharmacol.* **85**, Suppl., 226P.

Commerford, P. J. (1984). Selection and management of the recipient. In *Heart Transplantation: The Present Status of Orthotopic and Heterotopic Heart Transplantation* (D. K. C. Cooper and R. P. Lanza, Eds), pp. 15–22. MTP Press, Lancaster.

Cooper, D. K. C., Lanza, R. P., Boyd, S. T. and Barnard, C. N. (1983). Factors influencing survival following heart transplantation. *Heart Transplant.* **3**, 89–91.

Copeland, J. G., Emery, R. W., Levinson, M. M., Copeland, J., McAleer, M. J. and Riley, J. E. (1985). The role of mechanical support and transplantation in treatment of patients with end-stage cardiomyopathy. *Circulation* **72**, Suppl. 2, 7–12.

Daly, K., Richardson, P. J., Olsen, E. G. J., Morgan-Capner, P., McSorley, C., Jackson, G. and Jewitt, D. E. (1984). Acute myocarditis. Role of histological and virological examination in the diagnosis and assessment of immunosuppressive treatment. *Br. Heart J.* **51**, 30–35.

Dash, H., Johnson, R. A., Dinsmore, R. E. and Harthorne, J. W. (1977). Cardiomyopathic syndrome due to coronary artery disease. I: Relation to angiographic extent of coronary disease and to remote myocardial infarction. *Br. Heart J.*, **39**, 733–739.

Davies, M. J. and Pomerance, A. (1975). Surgical, traumatic and iatrogenic heart disease. In *The Pathology of the Heart* (A. Pomerance and M. J. Davies, Eds.), pp. 411–480. Blackwell, Oxford.

Davies, M. J., Woolf, N. and Robertson, W. B. (1976). Pathology of acute myocardial infarction with particular reference to occlusive coronary thrombi. *Br. Heart J.* **38**, 659–664.

Dec, G. W., Palacios, I. F., Fallon, J. T., Aretz, H. T., Mills, J., Lee, D. C-S. and Johnson, R. A. (1985). Active myocarditis in the spectrum of acute dilated cardiomyopathies. Clinical features, histologic correlates, clinical outcome. *New Engl. J. Med.* **312**, 885–890.

Dong, E., Stinson, E. B., Griepp, R. B., Coulson, A. S. and Shumway, N. E. (1973). Cardiac transplantation following failure of previous cardiac surgery. *Surg. Forum* **24**, 150–152.

Edwards, W. D. (1985). Current problems in establishing quantitative histopathologic criteria for the diagnosis of lymphocytic myocarditis by endomyocardial biopsy. In *Myocarditis and Related Disorders: Proceedings of the International Symposium on Cardiomyopathy and Myocarditis* (M. Sekiguchi, E. G. J. Olsen and J. F. Goodwin, Eds), pp. 138–142. Springer-Verlag, Tokyo.

English, T. A. H., Gristwood, R. W., Owen, D. A. A., Sampford, K. A. and Wallwork, J. (1986). Effects of dopamine on human ventricle *in vitro*: comparison with effects of isoprenaline, epinine and ibopamine. *Br. J. Pharmacol.* **87**, Suppl., 203P.

Factor, S. M. and Sonnenblick, E. H. (1985). The pathogenesis of clinical and experimental congestive cardiomyopathies: recent concepts. *Prog. Cardiovasc. Dis.* **27**, 395–420.

Fenoglio, J. J. (1982). The cardiomyopathies: diagnosis by endomyocardial biopsy. In *Endomyocardial Biopsy: Techniques and Application* (J. J. Fenoglio, Ed.), pp. 97–110. CRC Press Inc., Boca Raton.

Fenoglio, J. J., Ursell, P. C., Kellogg, C. F., Drusin, R. E. and Weiss, M. B. (1983). Diagnosis and classification of myocarditis by endomyocardial biopsy. *New Engl. J. Med.* **308**, 12–18.

Ferrans, V. J., Rodriguez, E. R. and McAllister, H. A. (1985). Granulomatous inflammation of the heart. In *Myocarditis and Related Disorders: Proceedings of the International Symposium on Cardiomyopathy and Myocarditis* (M. Sekiguchi, E. G. J. Olsen and J. F. Goodwin, Eds.), pp. 262–270. Springer-Verlag, Tokyo.

Figuera, D., Ardaiz, J., Martin-Judez, V., Pulpon, L. A., Pradas, G., Cuervas-Mons, V., Burgos, R., Arcas, M., Pardo, F., Cienfuegos, J. A., Turrion, V. S., Tellez, G. and Sanz-Ortega, E. (1986). Combined transplantation of heart and liver from two different donors in a patient with familial type IIa hypercholesterolaemia. *J. Heart Transplant.* **5**, 327–329.

Fleming, H. A. and Bailey, S. M. (1981). Sarcoid heart disease. Report of 197 United Kingdom cases with necropsy confirmation in 62. *J. Roy. Coll. Phys. Lond.* **15**, 245–253.

Frazier, O. H., Cooley, D. A., Painvin, A., Chandler, L. B. and Okereke, O. U. J. (1985). Cardiac transplantation at the Texas Heart Institute: comparative analysis of two groups of patients (1968–69 and 1982–83). *Ann. Thor. Surg.* **39**, 303–311.

Gallucci, V., Mazzucco, A., Faggian, G., Bortolotti, U., Stellin, G., Sorbara, C. and Dan, M. (1986). Orthotopic heart transplantation: initial clinical experience at the University of Padova. *Heart Transplant.* **5**, 50–51.

Hakim, M., White, D. J. G., Cory-Pearce, R., English, T. A. H. and Wallwork, J. (1985a) Is cyclosporine's nephrotoxicity related to its immunosuppressive effectiveness? *Heart Transplant.* **4**, 217–219.

Hakim, M., Wreghitt, T. G., English, T. A. H., Stovin, P. G. I., Cory-Pearce, R. and Wallwork, J. (1985b). Significance of donor-transmitted disease in cardiac transplantation. *Heart Transplant.* **4**, 302–305.

Halon, D. A., Sapoznikov, D., Lewis, B. S. and Gotsman, M. S. (1983). Localization of lesions in the coronary circulation. *Am. J. Cardiol.* **52**, 921–926.

Hassell, L. A., Fowles, R. E. and Stinson, E. B. (1981). Patients with congestive cardiomyopathy as cardiac transplant recipients. Indications for and results of cardiac transplantation and comparison with patients with coronary artery disease. *Am. J. Cardiol.* **47**, 1205–1209.

Henney, A. M. and Decker, R. S. (1987). Production of a factor by cultured human valves that is immunologically related to interleukin-1. *Cardiovasc. Res.* **21**, 21–27.

Henney, A. M., Dingle, J. T. and Decker, R. S. (1984). Effects of steroidal and non-steroidal drugs on the production of a cardiac catabolic factor by human and porcine heart valves. *Circulation* **70**, 150.

Henney, A. M., Parker, D. J. and Davies, M. J. (1982). Collagen biosynthesis in normal and abnormal human heart valves. *Cardiovasc. Res.* **16**, 624–630.

Jamieson, S. W., Oyer, P. E., Reitz, B. A., Baumgartner, W. A., Bieber, C. P., Stinson, E. B. and Shumway, N. E. (1981). Cardiac transplantation at Stanford. *Heart Transplant.* **1**, 86–91.

Joyce, L. D., Johnson, K. E., Pierce, W. S., DeVries, W. C., Semb, B. K. H., Copeland, J. G., Griffith, B. P., Cooley, D. A., Frazier, O. H., Cabrol, C., Keon, W. J., Unger, F., Bucherl, E. S. and Wolner, E. (1986). Summary of the world experience with clinical use of total artificial hearts as heart support devices. *J. Heart Transplant.* **5**, 229–235.

Just, H. and Schuster, H. P. (Eds) (1983). *Myocarditis Cardiomyopathy: Selected Problems of Pathogenesis and Clinic.* Springer-Verlag, Berlin.

Keogh, A., Baron, D. and Chang, V. (1987). The effect of blood pretransfusion on orthotopic cardiac transplantation. *Transplant. Proc.* **19**, 2503.

Keren, A., Billingham, M. E., Weintraub, D., Stinson, E. B. and Popp, R. L. (1985). Mildly dilated congestive cardiomyopathy. *Circulation* **72**, 302–309.

Kerwin, R. W., Dawbarn, D., Davies, G. J., Griffin, R., Yacoub, M. and Maseri, I. (1985). Immunohistochemical localisation of neuropeptide Y in single nerve fibres in fresh human heart. *Br. J. Pharmacol.* **85**, Suppl. 288P.

Koep, L. J., Paton, B. C., Terasaki, P. I. and Starzl, T. E. (1981). Hyperacute rejection of a transplanted human heart. *Transplantation* **32**, 71–72.

Laguens, R. P., Weinschelbaum, R. and Favaloro, R. (1979). Ultrastructural and morphometric study of the human heart muscle cell in acute coronary insufficiency. *Human Pathol.* **10**, 695–705.

Lanza, R. P., Campbell, E. M., Cooper, D. K. C., DuToit, E. D. and Barnard, C. N. (1983). The problem of the presensitized heart transplant recipient. *Heart Transplant.* **2**, 151–154.

Lanza, R. P. and Cooper, D. K. C. (1984). The management of chronic rejection: retransplantation. In *Heart Transplantation: The Present Status of Orthotopic and Heterotopic Heart Transplantation* (D. K. C. Cooper and R. P. Lanza, Eds), pp. 257–269. MTP Press, Lancaster.

Lautenschlager, I., Inkinen, K., Taskinen, E. and Hayry, P. (1984). The major histocompatibility complex antigens' distribution on cellular components of human and rat heart. *Heart Transplant.* **4**, 46–53.

Leger, J., Dechesne, C., Bouvagnet, P., Pons, F. and Leger, J. J. (1984). Characterisation and distribution of myosin variants in normal and pathological human hearts. *Eur. Heart J.* **5**, Suppl. F, 111–117.

Linder, J., Cassling, R. S., Rogler, W. C., Wilson, J. E., Markin, R. S., Sears, T. D. and McManus, B. M. (1985). Immunohistochemical characterization of lymphocytes in uninflamed ventricular myocardium. *Arch. Pathol. Lab. Med.* **109**, 917–920.

Lowry, P. J., Edwards, C. W. and Nagle, R. E. (1982). Herpes-like virus particles in myocardium of patient progressing to congestive cardiomyopathy. *Br. Heart J.* **48**, 501–503.

Lowry, P. J., Thompson, R. A. and Littler, W. A. (1985). Cellular immunity in congestive cardiomyopathy: hypersensitivity to cardiac antigens. *Br. Heart J.* **53**, 400–404.

Maron, B. J. and Roberts, W. C. (1979). Quantitative analysis of cardiac muscle cell disorganisation in the ventricular septum of patients with hypertrophic cardiomyopathy. *Circulation* **59**, 689–706.

Maron, B. J. and Roberts, W. C. (1981). Hypertrophic cardiomyopathy and cardiac muscle cell disorganisation revisited: relation between the two and significance. *Am. Heart J.*, **102**, 95–110.

Mason, J. W., Billingham, M. E. and Ricci, D. R. (1980). Treatment of acute inflammatory myocarditis by endomyocardial biopsy. *Am. J. Cardiol.*, **45**, 1037–1044.

O'Connell, J. B. and Gunnar, R. M. (1982). Dilated-congestive cardiomyopathy: prognostic features and therapy. *Heart Transplant.* **2**, 7–17.

Okada, R. and Wakafuji, S. (1985). Myocarditis in autopsy. In *Myocarditis and Related Disorders. Proceedings of the International Symposium on Cardiomyopathy and Myocarditis.*

(M. Sekiguchi, E. G. J. Olsen and J. F. Goodwin, Eds), pp. 23–29. Springer-Verlag, Tokyo.

Oldershaw, P. J., Brooksby, I. A. B., Davies, M. J., Coltart, D. J., Jenkins, B. S. and Webb-Peploe, M. M. (1980). Correlations of fibrosis in endomyocardial biopsies from patients with aortic valve disease. *Br. Heart J.* **44**, 609–611.

Olsen, E. G. J. (1979). The pathology of cardiomyopathies. A critical analysis. *Am. Heart J.* **98**, 385–392.

Olsen, E. G. J. (1980). Morphological evaluation (histologic, histochemical, and ultrastructural) of endomyocardial biopsies. In *Myocardial Biopsy. Diagnostic Significance* (H.-D. Bolte, Ed.), pp. 13–19. Springer-Verlag, Berlin.

Olsen, E. G. J. (1982). Myocardial disarray revisited. *Br. Med. J.*, **285**, 991–992.

Olsen, E. G. J. (1985a). Dilated (congestive) myopathy. Pathology, causes and relation to myocarditis. In *Heart Muscle Disease* (J. F. Goodwin, Ed.), pp. 57–74. MTP Press, Lancaster.

Olsen, E. G. J. (1985b). Histologic aspects of viral myocarditis and its diagnostic criteria. In *Myocarditis and Related Disorders. Proceedings of the International Symposium on Cardiomyopathy and Myocarditis* (M. Sekiguchi, E. G. J. Olsen and J. F. Goodwin, Eds), pp. 130–132. Springer-Verlag, Tokyo.

Parl, F., Gutstein, W. H. and Glasser, M. (1980). Relationship of small and large coronary artery disease to myocardial ischaemia. *Arch. Pathol. Lab. Med.* **104**, 70–74.

Pomerance, A. and Stovin, P. G. I. (1985). Heart transplant pathology: the British experience. *J. Clin. Pathol.* **38**, 146–159.

Ratcliff, N. B., Myles, J. L., McMahon, J. T., Golding, L., Hobbs, R., Rincon, G., Sterba, R. and Stewart, R. (1987). Myocyte injury in acute cardiac rejection and in lymphocytic myocarditis is similar and reversible. *Transplant. Proc.* **19**, 2568–2572.

Roberts, W. C. (1978). Cardiomyopathy and myocarditis: morphologic features. *Adv. Cardiol.* **22**, 184–198.

Roberts, W. C. and Ferrans, V. J. (1975). Pathologic anatomy of the cardiomyopathies. Idiopathic dilated and hypertrophic types, infiltrative types, and endomyocardial disease with and without eosinophilia. *Hum. Pathol.* **6**, 287–341.

Roberts, W. C., McAllister and Ferrans, V. J. (1977). Sarcoidosis of the heart: a clinicopathologic study of 35 necropsy patients (group 1) and review of 78 previously described necropsy patients (group 2). *Am. J. Med.* **63**, 86–108.

Rose, A. G. and Beck, W. (1985). Dilated (congestive) cardiomyopathy: a syndrome of severe cardiac dysfunction with remarkably few morphological features of myocardial damage. *Histopath.* **9**, 367–379.

Sanderson, J. E., Olsen, E. G. J. and Gatei, D. (1986). Peripartum heart disease: an endomyocardial biopsy study. *Br. Heart J.* **56**, 285–291.

Schuler, S., Warnecke, H. and Hetzer, R. (1987). Prevention of toxic side effects of cyclosporin in heart transplantation. *Transplant. Proc.* **19**, 2518–2521.

Sekiguchi, M., Olsen, E. G. J. and Goodwin, J. F. (Eds) (1985). *Myocarditis and Related Disorders: Proceedings of the International Symposium on Cardiomyopathy and Myocarditis.* Springer-Verlag, Tokyo.

Shapiro, L. M., Kleinebenne, A. and McKenna, W. J. (1985). The distribution of left ventricular hypertrophy in hypertrophic cardiomyopathy: comparison to athletes and hypertensives. *Eur. Heart J.* **6**, 967–974.

Shaw, B. W., Bahnson, H. T., Hardesty, R. L., Griffith, B. P. and Starzl, T. E. (1985). Combined transplantation of the heart and liver. *Ann. Surg.* **202**, 667–672.

Shelby, J., Fick, J., Kolegraff, R. J., Wakely, E. and Corry, R. J. (1985). Prolonged heart allograft survival induced by massive preoperative blood transfusions. *Transplant.* **40**, 334–336.

Silver, M. M. and Silver, M. D. (1983). Cardiomyopathies. In *Cardiovascular Pathology* (M. D. Silver, Ed.), pp. 489–516. Churchill Livingstone, New York.

Singer, D. R. J., Buckley, M. G., MacGregor, G. A., Khaghani, A., Banner, N. R. and Yacoub, M. (1986). Raised concentrations of plasma atrial natriuretic peptides in cardiac transplant recipients. *Br. Med. J.* **293**, 1391–1394.

Spiegelhalter, D. J. and Stovin, P. G. I. (1983). An analysis of repeated biopsies following cardiac transplantation. *Stats. Med.* **2**, 33–40.

Spry, C. J. F., Take, M. and Tai, P.-C. (1985). Eosinophilic disorders affecting the myocardium and endocardium: a review. In *Myocarditis and Related Disorders: Proceedings of the International Symposium on Cardiomyopathy and Myocarditis* (M. Sekiguchi, E. G. J. Olsen and J. F. Goodwin, Eds.), pp. 240–242. Springer-Verlag, Tokyo.

Szentpetery, S., Goldman, M. H., Woody, D., Salim, J., Mohanakumar, T. and Lower, R. (1984). Orthotopic cardiac transplantation in a Veterans Administration hospital. *Arch. Surg.* **119**, 390–393.

Tai, P.-C., Ackerman, S. J., Spry, C. J. F., Dunnette, S., Olsen, E. G. J. and Gleich, G. J. (1987). Deposits of eosinophil granule proteins in cardiac tissue of patients with eosinophilic endomyocardial disease. *Lancet* **1**, 643–647.

Tan, L. B. (1986). Cardiac pumping capability and prognosis in heart failure. *Lancet* **2**, 1360–1363.

Tanaka, M., Fujiwara, H., Onodera, T., Wu, D.-J., Hamashima, Y. and Kawai, C. (1986). Quantitative analysis of myocardial fibrosis in normals, hypertensive hearts, and cardiomyopathy. *Br. Heart J.* **55**, 575–581.

Tikkanen, I., Fyhrquist, F., Metsarinne, K. and Leidenius, R. (1985). Plasma atrial natriuretic peptide in cardiac disease and during infusion in healthy volunteers. *Lancet* **2**, 66–69.

Unverferth, B. J., Leier, C. V., Magorien, R. D. and Unverferth, D. V. (1983). Differential characteristics of myocardial nuclei in cardiomyopathy. *Hum. Pathol.* **14**, 974–983.

Vassall-Adams, P. R. (1983). Ultrastructure of the human atrioventricular conduction tissue. *Eur. Heart J.* **4**, 449–460.

Watson, D. C., Reitz, B. A., Oyer, P. E., Stinson, E. B. and Shumway, N. E. (1980). Sequential orthotopic heart transplantation in man. *Transplant.* **30**, 401–403.

Wigle, E. D. and Silver, M. D. (1978). Editorial: Myocardial fiber disarray and ventricular septal hypertrophy in asymmetrical hypertrophy of the heart. *Circulation* **58**, 398–402.

Wiseman, M. N. and Banim, S. (1987). 'Glue sniffer's' heart? *Br. Med. J.* **294**, 739.

Yacoub, M., Festenstein, H., Doyle, P., Martin, M., McCloskey, D., Awad, J., Gamba, A., Khaghani, A. and Holmes, J. (1987). The influence of HLA matching in cardiac allograft recipients receiving cyclosporine and azathioprine. *Transplant. Proc.* **19**, 2487–2489.

Yu, Z-X., Sekiguchi, M., Hiroe, M., Take, M. and Hirosawa, K. (1985). A comparative ultrastructural study on the nature of interstitial cell constituents in idiopathic myocarditis and myocardial infarction. In *Myocarditis and Related Disorders. Proceedings of the International Symposium on Cardiomyopathy and Myocarditis* (M. Sekiguchi, E. G. J. Olsen and J. F. Goodwin, Eds), pp. 154–158. Springer-Verlag, Tokyo.

Ariela Pomerance

11

Pathology of the Recipient Lung

INTRODUCTION

Heart–lung transplantation is now an accepted treatment for end-stage cardiorespiratory disease. The Stanford team began their human heart–lung programme early in 1981 and, up to 1 November 1986, had carried out 40 transplants, including 1 re-transplant. The two UK transplant centres, Papworth and Harefield, started heart lung transplantation in April 1984 and December 1983 and have treated 17 and 76 patients, respectively.

The majority of patients have had pulmonary vascular disease, either secondary to congenital heart disease or idiopathic (primary). Table 11.1 shows the types of respiratory disease in the patients operated on at these three centres.

Although the clinical progress of heart–lung transplantation has been fully recorded in the medical literature (Jamieson *et al.*, 1984; Burke *et al.*, 1986), the pathology of the recipient heart and lungs has received little attention. This is understandable since the diseases and pathological processes concerned, although perhaps uncommon outside specialized centres, are already adequately documented. The vascular changes of pulmonary hypertension have been well described, notably by Wagenvoort and Wagenvoort (1977) and Heath and Edwards (1958). Excellent descriptions of lung pathology in conditions like cystic fibrosis, rheumatoid disease, alpha-1 antitrypsin deficiency and fibrosing alveolitis are available in standard textbooks. Even obliterative bronchiolitis, which is now emerging as a major threat to long-term survival in lung transplant recipients, was well recognized many years before human transplantation became practicable (Lancet, 1982). Nevertheless, pathologists whose work includes material from a transplant centre are

TABLE 11.1
Heart–Lung Transplant Patients From Three Centres

	Stanford	*Papworth*	*Harefield*
No. of patients	39	17	74
Age range	15–45 yr	16–46 yr	2 months–55 yr
Sex	18 F, 21 M	13 F, 4 M	50 F, 24 M
LUNG PATHOLOGY			
Associated with congenital heart disease (patients)	20	6	36
Vascular disease without congenital heart disease (patients)	19	4	23
Parenchymal lung disease (patients)	—	7	15
Re-transplants (patients)	1	—	2

bound to be stimulated by the concentration of striking lung pathology which emerges.

This chapter is based on the findings in the 76 pairs of lungs replaced in the 74 patients who have undergone heart–lung transplants in Harefield hospital between December 1983 and November 1986.

Specimens are normally received in the laboratory already fixed by immersion in 10% formol-saline. Our practice is to take one block from each lobe of the lung and additional blocks from any localized abnormal areas. Sections are routinely stained with Miller's elastic and van Gieson stain, to show up muscle, fibrous tissue and elastic, as well as with the normal haematoxylin–eosin stains.

Vascular pathology is reported as recommended by Wagenvoort and Wagenvoort (1977) and Wagenvoort (1981), taking account of quantitative as well as qualitative changes, and the terminology used is that defined in the World Health Organization report on pulmonary hypertension (WHO, 1975).

The findings are most conveniently considered in two groups — patients requiring transplantation because of pulmonary vascular disease and those with essentially non-vascular end-stage pulmonary pathology.

PULMONARY VASCULAR DISEASE

The most common reason for heart–lung transplantation in our series, as at Stanford, has been pulmonary hypertension associated with congenital heart

TABLE 11.2
Pulmonary Vascular Pathology Associated With Congenital Heart Disease

POST-TRICUSPID SHUNTS			
Cardiac Abnormality	*No. of Patients*		*Lung Pathology*
VSD	10	PA*	4 cases with grade 3 changes 2 cases with grade 2 changes 4 cases with grade 1 changes
Double outlet ventricle	2	PA PA	1 case with grade 3 changes 1 case with grade 1 changes
Single ventricle	3	PA	All cases grade 3 changes
Atrioventricular canal	1	PA	Grade 3
Truncus arteriosus	2	PA	1 case with grade 1 changes 1 case with grade 2 changes
Transposition	1	PA	Grade 3
Aortopulmonary window	1	PA	Grade 3 changes
Patent ductus	5	PA	All cases grade 3 changes

PULMONARY ATRESIAS		
Other Cardiac Abnormality	*Previous Surgery*	*Lung Pathology*
Hypoplastic L. ventricle	Shunt and pulmonary valvotomy	Pulmonary venous hypertension. Marked arterial medial hyperplasia
Hypoplastic L. ventricle	Shunt	Plexogenic. Intimal fibrosis, arterial and venous
High VSD	Shunts ×3	Plexogenic. Fibroblastic occlusions, mainly venous
VSD	—	Intimal fibrosis, arterial and venous. Arterial dilatation
	—	Obliterative fibrosis, arterial and venous. Arterial dilatation
VSD and ASD	—	Obliterative fibrosis, arterial dilatation. Occasional plexiform lesions

WITH PULMONARY VENOUS OBSTRUCTION	
Cardiac Abnormality	*Lung Pathology*
VSD and supramitral ring	
Fibro-elastosis	Chronic venous hypertension and marked medial arterial hyperplasia
Single ventricle, mitral atresia	
TGA with tricuspid incompetence	
VSD and SVC draining into L. atrium	As above + plexiform lesions
VSD with L. side AV valve leak	

* Plexogenic arteriopathy

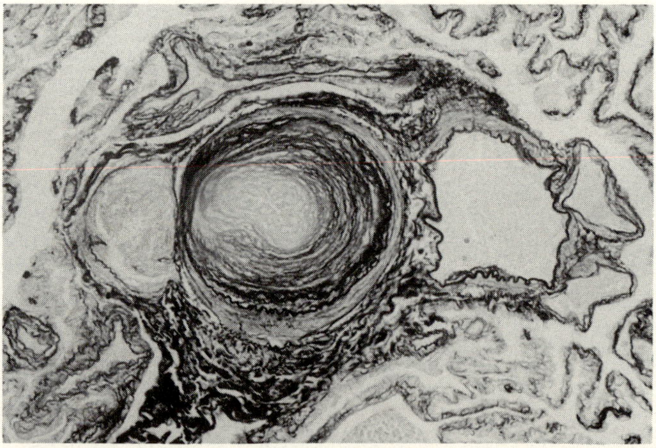

Fig. 11.1. *Concentric intimal fibrosis, characteristic of plexogenic pulmonary arteriopathy. The lumen of the small artery is occluded by concentric layers of fibrous tissue and material which stains as elastic. Elastic van Gieson × 100 approx.*

disease. The cardiac abnormality in the majority of these patients was a communication between systemic and pulmonary circulations at or distal to the level of the atrioventricular ring. Table 11.2 summarizes the abnormalities present in these patients.

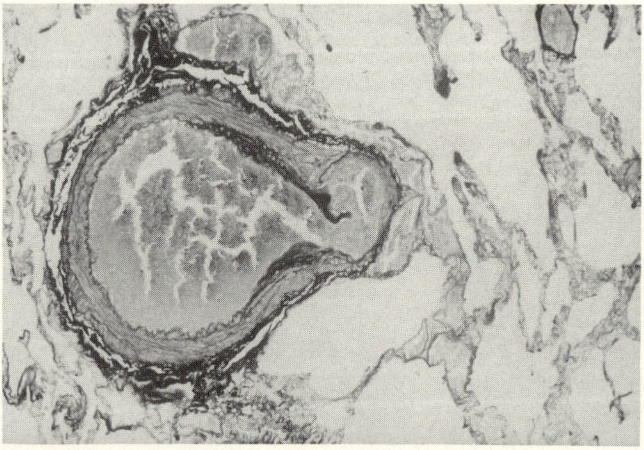

Fig. 11.2. *Plexiform lesions from a man with familial pulmonary hypertension, showing a small plexiform lesion apparently in continuity with a defect in the artery wall. Elastic van Gieson × 60 approx.*

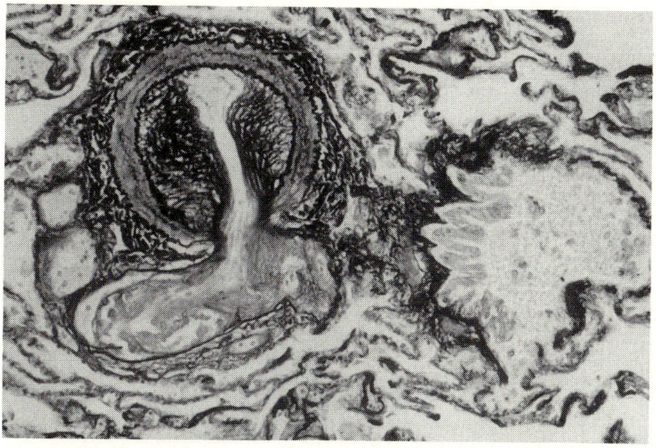

Fig. 11.3. *Plexiform lesions from a woman with primary pulmonary hypertension, also showing intimal fibrous proliferation at each side of the medial defect. Elastic van Gieson × 90 approx.*

Post-tricuspid shunts

Predictably, all the lungs in these cases showed vasoconstrictive disease with well-marked arterial medial hyperplasia and peripheral extension of muscle and elastic. Almost all also showed the vascular changes which are now termed plexogenic pulmonary arteriopathy (WHO, 1975; Wagenvoort and Wagenvoort, 1977) (Fig. 11.1). The term is derived from the characteristic

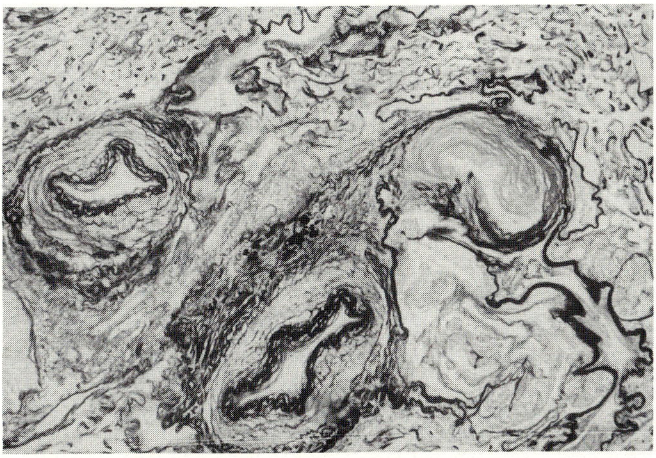

Fig. 11.4. *Plexiform lesions from a woman with congenital heart disease, showing marked hypertrophy of the walls of muscular arteries with elastic laminae in the media and adjacent angioma-like thin-walled vascular complexes. Elastic van Gieson × 60 approx.*

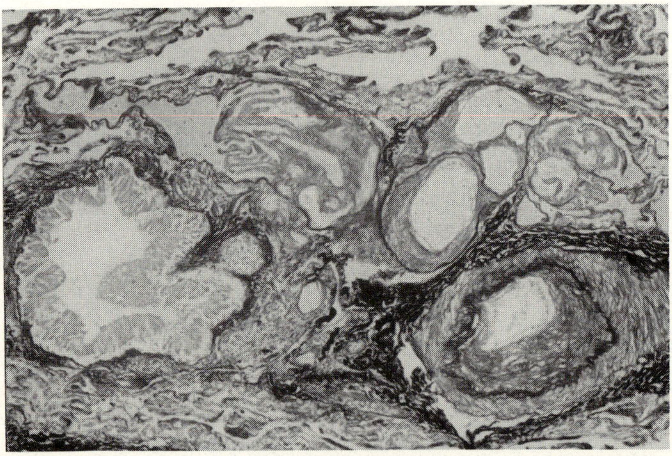

Fig. 11.5. *Plexiform lesions from a woman with primary pulmonary hypertension, showing a large angioma-like lesion between the artery and bronchial wall. The artery also shows eccentric intimal fibrosis. Elastic van Gieson × 60 approx.*

plexiform lesions (Figs 11.2–11.6). These consist of circumscribed angioma-like conglomerations of vascular channels, often with fibrin and irregular layers of granular material which stains as elastic. They are usually found adjacent to, or apparently arising from, small and medium calibre arteries,

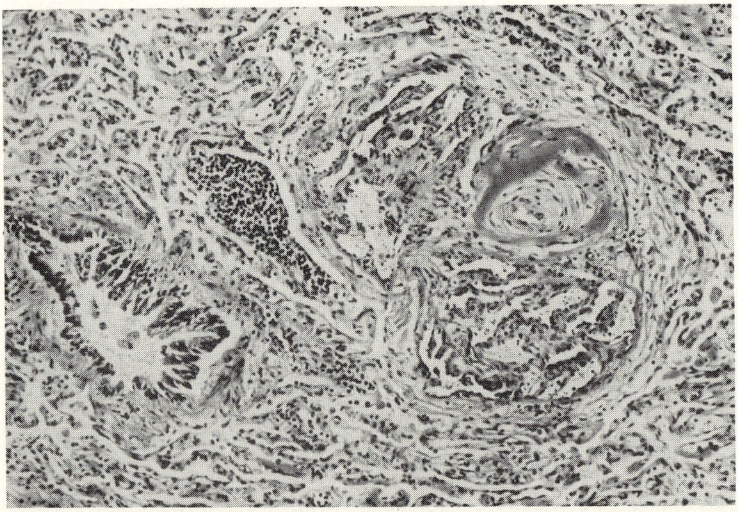

Fig. 11.6. *Fibrinoid change in a small artery adjacent to a plexiform lesion, from a child with congenital heart disease. Haematoxylin and eosin × 70 approx.*

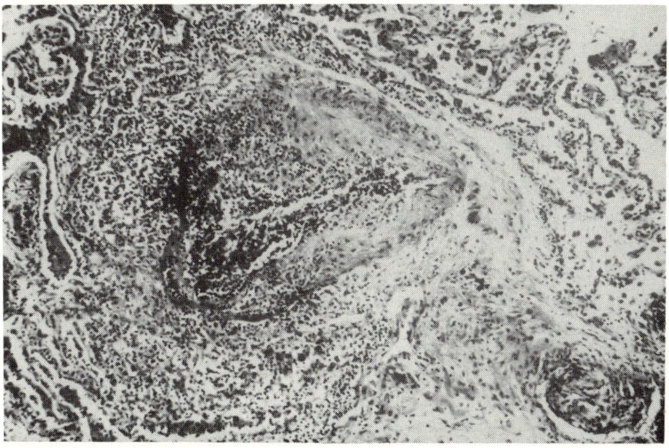

Fig. 11.7. *Arteritis in a young woman with familial primary pulmonary hypertension. Haematoxylin and eosin × 60 approx.*

often clearly in continuity with a defect in the arterial wall (Figs 11.2 and 11.3). Although their appearance suggests that they are micro-aneurysms, serial sectioning has shown that they actually arise in arterial branches just beyond their origin from the parent vessel, and that the thin-walled angiomatous component which is commonly present (Figs 11.4–11.6) is a post-stenotic dilatation of the branch beyond the lesion (Wagenvoort and Wagenvoort, 1977). Fibrinoid necrosis of the parent artery is often seen at the origin of the plexiform lesion and is probably the initiating event in the process which produces it. This leads to localized dilatation. Thrombosis occurs in the dilated section and organization and recanalization produces the network of spaces, endothelial cells, and material staining as elastic, which make up the plexiform lesion. All stages of this process were seen in our material. Arteritis was uncommon; it was seen in 3 cases only, involving occasional muscular pulmonary arteries in 2 (Fig. 11.7) and the main pulmonary artery in the other. This is perhaps unexpected in a series of cases with end-stage pulmonary hypertension and may well reflect the fact that only one block of tissue is normally processed from each lobe of the lungs.

Intimal fibrosis was also present in the majority of cases. In the arterial tree this varied from loose irregularly arranged cellular fibrous and fibroblastic tissue partly filling the lumen of small arteries (Fig. 11.5), and sometimes arterioles, to the very distinctive 'onion skin' concentric laminar fibrosis (Fig. 11.1), usually filling the lumen, which is also a feature of plexogenic pulmonary arteriopathy. Bands of fibrin were often clearly distinguishable in the fibrous 'laminae', together with layers of material which stained

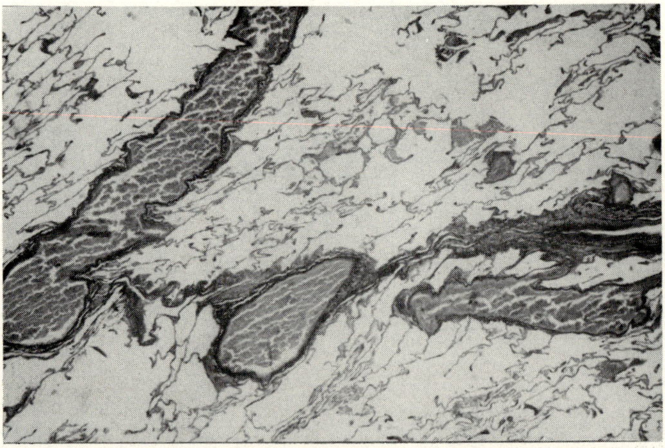

Fig. 11.8. *Dilatation lesions from the same patient as Fig. 11.2. Elastic van Gieson ×40 approx.*

strongly with elastic stains and which are apparently a stage in the organization of the fibrinous deposits. This form of concentric laminar fibrosis is also characteristic of plexogenic pulmonary arteriopathy, although it appears earlier than the plexiform lesions. We found no cases at the stage of concentric laminar fibrosis only, i.e. without concomitant plexiform lesions. This is clearly to be expected in patients whose pulmonary vascular disease is severe enough to require transplantation.

Dilatation and angiomatoid lesions (Fig. 11.8) were also seen in most of the patients. These lesions are the result of thinning of the media of small arteries, which become tortuous and may resemble thin-walled angiomas. Unlike plexiform lesions they are not associated with fibrinoid degeneration, and are thought to be another manifestation of post-stenotic dilatation.

Many patients also showed patchy intimal fibrous proliferation with obstruction of small peripheral vein branches by loose connective tissue. Most of these patients had been cyanosed, with high haemoglobin levels, and thrombotic changes in peripheral vessels were therefore to be anticipated.

Clinicopathological correlations

Studies in post-mortem and biopsy specimens of lung have not shown any correlation between the degree of plexogenic pulmonary arteriopathy and the severity or duration of symptoms (Wagenvoort and Wagenvoort, 1970). Since all our material was from patients with end-stage pulmonary vascular disease, there was no point in attempting to correlate pathology and severity of symptoms. We did, however, attempt to correlate pathology with duration of symptoms, site of shunt and rate of clinical deterioration. Proper

TABLE 11.3
Clinicopathological Correlations in Shunt-Associated Pulmonary Vascular Disease

Grade of Plexogenic Arteriopathy	*No. of patients*	*Site of Shunt*	*Average Age (yr)*
Grade 1	4	3 VSD	
		1 truncus	14
Grade 2	9	4 VSD	
		1 double outlet LV	
		1 AV canal	28.5
		1 truncus	
		2 PDA	
Grade 3	13	4 VSD	
		3 single ventricle	
		1 double outlet RV	18.8
		1 TGA	
		2 aortopulmonary window	
		2 PDA	

quantitation was not practicable in these specimens, but a crude grading was applied to the plexiform lesions:

Grade 1. Occasional lesions only, found with difficulty.
Grade 2. Lesions found easily but not numerous.
Grade 3. Lesions numerous.

The presence or absence of fibrinoid change and arteritis was also noted.

Most of the patients had numerous or at least easily found plexiform lesions. The 4 patients who had only grade 1 lesions were all under 20 years (average age 15). However, the average age of the 13 patients with grade 3 lesions was almost a decade less than those with grade 2 lesions (Table 11.3).

Fibrinoid change was more commonly associated with grade 3 plexiform pathology. It was seen in almost two-thirds of the lungs from this group and in one-third of the lungs with grade 2 lesions. There was only one example in the 4 cases with scanty, hard-to-find plexiform lesions.

Patients who had deteriorated rapidly while awaiting transplantation did not appear to have more fibrinoid degeneration or more severe plexogenic changes than the rest.

Only one of the 3 patients in whom arteritis was seen had deteriorated rapidly.

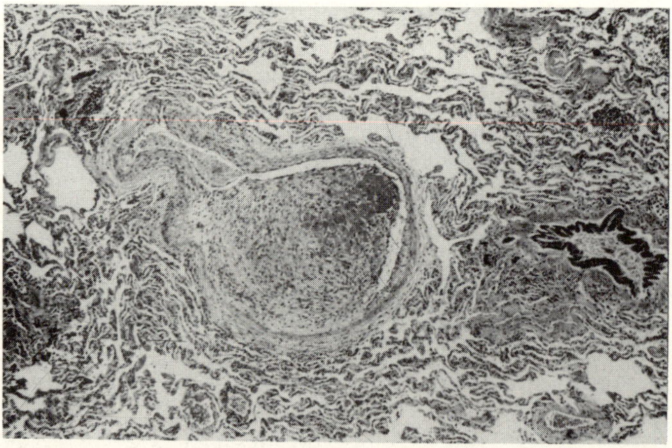

Fig. 11.9. *Intravascular thrombosis in a young man with pulmonary atresia. Haematoxylin and eosin ×25 approx.*

Pulmonary atresia

Pulmonary atresia needs to be considered separately from other congenital pathology. Apart from the obvious lesion in the main pulmonary outflow, quantitative morphometry has shown abnormal development of intrapulmonary vessels (Howarth and McCartney, 1980). Since the pulmonary flow is reduced, medial hypertrophy and plexiform lesions are not seen unless shunt operations have been carried out (Wagenvoort and Wagenvoort, 1977).

Three of the 6 patients with pulmonary atresia in the Harefield series had shunts, and plexogenic vascular changes were present in 2. The third had a small left ventricle and predominantly venous hypertensive pathology. The previously unoperated patients had thin dilated arteries, as would be expected, but the most striking histological feature was thrombotic and fibrous intimal proliferation (Figs 11.9 and 11.10). Table 11.2 summarizes the histological findings in these 5 patients.

Venous hypertensive changes

Changes due to raised pressure in the pulmonary venous system can be seen in any condition which interferes with pulmonary venous return, including, of course, chronic low-output cardiac failure. Alveolar haemorrhage, haemosiderosis and venous intimal fibrosis were therefore present to some degree in most of the lungs from patients with pulmonary vascular disease, although they were not the dominant abnormality.

Six cases had the changes of severe long-standing pulmonary venous hypertension only, and 2 others showed these changes together with plexi-

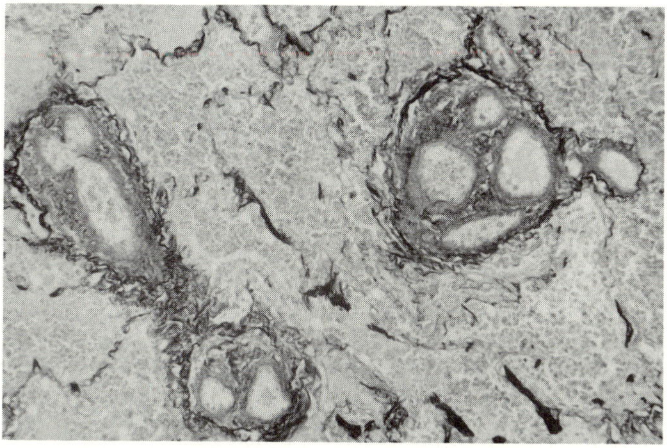

Fig. 11.10. *Recanalized thrombi in a young man with pulmonary atresia and gross polycythaemia. Elastic van Gieson × 80 approx.*

form lesions (Tables 11.2 and 11.3). In 4 patients these resulted from congenital abnormalities which raised left atrial pressure. Two had acquired atrioventricular valve incompetence in addition to congenital abnormalities and a further 2 had cardiomyopathic chronic left ventricular failure. The characteristic features in such cases are arterialized pulmonary veins, i.e. medial muscular hyperplasia and reduplication and re-orientation of elastic fibres resulting in veins whose structure resembles that of arteries

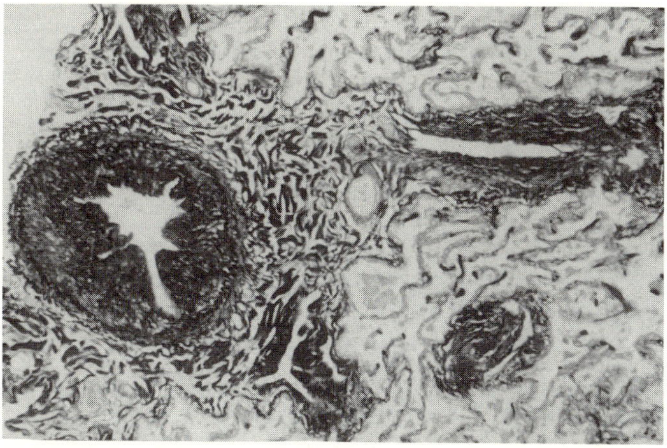

Fig. 11.11. *Venous pulmonary hypertensive changes. Arterialized vein. The largest vessel has well-defined and parallel elastic laminae. Marked intimal fibrous proliferation is also present. Elastic van Gieson × 80 approx.*

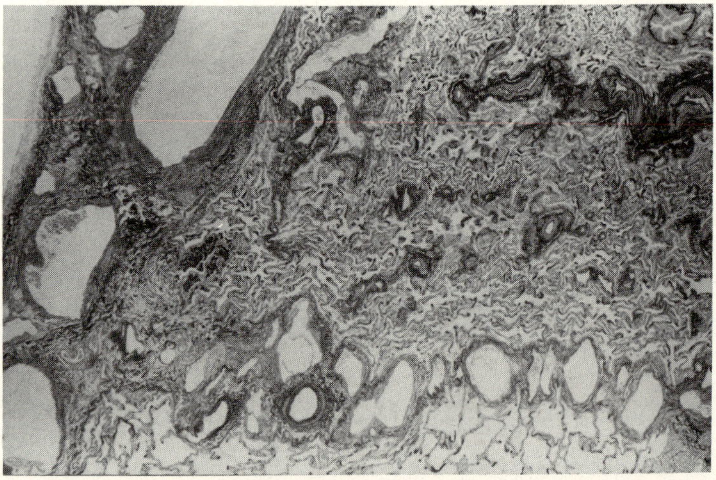

Fig. 11.12. *Venous pulmonary hypertensive changes. Gross dilatation of lymphatics under the pleura and in intrapulmonary fibrous septa. Arterialized veins and aggregated siderophages are also present. From a child with fibro-elastosis and hypoplastic left heart. Elastic van Gieson* × *30 approx.*

(Fig. 11.11). Intimal fibrosis is common. Dilated veins and lymphatics in the sub-pleural connective tissue and interlobar fibrous septa may be striking (Fig. 11.12) and haemosiderosis and focal interstitial fibrosis are almost always present. Arteries are also abnormal, with marked thickening of the media of muscular pulmonary arteries. This thickening is in part due to

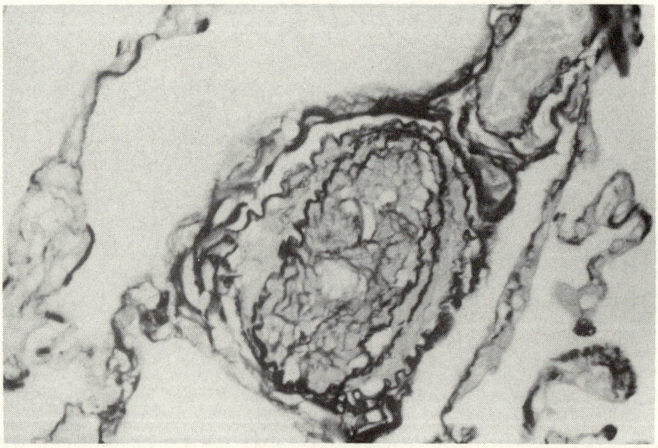

Fig. 11.13. *Longitudinal muscle fibres almost occluding a pulmonary arteriole. From the same patient as Fig. 11.12. Elastic van Gieson* × *200 approx.*

medial oedema and fibrosis (Wagenvoort and Wagenvoort, 1983). Eccentric intimal fibrosis and prominent longitudinal muscle bundles in the intima (Fig. 11.13) are also common.

Thrombo-embolic pulmonary hypertension

This form of pulmonary hypertension is characterized by patchy arterial intimal fibrous proliferation and fibrosis, usually eccentric, without evidence of plexogenic vascular pathology and usually without significant medial hypertrophy. Thrombi at varying stages of organization may be recognizable. Recanalized vessels with lumina divided by fibrous septa are characteristic of past thrombo-embolism (Fig. 11.10). Changes of this type were seen in 5 patients. The source of the emboli was clear from the past medical history in all cases (Table 11.4). Silent thrombo-embolism is also a well-recognized cause of clinically unexplained pulmonary hypertension (Wagenvoort and Wagenvoort, 1970; Wagenvoort, 1980; Howarth, 1983) and 2 of the 14 cases in this category in our series showed well-marked thrombo-embolic pathology. However, both also showed plexiform lesions and the concentric laminar type of intimal fibrosis, so are more appropriately classed as plexogenic primary pulmonary hypertension.

Unexplained (primary) pulmonary hypertension

The remaining 15 patients with end-stage pulmonary vascular disease in our series must be classified as 'unexplained' pulmonary hypertension (Table 11.4). Histopathological study of such cases usually shows one of three pictures — veno-occlusive disease, plexogenic pulmonary arteriopathy or evidence of thrombo-embolism unassociated with either veno-occlusive or plexogenic pathology (Wagenvoort and Wagenvoort, 1970; Wagenvoort, 1980). The preoperative diagnosis was veno-occlusive disease in 1 patient and primary pulmonary hypertension in the remainder. Histology, however, showed features of veno-occlusive disease in 5 of these cases.

Veno-occlusive disease

The essential pathology (Heath, Segal and Bishop, 1966; Wagenvoort and Wagenvoort, 1977) in veno-occlusive disease is partial or complete obliteration of the lumen of pulmonary veins and venules by connective tissue (Figs 11.14–11.16). Veins of any size may be affected. As in pulmonary venous hypertension, focal fibrosis, interstitial haemorrhage and haemosiderosis are usually present. The occluding connective tissue is typically of loose fibroblastic type, but may be dense collagen or any intermediate stage. Arterial involvement is also now recognized to be common (Wagenvoort, Wagenvoort and Takahashi, 1985; Hasleton, Ironside and Whittaker,

TABLE 11.4

Pulmonary Vascular Pathology Without Congenital Heart Disease

Aetiology		*Pathology*
Chronic LV failure	2 patients (COCM, ischaemic)	Marked chronic venous hypertensive changes
Iatrogenic kyphoscoliosis		Chronic venous hypertensive changes with marked fibroblastic proliferation
Thrombo-embolic	Source: shunt in R. atrium postoperative embolism ischaemic heart disease post-transfusion Associated with active TB	Fibroblastic and fibrous proliferation arteries and veins Recanalization lesions Fibroblastic occlusions including foreign material
Pulmonary veno-occlusive disease	6 patients	
	F 52 yr	Occlusion by loose fibroblastic tissue
	M 51	Occlusion by dense hyaline fibrous tissue
	F 13, 25, 30 yr	Occlusion by mixed fibrous/fibroblastic tissue
	M 46	
'Primary' plexogenic	9 patients (3 familial)	Grade 3 plexiform lesions, 7 cases Grade 1 plexiform lesions, 2 cases (2 with marked thrombo-embolic changes also)

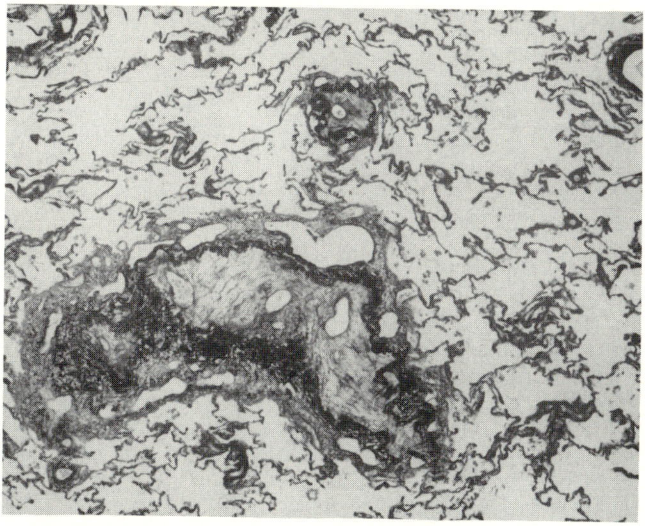

Fig. 11.14. *Veno-occlusive disease. Large and medium calibre veins almost entirely occluded by loose connective tissue. From a woman of 52 with a preoperative diagnosis of veno-occlusive disease. Elastic van Gieson ×40 approx.*

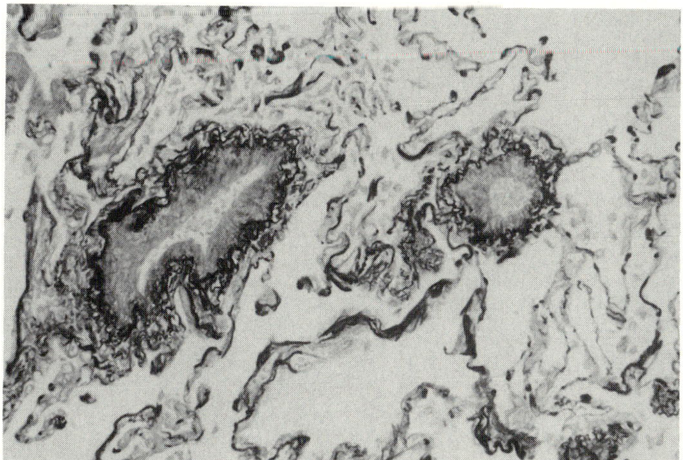

Fig. 11.15. *Veno-occlusive disease. Collagenous fibrous tissue partly filling medium calibre and small veins. From a man of 46 presenting with pulmonary hypertension of unknown cause. Elastic van Gieson ×85 approx.*

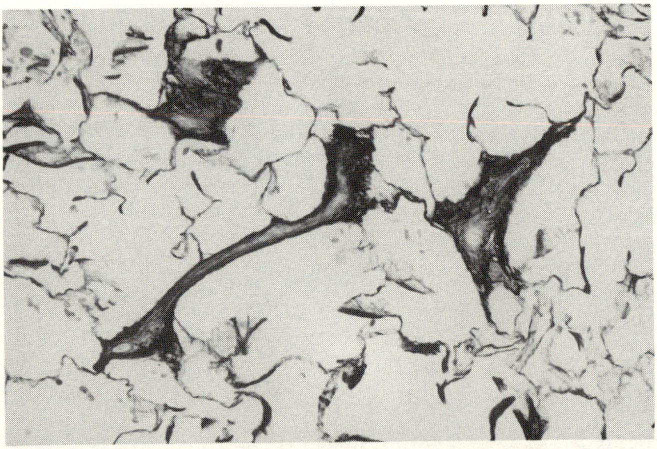

Fig. 11.16. *Veno-occlusive disease. Small veins occluded by mature fibrous tissue. From a 30-year-old woman with primary pulmonary hypertension. Elastic van Gieson × 70 approx.*

1986). Wagenvoort and colleagues found narrowed or obliterated pulmonary arteries in approximately half of their series of 26 patients with pulmonary veno-occlusive disease. Three of our cases had similar changes, including 1 patient with recent organizing thrombi (Fig. 11.17).

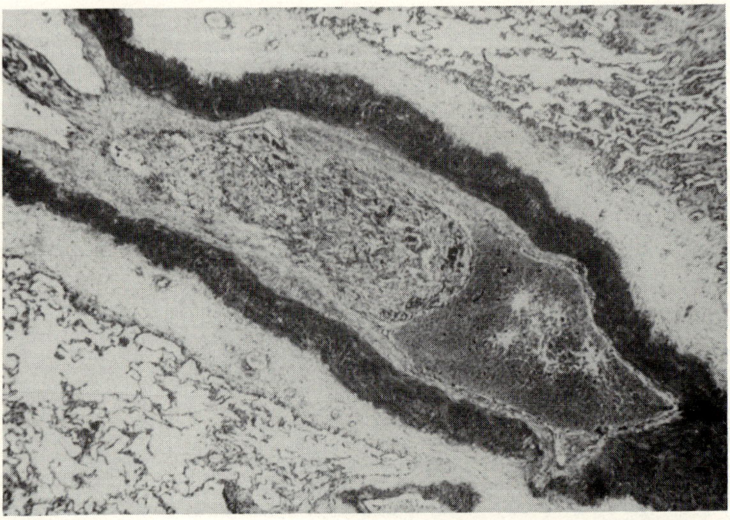

Fig. 11.17. *Veno-occlusive disease. Artery blocked by recent organizing thrombus. From the same patient as Fig. 11.14. Haematoxylin and eosin × 30 approx.*

TABLE 11.5
Familial Pulmonary Hypertension

Sex and Age	*Affected Family Members*	*Pathology*
F 5 yr	Sibling and cousin	Plexogenic grade 3 + mild chronic venous hypertensive changes
F 18 yr	Father and 2 siblings	Plexogenic grade 3 + moderate chronic venous hypertensive changes
M 30 yr	8 members in 3 generations	Plexogenic grade 3 + moderate chronic venous hypertensive changes

Pulmonary veno-occlusive disease is probably a non-specific pathological response to a variety of stimuli, rather than a single entity. Viral infections, toxins, hormonal factors and genetic influences have all been suggested as causes (see Wagenvoort, Wagenvoort and Takahashi, 1985). There were no apparent aetiological factors in most of our cases. One patient had required splenectomy for haemolytic anaemia. None of the others had any significant past medical history.

Idiopathic plexogenic pulmonary arteriopathy

The microscopic changes in this condition are identical to those of pulmonary hypertension associated with congenital shunts. Patients are usually young and female. The 7 females and 2 males in our series ranged in age from 3 to 34 years and included 3 with familial pulmonary hypertension. (Table 11.5). Most showed gross plexogenic arterial changes with numerous large, florid plexiform and angiomatoid lesions (Figs 11.2, 11.3 and 11.5). The exceptions were the youngest patient, where plexiform lesions were sparse, and one of the patients with well-marked thrombo-embolic changes, already mentioned. Plexiform lesions were scanty but present, as was concentric laminar fibrosis, justifying the inclusion of this young woman in the primary pulmonary hypertension group.

As its name indicates, primary plexogenic pulmonary hypertension is another form of pulmonary vascular disease whose aetiology is obscure. Informed opinion currently favours excessive vasoconstriction in susceptible individuals. It has been suggested that susceptibility may relate to inborn differences in pulmonary vascular muscle (Howarth, 1983). In susceptible individuals, hypoxia and some appetite suppressants are known precipitating agents. Neither of these appeared to be a factor in any of our patients.

TABLE 11.6
Non-vascular Pulmonary Disease

Pathology	*No. of Cases*
Mucoviscidosis	5
Alpha-1 antitrypsin deficiency	2 (1 also with foreign body granulomas from narcotic abuse)
Fibrosis due to past TB	1
associated with rheumatoid disease	1
idiopathic	2
Post-pneumonic	
staphylococcal	1
viral	1
Obliterative bronchiolitis	2 (10 and 14/12 post-transplant)
Diffuse pulmonary angiomatosis	1
Lymphangioleiomyomatosis	1

NON-VASCULAR PULMONARY DISEASE

Inflammatory lung diseases and idiopathic pulmonary fibrosis

In this group of patients, respiratory failure is the result of pulmonary parenchymal pathology. Vascular abnormalities are of relatively little practical significance. Our series (Table 11.6) included 5 patients with cystic fibrosis. All their lungs showed the gross infected tubular bronchiectasis typical of the final stages of this condition (Fig. 11.18). One patient had alveolar wall and focal interstitial fibrosis following staphylococcal pneumonia and another's symptoms followed a viral illness. One of the patients with thrombo-embolic pulmonary hypertension had active pulmonary tuberculosis with both caseating and miliary lesions.

Two patients had end-stage 'idiopathic' pulmonary fibrosis, with uniformly honeycomb cystic lungs. Both also had thrombo-embolic vascular changes.

Genetically determined lung disease

The 5 cases of cystic fibrosis have already been discussed in the section on inflammatory lung disease. The only other genetically determined lung abnormality represented was alpha-1 antitrypsin deficiency. This condition results in severe pan-acinar emphysema. The lungs macroscopically are soft and bulky with a 'soufflé-like' consistency. Microscopically they are indistin-

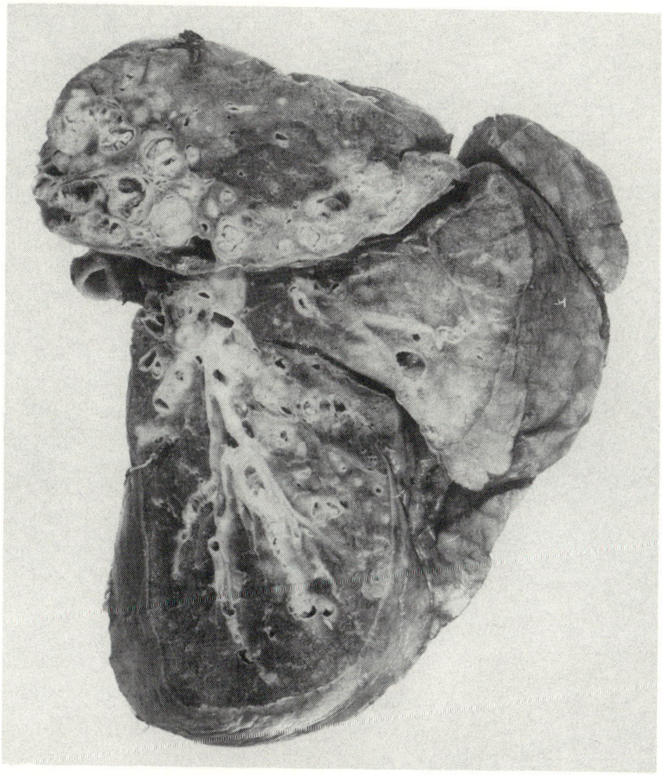

Fig. 11.18. *Lung from a case of cystic fibrosis. This gross degree of infected bronchiectasis was typical of all the 5 specimens.*

guishable from any other form of severe pan-acinar emphysema. One of the 2 patients with this condition also had multiple small foreign body granulomas (from intravenous narcotic abuse), which were clearly associated with thrombo-embolic lesions in small arteries and arterioles (Fig. 11.19).

Iatrogenic pulmonary disease

Obliterative bronchiolitis

Two patients were re-transplanted for progressive respiratory insufficiency 10 and 14 months after their original heart–lung transplants. The lungs in both cases showed the changes of obliterative bronchiolitis, a condition which has emerged as a major threat to long-term survival after heart–lung transplantation (Yousem, Burke and Billingham, 1985; Burke *et al.*, 1986). In the early stages, the bronchioles are filled with inflammatory debris and

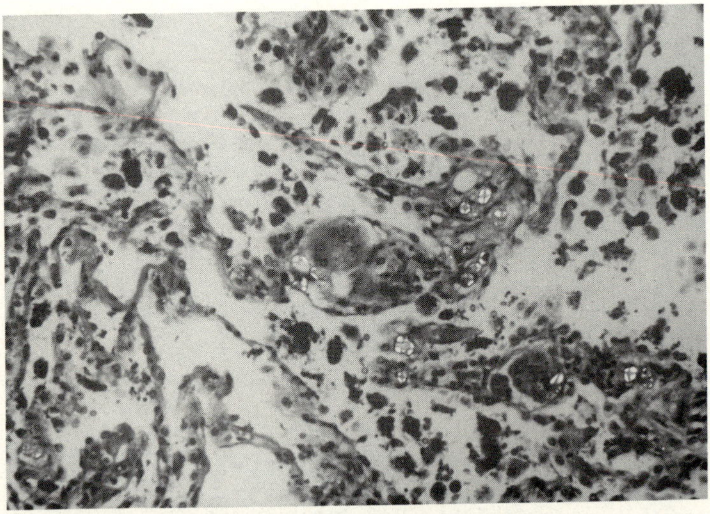

Fig. 11.19. *Granulomatous pulmonary disease and emphysema. The granulomas contain birefringent particles. From a narcotic addict with alpha-1 antitrypsin deficiency. Haematoxylin and eosin × 190 approx. (photographed through partly crossed prisms).*

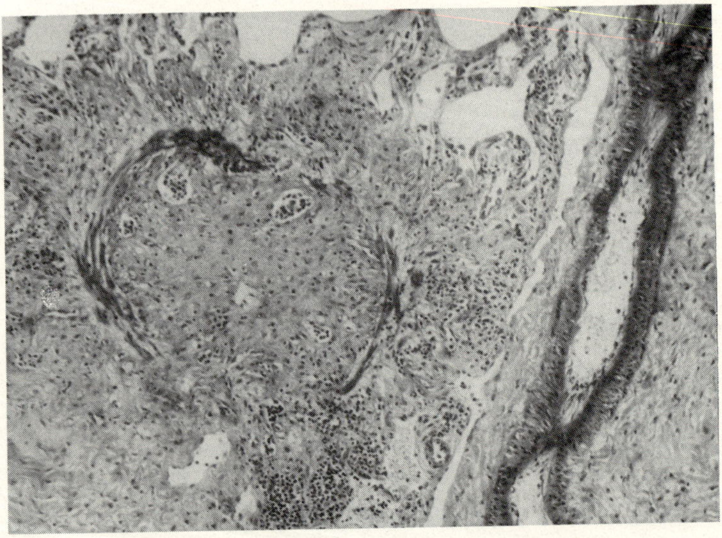

Fig. 11.20. *Post-transplant obliterative bronchiolitis, 10 months after transplant, showing occlusion of a bronchus by fibrous tissue. Haematoxylin and eosin × 50 approx.*

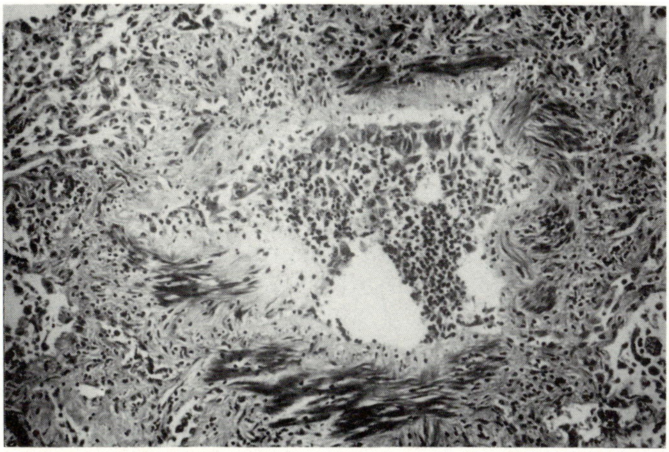

Fig. 11.21. *Post-transplant obliterative bronchiolitis, 14 months after transplant, showing loss of bronchial epithelium, with fibrinopurulent debris filling the lumen. Haematoxylin and eosin* ×45 *approx.*

granulation tissue and denuded of their epithelial lining. The inflammatory changes resolve, leaving bronchioles filled by fibrous tissue and only identifiable by their relation to arteries and with the use of elastic stains. Fibrous obliteration predominated in the patient re-transplanted at 10 months (Fig. 11.20) and more active inflammation in the later re-transplant patient (Fig. 11.21).

Obliterative bronchiolitis has developed in half of the 20 long-term survivors of heart–lung transplantation from the Stanford series, on average 11.2 months after surgery (Burke *et al.*, 1986). In addition to the bronchiolar pathology, the pulmonary vessels showed concentric intimal fibrosis (similar to that of post-transplant accelerated coronary atherosclerosis) in 6 of the 7 patients where lung tissue was available for histology. Similar changes were seen in an open lung biopsy specimen in 1 of our 2 cases, 14 months after transplantation. This patient died after re-transplantation and necropsy showed accelerated atherosclerosis in the coronary arteries, as was found in all 5 of the Stanford patients whose hearts were studied.

The association with vascular pathology of chronic rejection type suggests that post-transplant obliterative bronchiolitis may be a result of rejection. However, the bronchiolar changes are non-specific and have been described in a number of other conditions unrelated to transplantation (Lancet, 1982). An association with rheumatoid disease and fibrosing alveolitis has raised the possibility of an autoimmune response. Other suggestions have been increased susceptibility to infections and impaired mucus clearance due to denervation (Yousem, Burke and Billingham, 1985; McGregor *et al.*,

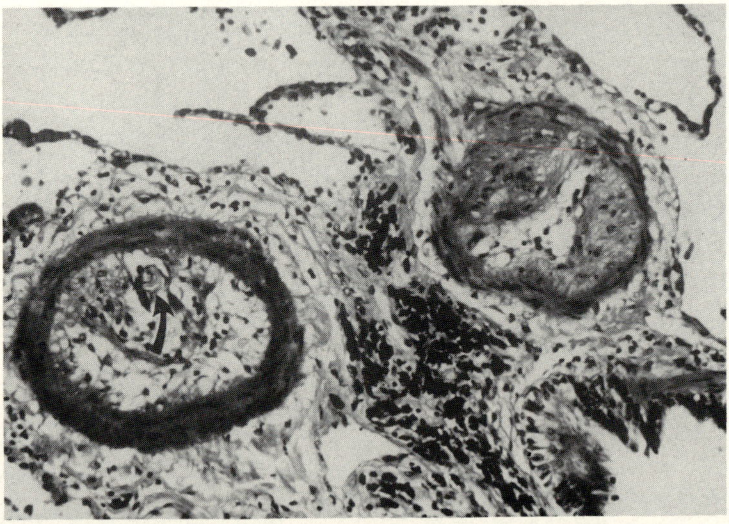

Fig. 11.22. *Thrombo-embolic pulmonary hypertension. Two arterioles are blocked by loose fibroblastic tissue and fibrin. Birefringent foreign material (arrowed) was also seen in other similarly sized and larger vessels. Haematoxylin and eosin* × *195 approx.*

1986). Immunosuppression itself is probably not a factor, since lung biopsies in other immunocompromised patients have not shown any significant incidence of obliterative bronchiolitis (Cockerill *et al.*, 1985), neither has it been a problem after lone cardiac transplantation. The explanation at present remains obscure.

Other iatrogenic pulmonary disease

Thrombo-embolic pathology in one patient was associated with relatively large birefringent foreign particles (Fig. 11.22), probably introduced via an intravenous drip. Radiotherapy for neuroblastoma in infancy was responsible for gross kyphoscoliosis and consequent venous hypertensive and hypoxic changes in 1 case.

MISCELLANEOUS RARITIES

One patient with pulmonary lymphangioleiomyomatosis and one child with diffuse pulmonary angiomatosis have had heart–lung transplants at Harefield.

Pulmonary lymphangioleiomyomatosis is characterized by irregular hyperplastic hamartomatous bundles of smooth muscle throughout the lungs, with obstruction to airways and lymphatics. It may occur as part of

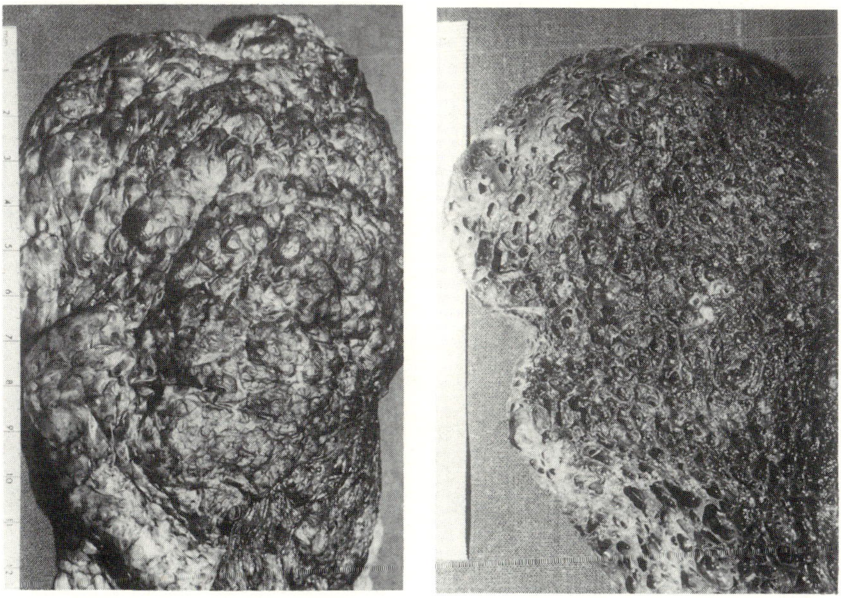

(a) (b)

Fig. 11.23a,b. *Pulmonary lymphangioleiomyomatosis. Pleural and cut surfaces of lung showing the typical appearance of lymphangioleiomyomatosis with multiple, rather uniform small cysts throughout the lungs.*

tuberous sclerosis or as an isolated condition, as in our case. Grossly (Figs 11.23a and 11.23b) the lungs showed multiple rather uniform small cysts with no significant fibrosis. Microscopy showed the features described by Corrin, Leibow and Friedman (1975) and Stovin *et al.* (1975) — localized foci of irregularly arranged smooth muscle bundles, emphysema and dilated vessels and lymphatics (Fig. 11.24). Wellens *et al.* (1985) have also carried out a heart–lung transplant on a young woman with lymphangioleiomyomatosis. This patient developed obliterative bronchiolitis 7 months after operation. However, our case is still well after 13 months.

In diffuse pulmonary angiomatosis, numerous thin-walled vascular channels are present in fibrous septa, perivascular connective tissue and subpleural tissue (Fig. 11.25), and may infiltrate the walls of pulmonary veins and arteries (Wagenvoort, Beetstra and Spikjer, 1978; Heath and Reid, 1985; Rowen *et al.*, 1986). In our case the angiomatosis also involved the pericardium, parietal and diaphragmatic pleura and peripancreatic tissue; the diaphragm was up to 2 cm thick and inflexible and this appeared responsible for the child's fatal postoperative respiratory failure.

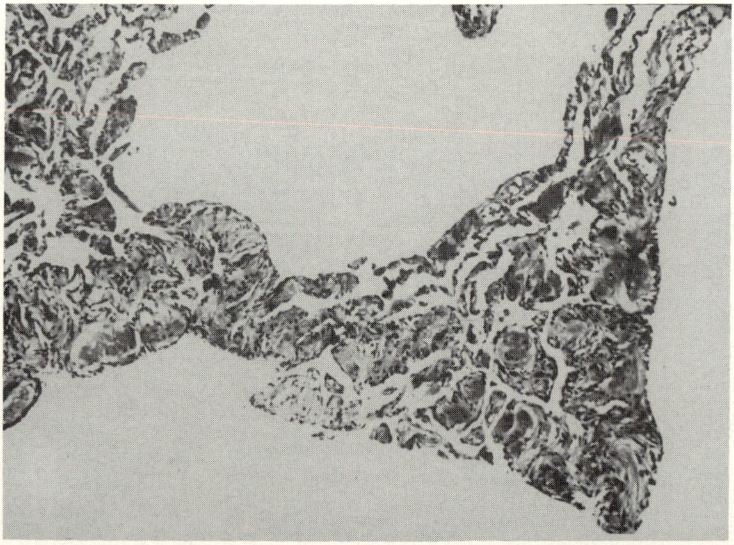

Fig. 11.24. *Pulmonary lymphangioleiomyomatosis. Microscopy shows irregular and nodular groups of smooth muscle fibres thickening alveolar septa. Haematoxylin and eosin × 30 approx.*

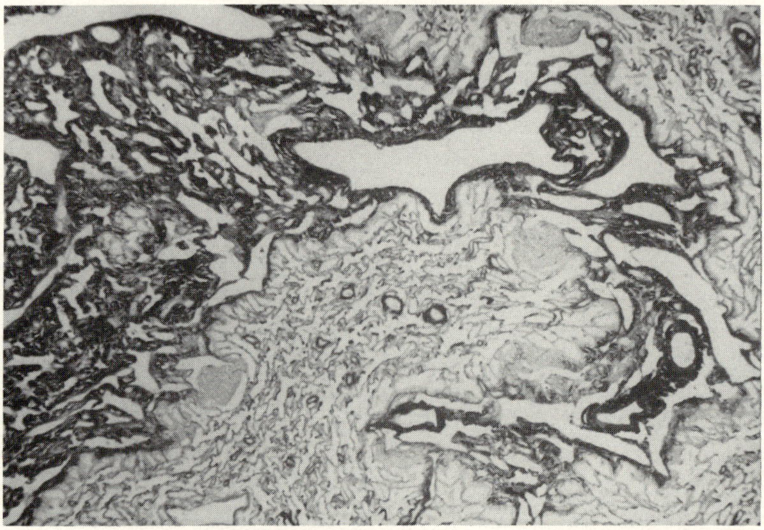

Fig. 11.25. *Diffuse pulmonary haemangiomatosis. Fibrous septa are replaced by angiomatous tissue. Elastic van Gieson × 30 approx.*

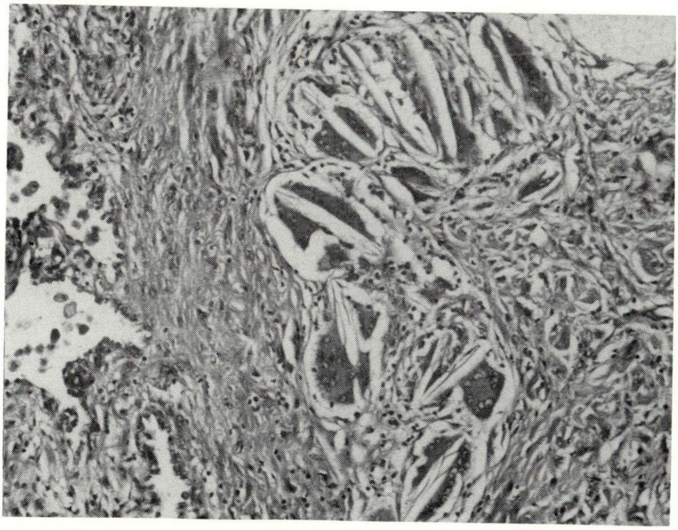

Fig. 11.26. *Cholesterol ester granuloma. Foreign body giant cells contain 'cigar-shaped' clefts. Haematoxylin and eosin × 120 approx.*

FAMILIAL PULMONARY HYPERTENSION

No specific pathology is associated with familial pulmonary hypertension. Familial veno-occlusive disease has been recorded (Wagenvoort, Wagenvoort and Takahashi, 1985; Hasleton, Ironside and Whittaker, 1986), as have the changes of primary plexogenic pulmonary hypertension (Wagenvoort and Wagenvoort, 1977.)

All 3 patients with familial pulmonary hypertension in our series showed plexogenic pulmonary vascular disease (see Table 11.5).

MISCELLANEOUS OBSERVATIONS

Cholesterol ester granulomas

Giant cell granulomatous foci are not uncommon in severe pulmonary hypertension. The foreign body giant cells contain needle-shaped clefts which have been identified as containing cholesterol palmitate or stearate (Glancy, Frazier and Roberts, 1968). These lesions have been reported only in association with pulmonary hypertension and must result from small haemorrhages. Eight patients in our series showed these cholesterol granulomas (Fig. 11.26). Five had plexogenic pulmonary hypertension, either

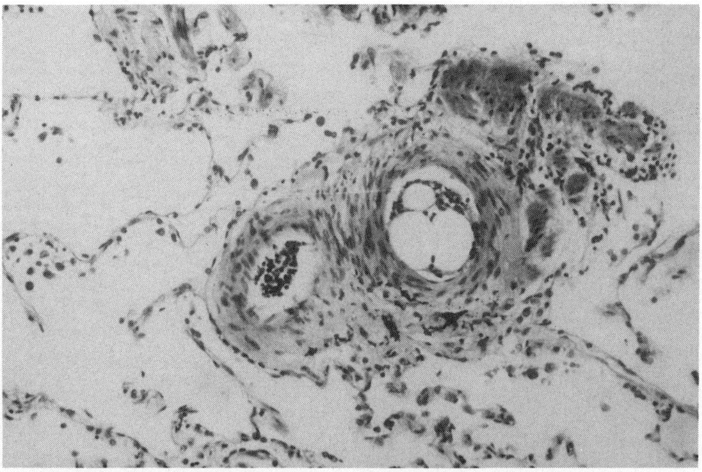

Fig. 11.27. *Bone marrow embolus consisting of fat and haemopoietic cells in a small pulmonary artery. Haematoxylin and eosin × 120 approx.*

primary or associated with congenital cardiac abnormalities, 2 had pulmonary fibrosis with associated vascular thrombosis and 1 thrombo-embolic pulmonary hypertension.

Pneumoliths

Four of our cases had small calcified or ossified foci of the type most often seen in patients with rheumatic mitral stenosis. These are also thought to result from small haemorrhages, but associated with chronic venous hypertension, which was the main pathological finding in 3 of the cases. The dominant pathology in the fourth case was severe plexogenic arteriopathy.

Micro-emboli

Particles of birefringent material were seen in 3 cases. This finding is not uncommon in patients who have been extensively investigated or had previous surgery and, in general, is of no significance (Wagenvoort and Wagenvoort, 1977). However, one of our cases of 'primary' pulmonary hypertension had thrombo-embolic disease centred around relatively large foreign particles (see Fig. 11.22). The history suggested that they had been introduced during intravenous therapy which preceded the pulmonary symptoms. The foreign material in another patient was a result of narcotic addiction (see Fig. 11.19). Small bone marrow emboli (Fig. 11.27) were observed in another 3 patients and are presumably a result of the sternotomy procedure.

REFERENCES

Burke C. M., Theodore, J., Baldwin, J. C., Tazelaar, H. D., Morris, A. J., McGregor, C., Shumway, N. E., Robin, E. D. and Jamieson, S. W. (1986). Twenty eight cases of human heart–lung transplantation. *Lancet* **i**, 517–519.

Cockerill, F. R., Wilson, W. R., Carpenter, H. A., Smith, T. F. and Rosenow, E. C. (1985). Open lung biopsy in immunocompromised patients. *Arch. Intern. Med.* **145**, 1398–1404.

Corrin, B., Leibow, A. A. and Friedman, P. J. (1975). Pulmonary lymphangioleiomyomatosis: a review. *Am. J. Pathol.* **79**, 348–382.

Glancy, D. L., Frazier, P. D. and Roberts, W. C. (1968). Pulmonary parenchymal cholesterol ester granulomas in patients with pulmonary hypertension. *Am. J. Med.* **45**, 198–210.

Hasleton, P. S., Ironside, J. W., Whittaker, J. S., Kelly, W., Ward, C. and Thompson, G. S. (1986). Pulmonary veno-occlusive disease. A report of 4 cases. *Histopathology* **10**, 933–944.

Heath, D. and Edwards, J. E. (1958). The pathology of hypertensive vascular disease. *Circulation* **18**, 533–547.

Heath, D. and Reid, R. (1985). Invasive pulmonary haemangiomatosis. *Br. J. Dis. Chest* **79**, 284–294.

Heath, D., Segal, N. and Bishop, J. (1966). Pulmonary veno-occlusive disease. *Circulation* **34**, 242–248.

Howarth, S. G. (1983). Primary pulmonary hypertension. *Br. Heart J.* **49**, 517–521.

Howarth, S. G. and McCartney, F. J. (1980). Growth and development of pulmonary circulation in pulmonary atresia with ventricular septal defect and major aortopulmonary collateral arteries. *Br. Heart J.* **44**, 14–24.

Jamieson, S. W., Stinson, E. B., Oyer, P. E., Reitz, B. A., Baldwin, J., Modry, D., Dawkins, K., Theodore, J., Hunt, S. and Shumway, N. E. (1984). Heart–lung transplantation for irreversible pulmonary hypertension. *Ann. Thorac. Surg.* **38**, 554–562.

Lancet (1982) Obliterative bronchiolitis. *Lancet* **i**, 603–604.

McGregor, C. G. A., Jamieson, S. W., Baldwin, J. C., Burke, C. M., Dawkins, K. D., Stinson, E. B., Oyer, P. E., Billingham, M. E., Zusman, D. R., Reitz, B. A., Morris, A., Yousem, S., Hunt, S. A. and Shumway, N. E. (1986). Combined heart–lung transplantation for end-stage Eisenmenger's syndrome. *J. Thorac. Cardiovasc. Surg.* **91**, 443–450.

Rowen, M., Thompson, J. R., Williamson, R. A. and Wood, B. J. (1986). Diffuse pulmonary haemangiomatosis. *Radiology* **127**, 445–451.

Stovin, P. G. I., Lum, L. C., Flower, C. D. R., Darke, C. S. and Beeley, M. (1975). The lungs in lymphangioleiomyomatosis and tuberous sclerosis. *Thorax* **30**, 497–509.

Wagenvoort, C. A. (1980). Lung biopsy specimens in the evaluation of pulmonary vascular disease. *Chest* **77**, 614–625.

Wagenvoort, C. A. (1981). Grading of pulmonary vascular lesions — a re-appraisal. *Histopathology* **5**, 595–598.

Wagenvoort, C. A., Beetstra, A. and Spikjer, J. (1978). Capillary haemangiomatosis of the lungs. *Histopathology* **2**, 401–406.

Wagenvoort, C. A. and Wagenvoort, N. (1970). Primary pulmonary hypertension. A pathologic study of the lung vessels in 156 clinically diagnosed cases. *Circulation* **42**, 1163–1184.

Wagenvoort, C. A. and Wagenvoort, N. (1977). *Pathology of Pulmonary Hypertension.* Wiley, New York.

Wagenvoort, C. A. and Wagenvoort, N. (1983). In *Cardiovascular Pathology* (M. D. Silver, Ed.), p. 698. Churchill Livingstone, New York.

Wagenvoort, C. A., Wagenvoort, N. and Takahashi, T. (1985). Pulmonary veno-occlusive disease: involvement of pulmonary arteries and review of the literature. *Hum. Pathol.* **16**, 1033–1041.

Wellens, F., Estenne, M., de Francquen, P., Goldstein, J., Leclerc, J. L. and Primo, G. (1985). Combined heart–lung transplantation for terminal pulmonary lymphangioleiomyomatosis. *J. Thorac. Cardiovasc. Surg.* **89**, 872–876.

WHO (1975). Primary pulmonary hypertension — Report of Committee. World Health Organisation, Geneva.

Yousem, S. A., Burke, C. M. and Billingham, M. E. (1985). Pathological pulmonary alterations in long-term human heart transplantation. *Hum. Pathol.* **16**, 911–923.

William A. Baumgartner

12

Practical Management of Cyclosporin A Following Transplantation

INTRODUCTION

Cyclosporin A is a cyclic peptide developed from crude extracts of Fungi Imperfecti, *Tolypocladium inflatum* Gams (Borel, 1982). It is purified chromatographically to a crystalloid powder that is insoluble in water but does dissolve slowly in lipids, such as olive oil. It was first reported to have immunosuppressive properties by Borel in 1972 (Borel *et al.*, 1976). The *in vitro* work was translated to experimental animal studies which demonstrated the immunosuppressive capabilities of the drug. Clinical studies were then conducted in both renal and extrarenal transplantation. Calne and colleagues reporting on the potency of cyclosporin, documented its immunosuppressive effect, and demonstrated its toxicity especially when combined with other immunosuppressive medications (Calne *et al.*, 1979). Starzl reported the successful use of cyclosporin in combination with prednisone for the immunosuppressive treatment of patients undergoing liver transplantation (Starzl *et al.*, 1980). Oyer *et al.* (1983) noted a significant increase in survival and decrease in complications in patients undergoing heart transplantation. Numerous studies have since recorded the efficacy of cyclosporin in both survival and quality of life for heart transplant recipients.

Considerable experience has been gained in the appropriate use of cyclosporin in cardiac transplantation. This chapter will outline particular characteristics and side effects unique to this drug and provide clinical information regarding its appropriate use for acute and chronic immunosuppression as well as in rejection in cardiac transplant recipients.

UNIQUE ASPECTS OF CYCLOSPORIN

In order to provide effective and efficacious management of heart transplant recipients, the transplant physician should be aware of the pharmacokinetics, drug monitoring capabilities, and interrelationships of cyclosporin with other drugs. The optimal use of cyclosporin remains elusive. There is considerable variation in protocols in time of initiation, dosage and appropriate combination of drugs, although all have the object of providing prophylaxis against cardiac rejection.

Drug characteristics

Cyclosporin is available in both oral and injectable forms. The oral solution contains cyclosporin in an olive and peglicol 5 oleate vehicle with 12.5% alcohol. The injectable form is mixed with polyoxyl 35 castor oil (Cremaphor EL) and 32.9% alcohol. Because of the possibility of leaching phthalates from commercial plastic bags, the intravenous administration should always be via glass bottles (Keown *et al.*, 1981). Since intramuscular delivery is both slow and unreliable, intravenous and oral administration are the preferred routes. The oral/intravenous equivalence of cyclosporin concentration is 3 : 1 (Kahan, 1987). The advantage of intravenous cyclosporin is in the avoidance of absorption problems that may occur in the early postoperative phase of transplantation. Bolus administration is not recommended because it results in unacceptably high blood levels. If cyclosporin is to be given intravenously, it should be a dose of 1–3 mg/kg per day as a continuous infusion. This creates a 'steady state', resulting in a lower incidence of renal dysfunction and other side effects.

Stewart *et al.* (1987) reported on the use of continuous intravenous infusion in the immediate postoperative phase after cardiac transplantation. The dose (2.8 ± 0.52 mg/kg) was adjusted to maintain blood levels of approximately 350 ng/ml (high-performance liquid chromatography) which resulted in diminished nephrotoxicity and no increase in rejection. We think this level is too high. We have used intravenous cyclosporin when complications following heart transplantation have resulted in the inability of the recipient to tolerate oral intake. An intravenous infusion of 1–2 mg/kg has resulted in blood levels between 75 and 150 ng/ml which have been adequate for prophylaxis against cardiac rejection.

The immunosuppressive protocol for renal transplantation utilized by Kahan (1987) consists of a continuous infusion of cyclosporin (2.5 mg/kg per day) to achieve levels of 150 ng/ml for 3 days before oral therapy is initiated. The use of continuous intravenous cyclosporin for extended periods has not been reported. The main disadvantage of intravenous cyclosporin is its potential for anaphylactoid reactions. The previously observed toxic reactions such as interstitial pulmonary oedema and convulsions may be more attributable to the carrier, Cremaphor (Kahan, 1987).

Methods of measurement and drug monitoring

Two methods for measuring cyclosporin concentration are available at the present time. A radioimmunoassay (RIA), performed by a kit distributed by Sandoz, detects both the parent compound as well as a group of cyclosporin-related metabolites (Niederberger, Schaub and Beveridge, 1980). To obtain uniform results, several important variables need to be controlled, including temperature and timing of sample storage, separation and transport, and the method and frequency of measurement of the standard curve. Although much of the clinical work utilizing the RIA assay has been with plasma or serum, it is recommended that whole blood be used. This obviates the variable of temperature. When temperature is lowered from 37°C to 21°C, cyclosporin rapidly diffuses from plasma into blood cells, thereby making plasma or serum determination suspect, depending on the temperature at the time of testing.

High-performance liquid chromatography (HPLC) is able to differentiate the parent compound from its metabolites (Donatsch *et al.*, 1981). The technique uses whole blood and is more time-consuming and complex than the RIA assay. However, if a clinical laboratory is experienced with the technique, reliable results can be obtained. The assay at the Johns Hopkins Hospital is conducted by the clinical laboratory which provides the service on weekdays and on weekends if necessary. Results have been uniform with acceptable variation in levels of an individual patient. Increasing information is being accumulated on the HPLC method as more heart transplant centres are incorporating it in their transplant programmes.

The optimal drug concentration of cyclosporin for prophylaxis against allograft rejection has evolved with experience. Since variation exists between assays and type of blood fraction being measured, multiple and sometimes confusing results have been reported. Table 12.1 summarizes the therapeutic ranges observed in clinical studies based upon two assays (RIA, HPLC), and two blood fractions (serum, whole blood). Nephrotoxicity has been demonstrated to occur in clinical renal transplantation when the serum trough level (RIA) exceeds 250 ng/ml (Kahan *et al.*, 1984). For cardiac transplantation, however, serum levels of 200–400 ng/ml (RIA) are considered appropriate for prophylaxis in the early postoperative period (Kahan *et al.*, 1987). Griffith *et al.* (1984) reported a whole blood level of 1000 ng/ml by RIA assay to be associated with nephrotoxicity in heart transplant recipients. Although there was not a statistically significant correlation between nephrotoxicity and whole blood cyclosporin levels of 1000 ng/ml, based

TABLE 12.1
Therapeutic Ranges of Cyclosporin in Heart Transplant Recipients

	Postoperative Levels (ng/ml)		
Assay/Blood Fraction	*Immediate*	*3 months*	*6 months*
RIA*/serum	200–400	75–150	50–150
RIA/whole blood	300–800	200–600	150–400
HPLC†/whole blood	150–400	—	75–150

* RIA, radioimmunoassay.
† HPLC, high-performance liquid chromatography.

upon their clinical findings, the target cyclosporin level was reduced to 750 ng/ml.

When using the RIA assay (whole blood), an immediate postoperative trough level of 300–800 ng/ml is considered therapeutic and generally non-toxic (Yee *et al.*, 1984a). The dose is gradually reduced to reach target levels of 150–400 ng/ml 6 months postoperatively (Kahan, 1987). A similar cyclosporin tapering scale is utilized with the RIA (serum) technique. In the early postoperative period, 200–400 ng/ml is the target value with gradual reduction to 75–150 ng/ml at 6 months (Keown *et al.*, 1982; Kahan, 1987). Less experience is available for the HPLC technique using whole blood. Our experience would suggest that a target level of 150–400 ng/ml is adequate for immunosuppression in the early postoperative phase (Baumgartner, Augustine and Borkon, 1987). Gradual reduction to 75–150 ng/ml at 6 months has not been associated with increased rejection and has resulted in fewer adverse reactions.

Pharmacokinetics

The oral bioavailability of cyclosporin averages 29% (Kahan, Reid and Newburger, 1983). This limited bioavailability has been attributed to poor gastrointestinal absorption in addition to extensive first-pass metabolism. Absorption is affected by numerous processes including ileus, diarrhoea or liver disease, as well as olive oil intolerance by the gastrointestinal tract.

Intravenous cyclosporin is distributed widely throughout the body. The greatest uptake is by the liver, probably related to its role in drug metabolism and excretion (Reid *et al.*, 1983). The second highest accumulation of cyclosporin is in the pancreas. This may have clinical relevance based upon both experimental evidence and clinical studies, demonstrating an increased incidence of pancreaticobiliary complications including cholelithiasis, glucose intolerance and pancreatitis after transplantation in patients immu-

TABLE 12.2
Cyclosporin–Drug Interactions

Effect	*Drug*
Acceleration of cyclosporin elimination	Rifampicin, phenytoin, phenobarbitone
Decreased cyclosporin elimination	Ketoconazole, erythromycin, frusemide in high doses
Increased nephrotoxicity	Amphotericin B, gentamicin, melphalan, trimethoprim, cimetidine

nosuppressed with cyclosporin (Kahan *et al.*, 1985; Hahn *et al.*, 1986; Lorber *et al.*, 1987). Fatty tissue represents the third major depot because of the lipophilic nature of the drug. Intermediate levels are found in the heart, lung, kidney and brain. Muscle and spinal cord contain the lowest levels.

In the liver, the cytochrome P450 system seems to be the primary mechanism of degradation (Kahan, 1985). Therefore, drugs that induce or compete for the cytochrome P450 system influence the blood or serum level of cyclosporin (Table 12.2). Drugs that induce cytochrome P450 activity and thereby accelerate cyclosporin elimination include rifampin, phenytoin and phenobarbitone. Drugs that compete for cytochrome P450 activity, thereby resulting in a decreased elimination of cyclosporin, include ketoconazole, frusemide in high doses and erythromycin. Since the breakdown of prednisone makes use of the same cytochrome P450 system, high doses of corticosteroid lead to a prolonged half-life of cyclosporin (Kahan *et al.*, 1986). Conversely, cyclosporin itself reduces prednisone clearance (Langhoff *et al.*, 1984).

In addition to these interactions, cyclosporin when combined with known nephrotoxic drugs can lead to an increased incidence of nephrotoxicity. These drugs include amphotericin B, gentamicin, melphalan, trimethoprim and cimetidine.

The half-life of cyclosporin has been demonstrated to be in the range of 7–9 h (Beveridge *et al.*, 1981; Kahan, 1986). The clearance of cyclosporin has been shown to be in the range of 12–15 ml/min per kg (Beveridge *et al.*, 1981; Langhoff *et al.*, 1984; Yee *et al.*, 1984b). Cyclosporin clearance varies with age. Children have shown a 40% higher drug clearance than adults, necessitating more frequent and higher doses (Kahan *et al.*, 1986; Lokiec, Fischer and Gluckman, 1987). These data have been accumulated in renal and bone marrow transplant patients, but nevertheless it is recommended that paediatric heart transplant patients be given cyclosporin in an initial dose of 15–35 mg/kg, with subsequent reduction based upon cyclosporin levels similar to that used in adults (Bailey *et al.*, 1986).

It has also been recognized that adults over the age of 45 require less cyclosporin because of a 30% decrease in the clearance of the drug (Kahan *et al.*, 1986). Cyclosporin drug clearance can also be altered by variation in hepatic function. Since the liver is the primary source for cyclosporin metabolism and excretion, elevations of bilirubin (>2 mg/dl) imply a reduction in drug clearance necessitating a reduction in cyclosporin dose (Yee *et al.*, 1984b).

PREOPERATIVE MANAGEMENT WITH CYCLOSPORIN

Numerous protocols addressing the role of cyclosporin in the postoperative and perioperative periods have been formulated. The advantage of any one protocol over others is not clear at this time. Data from the Registry of the International Society for Heart Transplantation presented at the most recent spring meeting suggested an increased survival in heart transplant recipients receiving 'triple drug' therapy, compared with patients receiving cyclosporin with one other immunosuppressive drug. Protocols from selected major institutions involved in heart transplantation are given below, illustrating the varied use of cyclosporin and its efficacy in the prophylaxis of allograft rejection. The advantages and disadvantages of each protocol in particular reference to cyclosporin are considered. Table 12.3 lists the preoperative management of cyclosporin according to individual institutions.

Finding a 22% incidence of acute renal failure after heart transplantation, McGiffin, Kirklin and Naftel (1985) changed their protocol by reducing the loading dose of oral cyclosporin to 0.5–1.0 mg/kg. Subsequent doses were gradually increased based upon cyclosporin blood levels. Rabbit antithymocyte globulin (RATG) was administered daily until therapeutic cyclosporin levels were achieved. They observed that a serum creatinine greater than 2.0 mg% within the year prior to heart transplantation and the need for inotropic support in the week before operation were associated with the development of acute renal failure. However, even in this high-risk group the modified protocol utilizing low-dose cyclosporin together with RATG avoided significant renal impairment. Similarly, Copeland *et al.* (1986) changed their cyclosporin protocol in January 1984 by omitting any cyclosporin until the third postoperative day, because of the toxic side effects they saw in the early postoperative period in their initial series of cyclosporin-treated recipients. Rabbit antithymocyte globulin was given by injection immediately following the operation and on the subsequent 2 days.

TABLE 12.3
Preoperative Immunosuppression for Heart Transplant Patients According to Institution

Institution	*Cyclosporin (mg/kg)*	*Reference*
University of Alabama	0.5–1.0	Copeland *et al.* (1986)
University of Arizona	None	Bailey *et al.* (1986)
Cleveland Clinic	None	Hardesty (1986)
Harefield Hospital	2–10	Yacoub *et al.* (1985); Yacoub (1986)
Johns Hopkins Hospital	6–10	Kahan *et al.* (1987)
La Pitié Hospital	None	McGiffin, Kirklin and Naftel (1985)
Medical College of Virginia	2–10	—
University of Minnesota/ Washington University, St. Louis	6–12	Yacoub *et al.* (1985)
University of Pittsburgh	None	Yee *et al.* (1984b); Griffith *et al.* (1985)
Stanford University	10–16	Kahan (1986)
Texas Heart Institute	14	Yacoub (1986)

Stewart *et al.* (1987) found that azotaemia requiring dialysis occurred in 3 out of 19 patients given cyclosporin as an intravenous bolus prior to transplantation. However, intravenous cyclosporin started immediately after transplantation did not lead to any significant increase in rejection or dialysis requirement. Yacoub, reporting his series of patients in which cyclosporin was given in an oral dose of 2–10 mg/kg depending upon the preoperative renal function (Yacoub, 1985; Yacoub *et al.*, 1986), saw no early incidence of azotaemia or acute renal failure. A similar protocol at the Medical College of Virginia has resulted in a significant decrease in postoperative renal dysfunction (personal communication).

The protocol at the Johns Hopkins Hospital consists of a titrated cyclosporin dose based upon preoperative renal function. If the creatinine is greater than 2.0 mg%, 6 mg/kg rather than 10 mg/kg of cyclosporin is administered as an oral dose (Baumgartner, Augustine and Borkon, 1987). The immunosuppressive regimen at La Pitié Hospital, Paris, avoids preoperative cyclosporin and initiates it on the second postoperative day (Cabrol *et al.*, 1985). Corticosteroids and azathioprine are begun prior to operation. The former is diminished to a low dose while the latter is stopped upon initiation of cyclosporin. This revised protocol has resulted in a 4-year actuarial survival of 80% for the last 76 patients undergoing transplantation.

'Triple therapy' was first applied clinically in heart transplantation by Bolman *et al.* (1987). In this protocol, cyclosporin is administered preoperatively in a dose of 6–12 mg/kg based upon preoperative renal function. Actuarial survival at 2 years was 83%. Serum creatinine was 1.3 ± 0.3

mg/dl at 1 month, 1.6 ± 0.4 mg/dl at 6 months, and 1.7 ± 0.4 mg/dl at 24 months. At the University of Pittsburgh, because dialysis was occasionally necessary during the first 10–14 days after transplantation, the immunosuppressive protocol was changed so that at present no cyclosporin is given preoperatively (Griffith *et al.*, 1985; Hardesty, 1986). Azathioprine was given preoperatively and continued until therapeutic levels of cyclosporin were achieved. In addition, RATG was given prophylactically for 5 days after transplantation. The present immunosuppressive protocol at Stanford University consists of the administration of cyclosporin preoperatively in an oral dose of 10–16 mg/kg based upon renal function, and azathioprine 4 mg/kg intravenously (Oyer, 1986). Frazier *et al.* (1985) gave 14 mg/kg by mouth prior to operation and then 2 mg/kg intravenously until the patient was able to take oral medication. Renal failure requiring dialysis occurred in 1 patient.

Although delaying the administration of cyclosporin until the early postoperative period may reduce the nephrotoxic effects, it may result in less than optimal immunosuppression. Schuler, Warnecke and Hetzer (1987) reported that starting treatment with 4 days of antilymphocyte serum–azathioprine–prednisone therapy was associated with decreased patient survival, prompting them to recommend initiating cyclosporin 24 h rather than 96 h postoperatively. We found that with assiduous monitoring of cyclosporin levels and serum creatinine, the oral cyclosporin dose can be effectively adjusted in the early postoperative period to give an adequate immunosuppression without a severe nephrotoxic effect (Baumgartner, Augustine and Borkon, 1987).

POSTOPERATIVE AND CHRONIC IMMUNOSUPPRESSION MANAGEMENT

A summary of the various immunosuppressive protocols appears in Table 12.4. Yacoub *et al.* (1985), who gave a combination of cyclosporin and azathioprine, reported that at the end of 1 year, 90% of the patients were not taking oral steroids and 80% had never had any. Long-term oral steroids were necessary in only 6 patients (3%). Actuarial survival at 1 and 3 years was 78% and 76%, respectively. The rejection rate was 2.8 episodes per patient.

Controversy still exists regarding the relation of cyclosporin levels to rejection. A recent article by Warnecke, Schueler and Hetzer (1987) observed that even a short decrease in the cyclosporin level below the therapeutic range (<150 ng/ml) may be dangerous. They recommended biopsy intervals of 10–12 weeks and treatment of the majority of rejection episodes with oral steroids.

TABLE 12.4
Present Immunosuppressive Regimen According to Selected Institutions

Institution	*Maintenance Immunosuppressive Protocol*	*Prophylactic ATG*
University of Alabama	Cyclosporin + prednisone	Yes
University of Arizona	Cyclosporin + prednisone	Yes
Cleveland Clinic	Cyclosporin + prednisone + azathioprine	No
Harefield Hospital	Cyclosporin + azathioprine	No
Johns Hopkins Hospital	Cyclosporin + prednisone + azathioprine	No
La Pitié Hospital	Cyclosporin + prednisone	Yes
Medical College of VA	Cyclosporin + azathioprine	Yes
University of Minnesota/ Washington University, St. Louis	Cyclosporin + prednisone + azathioprine	No
University of Pittsburgh	Cyclosporin + prednisone + azathioprine	Yes
Stanford University	Cyclosporin + prednisone + azathioprine	Yes
Texas Heart Institute	Cyclosporin + prednisone	No

Haverich *et al.* (1987), concerned about the potential side effects of cyclosporin in a two-drug regimen, switched to a four-drug regimen (RATG, low-dose prednisone, azathioprine and cyclosporin, 1 mg/kg per day increasing to 5–7 mg/kg per day). This protocol, however, was modified according to the patient's preoperative status and postoperative complications. Rejection was treated by steroids in the routine manner, except when it was also associated with a bacterial infection. In the latter case, RATG was substituted for prednisone. One-year actuarial survival using this individualized approach to immunosuppression was 80.5%.

The majority of the immunosuppressive protocols include intraoperative and early postoperative administration of intravenous steroids. All protocols looked to reduce the cyclosporin dose with the passage of time according to the levels mentioned earlier. In addition, there was a tendency to reduce steroids to a low maintenance dose (0.2–0.3 mg/kg) approximately 6 months after transplantation.

TREATMENT OF REJECTION

In the treatment of heart allograft rejection, cyclosporin was previously thought to be ineffective. This belief was a result of *in vitro* data and experimental findings (Homan *et al.*, 1980). However, reports of treatment of rejection with cyclosporin in renal allografts have demonstrated its efficacy (Margreiter *et al.*, 1983; Dickerman *et al.*, 1985). Margreiter and colleagues treated 8 consecutive kidney transplant recipients and 1 liver transplant recipient whose rejection was refractory to methylprednisolone treatment. Oral cyclosporin was initiated at a dose of 17 mg/kg per day for 2 weeks, then reduced to 15 mg/kg per day and tapered by 2 mg/kg per day every month until a maintenance dose of 7 mg/kg per day was reached. All 9 patients in this cyclosporin-treated group responded. No grafts were lost and, at the time of report, no further rejection was observed in any of the patients (Margreiter *et al.*, 1983).

Colon *et al.* (1987) conducted a trial to compare the efficacy of supplemental intravenous cyclosporin with intravenous bolus doses of corticosteroids to reverse moderate cardiac rejection. Patients received, in addition to their oral dose of cyclosporin, a supplemental infusion of 2 mg/kg per day for 7 days. This resulted in a 76% resolution of acute rejection episodes, similar to the 81% reversal rate observed in patients treated with high-dose (7 mg/kg) methylprednisolone. However, the infectious complications were significantly less in the cyclosporin-treated (23%) than in the steroid-treated group (50%). No significant acute or chronic nephrotoxicity or hepatoxicity was demonstrated in the cyclosporin-treated group of patients (Beveridge *et al.*, 1981).

TECHNIQUE OF CYCLOSPORIN REDUCTION OR CONVERSION TO AZATHIOPRINE

Before the initiation of triple-drug therapy, severe nephrotoxicity led to the conversion of treatment from cyclosporin to azathioprine, or a reduction of cyclosporin and addition of azathioprine to the regimen. A persistently elevated creatinine (>2–3 mg%) was the usual indication for a change of treatment. Hunt *et al.* (1987) reported on 'immunoconversion' from cyclosporin to azathioprine in 15 patients because of severe nephrotoxicity. Their protocol began with azathioprine 25 mg/day, and increased by 25 mg/day each week to either a maximum of 200 mg/day or until the white blood count fell below 6000. When the azathioprine dose had been stabilized, a right ventricular biopsy was obtained. If the biopsy showed no signs of rejection, the maintenance steroid dose was doubled and cyclosporin was stopped.

Follow-up biopsies were obtained 2 weeks after cessation of cyclosporin and monthly for 3 months. The biopsies of 8 out of 15 patients showed rejection during the 3-month surveillance period. However, none of these patients had clinical signs of cardiac rejection. The rejection cleared in half of these patients with oral steroid treatment, while half required high-dose methylprednisolone. Subsequently, 2 patients had multiple rejection episodes necessitating restoration of cyclosporin in a diminished dose. Three patients died after discontinuation of cyclosporin, but their deaths did not appear to be related to immunoconversion. The tendency for rejection following immunoconversion led Hunt *et al.* (1987) to conclude that cyclosporin should be reduced to a minimum but maintained, in addition to azathioprine and prednisone. The protocol for immunoconversion of patients at the Johns Hopkins Hospital is based upon a gradual reduction in cyclosporin (1–2 mg/kg) and the addition of azathioprine to achieve therapeutic levels determined by white blood count tolerance (white blood count ⩾5000). It is achieved over a 4-week period. Biopsies are obtained in the middle of the transition and upon completion. Rejection has been observed in approximately 50% of recipients. However, as in the Stanford data, no patient died as a result of immunoconversion.

SUMMARY

Experience in the proper use of cyclosporin in clinical transplantation continues to develop. This has led to a number of beneficial changes in the immunosuppressive protocols, contributing to increased survival in the majority of cardiac transplant programmes. The important principles to adhere to in treating a patient with cyclosporin are: assiduous monitoring of cyclosporin levels and serum creatinine during the early postoperative period; understanding of the mechanism of action, bioavailability, pharmacokinetics and interrelationships with other medications; and a triple or quadruple drug regimen in which the individual drug doses are reduced, thereby lessening the toxicity associated with each drug. Persistent and careful monitoring of these patients, including assessment of renal function and cyclosporin levels, and surveillance for infection, are mandatory, in order that they may continue to enjoy the benefits of this novel immunosuppressive agent.

REFERENCES

Bailey, L. L., Nehlsen-Cannarella, S. L., Doroshow, R. W., Jacobson, J. G., Martin, R. D., Allard, M. W., Hyde, M. R., Dang Bui, R. H. and Petry, E. L. (1986). Cardiac allotransplantation in newborns as therapy for hypoplastic left heart syndrome. *N. Engl. J. Med.* **315**, 949–951.

Baumgartner, W. A., Augustine, S., Borkon, A. M., Gardner, T. J. and Reitz, B. A. (1987). Present expectations in cardiac transplantation. *Ann. Thorac. Surg.* **43**, 585–590.

Beveridge, T., Gratwohl, A., Michot, F., Niederberger, W., Nüesch, E., Nussbaumer, K., Schaub, P. and Speck, B. (1981). Cyclosporin A: pharmacokinetics after a single dose in man and serum levels after multiple dosing in recipients of allogenic bone marrow grafts. *Curr. Ther. Res.* **30**, 5–18.

Bolman, R. M., Olivari, M. T., Saffitz, J., Sibley, R., Spadaro, J., Cance, C. and Elick, B. (1987). Current results with triple therapy for heart transplantation. *Transplant Proc.* **19,** 2490–2491.

Borel, J. F. (1982). The history of cyclosporin A and its significance. In *Cyclosporin A: Proceedings of an International Conference on Cyclosporin A* (D. J. G. White, Ed.), pp. 5–17. Elsevier Biomedical Press, Amsterdam.

Borel, J. F., Feurer, C., Gubler, H. U. and Stähelim, H. (1976). Biological effects of cyclosporin A: a new antilymphocyte agent. *Agents Act.* **6,** 468–475.

Cabrol, C., Gandjbakhch, I., Pavie, A., Cabrol, A., Mattei, M. F. and Leger, P. (1985). Heart transplantation in Paris at 'La Pitié' hospital. *J. Heart Transplant.* **4**, 476–480.

Calne, R. Y., Rolles, K., White, D. J. G., Thiru, S., Evans, D. B., McMaster, P., Dunn, D. C., Craddock, G. N., Henderson, R. G., Aziz, S. and Lewis, P. (1979). Cyclosporin A initially as the only immunosuppressant in 34 recipients of cadaveric organs: 32 kidneys, 2 pancreases, 2 livers. *Lancet*, **2**, 1033–1036.

Colon, R., Lorber, M. I., Frazier, O. H. *et al.* (1987). An alternative therapy for rejection in cardiac allograft recipients. *Transplant Proc.* (in press).

Copeland, J. G., Emery, R. W., Levinson, M. M., Icenogle, T. B., Riley, J. E., McAleer, M. J., Copeland, J. A. and Dietz, R. (1986). Cyclosporine: an immunosuppressive panacea? *J. Thorac. Cardiovasc. Surg.* **91**, 26–39.

Dickerman, R. M., Vergne-Marini, P., Long, D. L., Nesser, D. A. and Velez, R. L. (1985). The use of cyclosporine in treating acute allograft rejection. *Transplant Proc.* **17**, 78–80.

Donatsch, P., Abisch, E., Homberger, M., Traber, R., Trapp, M. and Voges, R. (1981). A radioimmunoassay to measure cyclosporin A in plasma and serum samples. *J. Immunoass.* **2**, 19–32.

Frazier, O. H., Cooley, D. A., Painvin, G. A., Chandler, L. B. and Okereke, O. U. (1985). Cardiac transplantation at the Texas Heart Institute: comparative analysis of two groups of patients (1968–1969 and 1982–1983). *Ann. Thorac. Surg.* **39**, 303–307.

Griffith, B. P., Hardesty, R. L., Trento, A. and Bahnson, H. T. (1985). Five years of heart transplantation in Pittsburgh. *J. Heart Transplant.* **4**, 489.

Griffith, B. P., Hardesty, R. L., Trento, A., Lee, A. and Bahnson, H. T. (1984). Targeted blood levels of cyclosporine for cardiac transplantation. *J. Thorac. Cardiovasc. Surg.* **88**, 952.

Hahn, H. J., Laube, F., Lucke, S., Klöting, I., Kohnert, K. D. and Warzock, R. (1986). Toxic effects of cyclosporine on the endocrine pancreas of Wistar rats. *Transplantation* **41**, 44–47.

Hardesty, R. L. (1986). Sequential Aza/CsA therapy with RATG and low-dose steroids for cardiac transplantation. *Transplant. Immunol. Lett.* **3**, 3.

Haverich, A., Frimpony-Boateng, K., Schafers, H. J., Wahlers, T., Fieguth, H. G., Herrmann, G., Wonigeit, K. and Borst, H. G. (1987). Individualized immunosuppression in heart transplant recipients. *Transplant Proc.* **19**, 2514–2515.

Homan, W. P., Fabre, J. W., Millard, P. R. and Morris, P. J. (1980). Effect of cyclosporin A upon second-set rejection of rat renal allografts. *Transplantation* **30**, 354–357.

Hunt, S. A., Stinson, E. B., Oyer, P. E., Billingham, M. E., Gamberg, P., Miller, J., Schroeder, J. S., Baldwin, J. C. and Shumway, N. E. (1987). Results of 'immunoconversion' from cyclosporine to azathioprine in heart transplant recipients with progressive nephrotoxicity. *Transplant Proc.* **19**, 2522–2524.

Kahan, B. D. (1985). Individualization of cyclosporine therapy using pharmacokinetics and pharmacodynamic parameters. *Transplantation* **40**, 457.

Kahan, B. D. (1986). The utility of pretransplant pharmacokinetic and pharmacodynamic profiling in clinical renal transplantation. *Transplant Proc.* **18**, 763.

Kahan, B. D. (1987). Immunosuppressive therapy with cyclosporine for cardiac transplantation. *Circulation* **75**, 40.

Kahan, B. D., Kramer, W. G., Wideman, C., Flechner, S. M., Lorber, M. I. and Van Buren, C. T. (1986). Demographic factors affecting the pharmacokinetics of cyclosporine estimated by radioimmunoassay. *Transplantation* **41**, 459–464.

Kahan, B. D., Kramer, W. G., Wideman, C. A., Frazier, O. H., Lorber, M. I., Williams, C., Flechner, S. M., Cooley, D. A. and Van Buren, C. T. (1987). Analysis of pharmacokinetic profiles in 232 renal and 87 cardiac allograft recipients treated with cyclosporine. In *Cyclosporine — Pharmacologic Aspects* (B. D. Kahan, Ed.), pp. 115–119. Grune and Stratton, New York.

Kahan, B. D., Reid, M. and Newburger, J. (1983). Pharmacokinetics of cyclosporine in human renal transplantation. *Transplant Proc.* **15**, 446.

Kahan, B. D., Van Buren, C. T., Flechner, S., Jarowenko, M., Yasumura, T., Rogers, A. J., Yoshimura, N., LeGrue, S., Drath, D. and Kerman, R. H. (1985). Clinical and experimental studies using cyclosporine in renal transplantation. *Surgery* **97**, 125–140.

Kahan, B. D., Wideman, C., Reid, M., Gibbons, S., Jarowenko, M., Flechner, S. and Van Buren, C. T. (1984). The value of serial serum trough cyclosporine levels in human renal transplantation. *Transplant Proc.* **16**, 1195–1199.

Keown, P. A., Stiller, C. R., Laupacis, A. L., Howson, W., Coles, R. Stawecki, M., Koegler, J., Carruthers, G., McKenzie, N. and Sinclair, N. R. (1982). The effects and side effects of cyclosporine: relationship to drug pharmacokinetics. *Transplant Proc.* **14**, 659–661.

Keown, P. A., Stiller, C. R., Ulan, R. A., Sinclair, N. R., Wall, W. J., Carruthers, G. and Howson, W. (1981). Immunological and pharmacological monitoring in the clinical use of cyclosporin A. *Lancet* **1**, 686–692.

Langhoff, E., Madsen, S., Olgaard, K. and Ladofoged, J. (1984). Clinical results and cyclosporine effects on prednisolone metabolism. *Kidney Int.* **26**, 642.

Lokiec, F., Fischer, A. and Gluckman, E. (1987). A safer approach to the clinical use of cyclosporine: the predose calculation. In *Cyclosporine — Pharmacologic Aspects* (B. D. Kahan, Ed.), pp. 194–199). Grune and Stratton, New York.

Lorber, M. I., Van Buren, C. T., Flechner, S. M., Williams, C. and Kahan, B. D. (1987). Hepatobiliary and pancreatic complications of cyclosporine therapy in 466 renal transplant recipients. *Transplantation* **43**, 35–40.

Margreiter, R., Huber, C., Spielberger, M. and Konig, P. (1983). Cyclosporine in the treatment of acute cadaveric kidney graft rejection refractory to high-dose methylprednisolone. *Transplantation* **36**, 203.

McGiffin, D. C., Kirklin, J. K. and Naftel, D. C. (1985). Acute renal failure after heart transplantation and cyclosporine therapy. *J. Heart Transplant.* **4**, 396.

Niederberger, W., Schaub, P. and Beveridge, T. (1980). High performance liquid chromatographic determination of cyclosporin A in human plasma and urine. *J. Chromatogr.* **182**, 454.

Oyer, P. E. (1986). Triple drug immunosuppressive therapy in cardiac transplantation. *Transplant. Immunol. Lett.* **3**, 3.

Oyer, P. E., Stinson, E. B., Jamieson, S. W., Hunt, S. A., Perlroth, M., Billingham, M. E. and Shumway, N. E. (1983). Cyclosporin in cardiac transplantation: a $2\frac{1}{2}$ year follow-up. *Transplant Proc.* **15**, 2546–2552.

Reid, M., Gibbons, S., Kwok, D., Van Buren, C. T., Flechner, S. and Kahan, B. D. (1983). Cyclosporine levels in human tissues of patients treated for one week to one year. *Transplant Proc.* **15**, 2434–2437.

Schuler, S., Warnecke, H. and Hetzer, R. (1987). Prevention of toxic side effects of cyclosporin in heart transplantation. *Transplant Proc.* **19**, 2518.

Starzl, T. E., Weil, R., Iwatsuki, J. T., Klintmalm, G., Schröter, G. P. J., Koep, L. J., Iwaki, Y., Terasaki, P. I. and Porter, K. A. (1980). The use of cyclosporin A and prednisone in cadaveric kidney transplantation. *Surg. Gynecol. Obstet.* **151**, 17–26.

Stewart, R. W., Rincon, G., Hobbs, R. E., Drogomir, G. E. and Golding, L. A. R. (1987). Intravenous cyclosporine immunosuppression for cardiac transplantation (Abstract). *J. Am. Coll. Cardiol.* **9**, 135A.

Warnecke, H., Schueler, S. and Hetzer, R. (1987). Late acute rejection after cardiac transplantation: incidence and treatment. *Transplant Proc.* **19**, 2504.

Yacoub, M. (1986). Cardiac transplantation with cyclosporine and azathioprine — double drug therapy. *Transplant. Immunol. Lett.* **3**, 2.

Yacoub, M., Alivizatos, P., Khaghani, A. and Mitchell, A. (1985). The use of cyclosporine, azathioprine, and antithymocyte globulin with or without low-dose steroids for immunosuppression of cardiac transplant patients. *Transplant Proc.* **17**, 221.

Yee, G. C., Kennedy, M. S., Storb, R. and Thomas, E. D. (1984a). Pharmacokinetics in bone marrow transplant patients. Comparison of two assay methods. *Transplantation* **38**, 511.

Yee, G. C., Kennedy, M. S., Storb, R. and Thomas, E. D. (1984b). Effect of hepatic dysfunction on oral cyclosporine pharmacokinetics in marrow transplant patients. *Blood* **64**, 1377.

David C. McGiffin, James R. Bonner, James K. Kirklin and David C. Naftel

13

Patterns of Infection and Management in Cardiac Transplantation

INTRODUCTION

Infection is an important cause of morbidity and mortality following cardiac transplantation. The major infectious disorders are caused by intracellular pathogens including bacteria, fungi, parasites and viruses, and result from suppression of cellular immunity necessary to prevent transplant rejection. This emphasizes the challenge of providing sufficient immunosuppression to achieve graft–host coexistence without excessively suppressing host defences.

Most patients have at least one infectious complication following transplantation. If proper treatment is not promptly initiated, many infections will follow a fulminant course, with rapid spread to multiple organ systems. With the variety of potential pathogens in the immunocompromised patient, aggressive pursuit of a specific cause is essential. Earlier recognition and better management of infectious complications (coupled with changes in immunosuppressive therapy) have contributed substantially to the overall improved survival in recent years.

PREDISPOSING FACTORS IN INFECTION

Immunosuppressive drugs

No matter what immunosuppressive manoeuvres are used following organ transplantation (including drugs, radiation or splenectomy), some alteration occurs in host defence mechanisms. It is the intensity of immunosuppression rather than the effects of specific agents that determines the kinds and frequency of infections.

Depression of polymorphonuclear leucocyte function results in increased susceptibility to bacterial infection. B-lymphocyte depression, and hence a reduction in antibody production, increases the risk of infection due to encapsulated bacteria, especially *Pneumococcus* and *Haemophilus influenzae*. When T-lymphocyte function is depressed, there is an increased likelihood of infection from certain viruses (herpes virus), certain bacteria (tubercle bacillus, *Listeria*), fungi, and protozoa (*Pneumocystis carinii* and *Toxoplasma*) (Rubin and Cosimi, 1982).

Corticosteroid administration has a widespread effect on host defences. A variety of alterations in neutrophil function occurs, and hence in the acute inflammatory response. A major consequence is reduced accumulation of neutrophils at the site of acute inflammation because of reduced chemotaxis (Wiener *et al.*, 1975). Circulating monocyte function is impaired (Rinehart *et al.*, 1975), and the ability of the monocyte macrophage system to clear foreign material is reduced (Atkinson, Schreiber and Frank, 1973). The number of circulating lymphocytes, both T and B cells, is reduced following corticosteroid administration (Yu *et al.*, 1974).

Antithymocyte globulin appears to be a more specific immunosuppressive agent than corticosteroid. Its administration markedly depresses T-cell levels and activity, but appears to leave B-cell reactivity intact (Thomas *et al.*, 1977). Furthermore, it does not appear to impair neutrophil or macrophage function (Dale, 1981).

Azathioprine inhibits cell replication by interfering with nucleic acid synthesis. The natural killer lymphoid subpopulation is reduced, and the primary antibody response is depressed (Fahey *et al.*, 1987). The neutrophil count is lowered. Although the specific effects of azathioprine on susceptibility to infection are not clear, some clinical experience suggests that viral infections are more common when the total daily dose exceeds 100–150 mg (A. D. Diethelm, 1986, personal communication).

Cyclosporin is a more specific immunosuppressive agent, in that its action appears largely confined to inhibition of the activation of T-lymphocytes, without suppression of the phagocytic function of the reticuloendothelial system (Lafferty, Borel and Hodgkin, 1984). It has no effect on polymorphonuclear leucocyte, macrophage or natural killer cell function. Although it depresses T-helper activity, there is relative sparing of T-suppressor function (Cohen *et al.*, 1984). Several studies have suggested a lower incidence of serious infection with a cyclosporin-based immunosuppressive programme (Griffith *et al.*, 1982; Oyer *et al.*, 1982; Dummer *et al.*, 1983; Barnhart *et al.*, 1985; Cabrol *et al.*, 1985; Dresdale *et al.*, 1985; Frazier *et al.*, 1985; Pennington, Sarafian and Swartz, 1985; Hoffin *et al.*, 1987). Hunt and colleagues from Stanford noted that the 90-day rate of non-fatal bacterial and fungal infections was reduced in the cyclosporin era to 47% (CL* 40–55%) compared with 71% (CL 64–78%) in the azathioprine era (Hunt, 1983).

Frazier *et al.* (1985) reported an actuarial freedom from infection at 18 months after transplantation of 6% for an azathioprine group and 24% for a cyclosporin group ($p < 0.05$). Copeland *et al.* (1986), however, found similar linearized infection rates (infections per patient-month) as between azathioprine and cyclosporin groups.

Weakened host defences

A number of factors other than drugs are known to alter immune competence and thus to increase susceptibility to infection after major surgery, and these factors are likely to be present in patients undergoing cardiac transplantation. Protein-calorie malnutrition causes a decrease in delayed hypersensitivity (Howard, 1980), and malnutrition is a feature of the cardiac cachexia (Blackburn *et al.*, 1977) present in many patients at the time of transplantation. Pulmonary oedema, which is frequently a component of the pre-transplant condition, has long been recognized as a predisposing factor to pulmonary infection (Robin and Thomas, 1954). Additionally, there is evidence that cardiac surgery itself may have a depressive effect on lymphocyte function (Park *et al.*, 1971; McLoughlin *et al.*, 1979; Roth *et al.*, 1981).

Entry of organisms through mucocutaneous barriers

The procedure of cardiac transplantation offers many opportunities for organisms to penetrate mucocutaneous barriers and cause infection. The normal defence mechanism of the respiratory tract can be disrupted by endotracheal intubation and by the presence of a nasogastric tube. This allows organisms that have colonized the pharynx to gain entry to the lungs and possibly the blood stream.

Similarly, the urinary tract epithelial barrier may be disrupted, facilitating urinary tract and blood stream infection. Because of the risk of infection from transurethral catheterization, the suprapubic route has been recommended by the Stanford group after cardiac transplantation (Baumgartner *et al.*, 1979). Transurethral catheterization is employed at the University of Alabama at Birmingham (UAB).

Intravenous and intra-arterial lines constitute an important source of local and systemic infection in immunosuppressed patients. Lack of meticulous asepsis in the care of these devices increases the risk of infection.

---

* CL, 70% confidence limits.

Patients with a prolonged and complicated convalescence after cardiac transplantation may develop decubitus lesions which are a potential source of bacterial septicaemia.

Additional factors

An important factor predisposing to post-transplant pulmonary infection is recent pre-transplant pulmonary infarction. In the early azathioprine experience at Stanford, 8 of 10 patients or 80% (CL 59–93%) with recent pulmonary infarction developed post-transplant infection at the site of the infarction, and 6 of these patients died as a consequence (Baumgartner *et al.*, 1979). In a recent series, the risk associated with pre-transplant pulmonary embolism was confirmed, 4 of 8 patients or 50% (CL 27–73%) developing pulmonary infection, but survival was somewhat better (Young *et al.*, 1985).

Heterotopic cardiac transplantation involves placing the donor heart in the right pleural space, and it has been reported from the extensive experience at Cape Town, South Africa, that there is invariably some collapse of the right lower lobe at the end of the procedure, re-expansion usually following within several days. Although there was no reported increase in the incidence of post-transplant pulmonary infection (Novitzky and Cooper, 1984), a limited experience with heterotopic heart transplantation at UAB has demonstrated persistent right lower lobe compression in several patients which could predispose to infection in long-term survivors.

INCIDENCE AND TIME-RELATED NATURE OF INFECTION

Infection after organ transplantation tends to occur in a predictable temporal sequence (Rubin, 1981). In the first month after surgery, infections with the usual nosocomial pathogens are most common, including staphylococci and Gram-negative bacilli. Opportunistic infections associated with deficient cellular immunity are rare in the early postoperative period, but begin about 1 month after transplantation and include infections acquired with the transplanted organ. The incidence of specific opportunistic infections varies somewhat among institutions depending on region (coccidioidomycosis, histoplasmosis), nosocomial factors (legionellosis, aspergillosis), and perhaps differences in immunosuppressive drug regimens. In the first 6 months, the most common opportunistic pathogens are those suspected of having a nosocomial origin (aspergillosis, legionellosis), endogenous reinfections (herpes viruses) or those acquired from the transplanted organ (cytomegalovirus, toxoplasmosis). Although the incidence of opportunistic infections decreases after 6 months, patients remain at risk as long as they are on immunosup-

TABLE 13.1
Cardiac Transplantation (UAB; 1981–July 1985, n = *63; Major Infections*—32 in 22 patients)*

Site	Organism	n	Deaths No.	Deaths %
Lung		19	2	11%
	Pneumococcus	2	0	
	Pseudomonas	2	0	
	Staphylococcus aureus	1	0	
	Mixed flora	3	0	
	Legionella	1	0	
	Nocardia	4	0	
	Mycobacterium	1	0	
	Aspergillus	4	2	
	Pneumocystis	1	0	
Mediastinal		2	0	0%
	Enterobacter	1	0	
	Staphylococcus aureus	1	0	
Gastrointestinal		2	1	50%
	(Cholecystitis)	1	0	
	Serratia marcescens	1	1	
Spine		1	0	0%
	Mixed flora	1	0	
Blood		4	0	0%
	Enterobacter	1	0	
	Klebsiella	1	0	
	Staphylococcus aureus	1	0	
	Candida	1	0	
Brain		1	1	100%
	Petriellidium boydii	1	1	
Blood plus other organs		3	1	33%
	Enterococcus	1	0	
	Listeria	1	0	
	Cytomegalovirus	1	1	
Total		32	5	16%

* Includes infections requiring hospital admission and treatment with intravenous antibiotics.

pressive therapy, particularly when it is increased as treatment for rejection episodes. Retinitis caused by cytomegalovirus (CMV) occurs even after 6 months (Egbert *et al.*, 1980; Pollard *et al.*, 1980), and infections depending on chance exposure to a pathogen such as listeriosis or cryptococcosis (Britt, Enzmann and Remington, 1981) can occur any time after transplantation.

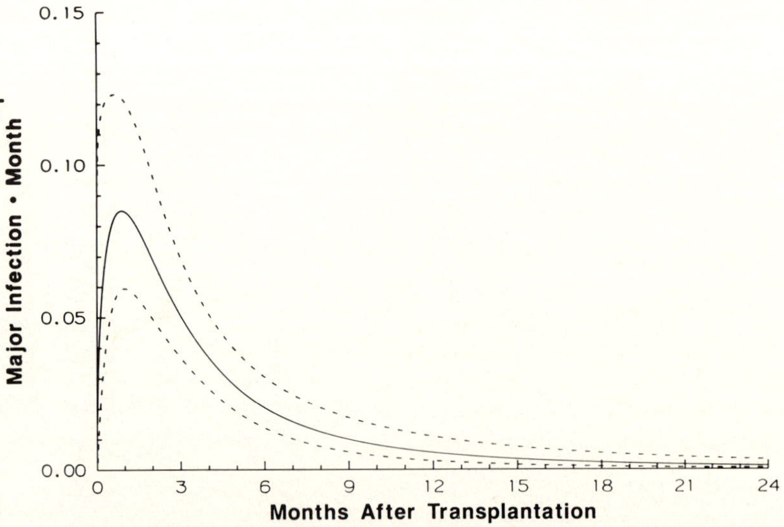

Fig. 13.1. *Hazard function (instantaneous risk of the event at all points in time after operation) for the first major infection following cardiac transplantation (UAB; 1981–July 1985;* n = *63). Time zero is the time of transplantation. Patients are censored after second transplantation (*n = *6). Dashed lines enclose the 70% confidence limits.*

Griffith *et al.* (1984) reported that 79% of the cyclosporin-treated patients followed for a mean of 9 months developed at least one infection. Reports (Cabrol *et al.*, 1985; Painvin *et al.*, 1985; Copeland *et al.*, 1986) from other centres confirm the high prevalence of infection in cardiac transplant recipients. In the UAB experience, including patients from both the azathioprine and the cyclosporin eras, 32 major infections developed in 22 of 63 patients undergoing cardiac transplantation (Table 13.1). The risk of infection at any time following cardiac transplantation is closely related to the magnitude of immunosuppression. Thus, the incidence of major infectious episodes per month is highest 1 month after transplantation (UAB) and decreases rapidly to a low level by about 9 months (Fig. 13.1). After the first 12 months, major infectious episodes are rare (Fig. 13.2). These findings have also been noted by others (Cooper *et al.*, 1981; Pennock *et al.*, 1982; Copeland *et al.*, 1984; Griffith, Hardesty and Bahnson, 1984; Halbrook *et al.*, 1985).

The relation between periods of augmented immunosuppression and infective episodes has been examined by Mason *et al.* (1976), who demonstrated that following the treatment of acute cardiac rejection in azathioprine patients, the incidence of infection rose from a level of 1.3 infections per 1000 patient-days to 3.6 per 1000 patient-days. Actuarial curves of freedom from

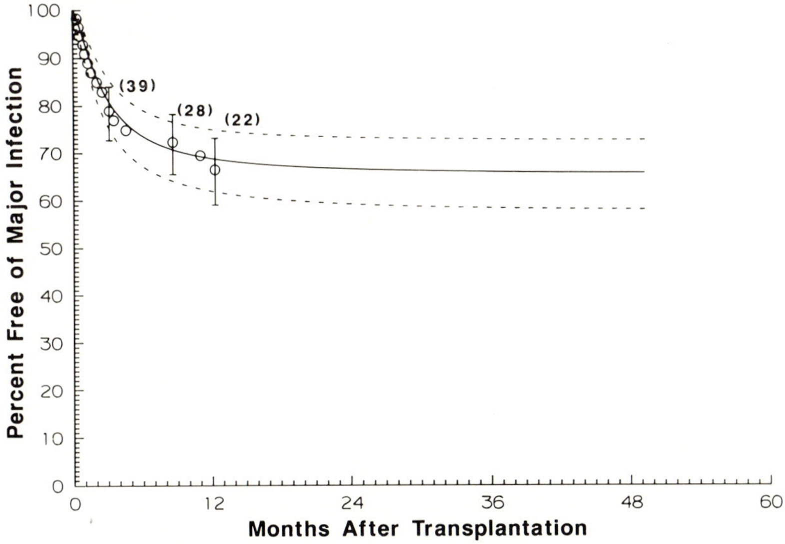

Fig. 13.2 *Freedom from the first major infection after cardiac transplantation (UAB; 1981–July 1985; n = 63). Time zero is the time of transplantation. Dashed lines enclose the parametric 70% confidence limits around the event-free estimate; circles represent individual patients undergoing an event, positioned actuarially, and the vertical bars represent the 70% confidence limits of the actuarial estimate; numbers in parentheses represent the number of patients at risk in the time interval.*

infection in patients treated for rejection and those not treated for rejection were significantly different 2 months after commencement of rejection therapy. Furthermore, if rejection episodes were treated only with increased doses of oral prednisone, the increase in the infection rate was smaller than when treatment included intravenous methylprednisolone and intramuscular antithymocyte globulin. In cyclosporin-treated patients, there was a higher incidence of infection among patients with severe rejection compared with those with no or lesser degrees of rejection (Dummer *et al.*, 1984).

At UAB, we have specifically analysed the freedom from major infection in relation to episodes of augmented immunosuppression (transplantation, acute rejection, or re-transplantation) (Fig. 13.3). The shape of the early part of the actuarial curves is strikingly similar whether time zero is the original transplant, re-transplantation, or the first, second or third episode of treated rejection (intravenous methylprednisolone ± rabbit antithymocyte globulin). In other words, the risk of developing a major infection is highest during the first 2–3 months following any period of major augmentation of immunosuppression.

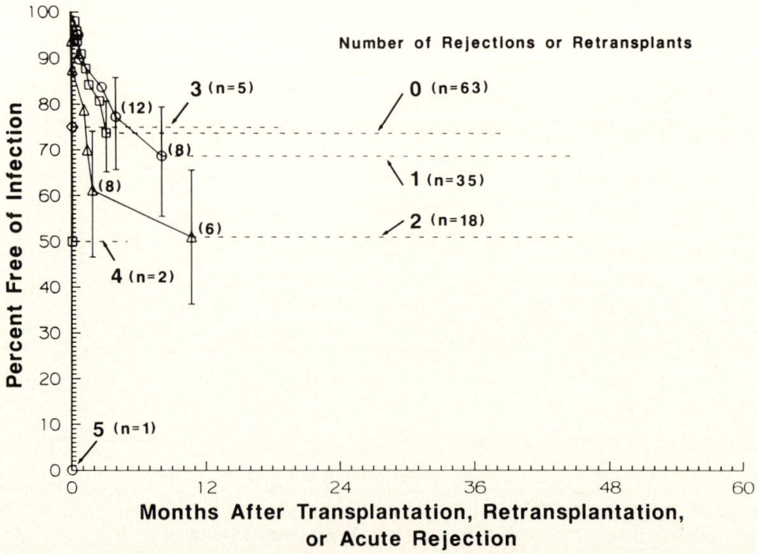

Fig. 13.3. *Actuarial freedom from the first major infection after one or more episodes of augmentation of immunosuppression (AI) (UAB; 1981–July 1985;* n = *63; patients experiencing major infection = 16). An episode of AI may be either treated rejection or re-transplantation. Group 0 (*n = *63) (squares) represents the study group after initial transplantation. Time zero is the time of initial transplantation. Patients are censored at the time of the first episode of AI. Group 1 (*n = *35) (circles) represents those patients with one episode of AI. Time zero is the time of the first episode of AI. Patients are censored at the second episode of AI. Group 2 (*n = *18) (triangles) represents those patients with two episodes of AI. Time zero is the time of the second episode of AI. Patients are censored at the third episode of AI. Group 3 (*n = *5), Group 4 (*n = *2) and Group 5 (*n = *1) are similarly defined. Dashed lines represent the longest additional follow-up of patients at the time of the last actuarial estimate.*

CONSEQUENCES OF INFECTION

Overall mortality

In the early Stanford (Baumgartner *et al.*, 1979) experience with azathioprine-treated cardiac transplant recipients, 60% of the deaths occurring in the first 3 postoperative months were due to infection, and after 3 months 42% of deaths occurring 4–65 months following transplantation were due to infection. Similarly, in the South African series, 39% of the overall mortality was attributed to infection (Cooper *et al.*, 1981).

In the UAB experience from 1981 to 1985, 21% (CL 13–31%) of deaths after cardiac transplantation were attributed to infection. Many infective episodes, however, were successfully treated. The mortality from a major infectious episode was 16% (5/32; CL 9–25%) (see Table 13.1).

Triggering of rejection

The temporal relationship between viral illnesses and the appearance of rejection in renal transplant recipients has been observed by many groups (Simmons *et al.*, 1970; Briggs *et al.*, 1972; Lopez *et al.*, 1974; Gabriel *et al.*, 1976; David *et al.*, 1982). Renal rejection has also been reported in association with bacterial infections (Byrd *et al.*, 1978). Possible mechanisms include non-specific stimulation of the immune system and cross-reactivity between antigens of the renal allograft and the infecting agent. To date this association has not been specifically described in heart transplant recipients, but it is likely that a similar capacity exists for triggering cardiac allograft rejection by an infecting agent.

Malignancy

Compared with the general population, immunosuppressed patients have a greatly increased likelihood of developing lymphoma (Hanto *et al.*, 1981b). Epstein–Barr virus (EBV), which is known to be excreted in the oropharynx of 47–87% of renal transplant recipients (Strauch *et al.*, 1974; Chang *et al.*, 1978) has been implicated in the aetiology of lymphoma in renal transplant recipients (Hanto *et al.*, 1981b; Hanto *et al.*, 1982). EBV is known to infect B cells selectively and cause a polyclonal B-cell proliferation (Robinson *et al.*, 1980). In some patients who have developed a polyclonal B-cell lymphoproliferative disorder, an autonomous monoclonal tumour may develop (Hanto *et al.*, 1981b). Lymphoproliferative disease has been described in cardiac transplant recipients, and the findings of EBV genome incorporated into the tumour-cell DNA in some of these patients, as well as elevated antibody titres to EBV, does suggest a causal relationship (Oyer *et al.*, 1984).

SPECIFIC ORGANISMS CAUSING INFECTION

Bacteria

Gram-positive cocci and Gram-negative bacilli

The lung is the most common site of infection after cardiac transplantation (Brooks and Remington, 1986). In the early postoperative period (1–2 weeks), the usual causes of nosocomial pneumonia predominate. Other common sites of early infection with Gram-positive cocci and Gram-negative rods are the urinary tract and the mediastinal wound (see Management of postoperative mediastinitis, p. 282). Particularly in the presence of indwelling venous catheters, Gram-positive or Gram-negative septicaemia may occur as in non-immunosuppressed patients.

Gram-negative enteric bacilli are the most common causative agents for early pneumonia, including *Escherichia coli, Klebsiella* sp., *Pseudomonas aeruginosa, Serratia marcescens, Proteus* sp., *Haemophilus influenzae* and *Enterobacter*. A number of Gram-positive pathogens may be involved in pulmonary infection, including *Pneumococcus, Enterococcus* and *Streptococcus* spp., but *Staphylococcus* occurs most frequently. Mixed infection with upper airway anaerobic flora can also cause postoperative pneumonia. Gram-negative bacillary infections tend to be acquired in hospital in the early post-transplant period, probably secondary to colonization of the pharynx. Factors known to promote pharyngeal colonization include: administration of antibiotics, prolonged hospitalization (Johanson, Pierce and Sanford, 1969), severe illness and consequent loss of normal pharyngeal clearance mechanisms (Johanson, Pierce and Sanford, 1969), and endotracheal intubation (Pierce and Sanford, 1974).

The radiological features in bacterial pulmonary infections are those of alveolar consolidation (Stinson *et al.*, 1971), but the appearances are not specific for any causative organisms (Matthay and Green, 1980).

The diagnosis of bacterial pneumonia is made by culture of sputum (usually via bronchoscopy to avoid contamination with organisms colonizing the upper airway) and blood.

Antibiotic therapy is based upon culture and sensitivity data and often involves a combination of drugs.

The outcome of therapy is generally good unless the infection is secondary to an opportunistic infection or the patient's overall condition is poor. At UAB, 8 transplant patients have been treated for Gram-positive or Gram-negative bacterial pneumonia, and all have survived (see Table 13.1).

Legionella

Legionella pneumophila, a Gram-negative bacillus, is a particularly important cause of pneumonia (England *et al.*, 1981; Muder, Yu and Zuravleff, 1983; Muder, Yu and Woo, 1986) in patients with compromised cell-mediated immunity. Patients remain at risk for this infection as long as they receive immunosuppressive therapy. Of importance to transplant centres is the finding that this ubiquitous organism has been detected in hospital air-conditioning machinery and shower units (Tobin *et al.*, 1980).

Renal transplants account for a high percentage of *Legionella* isolates in some series, and 50% of renal transplant patients developed *Legionella* infection during an outbreak at Wadsworth Medical Center (Haley *et al.*, 1979). Renal transplant patients have been identified as a high risk group for Legionnaires' disease (Marshall, 1981), and the occurrence of *Legionella* pneumonia has been linked to the dose of prednisone (Zeitler *et al.*, 1984). It is likely that as cardiac transplantation becomes more common these patients will also be increasingly recognized as a risk group. Indeed, Legionnaires' disease has been reported to be the most common cause of bacterial pneumonia in series of cardiac transplant patients at both Tucson (8 cases among 40 patients) (Fuller *et al.*, 1985) and Stanford (Brooks and Remington, 1986).

The site of infection is nearly always the lungs, but in the compromised host the presentation of legionellosis both clinically and radiologically is highly variable. The course may be an indolent, atypical pneumonia with a mildly troublesome dry cough, fever and chills; or fulminant with systemic signs of infection including rigors, mental changes, headache and diarrhoea. A variety of radiological changes are seen, including distal airspace disease in a segmental or lobar distribution (Storch, Sagel and Baine, 1981), bilateral disease, nodular or mass opacities with pleural effusions, and necrotizing pneumonia with cavitation (particularly common in compromised hosts) (Fuller *et al.*, 1985). Pulmonary fibrosis may occur (Cheung, 1980), with permanent radiological changes.

Diagnosis by serology or culture may be difficult. The serological diagnosis is complicated by the existence of multiple serotypes of *Legionella pneumophila* and the potential importance of other *Legionella* sp., particularly *L. bozemani* and *L. micdadei*. Serum immunofluorescent antibody studies often show a delayed response and results are never available immediately. Culture requires special media, results are often delayed, and overgrowth with organisms colonizing the respiratory tract is a problem even with semi-selective media. The urine antigen test has given both false negative and false positive results at our institution. Material obtained by lung biopsy, bronchoscopy or expectoration can be examined by direct immunofluorescent assay, but the test is difficult to perform and reported sensitivity varies from 25% to 80% (Edelstein, 1985). The histopathology of the bronchopneumonia in the absence of other known pathogens is considered specific by some, but special stains including the Dieterle silver stain are not always useful. New techniques involving either DNA probes or monoclonal antibody have shown promise (P. H. Edelstein, 1986, personal communication) in the examination of clinical specimens, but clinical experience is still limited.

The treatment of choice for legionellosis is erythromycin (Beaty, 1985) (Table 13.2). Initial high-dose intravenous treatment is followed by oral administration after the patient improves. Because of the high mortality in compromised hosts, some recommend the combination of rifampicin and erythromycin (Beaty, 1985; Fuller *et al.*, 1985). The potential toxicity of these agents emphasizes the importance of making a specific diagnosis whenever possible. Use of rifampicin may lead to decreased levels of cyclosporin (Langhoff, 1983; Daniels, Dover and Schachter, 1984), and conversely erythromycin may inhibit clearance of cyclosporin (Ptachcinski *et al.*, 1985; Martell *et al.*, 1986), so blood levels of cyclosporin must be followed closely

TABLE 13.2

Antibiotic Therapy of Opportunistic Infections After Cardiac Transplantation

Organism	*Common Sites*	*Antimicrobial Agent*	*Dose*	*Duration*
BACTERIA				
Legionella	Lung	Erythromycin*	4 g/d i.v.,	7 day
			then 2 g/day po	14 day
		± rifampicin*	600 mg/day po	21 day
Listeria	CNS	Ampicillin†	8 g/day i.v.	3–6 wk
monocytogenes	Blood	± gentamicin†	3–5 mg/kg per day i.v.	
Nocardia	Lung	Sulphasoxazole†	6 g/day po	6 mo
	Skin			
	CNS			
Mycobacterium	Lung	INH	300 mg/day po	9 mo
Tuberculosis		+ rifampicin*	600 mg/day po	
FUNGI				
Aspergillus	Lung	Amphotericin B	0.5–1.0 mg/kg per day i.v.	2–2.5 g
	CNS			Total systemic dose‡
Coccidioides	Lung	Amphotericin B	0.5–0.6 mg/kg per day i.v.	2–2.5 g‡
	CNS			
	Bone			
Cryptococcus	CNS	Amphotericin B	0.4 mg/kg per day	6 wk
	Lung	+ 5-flucytosine†	100 mg/kg per day	
Phycomyces	Sinus	Amphotericin B	0.8–1.0 mg/kg per day	2–3 g‡
	CNS			
Candida	Oral mucosa	Nystatin	500 000 units po q.i.d.	7 day‡
	Oesophagus	or ketoconazole*	400 mg po q.i.d.	
		or amphotericin B	10–20 mg/day i.v.	
	Systemic	Amphotericin B	0.4 mg/kg per day	‡

PROTOZOA				
Toxoplasma gondii	CNS	Pyrimethamine†	50 mg po b.i.d.,	2 day
	Eye		then 25–50 mg po q.i.d.	6 wk‡
	Liver	+ sulphadiazine†	4–6 g/day	6 wk‡
	Transplanted heart	± folinic acid	10 mg po q.i.d.	6 wk‡
		or folic acid	5 mg po q.i.d.	
Pneumocystis	Lung	Trimethoprim	20 mg/kg per day po or i.v. in 4 doses	3 wk
		+ sulphamethoxazole†	100 mg/kg per day po or i.v. in 4 doses	3 wk
VIRUSES				
CMV	Lung	None available		
	Systemic	DHPG		
	Retina	(investigational)		
	Liver			
	GI tract			
Herpes simplex	Oral/oesophageal	Acyclovir	1 g/d po in 5 doses	7–10 day
	Genital		or 5 mg/kg i.v. q 8 h	
	CNS	Acyclovir	10 mg/kg i.v. q 8 h	10 day‡
Varicella-zoster	Skin	Acyclovir	10 mg/kg i.v. q 8 h	7 day
	Systemic			7 day‡
EB virus	Lymphoid tissue	None available		

* Affects cyclosporin metabolism.
† Dose adjustment for renal failure.
‡ Total dose determined by clinical response.

in patients receiving either of these antibiotics. Because of the slow clinical response to treatment, delayed clearance of pulmonary infiltrates and the frequency of relapse, prolonged treatment of up to 6 months' duration has been advocated (Fuller *et al.*, 1985).

The overall reported mortality is 15–20%, but it is especially high (80%) among immunosuppressed patients who do not receive erythromycin (Meyer, 1983; Brooks and Remington, 1986). At UAB, 1 cardiac transplant patient has been treated for (and survived) *Legionella* pneumonia (see Table 13.1).

Listeria monocytogenes

This Gram-positive bacillus is an intracellular pathogen which is closely associated with infection in patients with deficient cell-mediated immunity. From 1968 to 1978, 22% of all reported cases of listeriosis occurred in renal transplant recipients (Nieman and Lorber, 1980), and this infection is now being reported as an important complication of cardiac transplantation (Britt, Enzmann and Remington, 1981; Griffin, Pope and Armstrong, 1983). In a Stanford series, listeriosis (4 cases) occurred both early and late after transplantation, and 1 of 2 late cases occurred shortly after treatment for rejection (Britt, Enzmann and Remington, 1981).

The condition is usually manifest as meningitis with or without encephalitis, but brain parenchymal disease alone and primary bacteraemia are also seen in compromised hosts (Stamm *et al.*, 1982).

Among renal transplant patients, approximately 50% of cases present with signs of acute meningitis (Stamm *et al.*, 1982), including fever, headaches, lethargy and signs of meningeal irritation. Seizures, focal neurological deficits and depression of consciousness are less common (Stamm *et al.*, 1982). However, immunocompromised patients with CNS involvement may have minimal neurological findings; meningismus is often lacking and the illness may be rapidly progressive with the development of focal neurological deficits.

CSF pleocytosis is usually marked and may be predominantly lymphocytic (Armstrong, 1985). The organism is easily grown on a variety of media, but may be misidentified as a non-pathogenic diphtheroid contaminant by inexperienced laboratory workers.

The therapy of choice is a combination of ampicillin and gentamicin (see Table 13.2). *Listeria* is usually resistant to third-generation cephalosporins. Nosocomial outbreaks with no identifiable environmental source have been reported in immunocompromised patients, and isolation precautions have been recommended for infected patients (Gantz *et al.*, 1975; Stamm *et al.*, 1982). Recurrence has been reported in compromised hosts and treatment for 3–6 weeks is therefore recommended.

The mortality is high in immunocompromised patients. Stamm *et al.* (1982) found a 26% overall mortality (27/102, CL 22–32%) in published cases of renal transplantation. The mortality was especially high (37%) with central nervous system (CNS) involvement. One patient at UAB was treated for (and survived) CNS and blood stream *Listeria* infection (see Table 13.1). That patient also developed acute cardiac failure and underwent emergency re-transplantation with long-term survival. Examination of the explanted heart showed multiple *Listeria* myocardial abscesses.

Nocardia

Nocardiosis is a bacterial infection most frequently occurring in association with deficient cell-mediated immunity. *Nocardia asteroides* is the usual organism.

The most frequent site of infection in cardiac transplant recipients is the lung (Krick, Stinson and Remington, 1975), but a number of other tissues may be secondarily involved, including skin, brain, kidneys and the skeletal system. In a study of cardiac transplant patients at Stanford over a 10-year period ending in 1978, *Nocardia* occurred in 13% of patients, with disease limited to the lung in 81% and with dissemination, primarily to skin and soft tissue, in the remainder (Simpson *et al.*, 1981).

Nocardia pulmonary infection usually presents with a non-productive cough, fever and malaise, and frequently runs a chronic course. Patients may be asymptomatic, the infection being detected on a routine chest radiograph. The pulmonary infiltrates can be lobar, segmental, nodular, cavitary or even miliary. *Nocardia* often produces a necrotizing infection in the compromised host. Soft-tissue abscesses, pustules or cellulitis may occur from dissemination of *Nocardia*, which emphasizes the importance of investigating infective skin lesions in immunosuppressed patients.

The diagnosis of nocardiosis can be made by finding the characteristic branching, filamentous, Gram-positive and weakly acid-fast organisms in sputum or other material. Although patients with nocardiosis sometimes produce purulent sputum, invasive techniques including transtracheal and transthoracic aspirates are often needed to make the diagnosis (Simpson *et al.*, 1981). *Nocardia* grows on most laboratory media, but growth is slow and routine sputum cultures are sometimes prematurely discarded. Growth on fungal media such as Sabouraud's is even slower and the decontamination procedures used for mycobacterial cultures may destroy *Nocardia*. However, if the laboratory is alerted to the possibility of *Nocardia* infection, the culture yield is high. The organisms can also be demonstrated on histological examination, provided appropriate stains such as the Brown and Brenn modification of the Gram stain or silver stains are used. Serological tests for *Nocardia* infection are not widely available, but a recently reported enzyme immunoassay showed promise in a limited number of patients (Angeles and

Sugar, 1987). Because of the frequency of CNS involvement in older series, a CT brain scan should probably be obtained in all cases of nocardiosis even in the absence of neurological findings.

Therapy should include drainage of extrapulmonary abscesses and administration of sulphonamides (Palmer, Davidson and Lusk, 1974) (see Table 13.2). In recent years, the combination of trimethoprim and sulphamethoxazole has been used to treat nocardiosis, and this combination may be preferred for patients with CNS involvement (Smego, Moeller and Gallis, 1983). Treatment of immunocompromised hosts should be continued for at least 6 months. Recovery of *Nocardia* on sputum culture probably warrants treatment of immunocompromised hosts even in the absence of radiological findings. A nosocomial outbreak of nocardiosis has been reported and infected patients should probably be isolated from immunocompromised hosts (Stevens *et al.*, 1981).

At UAB, 4 patients have been treated for *Nocardia* lung infection. There were no deaths attributable to the infection (0% mortality, CL 0–38%) (see Table 13.1).

Mycobacteria

Infection due to *Mycobacterium tuberculosis* or atypical mycobacteria is not common after transplantation, but has been described in cardiac (Cooper *et al.*, 1983; Reece *et al.*, 1984) and renal transplant recipients (Lloveras *et al.*, 1982). A single patient with *Mycobacterium tuberculosis* was reported from Cape Town (Cooper *et al.*, 1983), but most other reported cases have been atypical mycobacteria, most commonly *M. kansasii* (Brooks and Remington, 1986). Mycobacterial infections may occur late after transplantation and there is a strong association with preceding nocardiosis, as noted in 5 of 8 patients at Stanford who developed atypical mycobacterial infections in the azathioprine era (Brooks and Remington, 1986). No mycobacterial infections were seen in the first 3 years of cyclosporin use at Stanford (Brooks and Remington, 1986).

The lung is the most common site of infection, although extrapulmonary spread is occasionally seen.

Tuberculosis may present as reactivation of pulmonary disease or as disseminated infection. The diagnosis is made by finding the typical acid-fast bacilli in sputum or other material. Mycobacteria grow on most laboratory media, but growth is slow, often taking 3–6 weeks or longer.

Treatment with isoniazid (INH) and rifampicin is generally recommended for established infection (see Table 13.2). INH prophylaxis should usually be continued for 1 year in immunosuppressed patients with evidence of past tuberculous infection.

Among renal transplant recipients, the reported response to therapy has been generally excellent, with a cure rate exceeding 90% (Brooks and Remington, 1986). One patient developed atypical mycobacterial pulmonary infection at UAB and survived (see Table 13.1).

Fungi

Aspergillus

Aspergillosis has been the single most important invasive fungal infection in cardiac transplant patients. Twenty-one per cent of the 263 heart transplants performed at Stanford up to May 1983 developed aspergillosis (Baumgartner, 1983; Brooks and Remington, 1986). The incidence of this infection may have fallen since the introduction of cyclosporin, but aspergillosis remains an important cause of morbidity and mortality in this patient population. Infection is most commonly seen in the early months after transplantation when nosocomial exposure and immunosuppression are greatest. This organism is found throughout the environment, but of special importance are the reports of invasive aspergillosis occurring at the time of hospital reconstruction (Arnow *et al.*, 1978) or hospital air conditioning contamination (Burton *et al.*, 1972). Pulmonary infections may occur involving *Aspergillus* together with other organisms such as cytomegalovirus, *Myocobacteria* or *Nocardia* (Rubin and Cosimi, 1982).

The great majority of infections begin in the lungs, and the most common site of dissemination is the central nervous system, although virtually any organ may be involved. Invasive pulmonary aspergillosis has two important pathological processes—necrotizing bronchopneumonia, and pulmonary infarction as a result of invasion and occlusion of pulmonary vessels (Williams, 1976).

The clinical presentation of *Aspergillus* infection is frequently sudden and is characterized by fever, dyspnoea, non-productive cough and pleuritic pain. The clinical course ranges from an indolent disease to fulminant rapidly fatal infection. The usual radiographic finding is necrotizing patchy bronchopneumonia, but transplant patients sometimes show solitary or multiple pulmonary nodules. Although diffuse bilateral infiltrates are much less common, any type of pulmonary infiltrate may be encountered (Gurwith, Stinson and Remington, 1971). When CNS dissemination occurs, patients usually show signs of a brain abscess or meningo-encephalitis (Britt, Enzmann and Remington, 1981). The course may be fulminant with rapid progression from disorientation and confusion to coma, or indolent with the slow development of focal neurological deficits. Computerized tomographic (CT) brain scans show non-specific low-density lesions with minimal contrast enhancement (Aisner, Schimpff and Wiernik, 1977). Unfortunately, diagnosis is often difficult and requires invasive procedures. Aspergillosis can colonize the upper respiratory tract of immunocompromised hosts, and isolation of this fungus from expectorated sputum is not specific for invasive pulmonary infection

(Fisher *et al.*, 1981). The organism may be slow growing, and sputum culture may be negative in patients with invasive disease (Rinaldi, 1983). Serum antibody determination has not been clinically useful, and although tests for serum antigen are highly specific they are relatively insensitive (Shaffer, Kobayashi and Medoff, 1979; Weiner *et al.*, 1983). A better place to look for *Aspergillus* antigen may be material obtained by bronchoalveolar lavage (BAL). In one small series, radioimmunoassay in BAL fluid was found to be both highly specific and sensitive for the diagnosis of invasive aspergillosis (Andrews and Weiner, 1982). The diagnosis of CNS infection is also difficult since CT findings and the findings in cerebrospinal fluid are non-specific, and cerebrospinal fluid (CSF) does not yield the organism on culture (Britt, Enzmann and Remington, 1981). At present, definitive diagnosis usually depends on demonstrating the organism in pathological specimens obtained by lung biopsy, or needle aspiration of cerebral lesions.

Intravenous amphotericin B remains the only established treatment for invasive aspergillosis. The dose and duration of treatment are not well established. Treatment must be individualized according to patient response, but most cardiac transplant patients will require a total dose of at least 2 g (see Table 13.2). Since aspergillosis is frequently a nosocomial infection which has been associated with hospital renovation, transplant patients should be isolated from such activities (Arnow *et al.*, 1978).

The chance of survival depends on early diagnosis and treatment, before dissemination occurs. Despite early and aggressive treatment, the expected mortality is at least 50%. Among the 263 heart transplants performed at Stanford up to May 1983, 21% of the patients have had aspergillosis, and 57% of these infections were fatal (Baumgartner, 1983). At UAB, 4 patients have been treated for aspergillosis, with 2 deaths (see Table 13.1).

Coccidioidomycosis

This has been an important complication of immunosuppression for organ transplants in the endemic areas of the Southwestern United States (Cohen *et al.*, 1982). Self-limited primary pulmonary infection is a common affliction of normal hosts in endemic areas. Deficient cell-mediated immunity increases the risk of disseminated disease, which may occur soon after the primary infection, but in transplant patients is more commonly the result of reactivated infection. Coccidioidomycosis has been reported in only 3 cardiac transplant patients (Britt, Enzmann and Remington, 1981; Copeland *et al.*, 1984), but disseminated disease has been a significant problem in renal transplantation, and the incidence in cardiac transplantation can be expected to increase as the procedure becomes more common.

The lung is usually the primary site of infection. Common sites of dissemination include bone, joints, urinary tract and meninges. The clinical features of pulmonary disease are similar to those of aspergillosis.

Disseminated disease may be detected by culture of the slow-growing fungus from urine, bone marrow or cerebrospinal fluid. Sputum obtained by bronchoscopy is more likely to yield the organism than expectorated sputum (Cohen *et al.*, 1982). The cerebrospinal fluid usually shows pleocytosis (sometimes with eosinophils), elevated protein and a low glucose content. Serological tests are very helpful in diagnosis. Persistent or increasing titres of antibody detected by complement fixation or immunodiffusion, particularly in the absence or loss of skin test reactivity, are suggestive of disseminated disease, and complement fixing antibody is present in the cerebrospinal fluid of up to 95% of patients with meningitis (Stevens, 1985).

The treatment of choice is intravenous amphotericin B, with a total dose for disseminated disease of at least 2 g (see Table 13.2). Treatment of meningitis should include intrathecal or intraventricular amphotericin B. Antibody levels in serum and CSF may be helpful in following the response to therapy. Miconazole is an alternative therapeutic agent (Stevens, 1983).

The mortality associated with disseminated disease in the compromised host is high, even with treatment. Among renal transplant recipients, the mortality was 33% in pulmonary disease and exceeded 70% when disseminated disease was present (Cohen *et al.*, 1982; Brooks and Remington, 1986).

Phycomycosis

Phycomycosis involving both *Mucor* and *Rhizopus* has been reported rarely in cardiac transplant patients (Brooks and Remington, 1986), but is most commonly seen in patients with neoplastic disease or poorly controlled diabetes.

Phycomycosis usually begins in the nose and sinuses. Fungal invasion of blood vessels leads to ischaemic necrosis and spread to the orbit and CNS.

This rare infection should be suspected in a transplant patient who develops acute sinusitis, periorbital swelling or blood-tinged nasal drainage. Examination may disclose necrotic nasal turbinates, ophthalmoplegia, septal perforation, and the radiological changes of sinusitis with bone destruction.

Appropriate therapy includes intravenous amphotericin B and surgical debridement. The aggressive treatment of rhinocerebral phycomycosis using amphotericin B with or without surgery has resulted in reported survival rates of 44–85% among chronically debilitated patients (Lehrer *et al.*, 1980).

Cryptococcosis

The lung is the primary focus of infection in cryptococcosis, but pulmonary infection, even in the compromised host, is often asymptomatic and self-limited. Clinical disease usually reveals signs and symptoms of spread to the CNS, usually in the form of meningitis. Cryptococcal infection often develops late after cardiac transplantation, sometimes in association with the treatment of rejection episodes (Britt, Enzmann and Remington, 1981). Fever, headache and lethargy are the most common presenting complaints and rarely the illness may progress to seizures and focal neurological deficits (Rubin and Cosimi, 1982).

Examination of the cerebrospinal fluid usually shows a slight elevation in protein and a modest lymphocytic pleocytosis with or without low glucose levels. Organisms may be demonstrated in 50% of cases by direct examination with India ink, and tests for cryptococcal antigen in cerebrospinal fluid are positive in 90% of cases. The detection of cryptococci in any extraneural site requires investigation for CNS disease. Cerebrospinal fluid obtained from patients with deficient cell-mediated immunity should always be examined for cryptococcal antigen.

Treatment of cryptococcal meningitis requires at least 6 weeks with a combination of amphotericin B and 5-flucytosine (see Table 13.2) or 10 weeks of amphotericin B alone (Bennett *et al.*, 1979).

The reported mortality of cryptococcal CNS infection in 6 of 678 renal transplant patients over a 20-year period was 17% (1/6; CL 2–46%) (Tilney, Kohler and Strom, 1982).

Candidiasis

Candida is not infrequently isolated from patients after cardiac transplantation, and it is very important to make the distinction between colonization and invasive candidiasis. Invasive *Candida* infections are more closely associated with deficient phagocytosis than with deficient cell-mediated immunity, and deep-seated *Candida* infection is rare after cardiac transplantation.

The most common site of infection is the oral mucosa. Less commonly, the oesophagus may be involved. Rarely, *Candida* pneumonia or septicaemia occurs.

Oral candidiasis is characterized by pain and redness of the tongue and other parts of the buccal mucosa, together with a typical white exudate. *Candida* oesophagitis usually presents with painful dysphagia. Untreated, *Candida* oesophagitis may result in bleeding, perforation or dissemination. *Candida* pneumonia is rarely a primary infection, but has been described as a superinfection in renal transplant patients with bacterial or cytomegalovirus pneumonia (Ramsey and Rubin, 1980; Peterson *et al.*, 1982). *Candida* sepsis is generally seen in the setting of long-term indwelling venous catheters and broad-spectrum antibiotic administration for other infections.

The diagnosis of *Candida* oesophagitis is made by endoscopy. Biopsies of the oesophageal lesions must be obtained for histology and Gram staining since *Candida* oesophagitis can be confused with *Herpes simplex* and bacterial ulcers (Armstrong, 1981). Candidaemia may merely represent transient blood stream contamination as opposed to disseminated candidiasis originating from a site of invasive infection (Ellis and Spivack, 1967). The distinction is usually made on the clinical state of the patient, and the response to withdrawal of provocative factors such as intravenous lines and broad-spectrum antibiotics. Invasive *Candida* infection is unlikely if the patient is in good clinical condition and the candidaemia disappears on cessation of antibiotics and removal of intravenous lines.

The low incidence of invasive candidiasis in cardiac transplantation may be due, in part, to the frequent use of antifungal agents such as nystatin for the prevention and treatment of mucosal disease.

Oral nystatin provides effective prevention and treatment of mucosal infection with *Candida.* Invasive *Candida* sepsis requires amphotericin B for therapy (see Table 13.2), but there is generally an accompanying life-threatening condition and the outcome is usually fatal (Brooks and Remington, 1986).

Other fungal infections

Blastomycosis and histoplasmosis are important deep mycoses with a regional distribution and an increased incidence in immunocompromised hosts. The organisms have not been reported among cardiac transplant recipients, but histoplasmosis has been a significant problem in renal transplant patients in endemic areas, sometimes in association with community outbreaks (Wheat *et al.*, 1983).

Protozoa

Toxoplasma

Infection with *Toxoplasma gondii* has been a serious problem in heart transplant patients, and in many instances the organism appears to have been acquired with the donor heart (Ryning *et al.*, 1979; Hakim *et al.*, 1985). Recipients seropositive to *Toxoplasma* prior to transplantation frequently develop a rise in titre and even significant IgM antibody postoperatively without clinical disease. However, seronegative recipients of hearts from seropositive donors frequently (approximately 75%) develop clinical manifestations of *Toxoplasma* infection including hepatitis, retinitis, pneumonia, brain abscess and meningo-encephalitis. Seronegative recipients of hearts from seronegative donors generally remain seronegative and asymptomatic, further suggesting that donor organs are the most important route of disease transmission (Luft *et al.*, 1983).

When clinical infection occurs in immunocompromised hosts, CNS manifestations are most common (Ruskin, 1976; McLeod *et al.*, 1979; Britt, Enzmann and Remington, 1981). Patients present with meningitis, meningo-encephalitis or cerebral mass lesions with focal neurological deficits (Ruskin and Remington, 1976; Britt, 1981). Less commonly, pulmonary or hepatic involvement may occur.

Cerebrospinal fluid shows lymphocytic pleocytosis with protein elevation, and CT scan shows a mass lesion with contrast enhancement typical of brain abscess. Some patients, shown at autopsy to have microscopic evidence of diffuse encephalitis with *Toxoplasma* cysts, had no evidence of CNS infection during life (Britt, Enzmann and Remington, 1981). The diagnosis of toxoplasmosis in the immunocompromised host often depends on the demonstration of organisms in tissue, including material obtained by aspiration of CNS lesions and, particularly in cases acquired from the transplanted organ, endomyocardial biopsy (Rose *et al.*, 1983). If there is a clinical contra-indication to biopsy of suspected lesions, serological evidence of infection with a compatible clinical presentation may be sufficient indication for treatment (Luft *et al.*, 1983). Patients known to be seronegative prior to transplantation who receive hearts from seropositive donors should have frequent examinations for seroconversion or be given pyrimethamine prophylactically. Since severe disease is common in such patients and since clinical disease may be delayed long after seroconversion, some authorities recommend treatment at the time of seroconversion (Luft *et al.*, 1983).

The treatment of choice for toxoplasmosis in the compromised host is a combination of pyrimethamine and sulphadiazine (or trisulphapyrimidines) orally (see Table 13.2) until 4–6 weeks after resolution of clinical evidence of infection, which often means 6 months or longer. Since both of these antimicrobial agents are folic acid antagonists, bone marrow suppression is common, but may be prevented by concomitant administration of folinic acid. Theoretically, clinically important toxoplasmosis in cardiac transplantation could be largely prevented by screening donors and recipients for *Toxoplasma* antibody, but this is usually not feasible given the time limitations on surgery. Since toxoplasmosis can also be newly acquired by immunocompromised hosts, avoidance of known sources of infection, such as incompletely cooked meat and cat faeces, seems prudent.

Among seronegative patients who develop infection after receiving a heart from a seropositive donor, the mortality is high. In the Papworth series 2 of 3 such patients died as a result of their infection (67%; CL 24–97%) (Nagington and Martin, 1983; Brooks and Remington, 1986).

Pneumocystis carinii

Pneumocystis carinii pneumonia as an important infection risk in patients with deficient cell-mediated immunity. Clinical disease in most instances is the result of reactivation of latent infection (Hughes, 1984). Two-thirds of normal children develop antibodies to this organism by the age of 4 (Pifer *et al.*, 1978). Primary infection in some immunocompromised hosts is suggested by reports of nosocomial outbreaks (Singer *et al.*, 1975).

Infection is nearly always confined to the lungs. Patients usually present with fever, dry cough and tachypnoea. Chest radiographs usually show diffuse bilateral alveolar infiltrates most prominent in the perihilar areas and the lower lung fields (Michaelis *et al.*, 1976). Patients with radiographic changes are nearly always dyspnoeic and hypoxaemic. However, early in the disease, in spite of the presence of fever and dyspnoea, the chest radiograph may be normal (Michaelis *et al.*, 1976). This infection is almost always confined to the lung. Atypical presentations include the absence of fever, and radiographs showing nodules, mass lesions, pleural effusions, cavities or lobar infiltrates. Dissemination is very uncommon, but without treatment death occurs from respiratory failure.

Because the protozoa are usually within the alveoli and not present in the bronchi, the organism is rarely found in expectorated sputum, and diagnosis usually involves an invasive procedure such as open lung biopsy, transbronchial biopsy, bronchoalveolar lavage, endobronchial brushings or percutaneous needle aspiration or biopsy.

The important pathological feature of *Pneumocystis* pneumonia is an interstitial process involving thickening of the alveolar wall, hyperplasia of the cells lining the alveoli, and infiltrating plasma cells in the alveolar septae. The alveolar spaces become filled with an eosinophilic substance, which contains protozoa on staining with Gomori methenamine silver (Rubin and Cosimi, 1982). Serological tests are rarely helpful in the diagnosis.

Treatment involves the combination of trimethoprim and sulphamethoxazole or pentamidine (see Table 13.2). These agents are probably equally effective, and although trimethoprim–sulfonamide may contribute to the nephrotoxicity associated with cyclosporin (Thompson *et al.*, 1983; Nyberg *et al.*, 1984), this combination is usually preferred to pentamidine because of the numerous toxic effects associated with the latter agent. These include hypoglycaemia, hypotension, hepatitis and nephrotoxicity. Patients with active infection should be isolated from other immunocompromised hosts. Controversy exists regarding the prophylactic use of trimethoprim–sulphamethoxazole in transplant recipients. A significant decrease in the incidence of *Pneumocystis* pneumonia has been noted among bone marrow transplant recipients who receive prophylaxis (Winston *et al.*, 1979; Brooks and Remington, 1986) and possibly among renal transplant patients (Brooks and Remington, 1986). Among cardiac transplant patients receiving cyclosporin, the incidence of *Pneumocystis* has been low without prophylaxis (Brooks and Remington, 1986).

Despite therapy, the reported mortality for patients on immunosuppressive drugs is 25–30% (Hughes *et al.*, 1973, 1977).

Viruses

The most important viral infections seen in cardiac transplant patients are those caused by the herpes virus group including CMV, Epstein–Barr virus, varicella-zoster virus and herpes simplex virus. These are DNA viruses characterized clinically by long periods of asymptomatic latency with reactivation sometimes associated with deficient cell-mediated immunity, particularly during the first few months following transplantation when immunosuppression is maximal.

Cytomegalovirus

Cytomegalovirus (CMV) is an extremely common cause of infection in organ transplant patients, as it is in the general population. In the normal population, 80–90% are seropositive as they enter middle age (Rubin and Cosimi, 1982). Among transplant patients, CMV infection may be due to transmission of the virus with the donor heart, but more commonly it results from reactivation. In one study, all cardiac transplant patients with serological evidence of past infection prior to transplantation showed evidence of reactivation by viral shedding, and 60% developed four-fold titre rises in CMV antibody (Pollard *et al.*, 1982). Among patients seronegative prior to transplantation, 62% were found to be infected postoperatively. All patients with evidence of primary infection had received hearts from seropositive donors. In most studies of CMV in organ transplantation, primary infection was far more likely to produce clinical symptoms than reactivation (Peterson *et al.*, 1980; Ho, 1982), but both forms of infection may produce severe disease in patients receiving aggressive immunosuppressive therapy. Clinical manifestations of CMV infection are often associated with increases in immunosuppressive therapy (Peterson *et al.*, 1980), and conversely CMV infection itself is associated with depression of cell-mediated immunity (Oill *et al.*, 1977). The latter effect may be responsible for the known association between CMV infection and other opportunistic infections, particularly *Pneumocystis* pneumonia (Chatterjee *et al.*, 1978; Rand, Pollard and Merigan, 1978; Peterson *et al.*, 1980).

Clinical manifestations of CMV infection in the immunocompromised host include undifferentiated fever, pneumonitis, hepatitis, retinitis, gastroenteritis and a syndrome resembling infectious mononucleosis (Peterson *et al.*, 1980; Alford, 1985). Excepting retinitis, these manifestations are most common in the early post-transplant period. CMV pneumonia usually presents with diffuse bilateral interstitial or alveolar infiltrates and hypoxia, but atypical radiological findings including lobar and nodular infiltrates have been reported. Abnormalities of liver function tests are common in CMV infection, but hepatitis with typical histopathological changes is infrequent. Gastrointestinal manifestations of infection include oesophagitis, gastric and caecal ulcers, and haemorrhage from ulcerative caecitis. CMV retinitis is characterized by haemorrhage, exudates and sheathing of blood vessels with macular sparing (Egbert *et al.*, 1980; Pollard *et al.*, 1980). Retinitis may be asymptomatic or cause scotoma and blurred vision. The mononucleosis-like syndrome is characterized by fever, malaise, hepatosplenomegaly, and laboratory findings of leucopenia and atypical lymphocytes. In contrast to CMV-induced mononucleosis in normal hosts, lymphopenia and neutropenia rather than lymphocytosis is usually seen (Marker, Simmons and Balfour, 1981; Marker *et al.*, 1981).

The diagnosis of CMV infection can be very difficult. Titre rises of IgG complement-fixing antibodies, the appearance of IgM antibody, and shedding of the virus from the urinary or respiratory tract are all seen in the absence of clinical illness, and their significance in patients with particular symptoms is difficult to assess, since most manifestations of CMV infection can be seen with other opportunistic infections. Even viraemia can be seen without symptoms, although positive blood cultures may be more closely associated with true CMV disease than cultures from other sites. The diagnosis of CMV disease depends in most instances on demonstration of the typical histopathological changes in tissue. The recent development of monoclonal antibody and DNA probes may facilitate both the identification of virus in tissue, and the early detection of virus in culture (Meyerson, Hackman and Meyers, 1984; Spector *et al.*, 1984; Hackman *et al.*, 1985; Shuster *et al.*, 1985).

CMV infection does not respond to treatment with the antiviral agents at present available, although the newly introduced drug DHPG has been shown to be effective in several studies (Bach *et al.*, 1985; Felsenstein *et al.*, 1985; Icenogle *et al.*, 1986). Because of the central importance of CMV infection in organ transplantation, a number of preventive measures have been proposed including donor matching, passive immunization, vaccination, prophylactic interferon, and screening or special processing of blood products. The logistic problems of cardiac transplantation and the high prevalence of latent infections in the general population have made donor matching impracticable. Passive immunization with hyperimmune globulin has been shown to lessen the severity of CMV infection in recipients of bone marrow transplantation (Meyers *et al.*, 1983; Condie and O'Reilly, 1984). Vaccination with an attenuated strain of CMV has been studied in renal allograft recipients and has led to some amelioration of symptoms among patients undergoing primary infections (Marker, Simmons and Balfour, 1981; Marker *et al.*, 1981; Plotkin *et al.*, 1984). Prophylactic interferon given from the time of operation has also been shown to ameliorate the features of reactivation in seropositive renal transplant patients (Hirsch *et al.*, 1983). The use of seronegative blood products for seronegative recipients effectively prevents primary infection, but the logistics of blood support require that such designated blood products be reserved for patients at greatest risk, such as immunodeficient neonates (Onorato *et al.*, 1985). The use of leucocyte-poor blood products provides incomplete protection since leucocytes, the presumed cells of latency, are never totally removed (Lang *et al.*, 1977). The use of deglycerolysed blood may prevent infection by transfusion, but it is expensive (Brady *et al.*, 1984). The significance of primary and reactivation CMV infections in cardiac transplantation, and the relative importance of different vehicles of infection such as donor hearts and blood products, remain to be defined, and more data are needed on the efficacy, cost and potentially adverse effects of the various preventive measures.

The mortality rate of infection with CMV is difficult to establish, since CMV is frequently present with other serious infections. In one prospective study, the mortality among patients who were seronegative before transplantation (primary CMV) was 25% (2/8; CL 8–50%) (Pollard *et al.*, 1982). CMV can be cultured from lung tissue in approximately 40% of cardiac transplant recipients dying of other causes (Uys, Rose and Barnard, 1979).

Herpes simplex

The majority of cardiac transplant patients can be expected to be seropositive for herpes simplex virus and most of these individuals will shed the virus and develop herpetic lesions in the early months after transplantation (Rand *et al.*, 1976; Pollard *et al.*, 1982). Common sites of involvement include the mouth, genitalia and oesophagus. The typical lesions of herpes labialis or herpes genitalis are seen and lesions may extend and appear as deep necrotic ulcers. Severe stomatitis and oesophagitis are also seen. Disseminated infection with viraemia, hepatitis or CNS involvement is rare, but has been reported in renal transplant patients (Ho, 1977; Elliott *et al.*, 1980). Herpetic lesions in compromised hosts sometimes respond to the topical application of acyclovir, and intravenous acylovir (see Table 13.2) has been reported to promote relief of pain and healing of lesions in cardiac transplant patients (Chou, Gallagher and Merigan, 1981; Gold, 1987). Although the patient is often quite uncomfortable from the painful lesions, the outcome is rarely fatal.

Varicella-zoster

In one series, the incidence of reactivation infection with varicella-zoster virus was 22% among cardiac transplant patients observed for up to 2 years, the lesions beginning 4 weeks to 1 year after transplantation (Pollard *et al.*, 1982). Unusually prolonged and severe dermatomal lesions have been reported in cardiac transplant patients (Gallagher and Merigan, 1979).

Disseminated disease is always an indication for treatment with intravenous acyclovir (see Table 13.2) and cardiac transplant patients with dermatomal zoster should also receive acyclovir to prevent dissemination, reduce virus shedding and promote healing. Post-herpetic neuralgia remains a significant problem in these patients despite the use of effective antiviral agents. The mortality from varicella-zoster reported in one series was 12% (1/8; CL 2–36%) (Pollard *et al.*, 1982).

Epstein–Barr virus

This is another member of the herpes virus group which is capable of latency and reactivation. It is aetiologically associated with the infectious mononucleosis syndrome, as well as neoplastic disorders including Burkitt's lymphoma and nasopharyngeal carcinoma. In organ transplantation recipients, reactivation infection has been associated with a mononucleosis-like illness, often with associated leucopenia (Cheeseman *et al.*, 1980; Brooks and Remington, 1986). More important, however, is the link between this agent and the development of lymphoproliferative disorders in immunocompromised hosts (Hunt and Stinson, 1981; Hanto *et al.*, 1982; Cleary, Warnke and Sklar, 1984), which occur in 3–6% of cardiac transplant recipients (Penn, 1978; Cohen *et al.*, 1984). It is possible that immunosuppressive therapy leads to decreased EBV-specific cytotoxic T-cell memory, leading to polyclonal proliferation of latently infected B cells that sometimes progress to a monoclonal process (Hanto *et al.*, 1981a; Hanto *et al.*, 1982; Cleary, Warnke and Sklar, 1984). Clinically, these lymphoproliferative disorders are often extranodal and involve the CNS and gastrointestinal tract. Histopathologically, the disorder can present as non-specific reactive lymphoid hyperplasia, polymorphic diffuse B-cell lymphoma or immunoblastic sarcoma (Frizzera *et al.*, 1981; Hanto *et al.*, 1981b). The initial use of cyclosporin may have been associated with an increased incidence of lymphoproliferative disorders in cardiac transplants, but the relationship is unsubstantiated in current regimens using lower doses of cyclosporin (Cohen *et al.*, 1984).

SPECIAL PROBLEMS IN INFECTION FOLLOWING CARDIAC TRANSPLANTATION

Diagnostic approach to the radiological pulmonary infiltrate

The lungs are the most frequent site of infection in cardiac transplant recipients (Baumgartner *et al.*, 1979), and a wide variety of microbial pathogens is responsible. Clinical diagnosis is made difficult by the fact that many organisms can produce the same radiographic pattern, and atypical presentations are common. The fulminant course of many of these infections makes prompt diagnosis essential, particularly since the empirical use of antibiotics is complicated not only by the large number of potential pathogens but also by the significant toxicity associated with the use of many therapeutic agents. Expectorated sputum is usually inadequate for diagnosis, and the examination of specimens obtained by invasive techniques is often necessary. The fact that many of the most common pathogens are slow-growing microorganisms emphasizes the need for direct examination of specimens using a variety of histological stains and sometimes immunocytological techniques.

The methods used in the diagnosis of a specific pulmonary infection depend on a number of factors, including the rate of progression of the infection, the condition of the patient, familiarity with various diagnostic techniques, the location of the lung infiltrate and the presence or absence of a pleural effusion. Examination of expectorated sputum is a reasonable initial diagnostic step, but most patients cannot produce an adequate specimen and even with a good specimen the technique has a low yield. Interpretation of sputum culture results is made difficult by the potential for contamination with pathogens colonizing the upper airway, including *Pneumococci*, *Staphylococci*, anaerobes, Gram-negative bacilli and *Candida*. However, the presence of some pathogens in expectorated sputum can be taken as almost certain evidence of invasive lower respiratory tract infection, for example *Mycobacterium tuberculosis*, *Legionella* spp. and *Pneumocystis carinii*; and the presence of other organisms such as *Cryptococcus*, *Nocardia* and *Aspergillus* is at least highly suggestive of invasive lower tract disease. All of these pathogens grow slowly in culture, and even with carefully prepared Gram stains and special stains for *Pneumocystis*, fungi and mycobacteria, examination of expectorated sputum has a low diagnostic yield.

Because of the propensity for rapid progression of untreated pulmonary infection in the immunosuppressed patient, sampling of sputum or tissue at or near the site of intrapulmonary infection is essential. The initial and most important diagnostic procedure in most patients with a new radiological pulmonary infiltrate (in our opinion even if the patient is asymptomatic) is fibre-optic bronchoscopy (Lauver *et al.*, 1979). Bronchoscopy can be safely performed on patients receiving supplemental oxygen or assisted ventilation, including those requiring positive end-expiratory pressure. Although specimens obtained by bronchoscopy are also subject to contamination by upper airway secretions (Bartlett *et al.*, 1986), this can be substantially reduced with the use of a special telescoping brush system (in which the brush is protected by two catheters) and a polyethylene glycol plug (Wimberly, Falling and Bartlett, 1979). The proper use of such a system requires quantitative culturing of specimens (Pollock *et al.*, 1983); in the absence of quantitative bacteriology, rough quantitation can be obtained by examination of a Gram-stained specimen. Several studies have documented the excellent sensitivity and specificity of this system (Wimberly *et al.*, 1982; Pollock *et al.*, 1983; Chastre *et al.*, 1984). Although routine bronchial brushings, aspirates and washings obtained via bronchoscopy are always contaminated by upper airway secretions (Fossieck *et al.*, 1977), these specimens are still useful in the identification of certain pathogens such as *Legionella* and *Pneumocystis*. Transbronchial biopsy provides specimens which are also subject to contamination by upper respiratory flora, but has the advantage of providing lung parenchyma for observing cytopathic changes which may be helpful in interpreting the results of culture or serological studies. Transbronchial biopsy does increase the risk of fibre-optic bronchoscopy, particularly in patients with clotting disorders or those requiring ventilatory support (Cunningham *et al.*, 1977).

The technique of broncho-alveolar lavage (BAL) has been used extensively by research laboratories studying mechanisms of lung disease and is now gaining acceptance in the evaluation of pneumonia in the immunocompromised host (Stover *et al.*, 1984; Meden, Hall and Ahmad, 1985; Springmeyer *et al.*, 1986). During the procedure, the bronchoscope is wedged into a medium-sized bronchus of an involved segment of the lung, and repeated lavage is performed with small volumes of normal saline. Successful BAL usually produces 100–200 ml of fluid which can be used for culture, special stains and cytology. Studies have shown BAL to be an excellent method for the diagnosis of *Pneumocystis* pneumonia (Drew *et al.*, 1974; Kelley *et al.*, 1978; Ognibene *et al.*, 1984) and pulmonary haemorrhage (by demonstration of haemosiderin-laden macrophages) (Drew, Finley and Gold, 1977; Stover *et al.*, 1984), as well as viral, fungal and mycobacterial pneumonia (Stover *et al.*, 1984; Springmeyer *et al.*, 1986). This technique provides a true sampling of cells and secretions present in alveoli and it can be safely performed in patients with thrombocytopenia or other clotting disorders. Although usually well tolerated, BAL is commonly associated with transient temperature elevations and slight worsening of pulmonary infiltrates. A recent study showed BAL to be superior to transbronchial biopsy in the diagnosis of mycobacterial infection and better than routine bronchial washings in distinguishing colonization from tissue invasion with organisms of uncertain pathogenic significance such as *Aspergillus* and *Cryptococcus* (Stover *et al.*, 1984). BAL can also be used to diagnose neoplastic disease which can present with diffuse pulmonary infiltrates in the immunocompromised host. Since none of the diagnostic techniques performed with fibre-optic bronchoscopy is wholly satisfactory in terms of potential complications or diagnostic yield, several techniques should be incorporated into every procedure, provided the institution is capable of properly processing the specimens.

Other techniques used in the evaluation of pulmonary infiltrates in the immunocompromised host include transthoracic needle aspiration (Palmer, Davidson and Lusk, 1980) and transtracheal aspiration. Needle aspiration yields a very small amount of material, is subject to considerable sampling error (Springmeyer *et al.*, 1986), and has resulted in a serious complication rate in cardiac transplants (Mammana *et al.*, 1983). Transthoracic cutting-needle biopsy (Neff, 1972; Zavala and Bedell, 1972) may have a higher diagnostic yield but carries a high complication rate (Cunningham *et al.*, 1977; Matthay and Moritz, 1981). Transtracheal aspiration carries a significant risk of complication (Spencer and Beaty, 1972), is contraindicated in patients with bleeding disorders, and cannot be done on intubated patients.

Culture results on specimens obtained by transtracheal aspiration are difficult to interpret, since the trachea may become colonized with upper respiratory flora in severely ill patients (Bartlett, 1977), and there is often a discrepancy between the results of transtracheal aspiration and transthoracic needle aspiration (Davidson, Tempest and Palmer, 1976).

When the diagnosis cannot be established by other means, open lung biopsy is advisable (Leight and Michaelis, 1978; Satterfield and McLaughlin, 1979). Open lung biopsy can be performed through a limited incision; an anterior thoracotomy through the second intercostal space may be used for a diffuse process and a lateral thoracotomy for basilar disease (McElvein, 1985). The method of processing the tissue is very important. A recommended approach is to bisect the lung biopsy specimen and to send half to the bacteriology laboratory for appropriate cultures (aerobic, anaerobic, mycobacterial and fungal) and the other half for frozen section with smear preparations to look for *Pneumocystis carinii* and fungal hyphae, followed by rapid tissue fixation for permanent sections (McElvein, 1985; Potter *et al.*, 1985).

In summary, cardiac transplant patients found to have a new pulmonary infiltrate should be investigated with fibre-optic bronchoscopy unless examination of expectorated sputum provides a secure and prompt diagnosis. All patients should have a blood culture, and if there is a significant pleural effusion a thoracentesis should be performed. During bronchoscopy, specimens should be obtained by protected catheter brush followed by either routine bronchial washings or broncho-alveolar lavage. Finally, transbronchial biopsy should be done in patients with adequate platelet counts ($>50\,000/mm^3$) and clotting studies, or correctable coagulation disorders. Table 13.3 lists suggestions for processing specimens obtained during fibre-optic bronchoscopy. If a diagnosis cannot be established by bronchoscopy or needle aspiration, an open lung biopsy should be considered. Open lung biopsy has a high diagnostic yield (Greenman, Goodall and King, 1975; Leight and Michaelis, 1978; Johnston, Pizzo and Fauci, 1982; Haverkos *et al.*, 1983), but carries an important risk of complication in cardiac transplant patients (Baumgartner *et al.*, 1979). Rarely, in the face of rapid deterioration, empirical treatment with broad-spectrum antibiotics may be advisable before a definite diagnosis can be established.

Investigation of central nervous system infection

Although less common than pulmonary infection, CNS infections cause significant morbidity and mortality in cardiac transplantation (Stinson *et al.*, 1971; Britt, Enzmann and Remington, 1981; Cooper *et al.*, 1983; Dummer *et al.*, 1984). These infections commonly present with fever, headache and/or a change in mental state. A progressive course with development of focal neurological deficits is frequent, but nuchal rigidity is rare. Cardiac trans-

TABLE 13.3
Specimens Obtained During Fibre-Optic Bronchoscopy

Protected Catheter Brushing
- Gram stain
- Quantitative bacterial culture

Broncho-alveolar Lavage
- Cultures
- Routine bacterial
- Mycobacterial
- Legionella
- Fungal
- Viral
- Stains
  - Acid fast
  - PAS
  - Papanicolaou
  - Methenamine–silver
- DNA probes
  - Legionella
  - CMV
- Immunological studies
  - Legionella direct — fluorescent antibody
  - Aspergillus RIA
  - CMV indirect — immunofluorescence with monoclonal antibody

Transbronchial Biopsy
- Histological stains
  - Haematoxylin–eosin
  - Methenamine–silver
  - Brown and Brenn
  - Acid fast

plant patients presenting with confusion, disorientation, lethargy, a decreased level of consciousness, altered personality or affect, or a focal neurological deficit with or without fever, should have an emergency CT brain scan performed. If the CT scan shows a mass lesion, lumbar puncture is usually contraindicated and a neurosurgical consultation should be obtained. Most mass lesions require aspiration or open brain biopsy for diagnosis, and effective treatment of a brain abscess may require surgical drainage. If the CT scan is normal, a lumbar puncture should be performed and the cerebrospinal fluid cultured for bacteria, fungi and mycobacteria. Analysis of the CSF should include protein and glucose determination as well as cell count and differential, and slides should be prepared for Gram staining, acid-fast stain and India ink. Immunological studies include cryptococcal antigen determination and, in endemic areas, tests for complement-fixing antibody to coccidioidomycosis.

Management of postoperative mediastinitis

Serious and potentially fatal mediastinal infection occasionally occurs after cardiac transplantation (Barnard *et al.*, 1981; Pearl, Weiner and Dibbell, 1982; Copeland *et al.*, 1984; Trento *et al.*, 1984). This complication is recognized by the presence of fever, persistent chest pain, sternal instability, and a discharge from the wound which is usually serosanguineous. Occasionally, purulent drainage is the first manifestation. When the diagnosis is not apparent on physical examination of the wound, CT scan of the mediastinum may identify a retrosternal abscess (Kay *et al.*, 1983). The likelihood of a successful resolution is increased by early recognition.

The management options for this condition are to a large extent determined by the degree of sternal and mediastinal involvement. When mediastinal and sternal infection is minimal, management involves reopening of the wound, debridement of the sternum and mediastinum and reclosure over suction–irrigation tubes (Bryant, Spencer and Trinkle, 1969; Thurer *et al.*, 1974). Systemic antibiotics are administered and the mediastinum is irrigated for approximately 7 days with antibiotic solution or povidone-iodine (Thurer *et al.*, 1974). When mediastinal and sternal suppuration is extensive, it may be advisable to debride thoroughly and leave the wound packed open. When there is no evidence of a continuing infection, the wound is closed, usually employing a muscle flap (pectoralis major, latissimus dorsi, rectus abdominis) or an omental flap, to obliterate dead space (Pairolero and Arnold, 1984; Majure *et al.*, 1986).

In the UAB experience (1981–85), 2 of 63 patients (3%; CL 1–7%) developed postoperative mediastinitis. One was successfully managed with the closed irrigation technique, and the other patient underwent debridement. The wound was packed open, and subsequently closed with omental and bilateral pectoralis major flaps with a good result.

Fever of unknown origin

A study of the aetiology of fever in renal transplant recipients has been reported (Peterson *et al.*, 1981) and may provide insights for cardiac transplant recipients. Of 194 episodes of fever in 175 renal transplant recipients, 74% were attributed to infection, of which 55% were viral, 14% bacterial and 5% fungal. Allograft rejection accounted for 25% of febrile episodes.

Occasionally, transplant patients present with fever but no clear focus of infection despite a careful history, a thorough physical examination, and the results of routine laboratory studies and chest radiology. In this situation, non-infectious causes of fever such as thrombophlebitis, drug reactions, neoplasia and transplant rejection should be considered. New and old sites of intravenous fluid administration should be examined for evidence of phlebitis, and pulmonary thrombo-embolism should be considered in patients with fever and unexplained hypoxaemia, even in the absence of radiographic findings or pulmonary symptoms. Febrile reactions can occur after blood product transfusions, and drugs known to cause fever include many antimicrobials, anticonvulsants and anti-arrhythmics. Drug fever should be suspected when a patient appears clinically better than would be expected from the fever pattern. Defervescence from drug fever usually occurs within 48 h of stopping the responsible agent. Cardiac transplants are at increased risk of developing a lymphoma, and these tumours can produce fever and may have unusual extranodal presentations. Transplant rejection may rarely present with fever as the most prominent clinical finding and require endomyocardial biopsy for confirmation.

Fever may be the first sign of many of the opportunistic infections discussed in this chapter. Patients with fever but without localizing findings should be followed closely, particularly for the development of pulmonary signs and symptoms and changes in mental status. Both CMV and EB virus can cause a febrile mononucleosis syndrome in immunocompromised hosts, and CMV infection may produce a mild febrile illness with no specific laboratory or physical findings.

Most patients with undiagnosed fever should be admitted to hospital for observation and investigated with repeated examination and chest radiographs. They should have multiple blood cultures and serological studies for toxoplasma, CMV and EB virus. Patients who appear toxic or are haemodynamically unstable, particularly in the early postoperative period, should be treated with broad-spectrum antibiotics after cultures have been obtained. In most situations, however, empirical antibiotics should be withheld until a specific diagnosis is made.

PREOPERATIVE ASSESSMENT AND PREVENTIVE MEASURES

The preoperative assessment of prospective transplant recipients should aim to identify patients with active infection and include baseline studies that might help in the later diagnosis of possible infectious complications. Preoperative serological studies should include tests for toxoplasmosis, CMV, EB virus, hepatitis viruses and coccidioidomycosis (in endemic areas). A tuberculin skin test should be done in patients without a history of prior positive reactions. The preoperative period is also the optimal time to administer multivalent pneumococcal vaccine.

The most important preventive measure against early infection is scrupulous attention to asepsis by the surgeon, anaesthetist, perfusionist and scrub nurse. This applies not only to the surgical field, but also to the insertion of venous and arterial access devices, the bladder catheter and, as far as possible, the endotracheal tube.

Although the value of prophylactic antimicrobials has not been proven, numerous studies have suggested a benefit in cardiac surgery (Firor, 1967; Fong, Baker and McKee, 1979; Austin *et al.*, 1980) as well as renal transplantation (Tilney *et al.*, 1978). Particularly in view of the patient's immunosuppressed state, routine prophylactic antibiotics seem advisable.

At UAB, prophylactic perioperative antibiotics are given until the last indwelling line is removed, and also during percutaneous endomyocardial biopsy. Cefazolin (15 mg/kg up to a maximal dose of 1 g) is administered intravenously at induction and every 6 h thereafter until the last device is removed. Vancomycin is administered to patients with an immediate-type hypersensitivity reaction to penicillin or cephalosporins. Additional prophylaxis against candidiasis is administered in the form of nystatin oral suspension, 500 000 units (5 ml), gargled and swallowed every 6 h commencing on the second postoperative day (discontinued at 6 months). Patients also receive oral acyclovir (200 mg t.i.d. for 3 months) for prophylaxis against herpetic infections (Gold and Corey, 1987) and a combination of trimethoprim and sulphamethoxazole (cotrimoxazole) (1 regular strength tablet t.i.d. for 6 months) for prophylaxis against *Pneumocystis*. For patients undergoing endomyocardial biopsy, cefazolin (1 g) is given intravenously after insertion of an intravenous line just prior to biopsy. Cephradine (500 mg orally) is then administered every 6 h for 3 doses.

Although commonly practised, the benefit derived from reverse isolation nursing is controversial. Most infection in these patients is endogenously acquired rather than contracted from medical and nursing staff. Furthermore, enforcement of these procedures may have the unfortunate consequence of reducing clinical assessment of the patient, increasing the likelihood that important signs of rejection and infection might be overlooked. However, it is extremely important that the surgical wound, monitoring devices and intravenous lines are given special care.

At UAB, reverse isolation precautions are used while the patient is in the intensive care unit (usually for 3–7 days) following transplantation. There is limited access to the transplant room, and hand washing, gown, cap, mask, gloves and shoe coverings are required of all personnel entering the room. Intravenous and arterial access sites are treated with hydrogen peroxide and povidone-iodine ointment every 8 h and an occlusive dressing applied. Whenever possible, intravenous lines are changed every 48–72 h. All surgical wounds are painted with povidone-iodine every 8 h. No special laminar flow facilities are used. When out of the intensive care unit, the patient is placed in a private room without special isolation precautions. The patient does, however, wear mask, cap, gown and gloves when leaving the floor for radiography, physiotherapy or other special activities and procedures.

Isolation of certain organisms, notably *Legionella*, *Listeria monocytogenes* and *Pneumocystis carinii*, in a cardiac transplant unit should call for special precautions. *Listeria monocytogenes* has been isolated from urine, faeces and sputum of infected patients (Stamm *et al.*, 1982), and thus secretion and excretion precautions in patients with listeriosis are advisable. Airborne transmission of *Pneumocystis carinii* has been reported (Singer *et al.*, 1975) and hence isolation of infected patients should be practised. Cardiac transplant patients should also be kept separate from individuals with active infection, including family members with respiratory infections. Isolation from other immunocompromised hosts with active infection is especially important.

When transplant patients are ready to return home, they should be instructed to report promptly any symptoms of infection such as fever, weakness, shortness of breath, cough or diarrhoea. Any such features should be investigated immediately and routine follow-up is especially important during periods after treatment of acute rejection. Stable patients should be seen by a physician every 2 or 3 months, and a chest radiograph should be obtained at each visit. Transplant patients should receive annual vaccination for influenza.

In the paediatric transplant patient, routine childhood immunizations should be performed only with killed (not attenuated) vaccine, to avoid the small risk of producing active disease with live vaccine in the immunosuppressed patient.

ACKNOWLEDGEMENTS

We would like to thank Ms. Terri McVay for her excellent work in the preparation of the manuscript.

REFERENCES

Aisner, J., Schimpff, S. C. and Wiernik, P. H. (1977). Treatment of invasive aspergillosis: relation of early diagnosis and treatment to response. *Ann. Intern. Med.*, **86**, 539–543.

Alford, C. A. (1985). Cytomegalovirus infection. *Al. J. Med. Sci.*, **22**, 169–189.

Andrews, C. P. and Weiner, M. H. (1982). Aspergillus antigen detection in bronchoalveolar lavage fluid from patients with invasive aspergillosis and aspergillomas. *Am. J. Med.* **73**, 372–380.

Angeles, A. M. and Sugar, A. M. (1987). Rapid diagnosis of nocardiosis with an enzyme immunoassay. *J. Infect. Dis.* **155**, 292–296.

Armstrong, D. (1981). Fungal infections in the compromised host. In *Clinical Approach to Infection in the Compromised Host* (R. H. Rubin and L. S. Young, Eds), pp. 195–228. Plenum, New York.

Armstrong, D. (1985). *Listeria monocytogenes.* In *Principles and Practice of Infectious Disease*, 2nd edn (G. L. Mandell, R. G. Douglas and J. E. Bennett, Eds), pp. 1117–1182. Wiley, New York.

Arnow, P. M., Anderson, R. L., Mainous, P. D. and Smith, E. J. (1978). Pulmonary aspergillosis during hospital renovation. *Am. Rev. Resp. Dis.*, **118**, 49–53.

Atkinson, J. P., Schreiber, A. D. and Frank, M. M. (1973). Effects of corticosteroids and splenectomy on the immune clearance and destruction of erythrocytes. *J. Clin. Invest.*, **53**, 1509–1517.

Austin, T. W., Coles, J. C., Burnett, R. and Goldbach, W. (1980). Aortocoronary bypass procedures and sternotomy infections: a study of antistaphylococcal prophylaxis. *Can. J. Surg.* **23**(5), 483–485.

Bach, M. C., Bagwell, S. P., Knapp, N. P., Davis, K. M. and Hedstrom, P. S. (1985). 9-(1,3-Dihydroxy-2-propoxymethyl)guanine for cytomegalovirus infections in patients with the acquired immunodeficiency syndrome. *Ann. Intern. Med.*, **103**, 381–384.

Barnard, C. N., Barnard, M. S., Cooper, D. K. C., Curchio, C. A., Hassoulas, J., Novitsky, D. and Wolpowitz, A. (1981). The present status of heterotopic cardiac transplantation. *J. Thorac. Cardiovasc. Surg.* **81**, 433–439.

Barnhart, G. R., Hastillo, A., Goldman, M. H., Szentpetery, S., Wolfgang, T. C., Mohanakumar, T., Katz, M. R., Rider, S., Haurahan, J., Lower, R. and Hess, M. L. (1985). A prospective randomized trial of pretransfusion/azathioprine/prednisone versus cyclosporine/prednisone immunosuppression in cardiac transplant recipients: preliminary results. *Circulation* **72**, Suppl. 11, 227–230.

Bartlett, J. G. (1977). Diagnostic accuracy of transtracheal aspiration bacteriologic studies. *Am. Rev. Respir. Dis.* **115**, 777–782.

Bartlett, J. G., Alexander, J., Mayhew, J., Sullivan-Sigler, N. and Gorbach, S. L. (1986). Should fiberoptic bronchoscopy aspirates be cultured? *Am. Rev. Resp. Dis.* **114**, 73–78.

Baumgartner, W. A. (1983). Infection in cardiac transplantation. *Heart Transplant.* **3**(1), 75–80.

Baumgartner, W. A., Reitz, B. A., Oyer, P. E., Stinson, E. B. and Shumway, N. E. (1979). Cardiac homotransplantation. *Curr. Prob. Surg.* **16**, 1–61.

Beaty, H. N. (1985). *Legionella pneumophila* (Legionnaires' disease). In *Principles and Practice of Infectious Disease*, 2nd edn (G. L. Mandell, R. G. Douglas and J. E. Bennett, Eds), pp. 1306–1314, Wiley, New York.

Bennett, J. E., Dismukes, W. E., Duma, R. J., Medoff, G., Sande, M. A., Gallis, H., Leonard, J., Fields, B. T., Bradshaw, M., Haywood, H., McGee, Z. A., Cate, T. R., Cobbs, G. C., Warner, J. F. and Alling, D. W. (1979). A comparison of amphotericin B alone and combined with flucytosine in the treatment of cryptococcal meningitis. *N. Engl. J. Med.*, **301**, 126–131.

Blackburn, G. L., Gibbons, G. W., Bothe, A., Benotti, P. N., Harken, D. E. and

McEnany, T. M. (1977). Nutritional support in cardiac cachexia. *J. Thorac. Cardiovasc. Surg.* **73**(4), 489–496.

Brady, M. T., Milam, J. D., Anderson, D. C., Hawkins, E. P., Speer, M. E., Seavy, D., Bijou, H. and Yow, M. D. (1984). Use of deglycerolyzed red blood cells to prevent post-transfusion infection with CMV in neonates. *J. Infect. Dis.* **150**, 334–339.

Briggs, J. D., Timbury, M. C., Paton, A. M. and Bell, P. R. F. (1972). Viral infection and renal transplant rejection. *Br. Med. J.* **4**, 520–522.

Britt, R. H., Enzmann, D. R. and Remington, J. S. (1981). Intracranial infection in cardiac transplant recipients. *Ann. Neurol.* **9**(2), 107–119.

Brooks, R. G. and Remington, J. S. (1986). Transplant-related infections. In *Hospital Infections*, 2nd edn (J. V. Bennett and P. S. Brachman, Eds), pp. 581–618. Little, Brown, Boston, Mass.

Bryant, L. R., Spencer, F. C. and Trinkle, J. K. (1969). Treatment of median sternotomy infection by mediastinal irrigation with an antibiotic solution. *Ann. Surg.* **169**(6), 914–920.

Burton, J. R., Zachery, J. B., Bessin, R., Rathbun, H. K., Greenough, W. B., Sterioff, S., Wright, J. R., Slavin, R. E. and Williams, G. M. (1972). Aspergillosis in four renal transplant recipients: diagnosis and effective treatment with amphotericin B. *Ann. Intern. Med.* **77**, 383–388.

Byrd, L. H., Tapia, L., Cheigh, J. S., Aronian, J., Stenzel, K. H. and Rubin, A. L. (1978). Association between *Streptococcus fecalis* urinary infections and graft rejection in kidney transplantation. *Lancet* **2**, 1167–1169.

Cabrol, C., Gandjbakhch, I., Pavie, A., Cabrol, A., Mattei, M. F. and Leger, P. (1985). Heart transplantation in Paris, at 'La Pitié' Hospital. *Heart Transplant.* **4**(5), 476–480.

Chang, R. S., Lewis, J. P., Reynolds, R. D., Sullivan, M. J. and Neuman, J. (1978). Oropharyngeal excretion of Epstein-Barr virus by patients with lymphoproliferative disorders and by recipients of renal homografts. *Ann. Intern. Med.*, **88**, 34–40.

Chastre, J., Viau, F., Brun, P., Pierre, J., Dauge, M. C., Bouchama, A., Akesbi, A. and Gibert, C. (1984). Prospective evaluation of the protected specimens brush for the diagnosis of pulmonary infections in ventilated patients. *Am. Rev. Resp. Dis.* **130**, 924–929.

Chatterjee, S. N., Fiala, M., Weiner, J., Stewart, J. A., Stacey, B. and Warner, N. (1978). Primary cytomegalovirus and opportunistic infections. Incidence in renal transplant recipients. *J. Am. Med. Ass.*, **240**, 2446–2471.

Cheeseman, S. H., Henla, W., Rubin, R. H., Tolkoff-Rubin, N. E., Cosimi, B., Cantell, F., Winkle, S., Herrin, J. T., Black, P. H., Russell, P. H. and Hirsch, M. S. (1980). Epstein-Barr virus infection in renal transplant recipients: effects of antithymocyte globulin and interferon. *Ann. Intern. Med.* **93**, 39–42.

Cheung, M. T. (1980). Eight cases of Legionnaires' disease. *Can. Med. Ass. J.* **123**, 639–644.

Chou, S., Gallagher, J. G. and Merigan, T. C. (1981). Controlled clinical trial of intravenous acyclovir in heart transplant patients with mucocutaneous herpes simplex infections. *Lancet* **1**, 1392–1394.

Cleary, M. L., Warnke, R. and Sklar, J. (1984). Monoclonality of lymphoproliferative lesions in cardiac transplant recipients. *New Engl. J. Med.*, **310**, 477–482.

Cohen, I. M., Galgiani, J. N., Potter, D. and Ogden, D. A. (1982). Coccidiomycosis in renal replacement therapy. *Arch. Intern. Med.* **142**, 489–494.

Cohen, D. J., Loertscher, R., Rubin, M. F., Tilney, N. L., Carpenter, C. B. and Strom, T. B. (1984). Cyclosporine: a new immunosuppressive agent for organ transplantation. *Ann. Intern. Med.*, **101**, 667–682.

Condie, R. M. and O'Reilly, R. J. (1984). Prevention of CMV infection by prophylaxis with an intravenous hyperimmune native unmodified CMV globulin. Randomized trial in bone marrow recipients. *Am. J. Med.* **76**, 134–141.

Cooper, D. K. C., Lanza, R. P., Boyd, S. T. and Barnard, C. N. (1981). Factors influencing survival following heart transplantation. *Heart Transplant.* **3**(1), 86–91.

Cooper, D. K. C., Lanza, R. P., Oliver, S., Forder, A. A., Rose, A. G., Uys, C. J., Novitzky, D. and Barnard, C. N. (1983). Infectious complications after heart transplantation. *Thorax* **38**, 822–828.

Copeland, J. G., Emery, R. W., Levinson, M. M., Icenogle, T. B., Riley, J. E., McAleer, M. J., Copeland, J. A. and Dietz, R. (1986). Cyclosporine: an immunosuppressive panacea? *J. Thorac. Cardiovasc. Surg.* **91**, 26–39.

Copeland, J. G., Mammana, R. B., Fuller, J. K., Campbell, D. W., McAleer, M. J. and Sailer, J. A. (1984). Heart transplantation. Four years experience with conventional immunosuppression. *J. Am. Med. Ass.* **251**(12), 1563–1566.

Cunningham, J. H., Zavala, D. C., Corry, R. J. and Keim, L. W. (1977). Trephine air drill, bronchial brush, and fiberoptic transbronchial lung biopsies in immunosuppressive patients. *Am. Rev. Resp. Dis.* **115**, 213–220.

Dale, D. C. (1981). Defects in host defense mechanisms in compromised patients. In *Clinical Approach to Infection in the Compromised Host* (R. H. Rubin and L. S. Young, Eds), pp. 35–74. Plenum, New York.

Daniels, N. J., Dover, J. S. and Schachter, R. K. (1984). Interaction between cyclosporine and rifampicin. *Lancet* **2**, 639.

David, D. S., Millian, S. J., Whitsell, J. C., Schwartz, G. H., Riggio, R. R., Stenzel, K. H. and Rubin, A. L. (1982). Viral syndromes and renal homograft rejection. *Ann. Surg.* **175**(2), 257–259.

Davidson, M., Tempest, B. and Palmer, D. L. (1976). Bacteriologic diagnosis of acute pneumonia. *J. Am. Med. Ass.* **235**, 158–163.

Dresdale, A. R., Drusin, R. E., Lamb, J., Smith, C. R., Reemtsma, K. and Rose, E. A. (1985). Reduced infection in cardiac transplant recipients. *Circulation* **72**, Suppl. II, 237–240.

Drew, W. L., Finley, T. N. and Golde, D. W. (1977). Diagnostic lavage and occult pulmonary hemorrhage in thrombocytopenic immunocompromised patients. *Am. Rev. Resp. Dis.* **116**, 215–221.

Drew, W. L., Finley, T. N., Mintz, L. and Klein, Z. (1974). Diagnosis of PCP by bronchoalveolar lavage. *J. Am. Med. Ass.*, **230**, 713–715.

Dummer, J. S., Bahnson, H. T., Griffith, B. P., Hardesty, R. L., Thompson, M. E. and Ho, M. (1984). Infections in patients on cyclosporine and prednisone following cardiac transplantation. *Cyclosporine — Biological Activity and Clinical Applications* (B. D. Kahan, Ed.), pp. 563–565. Grune and Stratton, Orlando, Florida.

Dummer, J. S., Hardy, A., Poorsattar, A. and Ho, M. (1983). Early infections in kidney, heart, and liver transplant recipients on cyclosporine. *Transplantation* **36**, 259–267.

Edelstein, P. H. (1985). Legionella. In *Manual of Clinical Microbiology*, 4th edn (E. H. Lennette, A. Balows, W. J. Hausler and H. J. Shadomy, Eds), pp. 373–381. American Society for Microbiology, Washington DC.

Egbert, P. R., Pollard, R. B., Gallagher, J. G. and Merigan, T. C. (1980). Cytomegalovirus retinitis in immunosuppressed hosts. II. Ocular manifestations. *Ann. Intern. Med.* **93**, 664–670.

Elliott, W. C., Houghton, D. C., Bryant, R. E., Wicklund, R., Barry, J. M. and Bennett, W. M. (1980). *Herpes simplex* type I hepatitis in renal transplantation. *Arch. Intern. Med.*, **140**, 1656–1660.

Ellis, C. A. and Spivack, M. L. (1967). The significance of candidemia. *Ann. Intern. Med.* **67**(3), 511–522.

England, A. C., Fraser, D. W., Plikaytis, B. D., Tsai, T. F., Storch, G. and Broome, C. V. (1981). Sporadic legionellosis in the United States: the first thousand cases. *Ann. Intern. Med.* **94**, 164–170.

Fahey, J. L., Sarna, G., Gale, R. P. and Seeger, R. (1987). Immune interventions in disease. *Ann. Intern. Med.* **106**, 257–274.

Felsenstein, D., D'Amico, D. J., Hirsch, M. S., Neumeyer, D. A., Cederberg, D. M., deMiranda, P. and Schooley, R. T. (1985). Treatment of cytomegalovirus retinitis with 9-(2-hydroxy-1(hydroxymethyl)ethoxymethyl)guanine. *Ann. Intern. Med.* **103**, 377–380.

Firor, W. B. (1967). Infection following open-heart surgery, with special reference to the role of prophylactic antibiotics. *J. Thorac. Cardiovasc. Surg.* **53**(3), 371–378.

Fisher, B. D., Armstrong, D., Yu, B. and Gold, J. W. M. (1981). Invasive aspergillosis. Progress in early diagnosis and treatment. *Am. J. Med.* **71**, 571–577.

Fong, I. W., Baker, C. B. and McKee, D. C. (1979). The value of prophylactic antibiotics in aorta-coronary bypass operations. *J. Thorac. Cardiovasc. Surg.* **78**, 908–913.

Fossieck, B. E., Parker, R. H., Cohen, M. H. and Kane, R. C. (1977). Fiberoptic bronchoscopy and culture of bacteria from the lower respiratory tract. *Chest* **72**, 5–9.

Frazier, O. H., Cooley, D. A., Painvin, G. A., Chandler, L. B. and Okereke, O. U. J. (1985). Cardiac transplantation at the Texas Heart Institute: comparative analysis of two groups of patients (1968–1969 and 1982–1983). *Ann. Thorac. Surg.* **39**(4), 303–307.

Frizzera, G., Hanto, D. W., Gajl-Peczalska, J., Rosai, J., McKenna, R. W., Sibley, R. K., Holahan, K. P. and Lindquist, L. L. (1981). Polymorphic diffuse B-cell hyperplasias and lymphomas in renal transplant recipients. *Cancer Res.* **41**, 4262–4279.

Fuller, J., Levinson, M. M., Kline, J. R. and Copeland, J. (1985). Legionnaires' disease after heart transplantation. *Ann. Thorac. Surg.* **39**, 308–311.

Gabriel, R., Selwyn, S., Brown, D., Crossland, J. M., Loughridge, L. W., Morgan, M. N., Prosser, D. I. and Snow, M. (1976). Virus infections and acute renal transplant rejection. *Nephron* **16**, 282–286.

Gallagher, J. G. and Merigan, T. C. (1979). Prolonged herpes-zoster infection associated with immunosuppressive therapy. *Ann. Intern. Med.* **91**, 842–846.

Gantz, N. M., Myerowitz, R. L., Medeiros, A. A., Carrera, G. F., Wilson, R. E. and O'Brien, T. F. (1975). Listeriosis in immunosuppressed patients: a cluster of eight cases. *Am. J. Med.* **58**, 637–643.

Gold, D. and Corey, L. (1987). Acyclovir prophylaxis for herpes simplex virus infection. *Antimicrob. Agents. Chemother.* **31**(3), 361–367.

Greenman, R., Goodall, P. T. and King, D. (1975). Lung biopsy in immunocompromised hosts. *Am. J. Med.* **59**, 488–496.

Griffin, G. K., Pope, T. L. and Armstrong, P. (1983). Pittsburgh pneumonia agent in a cadaveric renal transplant recipient. *Clin. Nephrol.* **20**, 263–266.

Griffith, B. P., Hardesty, R. L. and Bahnson, H. T. (1984). Powerful but limited immunosuppression for cardiac transplantation with cyclosporine and low dose steroid. *J. Thorac. Cardiovasc. Surg.* **87**, 35–42.

Griffith, B. P., Hardesty, R. L., Deeb, G. M., Starzl, T. E. and Bahnson, H. T. (1982). Cardiac transplantation with cyclosporine A and prednisone. *Ann. Surg.* **196**(3), 324–329.

Gurwith, M. J., Stinson, E. B. and Remington, J. S. (1971). Aspergillus infection complicating cardiac transplantation. *Arch. Intern. Med.* **128**, 541–545.

Hackman, R. C., Myerson, D., Meyers, J. D., Shulman, H. M., Sale, G. E., Goldstein, L. C., Rastetter, M., Flournoy, N. and Thomas, E. D. (1985). Rapid diagnosis of cytomegalovirus pneumonia by tissue immunofluorescence with a murine monoclonal antibody. *J. Infect. Dis.* **151**, 325–329.

Hakim, M., Wreghitt, T. G., English, T. A. H., Stovin, P. G. I., Cory-Pearce, R. and Wallwork, J. (1985). Significance of donor-transmitted disease in cardiac transplantation. *Heart Transplant.* **4**(3), 302–306.

Halbrook, H., Stevens, L., Beckman, D., Hormuth, D., Fehrenbacher, J. and Herod, G. (1985). Heart transplantation at a private institution: a two year experience. *Heart Transplant.* **4**(3), 353–356.

Haley, C. E., Cohen, M. L., Halter, J. and Meyer, R. D. (1979). Nosocomial Legionnaires' disease: a continuing common source epidemic at Wadsworth Medical Center. *Ann. Intern. Med.* **90**, 583–586.

Hanto, D. W., Frizzera, G., Gajl-Peczalska, J., Purtilo, D. T., Klein, G., Simmons, R. L. and Najarian, J. S. (1981b). The Epstein-Barr virus (EBV) in the pathogenesis of post-transplant lymphoma. *Transplant. Proc.* **13**(1), 756–760.

Hanto, D. W., Frizzera, G., Gajl-Peczalska, K. J., Sakamoto, K., Purtilo, D. T., Balfour, H. H., Simmons, R. L. and Najarian, J. S. (1982). Epstein-Barr virus-induced B-cell lymphoma after renal transplantation. *N. Engl. J. Med.* **306**(15), 913–918.

Hanto, D. W., Sakamoto, K., Purtilo, D. T., Simmons, R. L. and Najarian, J. S. (1981a). The Epstein-Barr virus in the pathogenesis of post-transplant lymphoproliferative disorders. *Surgery* **90** (2), 204–213.

Haverkos, H. W., Dowling, J. N., Pasculle, A. W., Myerowitz, R. L., Lerberg, D. B. and Hakala, T. R. (1983). Diagnosis of pneumonitis in immunocompromised patients by open lung biopsy. *Cancer* **52**, 1093–1097.

Hirsch, M. S., Schooley, R. T., Cosimi, A. B., Russell, P. S., Delmonico, F. L.,

Tolkoff-Rubin, N. E., Herrin, J. T., Cantell, K., Farrell, M. L., Rota, T. R. and Rubin, R. H. (1983). Effects of interferon-alpha on cytomegalovirus reactivation syndromes in renal-transplant recipients. *New Engl. J. Med.* **308**, 1489–1493.

Ho, M. (1977). Virus infections after transplantation in man: brief review. *Arch. Virol.* **55**, 1.

Ho, M. (1982). Epidemiology of cytomegalovirus infection in man. In *Cytomegalovirus, Biology and Infection: Current Topics in Infectious Disease* (W. B. Greenough III and T. C. Merigan, Eds), pp. 79–104. Plenum Press, New York.

Hoffin, J. M., Potasman, I., Baldwin, J. C., Oyer, P. E., Stinson, E. B. and Remington, J. S. (1987). Infectious complications in heart transplant recipients receiving cyclosporine and corticosteroids. *Ann. Intern. Med.* **106**, 209–216.

Howard, R. J. (1980). Host defense against infection. Part II. *Curr. Prob. Surg.* **17**, 319–344.

Hughes, W. T. (1984). *Pneumocystis carinii* pneumonitis. *Chest* **85**, 810–813.

Hughes, W. T., Kuhn, R. N., Chaudhary, S., Feldman, S., Verzosa, M., Aur, R. J. A., Pratt, C. and George, S. L. (1977). Successful chemoprophylaxis for *Pneumocystis carinii* pneumonitis. *New Engl. J. Med.* **297**, 1419–1426.

Hughes, W. T., Price, R. A., Kim, H. K., Coburn, T. P., Grigsby, D. and Feldman, S. (1973). *Pneumocystis carinii* pneumonitis in children with malignancies. *J. Pediat.* **82**, 404–415.

Hunt, S. A. (1983). Complications of heart transplantation. *Heart Transplant.* **3**(1), 70–74.

Hunt, S. A. and Stinson, E. B. (1981). Cardiac transplantation. *Ann. Rev. Med.* **32**, 213–220.

Icenogle, T. B., Peterson, E., Ray, G., Mimrick, L. and Copeland, J. G. (1986). DHPG effectively treats cytomegalovirus infection in heart and heart–lung transplant patients: a preliminary report. *J. Heart Transplant.* **5**, 371.

Johanson, W. G., Pierce, A. K. and Sanford, J. P. (1969). Changing pharyngeal bacterial flora of hospitalized patients: emergence of Gram-negative bacilli. *New Engl. J. Med.* **281**(21), 1137–1140.

Johnston, M. R., Pizzo, P. A. and Fauci, A. S. (1982). Thoracic mass lesions in immuno-incompetent patients. *Chest* **82**, 164–167.

Kay, H. R., Goodman, L. R., Teplick, S. K. and Mundth, E. D. (1983). Use of computed tomography to access mediastinal complications after median sternotomy. *Ann. Thorac. Surg.* **36**, 706–714.

Kelley, J., Landis, J. N., Davis, G. S., Trainer, T. D., Jakab, G. J. and Green, G. M. (1978). Diagnosis of pneumonia due to pneumocystis by subsegmental pulmonary lavage via the fiberoptic bronchoscope. *Chest* **74**, 24–28.

Krick, J. A., Stinson, E. B. and Remington, J. S. (1975). Nocardia infection in heart transplant patients. *Ann. Intern. Med.* **82**, 18–26.

Lafferty, K. J., Borel, J. F. and Hodgkin, P. (1984). Cyclosporine-A (CsA): models for the mechanism of action. *Cyclosporine: Biological Activity and Clinical Applications* (B. D. Kahan, Ed.), pp. 26–31. Grune and Stratton, Orlando, Florida.

Lang, D. J., Ebert, P. A., Rodgers, B. M., Boggess, H. P. and Rixse, R. S. (1977). Reduction of post-perfusion cytomegalovirus-infections following the use of leukocyte depleted blood. *Transfusion* **17**, 391–395.

Langhoff, E. and Madsen, S. (1983). Rapid metabolism of cyclosporine and prednisone in kidney transplant patients receiving tuberculostatic treatment. *Lancet* **2**, 1031.

Lauver, G. L., Hasan, F. M., Morgan, R. B. and Campbell, S. C. (1979). The usefulness of fiberoptic bronchoscopy in evaluating new pulmonary lesions in the compromised host. *Am. J. Med.* **66**, 580–585.

Lehrer, R. I., Howard, D. H., Sypherd, P. S., Edwards, J. E., Segal, G. P. and Winston, D. J. (1980). Mucormycosis. *Ann. Intern. Med.* **93**(1), 93–108.

Leight, G. S. and Michaelis, L. L. (1978). Open lung biopsy for the diagnosis of acute, diffuse pulmonary infiltrates in the immunosuppressed patient. *Chest* **73**, 477–482.

Lloveras, J., Peterson, P. K., Simmons, R. L. and Najarian, J. S. (1982). Mycobacterial infections in renal transplant recipients: seven cases and a review of the literature. *Arch. Intern. Med.* **142**, 888–892.

Lopez, C., Simmons, R. L., Mauer, S. M., Najarian, J. S., Good, R. A. and Gentry, S. (1974). Association of renal allograft rejection with virus infections. *Am. J. Med.* **56**, 280–289.

Luft, B. J., Naot, Y., Araujo, F. G., Stinson, E. B. and Remington, J. S. (1983). Primary and reactivated toxoplasma infection in patients with cardiac transplant. *Ann. Intern. Med.* **99**, 27–31.

Majure, J. A., Albin, R. E., O'Donnell, R. S. and Arganese, T. J. (1986). Reconstruction of the infected median sternotomy wound. *Ann. Thorac. Surg.* **42**, 9–12.

Mammana, R. B., Petersen, E. A., Fuller, J. K., Siroky, K. and Copeland, J. G. (1983). Pulmonary infections in cardiac transplant patients: modes of diagnosis, complications, and effectiveness of therapy. *Ann. Thorac. Surg.* **36**, 700–705.

Marker, S. C., Howard, R. J., Simmons, R. L., Kalis, J. M., Connelly, D. P., Najarian, J. S. and Balfour, H. H. (1981). Cytomegalovirus infection: a quantitative prospective study of 320 consecutive renal transplants. *Surgery* **89**, 660–671.

Marker, S. C., Simmons, R. L. and Balfour, H. H. (1981). CMV vaccine in renal allograft recipients. *Transplant Proc.* **13**, 117–119.

Marshall, W., Foster, R. S. and Winn, W. (1981). Legionnaires' disease in renal transplant patients. *Am. J. Surg.* **141**, 423–429.

Martell, R., Heinrichs, D., Stiller, C. R., Jenner, M., Keown, P. A. and Dupre, J. (1986). The effects of erythromycin in patients treated with cyclosporine. *Ann. Intern. Med.* **104**, 660–661.

Mason, J. W., Stinson, E. B., Hunt, S. A., Schroeder, J. S. and Rider, A. K. (1976). Infections after cardiac transplantation: relation to rejection therapy. *Ann. Intern. Med.* **85**, 69–72.

Matthay, R. A. and Greene, W. H. (1980). Pulmonary infections in the immunocompromised patient. *Med. Clin. N. Am.* **64**(3), 529–551.

Matthay, R. A. and Moritz, E. D. (1981). Invasive procedures for diagnosing pulmonary infection: a critical review. *Clin. Chest Med.* **2**(1), 3–18.

McElvein, R. B. (1985). Open lung biopsy versus empirical antibiotic therapy in the immunosuppressed patient. *Ann. Thorac. Surg.* **40**(5), 419–420.

McLeod, R., Berry, P. F., Marshall, W. H., Hunt, S. A., Ryning, F. W. and Remington, J. S. (1979). Toxoplasmosis presenting as brain abscesses. *Am. J. Med.* **67**, 711–714.

McLoughlin, G. A., Wu, A. V., Saporoschetz, I., Nimberg, R. and Mannick, J. A. (1979). Correlation between anergy and a circulating immunosuppressive factor following major surgical trauma. *Ann. Surg.* **190**(3), 297–304.

Meden, G., Hall, G. S. and Ahmad, M. (1985). Retrieval of microbiological specimens through the fiberoptic bronchoscope. *Cleve. Clin. Q.* **52**, 495–502.

Meyer, R. (1983). Legionella infections: a review of five years of research. *Rev. Infect. Dis.* **5**(2), 258–278.

Meyers, J. D., Leszczynski, J., Zaia, J. A., Flournoy, N., Newton, B., Snydman, D. R., Wright, G. G., Levin, M. J. and Thomas, E. D. (1983). Prevention of CMV infection by cytomegalovirus immune globulin after marrow transplantation. *Ann. Intern. Med.* **98**, 442–446.

Meyerson, D., Hackman, R. C. and Meyers, J. D. (1984). The diagnosis of cytomegalovirus pneumonia by in situ hybridization. *J. Infect. Dis.* **150**, 272–277.

Michaelis, L. L., Leight, G. S., Powell, R. D. and DeVita, V. T. (1976). *Pneumocystis pneumonia*: the importance of early open lung biopsy. *Ann. Surg.* **183**(3), 301–306.

Muder, R. R., Yu, V. L. and Woo, A. H. (1986). Mode of transmission of *Legionella pneumophila. Arch. Intern. Med.* **146**, 1607–1612.

Muder, R. R., Yu, V. L. and Zuravleff, J. J. (1983). Pneumonia due to Pittsburgh pneumonia agents: new clinical perspective with a review of the literature. *Medicine* **62**, 120–128.

Nagington, J. and Martin, A. L. (1983). Toxoplasmosis and heart transplantation. *Lancet* **2**, 679.

Neff, T. A. (1972). Percutaneous trephine biopsy of the lung. *Chest* **61**, 18–23.

Nieman, R. E. and Lorber, B. (1980). Listeriosis in adults: a changing pattern. Report of eight cases and review of the literature. *Rev. Infect. Dis.* **2**(2), 207–227.

Novitzky, D. and Cooper, D. K. C. (1984). The surgical techniques of orthotopic and heterotopic heart transplantation. In *Heart Transplantation* (D. K. C. Cooper and R. P. Lanza, Eds), pp. 103–127. MTP Press, Lancaster.

Nyberg, G., Gabel, H., Althoff, P., Bjork, S., Herlitz, H. and Brynger, H. (1984). Adverse effect of trimethoprim on kidney function in renal transplant patients. *Lancet* **2**, 394–395.

Ognibene, F. P., Shelhamer, J., Gill, V., Macher, A. M., Loew, D., Parker, M. M., Gelmann, E., Fauci, A. S., Parrillo, J. E. and Masur, H. (1984). The diagnosis of PCP in patients with AIDS using subsegmental bronchoalveolar lavage. *Am. Rev. Resp. Dis.* **129**, 929–932.

Oill, P. A., Fiala, M., Schofferman, J., Byfield, P. A. and Guze, L. B. (1977). Cytomegalovirus mononucleosis in a healthy adult. *Am. J. Med.* **62**, 413–417.

Onorato, I. M., Morens, D. M., Martone, W. J. and Stansfield, S. K. (1985). Epidemiology of cytomegaloviral infections: recommendations for prevention and control. *Rev. Infect. Dis.* **7**(4), 479–497.

Oyer, P. E., Stinson, E. B., Jamieson, S. W., Hunt, S. A., Perlroth, M., Billingham, M. and Shumway, N. E. (1984). Cyclosporine in cardiac transplantation: a $2\frac{1}{2}$ year follow-up. In *Cyclosporine: Biological Activity and Clinical Applications* (B. D. Kahan, Ed.), pp. 330–336. Grune and Stratton, Orlando, Florida.

Oyer, P. E., Stinson, E. B., Jamieson, S. W., Hunt, S., Reitz, B. A., Bieber, C. P., Schroeder, J. S., Billingham, M. and Shumway, N. E. (1982). One year experience with cyclosporine A in clinical heart transplantation. *Heart Transplant.* **1**(4), 285–290.

Painvin, G. A., Okereke, O. U. J., Frazier, O. H., Kahan, B. D., VanBuren, C. T. and Cooley, D. A. (1985). Cardiac transplantation: current results of cyclosporine-treated patients at the Texas Heart Institute. *Transplant. Proc.*, **17**(1), 223–224.

Pairolero, P. C., and Arnold, P. G. (1984). Management of recalcitrant median sternotomy wounds. *J. Thorac. Cardiovasc. Surg.* **88**, 357–364.

Palmer, D. L., Davidson, M. and Lusk, R. (1974). Diagnostic and therapeutic considerations in *Nocardia asteroides* infections. *Medicine* **53**, 391–399.

Palmer, D. L., Davidson, M. and Lusk, R. (1980). Needle aspiration of the lung in complex pneumonias. *Chest* **78**, 16–21.

Park, S. K., Brody, J. I., Wallace, H. A. A. and Blakemore, W. S. (1971). Immunosuppressive effect of surgery. *Lancet* **1**, 53–55.

Pearl, S. N., Weiner, M. A. and Dibbell, D. G. (1982). Sternal infection after cardiac transplantation. Successful salvage utilizing a variety of techniques. *J. Thorac. Cardiovasc. Surg.* **83**, 632–634.

Penn, I. (1978). Malignancies associated with immunosuppressive or cytotoxic therapy. *Surgery* **83**(5), 492–502.

Pennington, D. G., Sarafian, J. and Swartz, M. (1985). Heart transplantation in children. *Heart Transplant.* **4**(4), 441–445.

Pennock, J. L., Oyer, P. E., Reitz, B. A., Jamieson, S. W., Bieber, C. P., Wallwork, J., Stinson, E. B. and Shumway, N. E. (1982). Cardiac transplantation in perspective for the future. Survival, complications, rehabilitation and cost. *J. Thorac. Cardiovasc. Surg.* **83**, 168–177.

Peterson, P. K., Balfour, H. H., Fryd, D. S., Ferguson, R. M. and Simmons R. L. (1981). Fever in renal transplant recipients: causes, prognostic significance and changing patterns at the University of Minnesota Hospital. *Am. J. Med.* **71**, 345–351.

Peterson, P. K., Balfour, H. H., Marker, S. C., Fryd, D. S., Howard, R. J. and Simmons, R. L. (1980). Cytomegalovirus disease in renal allograft recipients: a prospective study of the clinical features, risk factors, and impact on renal transplantation. *Medicine* **59**, 283–300.

Peterson, P. K., Ferguson, R., Fryd, D. S., Balfour, H. H., Rynasiewicz, J. and Simmons, R. L. (1982). Infectious diseases in hospitalized renal transplant recipients. A prospective study of a complex and evolving problem. *Medicine* **61**, 360–372.

Pierce, A. K. and Sanford, J. P. (1974). Aerobic Gram-negative bacillary pneumonias. *Am. Rev. Resp. Dis.* **110**, 647–658.

Pifer, L. L., Hughes, W. T., Stagno, S. and Woods, D. (1978). *Pneumocystis carinii* infection: evidence for high prevalence in normal and immunosuppressed children. *Pediatrics* **61**(1), 35–41.

Plotkin, S. A., Friedman, H. M., Fleisher, G. R., Dafoe, D. C., Grossman, R. A., Smiley, M. L., Starr, S. E., Wlodaver, C., Friedman, A. D. and Barker, C. F. (1984). Towne-vaccine-induced prevention of cytomegalovirus disease after renal transplantation. *Lancet* **2**, 528–530.

Pollard, R. B., Arvin, A. M., Gamberg, P., Rand, K. H., Gallagher, J. G. and Merigan, T. C. (1982). Specific cell-mediated immunity and infections with herpes viruses in cardiac transplant recipients. *Am. J. Med.* **73**, 679–687.

Pollard, R. B., Egbert, P. R., Gallagher, J. G. and Merigan, T. C. (1980). Cytomegalovirus retinitis in immunosuppressed hosts. *Ann. Intern. Med.* **93**, 655–664.

Pollock, H. M., Hawkins, E. L., Bonner, J. R., Sparkman, T. and Bass, J. B. (1983). Diagnosis of bacterial pulmonary infections with quantitative protected catheter cultures obtained during bronchoscopy. *J. Clin. Microbiol.* **17**, 255–259.

Potter, D., Pass, H. I., Brower, S., Macher, A., Browne, M., Thaler, M., Cotton, D., Hathorn, J., Wesley, R., Longo, D., Pizzo, P. and Roth, J. A. (1985). Prospective randomized study of open lung biopsy versus empirical antibiotic therapy for acute pneumonitis in non-neutropenic cancer patients. *Ann. Thorac. Surg.* **40**(5), 422–428.

Ptachcinski, R. J., Carpenter, B. J., Burckart, G. J., Venkataramanan, R. and Rosenthal, J. T. (1985). Effect of erythromycin on cyclosporine levels. *New Engl. J. Med.* **313**, 1416–1417.

Ramsey, P. G., Rubin, R. H., Tolkoff-Rubin, N. E., Cosimi, A. B., Russill, P. S. and Greene, R. (1980). The renal transplant patient with fever and pulmonary infiltrates: etiology, clinical manifestations, and management. *Medicine* **59**(3), 206–222.

Rand, K. H., Pollard, R. B. and Merigan, T. C. (1978). Increased pulmonary superinfections in cardiac transplant patients undergoing primary cytomegalovirus infection. *N. Engl. J. Med.* **298**, 951–953.

Rand, K. H., Rasmussen, L. E., Pollard, R. B., Arvin, A. and Merigan, T. C. (1976). Cellular immunity and herpes virus infections in cardiac transplant patients. *New Engl. J. Med.* **296**(24), 1371–1377.

Reece, I. J., Painvin, G. A., Zeluff, B., Chandler, L. B., Okereke, O. U. J., Gentry, L. O., Cooley, D. A. and Frazier, O. H. (1984). Infection in cyclosporine-immunosuppressed cardiac allograft recipients. *Heart Transplant.* **3**(3), 239–242.

Rinaldi, M. G. (1983). Invasive aspergillosis. *Rev. Infect. Dis.* **5**, 1061.

Rinehart, J. J., Sagone, A. L., Balcerzak, S. P., Ackerman, G. A. and LoBuglio, A. F. (1975). Effects of corticosteroid therapy on human monocyte function. *N. Engl. J. Med.* **292**(5), 236–241.

Robin, E. D. and Thomas, E. D. (1954). Some relations between pulmonary edema and pulmonary inflammation (pneumonia). *Arch. Intern. Med.* **93**, 713–724.

Robinson, J. E., Brown, N., Andiman, W., Halliday, K., Franke, U., Robert, M. F., Andersson-Anvert, M., Horstmann, D. and Miller, G. (1980). Diffuse polyclonal B-cell lymphoma during primary infection with Epstein-Barr virus. *New Engl. J. Med.*, **302**(33), 1293–1297.

Rose, A. G., Uys, C. J., Novitzky, D., Cooper, D. K. C. and Barnard, C. N. (1983). Toxoplasmosis of donor and recipient hearts after heterotopic cardiac transplantation. *Arch. Path. Lab. Med.* **107**, 368–373.

Roth, J. A., Golub, S. H., Cukingnan, R. A., Brazier, J. and Morton, D. L. (1981). Cell-mediated immunity is depressed following cardiopulmonary bypass. *Ann. Thorac. Surg.* **31**(4), 350–356.

Rubin, R. H. (1981). Infection in the renal transplant patient. In *Clinical Approach to*

Infection in the Compromised Host (R. H. Rubin and L. S. Young, Eds), pp. 553–605. Plenum, New York.

Rubin, R. H. and Cosimi, A. B. (1982). Infection in the immunocompromised host. In *Surgical Infectious Diseases* (R. L. Simmons and R. J. Howard, Eds), pp. 1101–1123. Appleton-Century-Crofts, New York.

Ruskin, J. and Remington, J. S. (1976). Toxoplasmosis in the compromised host. *Ann. Intern. Med.* **84**, 193–199.

Ryning, F. W., McLeod, R., Maddox, J. C., Hunt, S. and Remington, J. S. (1979). Probable transmission of *Toxoplasma gondii* by organ transplantation. *Ann. Intern. Med.* **90**, 47–49.

Satterfield, J. R. and McLaughlin, J. S. (1979). Open lung biopsy in diagnosing pulmonary infiltrates in immunosuppressed patients. *Ann. Thorac. Surg.* **28**(4), 359–362.

Shaffer, P. J., Kobayashi, G. S. and Medoff, G. (1979). Demonstration of antigenemia in patients with invasive aspergillosis by solid phase (protein A-rich *Staphylococcus aureus*) radioimmunoassay. *Am. J. Med.* **67**, 627–630.

Shuster, E. A., Beneke, J. S., Tegtmeier, G. E., Pearson, G. R., Gleaves, C. A., Wold, A. D. and Smith, T. F. (1985). Monoclonal antibody for rapid laboratory detection of CMV infection: characterization and diagnostic application. *Mayo Clin. Proc.* **60**, 577–585.

Simmons, R. L., Weil, R., Tallent, M. B., Kjellstrand, C. M. and Najarian, J. S. (1970). Do mild infections trigger the rejection of renal allografts? *Transplant. Proc.* **2**(3), 419–423.

Simpson, G. L., Stinson, E. B., Egger, M. J. and Remington, J. S. (1981). Nocardial infections in the immunocompromised host: a detailed study in a defined population. *Rev. Infect. Dis.* **3**(3), 492–507.

Singer, C., Armstrong, D., Rosen, P. P. and Schottenfield, D. (1975). *Pneumocystis carinii* pneumonia: a cluster of 11 cases. *Ann. Intern. Med.* **82**(6), 772–777.

Smego, R. A., Moeller, M. B. and Gallis, H. A. (1983). Trimethoprim-sulfamethoxazole therapy for nocardia infections. *Arch. Intern. Med.* **143**, 711–718.

Spector, S. A., Rua, J. A., Spector, D. H. and McMillan, R. (1984). Rapid detection of cytomegalovirus in clinical specimens by DNA–DNA Hy. *J. Infect. Dis.* **150**, 121–126.

Spencer, C. D. and Beaty, H. N. (1972). Complications of transtracheal aspiration. *New Engl. J. Med.* **286**, 304–306.

Springmeyer, S. C., Hackman, R. C., Holle, R., Greenberg, G. M., Weems, C. E., Myerson, D., Meyers, J. D. and Thomas, E. D. (1986). Use of bronchoalveolar lavage to diagnose acute diffuse pneumonia in the immunocompromised host. *J. Infect. Dis.* **154,** 604–610.

Stamm, A. M., Dismukes, W. E., Simmons, B. P., Cobbs, G. C., Elliott, A., Budrich, P. and Harmon, J. (1982). Listerosis in renal transplant recipients: report of an outbreak and review of 102 cases. *Rev. Infect. Dis.*, **4**, 665–682.

Stevens, D. A. (1983). Miconazole in the treatment of coccidiomycosis. *Drugs* **26**, 347.

Stevens, D. A. (1985). *Coccidioides immitis*. In *Principles and Practice of Infectious Disease*, 2nd edn (G. L. Mandell, R. G. Douglas and J. E. Bennett, Eds), pp. 1485–1493. Wiley, New York.

Stevens, D. A., Pier, A. C., Beaman, B. L., Morozumi, P. A., Lovett, I. S. and Houang, E. T. (1981). Laboratory evaluation of an outbreak of nocardiosis in immunocompromised hosts. *Am. J. Med.* **71**, 928–934.

Stinson, E. B., Bieber, C. P., Griepp, R. B., Clark, D. A., Shumway, N. E. and Remington, J. S. (1971). Infectious complications after cardiac transplantation in man. *Ann. Intern. Med.* **74**(1), 22–36.

Storch, G. A., Sagel, S. S. and Baine, W. B. (1981). The chest roentgenogram in sporadic cases of Legionnaires' disease. *J. Am. Med. Ass.* **245**, 587–590.

Stover, D. E., Zaman, M. B., Hajdu, S. I., Lange, M., Gold, J. and Armstrong, D. (1984). Bronchoalveolar lavage in the diagnosis of diffuse pulmonary infiltrates in the immunosuppressed host. *Ann. Intern. Med.* **101**, 1–7.

Strauch, B., Andrews, L. L., Siegel, N. and Miller, G. (1974). Oropharyngeal excretion of Epstein-Barr virus by renal transplant recipients and other patients treated with immunosuppressive drugs. *Lancet* **1**, 234–237.

Thomas, F., Thomas, J., Mendez, G., Lower, R. and Lee, H. M. (1977). Differential effects of immunosuppressive drugs on human T, B, and K lymphocytes. *Transplantation* **24**(6), 435–441.

Thompson, J. F., Chalmers, D. H. K., Hunnisett, A. G. W., Wood, R. F. M. and Morris, P. J. (1983). Nephrotoxicity of trimethoprim and cotrimoxazole in renal allograft recipients treated with cyclosporine. *Transplantation* **36**, 204–206.

Thurer, R. J., Bognolo, D., Vargas, A., Isch, J. H. and Kaiser, G. A. (1974). The management of mediastinal infection following cardiac surgery: an experience utilising continuous irrigation with povidone-iodine. *J. Thorac. Cardiovasc. Surg.* **68**(6), 962–968.

Tilney, N. L., Kohler, T. R. and Strom, T. B. (1982). Cerebromeningitis in immunosuppressed recipients of renal allografts. *Ann. Surg.* **195**, 104.

Tilney, N. L., Strom, T. B., Vineyard, G. C. and Merril, J. P. (1978). Factors contributing to the declining mortality rate in renal transplantation. *New Engl. J. Med.* **299**(24), 1321–1325.

Tobin, J. O. H., Beare, J., Dunnill, M. S., Fisher-Hoch, S., French, M., Mitchell, R. G., Morris, P. J. and Muers, M. F. (1980). Legionnaires' disease in a transplant unit: isolation of the causative agent from shower baths. *Lancet* **ii**, 118–121.

Trento, A., Dummer, G. S., Hardesty, R. L., Bahnson, H. T. and Griffith, B. P. (1984). Mediastinitis following heart transplantation: incidence, treatment, and results. *Heart Transplant.* **3**(4), 336–340.

Uys, C. J., Rose, A. G. and Barnard, C. N. (1979). The pathology of human cardiac transplantation: an assessment after 11 years experience at Groote Schuur Hospital. *S. Afr. Med. J.* **56**, 887–896.

Weiner, M. H., Talbot, G. H., Gerson, S. L., Filice, G. and Cassileth, P. A. (1983). Antigen detection in the diagnosis of invasive aspergillosis. *Ann. Intern. Med.* **99**, 777–782.

Wheat, L. J., Smith, E. J., Sathapatayavongs, B., Batteiger, B., Filo, R. S., Leapman, S. B. and French, M. V. (1983). Histoplasmosis in renal allograft recipients: two large urban outbreaks. *Arch. Intern. Med.* **143**, 703–707.

Wiener, S. L., Wiener, R., Urivetzky, M., Shafer, S., Isenberg, H. D., Janov, C. and Meilman, E. (1975). The mechanism of action of a single dose of methylprednisolone on acute inflammation *in vivo*. *J. Clin. Invest.* **56**, 679–689.

Williams, D. M., Krick, J. A. and Remington, J. S. (1976). Pulmonary infection in the compromised host. *Am. Rev. Resp. Dis.* **114**, 359–394.

Wimberley, N. W., Bass, J. B., Boyd, B. W., Kirkpatrick, M. B., Serio, R. A. and Pollock, H. M. (1982). Use of a bronchoscopic protected catheter brush for the diagnosis of pulmonary infections. *Chest* **81**, 556–562.

Wimberley, N. W., Faling, L. J. and Bartlett, J. G. (1979). A fiberoptic bronchoscopy technique to obtain uncontaminated lower airway secretions for bacterial culture. *Am. Rev. Resp. Dis.* **119**, 337–343.

Winston, D. J., Gale, R. P., Mayer, D. V. and Young, L. S. (1979). Infectious complications of human bone marrow transplantation. *Medicine* **58**, 1.

Young, J. N., Yazbeck, J., Esposito, G., Mankad, B., Townsend, E. and Yacoub, M. (1985). The influence of acute preoperative pulmonary infarction on the results of cardiac transplantation. *Heart Transplant.* **4**(6), 600.

Yu, D. T. Y., Clements, P. J., Paulus, H. E., Peter, J. B., Levy, J. and Barnett, E. V. (1974). Human lymphocyte subpopulations: effect of corticosteroids. *J. Clin. Invest.* **53**, 565–571.

Zavala, D. C. and Bedell, G. N. (1972). Percutaneous lung biopsy with a cutting needle: an analysis of 40 cases and comparison with other biopsy techniques. *Am. Rev. Resp. Dis.* **106**, 186–193.

Zeitler, R., Helms, C., Hall, N., Goeken, N., Anderson, G. and Corry, R. (1984). Legionnaires' disease in renal transplant recipients. In *Legionnella, Washington DC: Proceedings of the 2nd International Symposium on Legionella* (C. Thornsberry, Ed.), pp. 234–235, Washington DC, American Society for Microbiology.

Bernhard M. Kemkes

14

Non-invasive Assessment Methods to Detect Rejection Following Cardiac Transplantation

INTRODUCTION

Despite increased survival in transplanted patients and improvements in immunosuppressive therapy, infection and rejection still remain the main causes of death after heart transplantation (Kaye, 1987).

Acute cardiac rejection is characterized histologically by a diffuse infiltration of mononuclear cells and oedema of the myocardium, in late stages accompanied by haemorrhage and myocyte necrosis. It is essential to detect acute cardiac rejection before the onset of focal necrosis, since early treatment may result in full reversal of the inflammatory changes. Therefore, acute rejection of a cardiac allograft requires prompt and accurate diagnosis before the occurrence of clinically detectable deterioration of left ventricular function.

Endomyocardial biopsy has been considered to be the most reliable means of diagnosing transplant rejection, especially in view of a very low complication rate. However, this method is invasive and inconvenient and cannot be performed daily. The subsequent pathological diagnosis involves the preparation time of the biopsy material, which could delay institution of therapy for 12–24 h. Non-invasive techniques to supplement endomyocardial biopsy in the diagnosis of rejection are therefore desirable.

The methods of early diagnosis of allograft rejections depend, to a large extent, on the effects of immunosuppressive therapy. Following the introduction of cyclosporin A as an immunosuppressive agent, many of the previously valuable non-invasive parameters of cardiac rejection became unreliable. Although rejection episodes occur with similar frequency in cyclosporin-treated patients, whether in combination with azathioprine or low-dose corticoids as in conventionally immunosuppressed patients, their degree of severity is not as great as in the latter. Consequently, clinical parameters lose their validity.

CYTO-IMMUNOLOGICAL MONITORING OF THE PERIPHERAL BLOOD

The change in the recipient's immune system's tolerance to an allograft is reflected by changes in the peripheral blood lymphocyte population. The onset of rejection is manifested by signs of peripheral blood leucocyte activation. Until 1980, when patients were treated with conventional immunosuppressive therapy, the monitoring of circulating T lymphocytes was possible by means of the E-rosette assay (Lay, Mendez and Bianco, 1971; Jondal, Holm and Wigzell, 1972; Oyer *et al.*, 1979). However, this method became unreliable after the introduction of cyclosporin as the main immunosuppressive agent.

The development of methods for the early diagnosis of acute rejection episodes, using qualitative analysis of peripheral lymphocytes and their subsets, was attempted at the University of Munich (Hammer *et al.*, 1984; Reichenspurner *et al.*, 1984) Cyto-immunological monitoring is performed daily for the first 3 weeks after heart transplantation. The cyto-immunological monitoring consists of two steps (Fig. 14.1):

(1) A routine method, which gives general information about the appearance of activated cells in the peripheral blood.
(2) A differential diagnostic test for discrimination between acute rejection and infection.

Technique

The leucocytes in 1 mm^3 of the patient's heparinized blood are counted and a blood smear is prepared. Mononuclear cells (lymphocytes and monocytes) are obtained from the remainder of the specimen by centrifugation over a Ficoll Hypaque Gradient. Some of these cells are spread onto microscopic slides using a cytocentrifuge and then stained with panoptic leucocyte staining by the method of Pappenheim. The remaining cells are labelled with

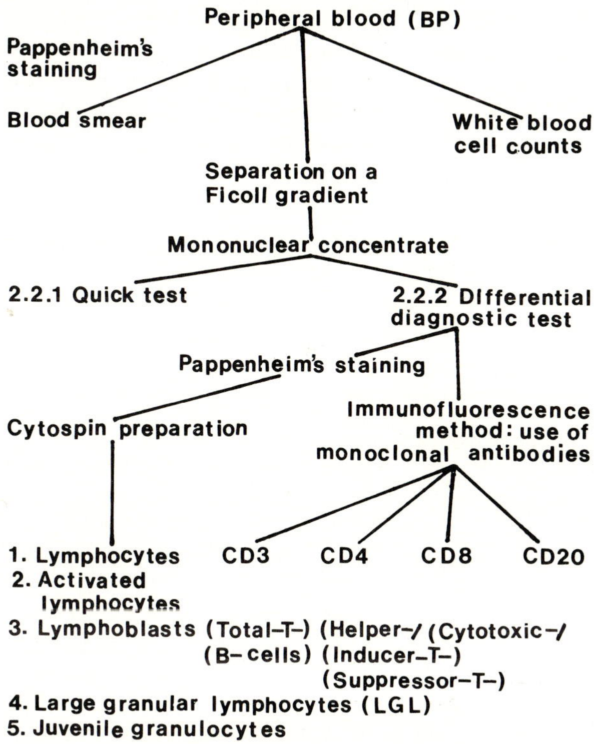

Fig. 14.1. *Schematic of laboratory analysis.*

monoclonal antibodies against T lymphocytes (OKT 3, Orthoclon Inc., Raritan, New Jersey, USA); T-helper/inducer cells (OKT 4) and T-suppressor/cytotoxic cells (OKT 8). The percentages of these cells are then determined under the fluorescent microscope or with the help of a computer-controlled cell analysis instrument — the fluorescence activated cell sorter (FACS).

The lymphocytes are separated under the light microscope according to their degree of activation into normal lymphocytes, activated lymphocytes and lymphoblasts. If more than 1 blast or more than 50 activated lymphocytes/mm^3 are present, the mononuclear cell pattern of a patient is described as being 'activated' in the sense of an acute inflammatory process. The reliability of lymphoblast counts of two observers at our institution showed nearly perfect concordance (correlation coefficient of 0.99). Therefore, cyto-immunological monitoring can be compared with the established method of endomyocardial biopsy (Klanke *et al.*, 1987).

An examination of 50 consecutive heart transplant patients showed activation of the peripheral lymphocytes in 95% of the acute rejections proved by endomyocardial biopsy. This result was confirmed by other transplantation centres including Stanford University (Hetzer *et al.*, 1985; Bleese *et al.*, 1985; Kasischke *et al.*, 1986; Borleffs, Jambroes and Prenger, 1987). Specificity was 72% (with 28% false-positive results), because infections also cause activation in the cell pattern of cyto-immunological monitoring.

If regularly used, this method permits a controlled use of endomyocardial biopsies. In Munich, a saving as high as 75% in myocardial biopsies, which would otherwise have been routinely performed in patients examined during the early postoperative phase, could be attributed to this test. However, endomyocardial biopsy remains irreplaceable in the therapeutic control of rejection reactions, because corticosteroids used for rejection therapy may give the illusion of peripheral decrease in lymphocyte activation.

ELECTROCARDIOGRAPHY

Changed QRS voltage in the surface ECG is almost insignificant in a patient treated with cyclosporin. The sensitivity of this method in diagnosing acute rejection is only 37%, although the specificity is 92% (Dawkins *et al.*, 1984).

There are, however, some new and promising methods regarding the use of ECG for the diagnosis of cardiac rejection. An epicardial ECG was obtained daily in a patient with an implanted pacemaker at the Medical School of Hannover (Warnecke *et al.*, 1985). The amplitude of the QRS complex was correlated with the results obtained by myocardial biopsy. There was a correlation between decreased amplitude and rejection reaction in 89% of the 50 patients examined; specificity was 96%.

This simple, telemetric method may be carried out daily. The necessary implantation of a pacemaker is the only disadvantage.

FOURIER ANALYSIS OF THE ELECTROCARDIOGRAM

As an alternative approach for the non-invasive detection of acute rejection, the Munich group analysed the frequency content of the QRS complex and ST segment of surface ECG recordings by fast Fourier transformation (FFT), a powerful analytic algorithm which reveals changes in the surface ECG invisible in the routine electrocardiogram (Haberl *et al.*, 1987).

Two well-defined surface ECG recordings were analysed by FFT (Blackman Harris window, 512 points) after low-noise, high-gain amplification (filter setting 0.5–300 Hz) each day for 4–6 weeks after heart transplantation in 40 patients.

Thirty-six acute rejection crises requiring treatment were diagnosed by cyto-immunological monitoring and endomyocardial biopsy. Single beat analysis of the QRS by FFT revealed a progressive change of the spectral morphology (increase of the frequency content between 70 and 110 Hz) on the days of rejection (33 out of 36 cases). At the same times the frequency content of the ST segment (300 msec) decreased between 10 and 30 Hz. The ECG did not change during these periods in most patients. After treatment of the rejection episodes, the frequency spectra of the QRS and ST segment returned to normal within 1–2 weeks. False-positive results were seen in 2 cases of mediastinitis.

QRS voltage decreased more than 20% in 18 out of 36 rejection crises and in 30 cases without rejection. The frequency spectra were constant in patients after heart transplantation without rejection and in patients after cardiac surgery but not transplantation. Electrophysiological changes, such as reduction of QRS amplitude, have been shown to be inconstantly correlated with acute rejection, and were too variable for therapeutic decisions. The causes of failure might include changes of skin–electrode impedance (Berson and Pipberger, 1968), circadian rhythms (Losman *et al.*, 1981), deviation of heart axes, pericardial effusion, chest wall oedema from steroid administration and development of fibrous scar tissue around the heart.

Our results indicate that Fourier transformation of the ECG, but not QRS amplitude, offers promise for non-invasive detection of acute rejection after heart transplantation and thus may reduce the number of necessary biopsies.

ECHOCARDIOGRAPHIC DIAGNOSIS OF CARDIAC REJECTION

Several approaches to the detection of heart transplant rejection with ultrasound have been reported in the literature, including the determination of left ventricular posterior wall thickness (Schroeder *et al.*, 1969; Popp *et al.*, 1971; Paulsen *et al.*, 1985), of left ventricular mass from M-mode (Sagar *et al.*, 1981; Dubroff *et al.*, 1984; Paulsen *et al.*, 1985) or 2-D-echocardiograms (Clark *et al.*, 1983; Nowygrod *et al.*, 1983) and of the isovolumic relaxation period (Dawkins *et al.*, 1985) as well as measurements of the intensity and the cyclic changes of myocardial echoes (Burckhardt, 1978; Wear *et al.*, 1986; Chandrasekaran *et al.*, 1987). However, most of the echocardiographic parameters of cardiac function remain within normal limits during rejection episodes in cyclosporin-treated patients, although a measurable change in comparison to control values might occur in the individual patient.

New methods (Angermann *et al.*, 1987) of computerized frame-by-frame evaluation of the endocardial border in two-dimensional echocardiographic short-axis views allow the measurement of left ventricular cross-sectional area throughout the cardiac cycle and the assessment of dynamic functional changes in the heart (Fig. 14.2). If, besides the measurement of left and right

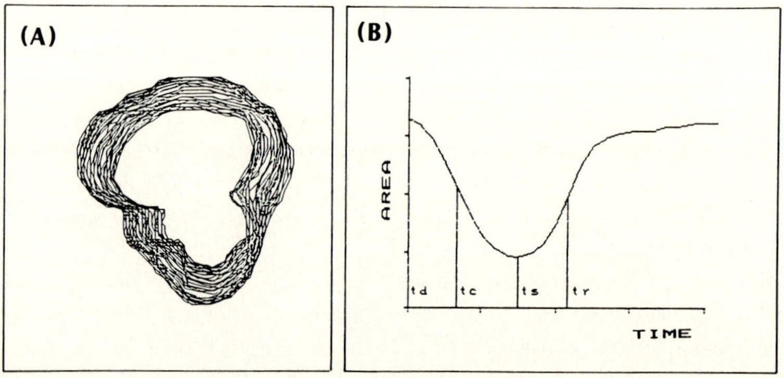

Fig. 14.2. *Computerized frame-by-frame evaluation of the endocardium in short axis views. (A) Endocardial borders of a whole cardiac cycle after automated edge detection. (B) Graphic display of cross-sectional area as a function of time: x-axis, time from QRS; y-axis, short axis cross-sectional area.*

ventricular wall thickness and isovolumic relaxation time, these new techniques are employed for follow-up studies in cardiac transplant recipients, alterations of the left ventricular cross-sectional area and of the rate and time course of left ventricular contraction and relaxation during rejection episodes may be objectively assessed.

An echocardiographic follow-up study of 45 cardiac transplant recipients at Munich University, in which the examination techniques were strictly standardized and computerized frame-by-frame edge detection in two-dimensional short axis cross-sections was employed for data analysis, was carried out (Angermann *et al.*, 1986). During mild rejection episodes, left ventricular cross-sectional area was found to decrease in comparison to

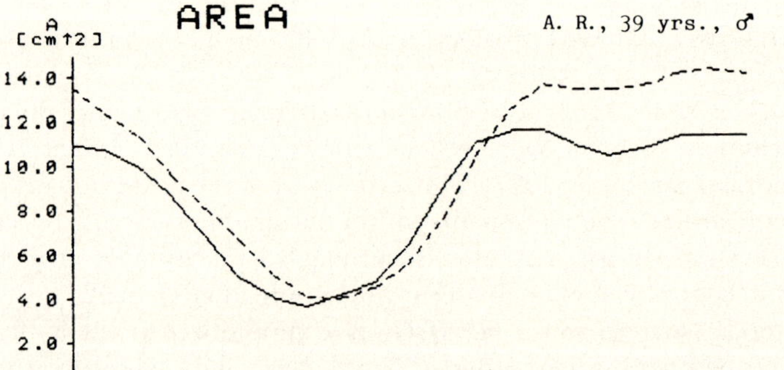

Fig. 14.3. *Area curves of the left ventricular short axis cross-section after orthotopic cardiac transplantation. Broken line, no rejection; Solid line, mild rejection. See text for further details.*

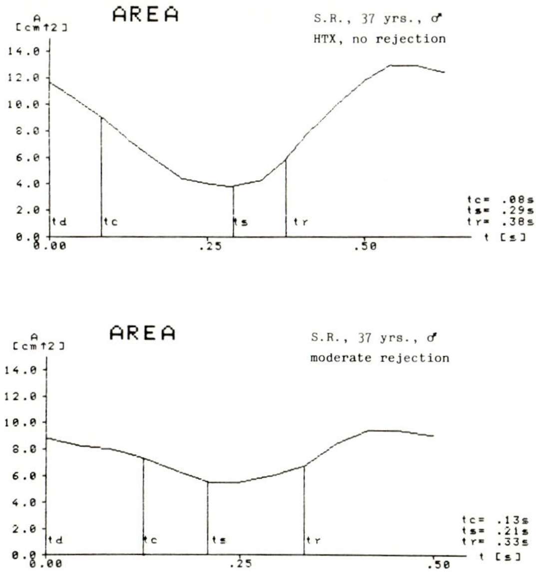

Fig. 14.4. *Area curves of the left ventricular short axis cross-section after orthotopic cardiac transplantation. Top, no rejection; bottom, moderate rejection. See text for further details.*

control values, while the pattern of contraction and relaxation remained unchanged (Fig. 14.3). During moderate rejection, an additional decrease in the extent and velocity of systolic area change and the diastolic relaxation velocity occurred (Fig. 14.4). As the measured values of cardiac function parameters often remained within the normal range during acute rejection, the diagnosis could only be made by comparison to the reference echocardiogram, which had been obtained at a time when rejection was ruled out histologically.

When all examined parameters were included in the diagnosis, 32 of the 36 rejection episodes diagnosed by biopsy, including all requiring treatment, could also be recognized by echocardiography. However, the severity of the rejection process, as determined by the histological findings, could not be reliably predicted from the echocardiogram. There were two false positives, both in patients who developed left ventricular hypertrophy postoperatively. The differential diagnosis of an increase in wall thickness, with concomitant change of the diastolic properties of the left ventricle, may require endomyocardial biopsy in the individual patient.

Echocardiographic changes usually reverse when rejection is resolving after treatment. In our experience, persistent changes of cardiac function have been a poor prognostic sign, as one of three patients with this phenomenon died from recurrent episodes of acute rejection and two others developed chronic cardiac rejection.

In summary, when echocardiographic examination techniques are strictly standardized and, in addition to conventional measurements of left ventricular wall thickness and isovolumic relaxation time, frame-by-frame evaluation of two-dimensional echocardiographic short axis cross-section is employed, functional changes accompanying acute rejection may be recognized by serial studies. This allows a non-invasive diagnosis, although not for a reliable prediction of the severity of acute rejection in individual patients. Mild rejections, not requiring treatment, may not always be detected, but evaluation of several echo parameters improves the diagnostic accuracy. Echocardiography, together with other newly developed non-invasive techniques, may provide the means to a safe decrease in biopsy frequency even in patients on cyclosporin.

RADIONUCLIDE SCANNING

As a further non-invasive method of diagnosing cardiac rejection, radionuclide scanning of the heart has been used (Novitzky *et al.*, 1984). Acute rejection leads to cellular infiltration and interstitial oedema of the myocardium as well as to myocyte necrosis. These inflammatory processes cause deterioration of myocardial function and, in particular, loss of compliance. The changes in volume and function are measured by radionuclide scanning. In this method, donor red blood cells are incubated with 25 mCi technetium-99m pertechnetate and reinjected via a peripheral vein. Scanning commences after 10–15 min of equilibration of radioactivity; the gamma camera is placed in the LAO position in order to facilitate an apical view of the donor left ventricle. This technique is called multigated (MUGA) blood pool scanning.

By this technique, ejection fraction, end-diastolic volume, end-systolic and stroke volume are calculated. The results were compared with those obtained by simultaneous endomyocardial biopsy. The decreased stroke volume showed the highest correlation with acute transplant rejection. The same applied to the cardiac output, which was explained mainly by the changed stroke volume rather than decreased heart rate. Changes in end-diastolic and end-systolic left ventricular volumes showed a lesser degree of correlation, and changes in ejection fraction showed no correlation.

Radionuclide scanning is non-invasive and may be carried out with a mobile camera in the isolation ward. Results are obtained within an hour.

The Munich group used 'first pass radionuclide scintigraphy' to diagnose chronic rejection episodes and for assessment of left ventricular function in transplanted hearts (Schad *et al.*, 1986). Examination under stress turned out to be indispensable for early detection of poor global and regional left ventricular function. At present, the fastest and easiest non-invasive technique to study global and regional LV function is radionuclide scintigraphy (Kemkes *et al.*, 1987).

DETERMINATION OF NEOPTERINES AS BIOCHEMICAL MARKERS OF ACUTE REJECTION EPISODES

Neopterines are pteridine derivates and are found in stimulated cultures of activated lymphocytes. Inflammatory processes as well as acute rejection episodes lead to the activating of lymphocytes and thus to increased release of this substance in the urine.

The groups at the Universities of Innsbruck and Vienna found a sensitivity of 95% in the diagnosis of acute rejection episodes (Margreiter *et al.*, 1983; Havel *et al.*, 1986). The disadvantage of this method is its lack of specificity. Viral infections also cause activation of lymphocytes and thus neopterine release. Therefore, a differentiation between various inflammatory processes and acute rejection is not possible, in contrast to cyto-immunological monitoring. Increased levels of neopterines in serum and urine can be an indicator for acute rejection only if inflammatory processes can be excluded.

IMMUNE MONITORING OF INTERLEUKIN-2-RECEPTORS

At the University of St. Louis, USA, interleukin-2-receptors as surface markers of lymphocyte activation of T-cell subsets from peripheral blood were studied by two-colour flow cytometry for correlation with endomyocardial biopsies (Miller *et al.*, 1986). The test was considered positive if either the percentage of T_4 cells positive for interleukin-2-receptor was more than 20% of the total T_4 cells or the absolute count was more than 120 cells/ml. These criteria were highly correlated with grade II biopsies according to the modified Stanford classification or with proven bacterial or viral infections.

Results obtained within 5 weeks after heart transplantation showed a sensitivity of 78% (70% for rejection only) and a specificity of 97%. The sensitivity of these tests was 75% (50% for rejection only) after 5 weeks, but the specificity remained at 97%.

The use of these surface markers may improve the monitoring of immunosuppression. The disadvantage of this method is that the number of

T_4/interleukin-2-receptor cells differs according to the serum levels of cyclosporin.

BETA-2-MICROGLOBULIN SECRETION

Beta-2-microglobulin is found in non-covalent association as the invariate small subunit of the major histocompatibility complex (MHC), class I. Certain lymphoid cell types, such as thymocytes, express beta-2-microglobulin in considerable excess over MHC glycoprotein (Messner, 1984). Such lymphocytes, exhibiting high levels of beta-2-microglobulin expression, have high natural killer cell activity. Beta-2-microglobulins are present in serum, urine and cerebrospinal fluids.

At Vienna University, levels of beta-2-microglobulin were found to be elevated during acute rejection. Beta-2-microglobulin changes were indicative of acute rejection, infections and renal failure. According to its pathophysiology, an increasing serum level of beta-2-microglobulin should parallel transplant rejection.

The tubular injury induced by cyclosporin, however, leads to diminished tubular reabsorption and hence to elevated urinary excretion of renal metabolized beta-2-microglobulin. Serum levels of beta-2-microglobulin are closely correlated to serum creatinine and are used in the diagnosis of renal tubular disease (Goebel *et al.*, 1983). High amounts of serum beta-2-microglobulin are also found in lymphoproliferative disorders. Production of beta-2-microglobulins by lymphoid cells is enhanced by mitogens, by the Epstein–Barr virus (Hammarström and Smith, 1985) and by interferon (Grönberg, Kiessling and Fiers, 1985).

EXPERIMENTAL STUDIES FOR ASSESSMENT OF CARDIAC ALLOGRAFT REJECTION

Besides these clinically established non-invasive methods, a number of experimental investigations is under way. In these experiments, the applicability of magnetic resonance imaging and proton relaxation times (Sasaguri *et al.*, 1984; Walpoth *et al.* 1984; Aherne *et al.*, 1986; Eugene *et al.*, 1986), the use of indium-111-labelled cells for measurement of cellular dynamics (Oluwole *et al.*, 1981; Wang *et al.*, 1982) as well as antimyosin monoclonal antibodies (Hall *et al.*, 1986; Sasaki *et al.*, 1987) were tested. Both antimyosin antibody and phosphorous nuclear magnetic spectroscopy detected changes consistent with mild to moderate rejection.

T_2 relaxation time can provide an index of severity of interstitial oedema and mononuclear cell infiltration in cases that have not progressed to myocytolysis.

Magnetic resonance imaging of cardiac transplants has been proposed for detection of increased cellular and interstitial oedema, myocardial necroses and haemorrhage accompanying acute allograft rejection (Aherne *et al.*, 1986). However, limited availability and the problems with monitoring of critically ill patients in a high magnetic field outside the isolation unit are current disadvantages.

Antimyosin monoclonal antibody uptake correlated with the severity of rejection based on septal biopsy interpretation. The use of indium-111-labelled cells (leucocytes and platelets) (Farowaz *et al.*, 1984) seems to be suited for studying the kinetics and detection of allograft rejection (Oluwole *et al.*, 1981; Wang *et al.*, 1982). However, until clinical data using magnetic resonance imaging are available (Wisenberg *et al.*, 1987), these methods are still experimental and not yet available for routine clinical purposes. In particular, many technical problems have still to be resolved.

Further investigation into the mechanism of injury in rejection, particularly regarding the metabolic changes, would have great potential for elucidation of immunological mechanics and ideally could translate into clinical benefit for transplant patients. All these experimental methods have yet to have their clinical reliability established.

REFERENCES

Aherne, T., Tscholakoff, D., Finkbeiner, W., Sechtem, U., Deragin, N. and Yee, E. (1986). Magnetic resonance imaging of cardiac transplants: the evaluation of rejection of cardiac allografts with and without immunosuppression. *Circulation* **74**, 145.

Angermann, C. E., Hart, R. J., Spes, C. H., Zwehl, W., Marquart, M. and Schmid, D. (1987). Computerized quantitative evaluation of the endocardium in serial two-dimensional echocardiograms of the left ventricular short axis. *Computers in Cardiology*, IEEE, Leuven, in press.

Angermann, Ch., Schott, L., Hart, R. J., Reichenspurner, H., Kemkes, B. M., Zwehl, W., Gokel, J. M. and Theisen, K. (1986). Echo monitoring of heart transplant recipients: acute and long-term results and assessment of complications. *Heart Transplant.* **5**, 397.

Berson, A. S., and Pipberger, H. V. (1968). Skin–electrode impedance problems in electrocardiography. *Am. Heart J.* **76**, 514.

Bleese, N., Arndt, R., Delling, G., Kasischke, D., Rodewald, G., Rödiger, W., Schäfer, H. and Bleese, E. (1985). Neue Aspekte der Rejectionsdiagnostik und -therapie nach orthotoper Herztransplantation. *Thorac. Cardiovasc. Surg.* **33**, 91.

Borleffs, J. U., Jambroes, G. and Prenger, K. B. (1987). Cytoimmunologic monitoring and endomyocardial biopsies in patients after heart transplantation. *Heart Transplant.* **6**, 370.

Burckhardt, C. B. (1978). Speckle in ultrasound B-mode scans. *Trans. Son. Ultrason.* **25**, 1–6.

Chandrasekaran, K., Bansol, R. C., Grunleaf, J. F., Hauch, A., Seward, J. B., Tajik, A. J. and Bailey, L. L. (1987). Early recognition of heart transplant rejection by backscatter analysis from serial 2D-ECHO in a heterotopic transplant model. *Heart Transplant.* **6**, 1.

Clark, M. B., Spotnitz, H. M., Dubroff, J. M., Wong, C. Y. H., Vayda, J. L., Costello, D., Drusin, R., Rose, E. A. and Reemtsma, K. (1983). Acute rejection after cardiac transplantation: detection by two-dimensional echocardiography. *Surg. Forum* **34**, 248–250.

Dawkins, K. D., Haverich, A., Aziz, S., Billingham, M. E., Jamieson, S. W. and Gibson, D. G. (1985). Detection of acute rejection using color echocardiography (Abstract) A. *Circulation* **72**, Suppl. III, 207.

Dawkins, K. D., Oldershaw, P. J., Billingham, M. E., Hunt, S. A., Oyer, P. E., Jamieson, S. W., Popp, R. L., Stinson, E. B. and Shumway, N. E. (1984). Changes in diastolic function as a noninvasive marker of cardiac allograft rejection. *Heart Transplant.* **3**, 286.

Dubroff, J. M., Clark, M. B., Wong, C. Y. H., Spotnitz, H. M., Fenoglio, J. J., Rose, E. A. and Reemtsma, K. (1984). Changes in left ventricular mass associated with onset of acute rejection after cardiac transplantation. *Heart Transplant.* **3**, 105–109.

Eugene, M., Lechat, P., Hadgisky, P., Teillac, A., Grosgogeat, Y. and Cabrol, C. (1986). Nuclear magnetic resonance and proton relaxation times in experimental heterotopic heart transplantation. *Heart Transplant.* **5**, 41.

Farowaz, R. A., Iga, C., Hardy, M. A. *et al.* (1984). Diagnosis of allograft rejection with indium-111 labeled platelets in cyclosporin treated rats. *J. Nucl. Med.* **25**, 80.

Goebel, F., Schmeidl, H., Fueßl, H. and Vogel, S. (1983). Zur Früherkennung der Nephropathie: Beta-2-Microglobulin im Serum. *Klin. Wschr.* **61**, 1209.

Grönberg, A., Kiessling, R. and Fiers, W. (1985). Interferon is a strong modulator of NK susceptibility and expression of β-m but not of transferrin receptors of K 5622 cells. *Cell. Immunol.* **95**, 195.

Haberl, R., Weber, M., Reichenspurner, H., Kemkes, B. M., Osterholzer, G., Anthuber, M. and Steinbeck, G. (1987). Frequency analysis of the surface electrocardiogram for recognition of acute rejection after orthotopic transplantation in man. *Circulation* **76**, 102–108.

Hall, T. S., Baumgartner, W. A., Borkon, A. M., LaFrance, N. D., Traill, T. A., Norris, S., Hutchins, G. M., Brawn, J. and Reitz, B. A. (1986). Diagnosis of acute cardiac rejection with antimyosin monoclonal antibody, phosphorous nuclear magnetic resonance imaging, two-dimensional echocardiography, and endocardial biopsy. *Heart Transplant.* **5**, 419–424.

Hammarström, L. and Smith, C. (1985). β_2-microglobulin secretion from lymphoid cells: a study at the cellular level. *Med. Microbiol. Immunol.* **174**, 59.

Hammer, C., Reichenspurner, H., Ertel, W., Lersch, C., Plahl, M., Brendl, W., Reichart, B., Überfuhr, P., Weiz, A., Kemkes, B. M., Reble, B., Funccius, W. and Goke, M. (1984). Cytological and immunologic monitoring of cyclosporine-treated human heart recipients. *Heart Transplant.* **3**, 228.

Havel, M. P., Laczkovics, A. M. D., Preiss, P. S., Müller, M. M. and Wolner, E. (1986). Neopterin as a new marker to detect acute rejection after heart transplantation. *Heart Transplant.* **4**, 594.

Hetzer, R., Warnecke, H., Schüler, S., Süthoff, U., Frimpong, K., Lang, W., Wonnigeit, K., Schaps, D., Herrmann, G. and Borst, H. G. (1985). Herztransplantation — Ein klinischer Erfahrungsbericht. *Münch. Med. Wschr.* **127**, 359.

Jondal, M., Holm, G. and Wigzell, H. (1972). Surface markers on human T and B lymphocytes. *J. Exp. Med.* **136**, 207.

Kasischke, D., Bleese, N., Jamieson, S. W. and Billingham, M. E. (1986). The validation of cytological and immunological monitoring of cyclosporine treated human heart recipients. *Heart Transplant.*, in press.

Kaye, M. (1987). The Registry of the International Society for Heart Transplantation: Fourth Official Report 1987. *Heart Transplant.* **6**, 63.

Kemkes, B. M., Reichenspurner, H., Osterholzer, G., Anthuber, M., Schad, N., Maccio, A., Erdmann, E. and Rienmüller, R. (1987). First pass radionuclide scintigraphy for long-term follow up after heart and heart–lung transplantation. *Transplant. Proc.* **19**, 2543.

Klanke, D., Hammer, C., Kemkes, B. M., Dirschedl, P. and Krombach, F. (1987). Sensitivity and specificity of the cyto-immunological monitoring (CIM) in correlation to endomyocardial biopsies (EMB) in heart transplanted patients. *Transplant. Proc.* **19**, in press.

Lay, W. H., Mendez, N. F. and Bianco, F. (1971). Binding of sheep red blood cells to a large population of human T-lymphocytes. *Nature* **230**, 531.

Losman, J. G., McDonal, J., Levine, H. D., Campbell, C. D. and Replogle, R. L. (1981). The variation of the electrocardiographic voltage during the day in normal adult subjects. *Heart Transplant.* **1**, 37.

Margreiter, R., Fuchs, D., Hansen, A., Huber, C., Reibenegger, G., Spielberger, M. and Wachter, H. (1983). Neopterine as new biochemical marker for diagnosis of allograft rejection. *Transplantation* **36**, 650.

Messner, R. (1984). β_2-m: an old molecule assumes a new look. *J. Lab. Clin. Med.* **104**, 141.

Miller, L. W., Roodman, S. T., Tsai, C., Pennington, D. G., Kauter, K. and McBride, L. (1986). Immune monitoring of interleukin-2-receptors (IL2R) in heart transplantation. *Heart Transplant.* **5**, 377.

Novitzky, D., Bouiaszczuk, J., Cooper, D. K. C., Isaacs, S., Rose, A. G., Smith, J. A., Uys, C. J., Barnard, C. N. and Fraser, R. (1984). Prediction of acute cardiac rejection using radionuclide techniques. *S. A. Med. J.* **65**, 5.

Nowygrod, R., Spontnitz, H. M., Dubroll, J. M., Hardy, M. A. and Reemtsma, K. (1983). Organ mass: an indicator of heart transplant rejection. *Transplant. Proc.* **15**, 1225–1228.

Oluwole, S., Wang, T., Fawwaz, R. A., Satabe, K., Nowygrod, R., Reemtsma, K. and Hardy, M. A. (1981). Use of iridium-111-labelled cells in measurement of cellular dynamics of experimental cardiac allograft rejection. *Transplantation* **31**, 51–55.

Oyer, P. E., Stinson, E. B., Bieber, C. P., Reitz, B. A., Raney, A. A., Baumgarnter, W. A. and Shumway, N. E. (1979). Diagnosis and treatment of acute cardiac allograft rejection. *Transplant Proc.* **16**, 296.

Paulsen, W., Magid, N., Sagar, K., Hastillo, A., Wolfgang, T. C., Lower, R. R. and Hess, M. L. (1985). Left ventricular function of heart allografts during acute rejection. An echocardiographic assessment. *Heart Transplant.* **4**, 525–529.

Popp, R. L., Schroeder, J. S., Stinson, E. B., Shumway, N. E. and Harrison, D. C. (1971). Ultrasonic studies for the early detection of acute cardiac rejection. *Transplantation* **11**, 543–550.

Reichenspurner, H., Ertel, W., Hammer, C., Lersch, C., Reichart, B., Überfuhr, P., Welz, A., Reble, B., Kemkes, B. M. and Gokel, J. M. (1984). Immunologic monitoring of heart transplant patients under cyclosporine immunosuppression. *Transplant Proc.* **16**, 1251.

Sagar, K. B., Hastillo, A., Wolfgang, T. C., Lower, R. R. and Hess, M. L. (1981). Left ventricular mass by M-mode echocardiography in cardiac transplant patients with acute rejection. *Circulation* **64**, Suppl. II, 216–220.

Sasaguri, S., LaRaia, P. J., Fallon, J. T., Aylesworth, C. A., Brady, T. J. and Buckley, M. J. (1984). Early detection of cardiac allograft rejection using proton nuclear magnetic resonance. *Circulation*, Suppl. II, **70**, 165.

Sasaki, H., Sada, M., Nishimura, T., Kavazoe, K. and Fugita, T. (1987). T_2-Relaxation time imaging and 111 In-antimyosin fab. RI imaging in canine heterotopic heart transplantation. *Heart Transplant.* **6**, 390.

Schad, N., Kemkes, B. M., Ciavolella, M., Maccio, A., Reichenspurner, H., Osterholzer, G. and Reichart, B. (1986). Non-invasive assessment of left ventricular function with first pass angiography in transplanted hearts. *Cardiologia* **31**, 111.

Schroeder, J. S., Popp, R. L., Stinson, E. B., Dong, E., Shumway, N. E. and Harrison, D. C. (1969). Acute rejection following cardiac transplantation. Phonocardiographic and ultrasound observations. *Circulation* **60**, 155–164.

Walpoth, B., McGregor, C. G., Aziz, S., Billingham, M. E., Jardetzky, N. W., Jardetzky, O., Jamieson, S. W. and Shumway, N. E. (1984). Assessment of myocardial rejection by nuclear magnetic resonance (31 P NMR). *Circulation*, Suppl. II, **70**, 165.

Wang, T. S. T., Oluwole, S., Fawwaz, R. A., Wolff, M., Kuromoto, N., Satake, K., Hardy, M. A. and Alderson, P. O. (1982). Cellular basis for accumulation of In^{111}-labeled leukocytes and platelets in rejection of cardiac allografts: concise communication. *J. Nucl. Med.* **23**, 993–997.

Warnecke, H., Hetzer, R., Schüler, S., Goetze, H. J., Schäfers, H. J., Blazek, J., Meyer, U. D., Stüthoff, U. and Borst, H. G. (1985). Das intramyokardiale Elektrokardiogramm zur nicht-invasiven Abstoßungsdiagnostik nach Herztransplantation. *Thorac. Cardiovasc. Surg.* **33**, 44.

Wear, K. A., Schnittger, I., Director, B. A., Dawkins, K. D., Haverich, A., Billingham, M. E., Jamieson, S. W. and Popp, R. L. (1986). Ultrasonic characterization of acute cardiac rejection from temporal evolution of echocardiograms. *Heart Transplant.* **5**, 424–429.

Wisenberg, G., Pflugfelder, P. W., Kostuk, W. J., McKenzie, F. N. and Prato, F. S. (1987). Diagnostic applicability of magnetic resonance imaging in assessing human cardiac allograft rejection. *Am. J. Cardiol.* **60**, 130–136.

P. G. I. Stovin

15

Monitoring of Cardiac Rejection by Endomyocardial Biopsy

INTRODUCTION

History

From the standpoint of this chapter, heart transplantation in man started when Barnard (1967) performed the first successful orthotopic operation. At that time, the only methods for monitoring the state of the transplanted organ were clinical assessment of the patient and the ECG which proved to be relatively insensitive procedures.

The next major advance was the introduction of transvenous endomyocardial biopsy in 1972 by Caves *et al.* (1973a) at Stanford. This proved to be a more sensitive way of diagnosing rejection and it allowed detection up to 4 days earlier than by clinical methods.

A second advance was made by the Stanford group with the introduction of anti-thymocyte globulin, and of T-cell monitoring using the sheep erythrocyte rosetting technique (Bieber *et al.*, 1977; Griepp *et al.*, 1977). These changes delayed the time of the first rejection episode and reduced the frequency of rejection episodes. Sheep cell rosetting provided a functional method of monitoring the dose of an immunosuppressive agent before it had produced toxic effects. Up to this time, the only monitoring of the effect of the azathioprine and steroid used in immunosuppression had been the effect on the platelet and white cell counts in the peripheral blood.

With the introduction of cyclosporin (Cy) in 1980 (Oyer *et al.*, 1983) a further improvement in patient survival was achieved, even though hypertension and renal impairment proved to be complications of this therapeutic agent. The effect of Cy on the heart will be discussed later, and in this connection the introduction of heterotopic heart transplantation by Barnard in 1974 (Cooper *et al.*, 1980) has yielded some interesting observations. Although the determination of blood levels of Cy is useful in controlling the dosage of this drug, the blood level does not accurately reflect the functional level of immunosuppression (Hakim *et al.*, 1985a).

Although there is need for further refining of the use of immunosuppressive drugs singly or in combination, this chapter will discuss endomyocardial biopsy in the assessment of rejection in heart transplantation, and will touch on the evaluation of different therapeutic regimens. At present, myocardial biopsy provides the standard for assessing the degree of rejection occurring in the heart, against which other methods of assessment are judged; these other methods are discussed in Chapter 14.

Aims of transplant patient management

After the successful completion of the operation there are two principal risks for the patient. First, there is rejection of the donor heart if the immunosuppression has been inadequate, and secondly, if the immunosuppression has been excessive there is a very real risk of serious and even lethal infection and of malignancy. The success of any immunosuppressive regimen can therefore be crudely assessed if the mortality from each of these two main causes is about equal. However, patients vary in both their responsiveness to immunosuppressive drugs and in their reactivity to the immunological stimulus of an alien organ. Thus, improvements in transplant survival are likely to come from methods for recognizing individual patients at the ends of the reactivity scale, so that treatment and monitoring schedules can be more effectively planned. We have found that if the first biopsy taken between days 7 and 12 after transplantation shows moderate or severe rejection, then there is only a 36% chance of surviving 1 year. This compares with a 77% chance of surviving 1 year for those with lesser degrees of rejection.

At this stage it must be pointed out that the term 'rejection episode' has been used in two different senses by different people. Billingham and coworkers (Imakita, Tazelaar and Billingham, 1986) use the term to mean any episode of increasing severity of cellular infiltration which may resolve spontaneously or require increased immunosuppression. Most clinicians and surgeons restrict the term to an episode of moderate or severe rejection that has necessitated an increase of immunosuppression.

MYOCARDIAL BIOPSY

Handling the specimen

The technique of percutaneous endomyocardial biopsy has been described by Caves *et al.* (1973b) and the method and results with the Caves–Shultz bioptome were described by Caves *et al.* (1975). This bioptome has a larger bite than the Sakakibara–Konno or the King's bioptomes and therefore yields a better sample for histological examination without any greater discomfort or hazard to the patient. The technique for taking endomyocardial biopsies from patients with a heterotopic heart transplant has been described by Cooper *et al.* (1982).

The easiest method for extracting the specimen from jaws of the bioptome without squeezing or contaminating it, is to use a sterile fine venipuncture needle that can be put with the specimen into the laboratory container, or onto a glass slide for cytology. Occasionally, the needle may transfix the specimen, producing a small hole in the final sections.

For the routine assessment of rejection, three or four specimens are immersed in 10% buffered formol-saline solution. Additional biopsies can be put into buffered glutaraldehyde for electron microscopy (Uys and Rose, 1983) or into liquid nitrogen with or without a cryopreservative for immunological (Rose *et al.*, 1984; Weintraub, Masek and Billingham, 1985) or for functional studies (Darracott-Cankovic *et al.*, 1984, 1987). Impression smears may be made for cytological examination before fixing the biopsy specimens (Topalidis *et al.*, 1986). These smears can be examined sooner than the histological sections. Lymphocytes from tissue culture of the biopsy have been used in a primed lymphocyte test to assess their alloreactivity (Duquesnoy *et al.*, 1987).

The routine biopsies are processed through alcohol, trichlorethylene and wax on a 2 h cycle (Autotechnicon Ultra 2 or Shandon Hypercentre). The 3–5 specimens from one patient are embedded together and then serially sectioned with successive short ribbons mounted on 10 glass slides. Slides 1, 5 and 10 are stained with the usual haematoxylin and eosin or (author's preference) with haematoxylin, phloxin and saffron (HPS). Slide 4 is stained with methyl green and pyronin (MGP), and slide 6 with Masson's trichrome (MT). Figure 15.1 shows a typical set of routine sections which provide a reasonable survey through the biopsy material. The remaining slides are available for further stains as necessary. The reasons for preferring serial sections to step sections will become evident later.

Histological assessment of the rejection processes

Typically, the transplant rejection reaction is a T-cell-mediated one (Rabin, 1983; Rose *et al.*, 1984; Weintraub, Masek and Billingham, 1985). The

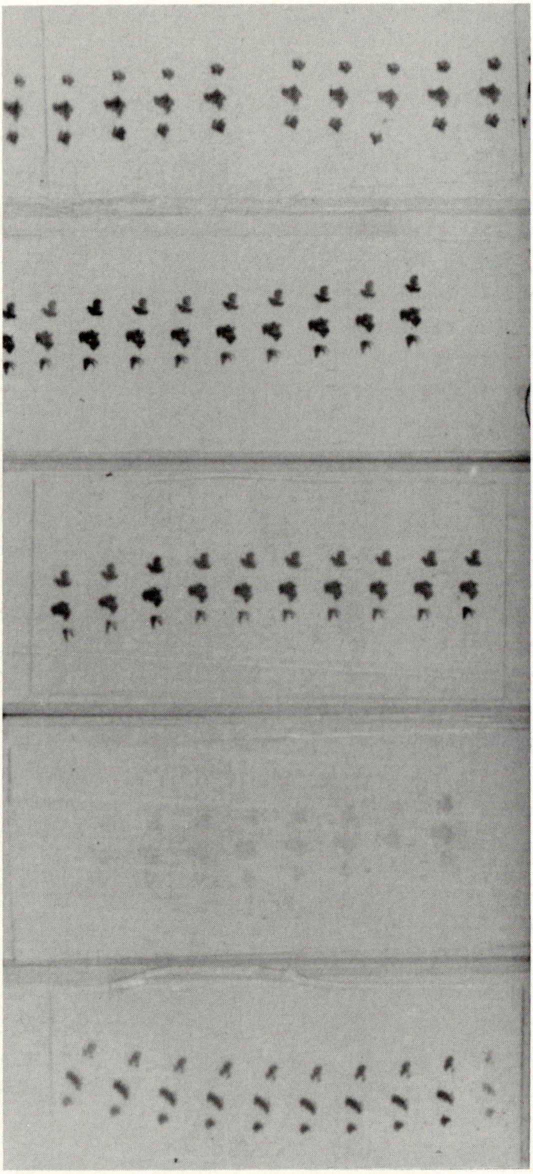

Fig. 15.1. *Set of routine biopsy sections. For details see text.*

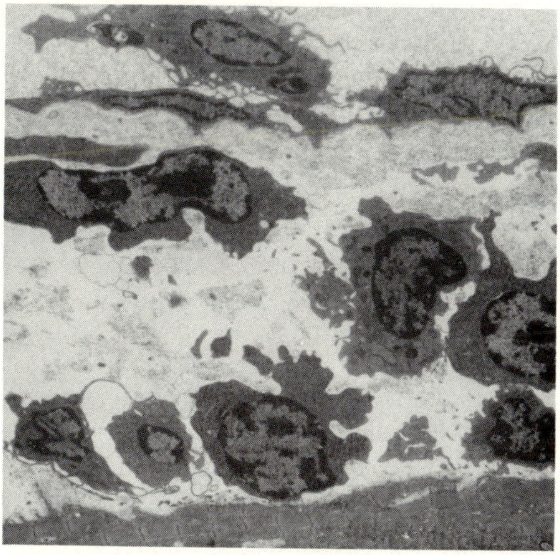

Fig. 15.2. *Early rejection; interstitial lymphocytes reacting with each other rather than with the myocytes (bottom) or vascular endothelium (top) where a macrophage appears to be seeking a space between the endothelial cells to escape from the lumen. ×2660.*

details of rejection immunology have been discussed in Chapter 2. The host's lymphocytes reach the donor heart by migrating from the interstitial capillaries. These lymphocytes react closely with each other (Fig. 15.2) before making contact with and damaging the myocytes. This early phase of rejection is multifocal and shows small pericapillary accumulations of lymphocytes widely scattered through the myocardium. Duquesnoy *et al.* (1987) observed that the infiltrates of lymphocytes directed against class II antigens tended to be more focal and those directed against class I antigens more diffuse.

Rose, Losman and Barnard (1970) and Billingham (1979) have shown that the rejection reaction is fairly uniformly and equally distributed between the two sides of the heart. Stovin and Hewitt (1986) have shown that the conducting tissue of the heart is also involved in the rejection reaction, although the valves, coronary veins and pulmonary trunk and aorta are rarely and minimally involved (Pomerance and Stovin, 1985). While on immunotherapy not all foci are of the same degree of activity and some may be regressing whereas others are progressing. The MGP stain is useful for demonstrating the degree of activity, which is proportional to the number of pyroninophilic cells present. If the immunosuppression is not quite adequate the infiltrate will tend to progress both in intensity of the lymphocytic reaction and also in the frequency of the foci in the myocardium. Besides the migration of lymphocytes from the capillaries there is also fluid leak with the formation of interstitial oedema. Myocyte damage is a relatively late event.

It usually affects one or a few adjacent cells, and is accompanied by the lymphocytic infiltrate.

Herskowitz *et al.* (1987) reported that interstitial oedema and lymphocytic infiltration of vessel walls with extension of the infiltrate into the myocardium, either singly or together, were predictors of myocyte damage in the following one or two biopsies. Occasionally, the cell-mediated rejection reaction is accelerated, especially in patients being re-transplanted for acute rejection of their first heart (Lanza *et al.*, 1983). The rejection reaction is said to evolve more slowly under Cy than under the older conventional immunosuppression (Billingham, 1986). However, we have encountered rapidly evolving severe rejection in patients on Cy therapy.

Variants on the above basic pattern are found, particularly if the coronary arteries and arterioles are involved by rejection. Hess *et al.* (1983) have indicated that this arterial lesion may be due to cytotoxic B-cell antibodies directed against HLA-DR rather than due to T lymphocytes. In these circumstances, vascular occlusions will produce ischaemic vacuolation or even necrosis of groups of myocytes, which attract secondarily a lymphocytic and neutrophilic response. This process is seen mostly in the epicardial arteries, takes a number of months or years to produce clinical disturbances, and is therefore usually referred to as chronic rejection. The transplanted heart, being denervated, is incapable of manifesting angina.

Very occasionally, a different type of rejection may be encountered. This consists of swelling of the intramyocardial vascular endothelium, and intravascular thrombi of red and/or white cells (Fig. 15.3). There is no or absolutely minimal interstitial lymphocytic infiltrate and it is usually an acute,

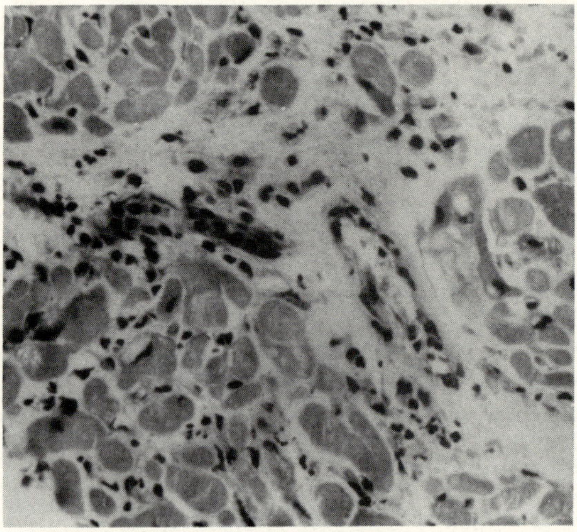

Fig. 15.3. *Intravascular cellular aggregates and endothelial cell swelling. HPS × 400.*

TABLE 15.1
Acute Vascular Rejection Deaths (1.1.79–30.6.86)

Case No.	*Survival (days)*	*Transfusion*	*Pregnancy*	*Non-identical Blood Groups ABO*	*Rh*	*Antibody*
106	6		+	+		
84*	6	11 d				
63	9			+	+	
82*	11					
43	11		?		(+)	
52†	13	36 m				
41	24	60 m				
15	51	11 m			+	E
105	64		+	+		
Total 9	22 M	4	2	3	3	1

* Same case re-transplanted.
† Re-transplanted for acute cellular rejection.
( ) = not compatible in blood transfusion terms.
E, rhesus group E antibody; M, mean survival.

serious and often lethal event occurring in the first 3 weeks after transplantation. In our experience there has been a relatively high incidence of this acute vascular type of rejection in women (Table 15.1). Women form only 1 in 17 of our heart transplant patients, but one-third of this acute vascular rejection group. Hyperacute rejection with antibodies against HLA-ABC antigens has been reported by Weil *et al.* (1981) and with vascular endothelial cell antibody by Brasile *et al.* (1985).

How many biopsies to take and when

As the rejection reaction is fairly uniformly distributed through the myocardium, the source of the myocardial biopsies is unimportant. Because the right ventricle is technically easy of access, the diagnosis of rejection is based on sampling this chamber. In view of the multifocal nature of the rejection process, there is a sampling error, which is reduced progressively with increasing number of samples. This was studied by Spiegelhalter and Stovin (1983), who found that four readable biopsies were necessary to reduce the chance of missing a moderate rejection reaction to 2%. For three biopsies, the chance of missing a lesion was 5%. These data were derived from the relatively large bite of the Caves–Schultz bioptome. More samples will obviously be required if the smaller Olympus or King's bioptomes are used. The number of these smaller biopsy bites must be increased to at least five (Baandrup, Florio and Olsen, 1982).

Not all the biopsies are readable, as some may include previous biopsy sites, tricuspid chordal tissue, endocardium only or epicardial fat. On occasions the bioptome can be in the coronary sinus or liver yet appear to be in the right ventricle on single plane radiological monitoring. The number of biopsy bites taken may amount to nearly 100 over the transplant patient's life. However, such is the size of the ventricle in comparison to the size of the biopsy that it is often very difficult to be certain of seeing more than a couple of scars at necropsy. There is therefore no need to worry about taking multiple bites at the biopsy session. There is, however, some suggestion that the taking of up to 8 bites at a session may increase the incidence of biopsies from previous sites up to 69% (Sibley *et al.*, 1986). Because of the postoperative pericardial adhesions, there is no risk of tamponade following penetration of the right ventricular myocardium and indeed epicardial fat is occasionally found in a biopsy bite.

With orthotopic heart transplantation, the heart must be protected from any damaging degree of rejection because there is no back-up similar to dialysis for renal patients, although the artificial heart may be of temporary help (Joyce *et al.*, 1986). The situation is slightly different for heterotopic heart transplantation in that the patient's own failing heart is retained and can provide some back-up should the donor heart fail (Cooper *et al.*, 1980). It is therefore necessary to take advantage of the ability of the biopsy to detect rejection earlier than other clinical or ECG methods.

Endomyocardial biopsies can be taken at the most likely times of rejection, which are mainly in the early weeks after the operation. A basic schedule arranges for the first biopsy at about 8–10 days after operation. After this, biopsies are taken at 10–15-day intervals over the first 6 weeks, followed by another 6 weeks of biopsies at 20-day intervals. After this, until the first anniversary, biopsies are done at the fourth and sixth months, and thereafter on an annual basis. Warnecke, Schueler and Hetzer (1987) have advocated biopsies every 10–12 weeks in the second year, as 16% of them produce positive results. Obviously if there are clinical suspicions of acute rejection, then biopsies are taken as a matter of urgency. These suspicions include fever, dysrhythmia, drop in summated ECG voltages, increasing weight, oedema and dyspnoea.

The biopsy schedule outlined above is not fixed, but is a balance struck between the number of patients being monitored and the available resources for undertaking the monitoring. In assessing resolution of a rejection episode, it is unlikely that biopsies at less than 3-day intervals will show any detectable change. However, if an evolving rejection is suspected but the first biopsy is equivocal, a repeat biopsy the following day may well be diagnostic. It is very likely that the methods of monitoring rejection described in Chapter 14 will prove to be better guides as to when to take a biopsy than reliance on a standard routine.

Grading of rejection severity

Although the rejection reaction is a continuous spectrum from no rejection to severe lethal rejection, it is useful to have a grading system. The most widely used is that of Billingham which was introduced by Caves *et al.* (1974) in which the rejection reaction was graded as mild, moderate or severe. Later, she modified the grading system by adding a 'resolving' category (Billingham, 1979). The essential feature of the moderate grade is the presence of damaged myocytes, while in the severe grade neutrophils are present and there may also be interstitial haemorrhages in addition to the myocyte necrosis. Rose *et al.* (1978) used a 9-point scale to grade rejection, points 3, 6 and 9 corresponding to Billingham's mild, moderate and severe grades at their upper ends. Stovin (1984) made a slight modification to Billingham's 1979 grading by introducing a minimal rejection grade, feeling that this might give some reassurance against over-immunosuppression.

Ueda *et al.* (1985) studied 13 parameters in heterotopically transplanted hearts in rats, grading each parameter on a 0–3 + or 4 + scale in order to see which were the more important. The results, while similar to the human experience, differed in showing an early infiltration of veins and arteries. However, these animals were immunosuppressed only for a short time after the operation, at which the donor heart was connected to the abdominal aorta and IVC. The lack of continuous immunosuppression and the different vascular connections may account for the venous and arterial reactions in the rats, which are only rarely seen in man.

Other systems used in man have been described by Cooper *et al.* (1982), Sibley *et al.* (1986) and Ratliff *et al.* (1987). Cooper *et al.* (1982) used a summation of the individual 0–3 scores on each of 5 histological features, a score of 2.5–4 indicating moderate rejection and any score over 4 representing severe rejection. With such a small scoring margin between mild and serious degrees of rejection, there seems little point in using a rather complex scoring system. Ratliff *et al.* (1987) have used a 7-point scale and regard the myocyte damage as reversible and recommend plastic embedded sections for its detection. The scoring of cytological preparations is given by Topalidis *et al.* (1986) and depends on the recognition of damaged myocytes for the diagnosis of moderate rejection. In contrast to other workers, Sibley *et al.* (1986) found myocyte necrosis difficult to assess and preferred to rely on the intensity of the lymphocytic infiltrate to grade the severity of rejection.

The grading system of Margaret Billingham as modified by Pomerance

TABLE 15.2
Diagnostic Grades of Acute Cell-Mediated Rejection as Seen in Endomyocardial Biopsies*

Grade	*Microscopical Features*
Minimal	A few pyroninophilic cells, either endocardial or interstitial, present in only a few adjacent sections; the biopsy otherwise normal
Mild	Scattered foci of interstitial, perivascular or endocardial pyroninophilic mononuclear cells in many sections. Interstitial oedema. No damage to myocytes
Moderate	More intense infiltration than in mild grade, with damage to single or small groups of myocytes
Severe	Increased cellular infiltration with neutrophils or haemorrhages or both. Larger groups of myocytes showing damage
Resolving	Remaining mononuclear cells are smaller and mostly non-pyroninophilic. Decreasing cellular infiltrate may be accompanied by or replaced by active fibrosis, scarring and lipochrome pigment in macrophages

* Based on Pomerance and Stovin (1985).

and Stovin (1985) is shown in Table 15.2 and the histological appearances are illustrated in Figs 15.4–15.9.

The determination of myocyte necrosis is a crucial feature in the diagnosis of the level of rejection which requires some modification of the immunosuppression. Reemtsma *et al.* (1985) and Herskowitz *et al.* (1987) have recommended that two pathologists should agree on the presence of myocyte damage before accepting the diagnosis of moderate rejection. Care has to be exercised that cells overlapping the myocyte are not interpreted as within the myocyte. Cells within a myocyte are certain evidence that it is damaged. This diagnostic problem is resolvable if serial sections are available. Serial sections also help to distinguish genuine fragmentation of the myocyte from pseudo-fragmentation, which is really oblique cutting of myocytes that are twisted or distorted by the interstitial oedema. Contraction bands can also give a false appearance of myocyte damage. These are in reality good indicators of well-functioning muscle and if they are absent from the biopsy, one should suspect ischaemic damage.

Billingham (1979) advocates Masson's trichrome stain for detecting myocyte damage. Graham and Paplanus (1985) advocated the use of fluor-

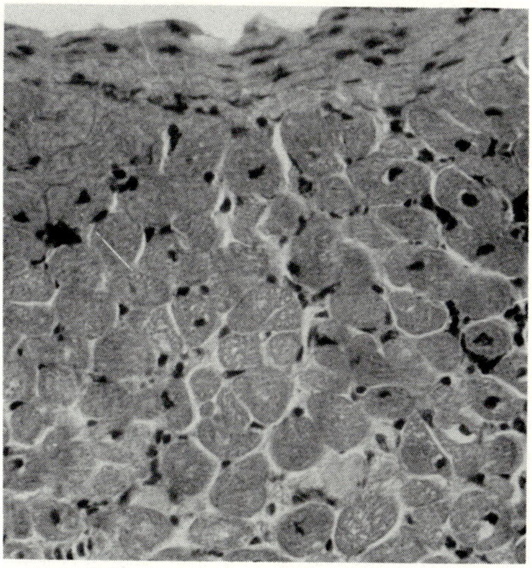

Fig. 15.4 *Minimal rejection. Endocardium at top. A few dark lymphocytes present in the position of the perimyocyte capillaries. HPS ×270.*

escence for detecting early myocyte damage in rejection. Al-Rufaie, Florio and Olsen (1983) showed that fluorescence was comparable in specificity and sensitivity to the haematoxylin-basic fuchsin–picric acid (HBFP) method for detecting early myocardial infarction. The advantage of the fluorescence method is that it is done on the same haematoxylin and eosin stained sections as the routine light microscopy and does not depend on the very carefully controlled conditions required to get reproducible results with the Masson or HBFP stains.

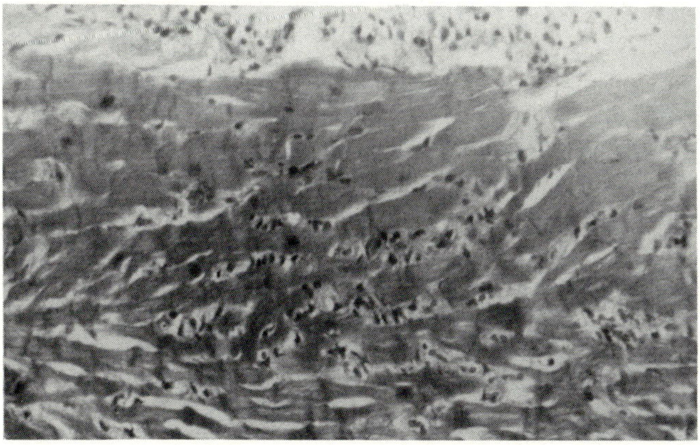

Fig. 15.5. *Mild rejection. Lymphocytic infiltrate focally in myocardium and in the endocardium (top). HPS ×225.*

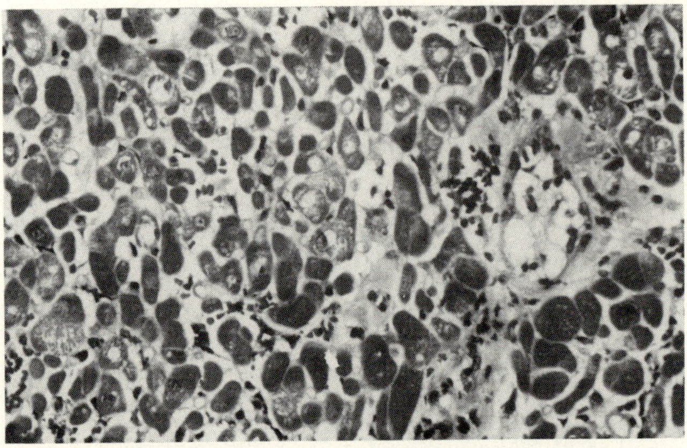

Fig. 15.6. *More cellular but still mild rejection. HPS ×290.*

Because rejection is not absolutely uniformly distributed throughout the myocardium, it is necessary to report the rejection grade for each separate biopsy. In this way, the clinician has an indication of not only the maximum and minimum intensity of the rejection but also the degree of uniformity of its distribution. As part of a research project (Daracott-Cankovic *et al.*, 1984), we have had occasion to examine 751 biopsies separately and independently from the routine biopsies. In 30 instances, moderate rejection, which had not been evident in the three biopsies taken for the routine histology, was found.

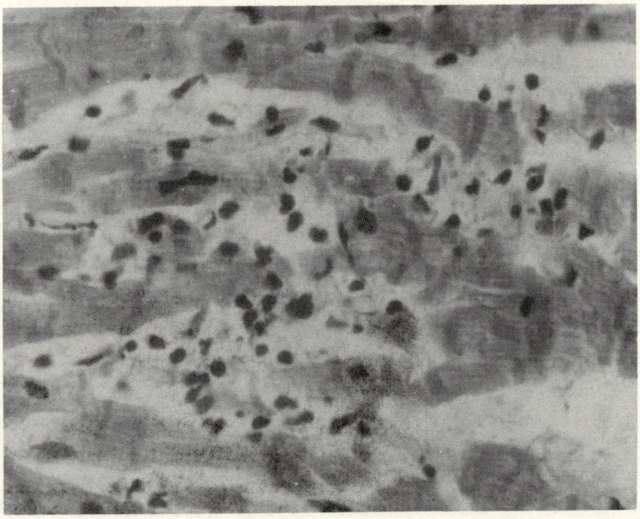

Fig. 15.7. *Moderate rejection. Note the occasional lymphocyte within a myocyte and the disruption of a few myocytes. HPS ×510.*

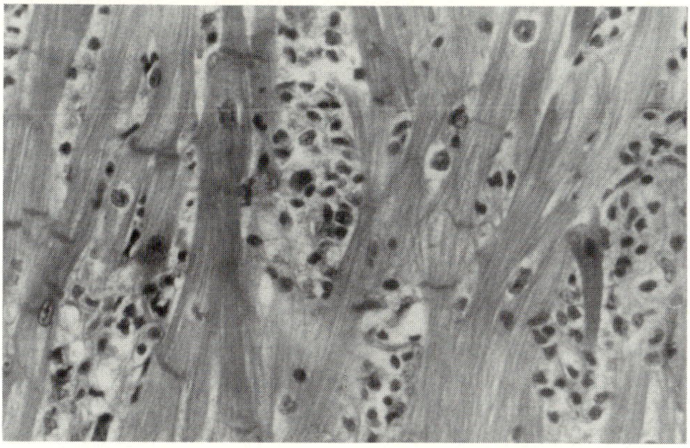

Fig. 15.8. *Severe rejection. This is similar to Fig. 15.7 but neutrophils are present. H & E ×345.*

In only 2 out of the 30 instances had immunosuppression been increased on clinical suspicion. The remaining 28 had no alteration to their therapy. These 26 patients (Table 15.3) did no worse than the 95 with the 721 concordant biopsies. Thus it would seem that an increase in immunosuppression may possibly not be necessary unless half or more of the biopsies show the presence of moderate rejection. However, the finding of severe rejection or of vascular rejection is an urgent indication for a major increase in immunosuppression.

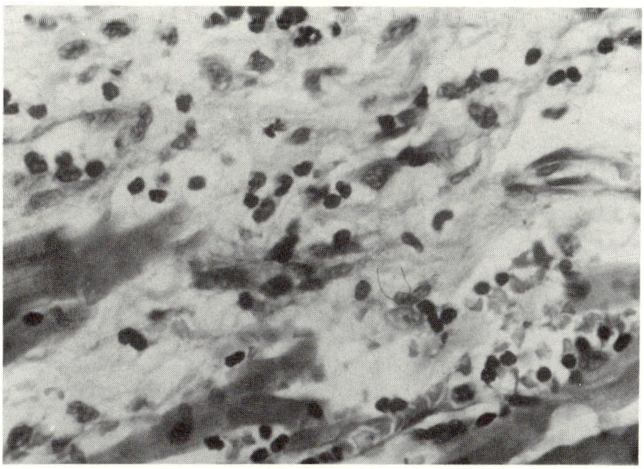

Fig. 15.9. *Severe rejection showing neutrophils, a small interstitial haemorrhage (lower right) and a damaged vessel (in centre). HPS ×410.*

TABLE 15.3
Missed Moderate Rejection Detected on Late Reported Fourth Biopsy Bite

Group	*Patients*	*Biopsy Occasions*
A. Moderate rejection present but missed on the 3 bites reported	26	30
Not treated	24	28
Surviving (121–1274 days)	22	
B. Moderate rejection not missed on the 3 bites reported	95	721
Surviving (121–2283 days)	70	
Total	121	751

Although this chapter is not primarily concerned with heart–lung transplantation, it is of interest that the endomyocardial biopsies of heart–lung transplant recipients have shown noticeably less severe grades of rejection than their heart transplant contemporaries (Table 15.4). Imakita, Tazelaar and Billingham (1986) have also observed this phenomenon. Prop *et al.* (1985) have demonstrated experimentally in rats reasons why the lungs reject more actively than the heart, relating it mainly to the amount of immunologically active material in the lung compared with the heart. Alternatively, it may be that the immunologically activated T cells get taken up by the transplanted lungs before they reach the heart.

TABLE 15.4
Effect of Transplanted Lung on Heart Rejection Grade

	Heart–Lung Transplant	*Heart Transplant*
No. of cases	11	11
No. of biopsies	76	85
Rejection grade:		
none	34	15
minimal	27	22
mild	14	39
moderate	1	9
severe	0	0

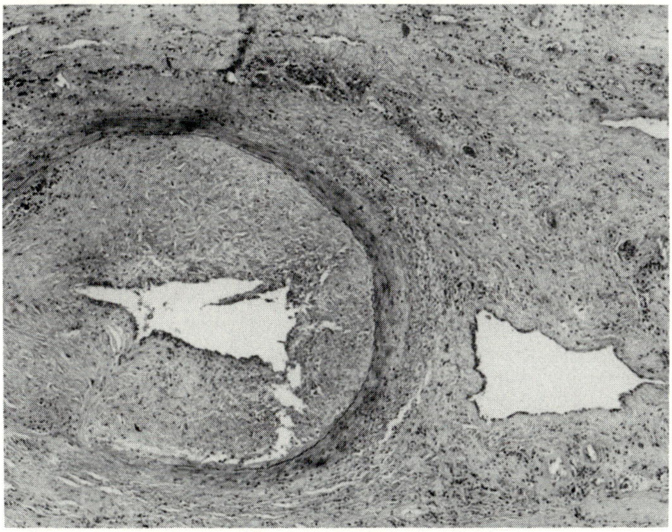

Fig. 15.10. *Chronic rejection. Note the severe stenosis of the epicardial coronary artery without intimal change in the accompanying thin-walled vein. El & vG ×55.*

Chronic vascular rejection affects the epicardial coronary arteries and as such is not amenable to direct biopsy assessment. This does not mean that it is not an important cause of donor organ failure, only that its early diagnosis is very difficult. As the arteries are affected by a fairly uniform intimal fibrocellular thickening along their length, it is the small (1–2 mm diameter) branches (Figs 15.10 and 15.11) that are proportionately more severely narrowed than the main named branches. This means that angiographic visualization is not easy and chronic rejection has to be inferred from slow flow of the contrast medium. In endomyocardial biopsies, the inference can be drawn from grouped areas of ischaemic vacuolation or loss of contraction band formation. Functional histological studies (Darracott-Cankovic *et al.*, 1984) may prove to be the most sensitive method for detecting chronic rejection. It is not known at present if this chronic rejection reaction is related to the development of accelerated atheroma in the coronary arteries. Hess *et al.* (1983) have related the development of accelerated atheroma to the combination of hyperlipidaemia and cytotoxic B-cell antibodies.

Over-immunosuppression

Emphasis has so far been placed on the detection of, and assessing the severity of, rejection. However, it is important to avoid over-immunosuppression of the patient. The endomyocardial biopsy can at times give some useful

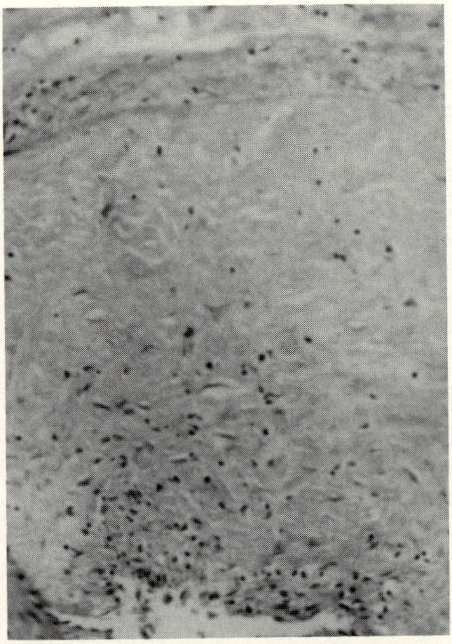

Fig. 15.11. *Chronic rejection with still continuing lymphocytic infiltrate on the inner aspect of the grossly thickened intima. HPS ×140.*

clues. The absence of any sign of rejection in all the biopsy bites is one such clue. Serial sections are necessary so that the occasional very small scattered focus of minimal rejection is not missed.

Over-immunosuppression may result from over-enthusiastic reporting of grade of rejection. Recently, Billingham (1986) has drawn attention to a particular type of florid tumour-like lymphocytic endocardial infiltrate (Fig. 15.12) that is not accompanied by an equally intense myocardial infiltrate in any of the biopsy bites. Like her, we have seen this phenomenon in Cy-treated patients. It does not seem to be associated with clinical symptoms or signs of rejection, and it clears without special treatment. Usually at the base of this type of lesion there is a minimal degree of infiltration of the myocardium, with apparent disruption of one or two myocytes. The nature of this lesion is uncertain, but it would seem unwise to grade it as a moderate rejection. For ease of reference, Billingham refers to it as the 'Quilty effect', after the first patient to show it (M. E. Billingham, personal communication, 1986).

If there is any evidence of an infection in the myocardium, it is likely that the patient is over-immunosuppressed, and any inflammatory cellular infiltrate is most likely to be a reaction to the infection and not to rejection. Lymphomas are also evidence of over-immunosuppression and they may

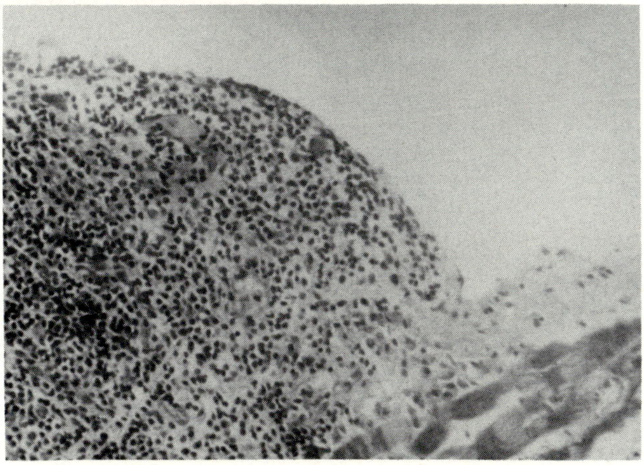

Fig. 15.12. *Endocardial tumour-like lymphocytic infiltrate of the 'Quilty' effect. HPS ×150.*

involve the heart. Neither infection nor lymphoma has been implicated in the nodular endocardial 'Quilty' infiltrate (Billingham, 1986), although in one of our patients who has an Epstein–Barr virus infection with a lymphoma, there was a tumour-like endocardial lymphomatous infiltrate that cleared after treatment with acyclovir. The cells in this infiltrate were quite obviously not the mature lymphocytes of the benign 'Quilty' change.

The characteristic nuclear changes of cytomegalovirus (CMV) or the intracytoplasmic cysts of *Toxoplasma* (Figs 15.13 and 15.14) are diagnostic.

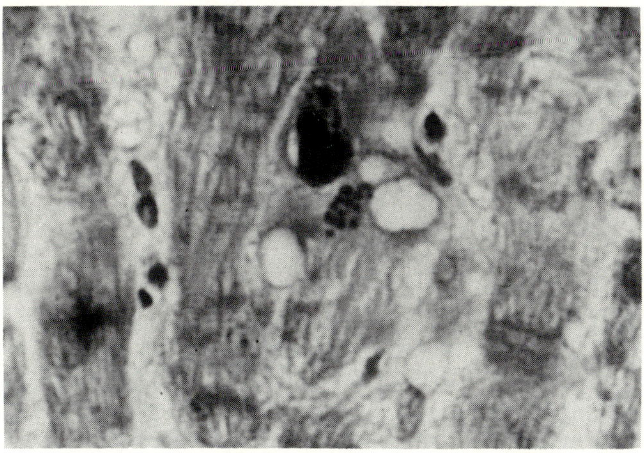

Fig. 15.13. *CMV intranuclear inclusion with clump of haematoxyphil granules below the nucleus. These are too large to be* Toxoplasma, *from which this patient also suffered. Note the absence of inflammatory cellular reaction. HPS ×700.*

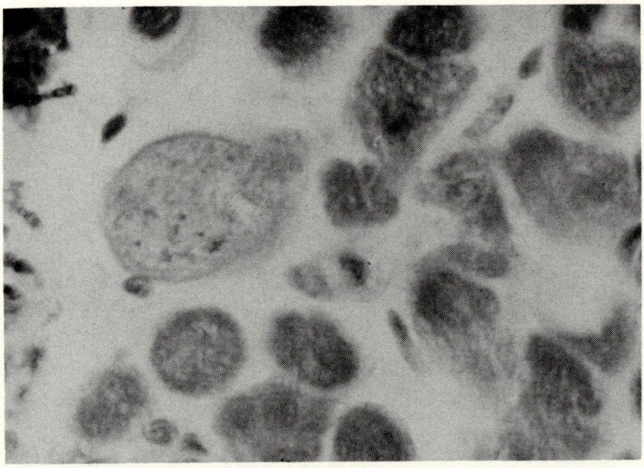

Fig. 15.14. Toxoplasma *cyst. Same biopsy as Fig. 15.13. HPS* × *700.*

This requires diligent searching of all the serial sections made from each biopsy bite, because an infected nucleus or a cyst may well only be present in two adjacent serial sections. A histological indicator for undertaking this intensive search is the finding of damaged myocytes that are not accompanied by an inflammatory cellular reaction. In the discussion on the rejection process, it was pointed out that myocyte damage is the result of a developed rejection reaction. In the case of myocardial infection, the myocyte damage often precedes the inflammatory reaction and in a part of the biopsy one may be lucky enough to see this clue. Other clues to possible *Toxoplasma* infection are interstitial eosinophils and the presence of fibrotic replacement of occasional individual myocytes (McGregor *et al.*, 1984).

In most cases it seems likely that the infection is transmitted with the donor heart (Hakim *et al.*, 1985b) because before transplantation antibodies to the infecting organism are present in the donor but not in the recipient. The possibility that the infection has been transmitted in the transfused blood is not absolutely excluded, but is unlikely (McGregor *et al.*, 1984). These infections usually occur in the period 20–120 days after the operation. There may well be other organisms besides CMV and *Toxoplasma* that can be transmitted with the donor heart, but these two are the best established.

When appropriate treatment for infection with over-immunosuppression has been given, it is necessary to take biopsies to see if rejection is occurring, or if the infection is not responding. This is a difficult histological problem. The amount of cell damage and the intensity and nature of the cellular infiltrate has to be compared very critically with that found in the biopsies at the time of diagnosis. As a working hypothesis, if the necrosis has increased but the cellular element has stayed about the same, then the infection is still active. If the reverse holds, then rejection is likely.

Stovin (1984) raised the possibility that some viral infections of the myocardium might mimic moderate rejection histologically. With further experience, no evidence has emerged to link either primary or reactivated CMV infection with a moderate rejection reaction. However, in a few cases the serological evidence of active infection has followed energetic treatment of moderate rejection.

An important indicator of over-immunosuppression is respiratory opportunistic infection. The infecting organisms and the methods of making the diagnosis have been reviewed by Warren and Newsom (1984) and Matthay and Moritz (1981), and are discussed in Chapter 13.

Cyclosporin effect

Billingham (1981, 1986) has drawn attention to a fine interstitial oedema with cellular infiltration, progressing to an interstitial fibrosis, which is seen in Cy-treated patients but not in those treated before the introduction of this drug. Further, there is the tumour-like endocardial lymphocytic infiltrate of benign nature that has been seen only in Cy-treated patients. Interestingly, Pomerance and Stovin (1985) and Karch and Billingham (1985) have each reported that in heterotopic transplantation it is only the donor and not the recipient heart that has shown the Cy type of fine interstitial fibrosis. This may in fact be related to the slow resolution of rejection seen with Cy (Billingham, 1986). It is probable that this fine fibrosis is not due primarily to the lymphatic obstruction, as the change was not seen in transplanted hearts prior to the introduction of Cy.

Our own studies (P. G. I. Stovin and T. A. H. English, 1987) show that a mild degree of interstitial oedema is seen more frequently with Cy than with the earlier anti-rejection regimens. This oedema is augmented by the oedema of rejection (Table 15.5). An occasional neutrophil may also be present in the Cy oedema. In our experience, eosinophils have been seen more often in patients receiving anti-thymocyte globulin (ATG) than in those given Cy. On the other hand, Billingham has encountered eosinophils as an apparent response to Cy or in the inflammatory response to *Toxoplasma* infection.

The slow course of resolution of rejection, and the development of interstitial fibrosis after about 6 months on Cy immunosuppression, have also been reported by Devineni *et al.* (1983). Billingham (1986) has also commented on the slow evolution of rejection under Cy treatment. However, we have experienced a few cases of rapidly progressing cellular rejection with this drug. These different experiences may be due to different methods of assessing therapeutic Cy levels in the blood.

TABLE 15.5
*Effect of Cyclosporin on Heart Weight**

Group	Non-cyclosporin No.	Non-cyclosporin Weight	Cyclosporin No.	Cyclosporin Weight
Liver transplants (patient's own heart)	4	242 (200–310)	5	341 (219–440)
Heart transplants:				
non-rejectors	8	405 (240–510)	15	483 (310–650)
rejectors	13	483 (360–670)	23	554 (380–800)

* Mean heart weight in grams (range). The differences in heart weights between all pairs of Cy and non-Cy and between rejectors and non-rejectors in each treatment category are significant, $p < 0.05$.

That different Cy therapeutic regimens do have different effects has been documented for the rejection histology (Imakita, Tazelaar and Billingham, 1986) and for the neurological complications of heart transplantation (Warnecke *et al.*, 1987).

PROBLEMS FROM MULTIPLE BIOPSIES

Previous biopsy sites

With the repeated endomyocardial biopsies it is not surprising that from time to time a current biopsy includes part of a previous biopsy site and this event is more likely, reaching 69%, if up to 8 bites are taken at a session (Sibley *et al.*, 1986). It is important to recognize this and not mistake the traumatic cellular reaction and damaged myocytes for moderate or severe rejection, or for infection. Generally, the immediately sub-endocardial myocytes are arranged parallel to the endocardial surface and there is a thin layer of well-ordered collagen fibrils in the endocardium. Fibrin is seen in or on the endocardial collagen, with some swelling, haemorrhage and disruption if the biopsy is from the same site as another biopsy at the same session. The thrombus-filled biopsy site becomes organized, and a variable degree of cellular infiltrate is found in the proliferating fibroblasts. This infiltrate has a predominance of lymphocytes, which show an appreciable degree of pyroninophilia. As organization proceeds, the lymphocytes decrease and macrophages with some haemosiderin and lipofuchsin pigment in their cytoplasm become more evident. Finally, a fibrotic scar is left. The myocytes will

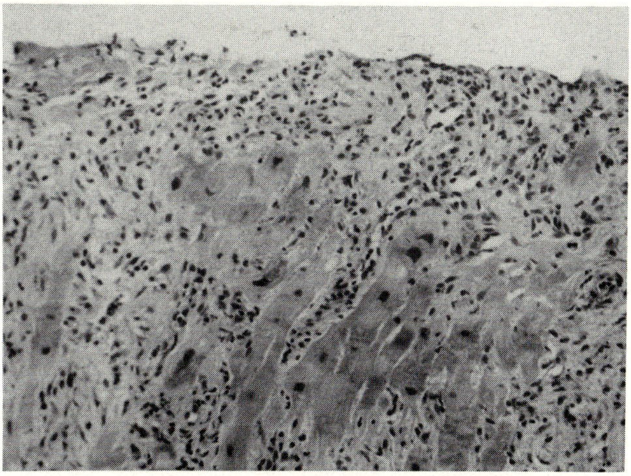

Fig. 15.15. *Previous biopsy site. Damaged endocardium at top with myocytes appearing to run into the re-forming endocardium. The lymphocytic infiltrate cannot be interpreted as rejection. HPS ×125.*

now, because the superficial layer has been removed, show an appearance of running into the repaired endocardium (Fig. 15.15).

Because the cellular infiltrate is predominantly lymphocytic, and because the biopsy bites are often of uncertain orientation, previous biopsy sites pose a diagnostic difficulty. Serial sections very materially help to resolve this difficulty by allowing one to follow the lesion until it reaches the endocardial surface. They may also show the tell-tale endocardial fibrin or arrangement of myocytes running perpendicularly into the endocardial surface.

In occasional patients, the bioptome has a marked tendency to contact the same site, so that every third bite may be from a previous site (Stovin, 1984). Usually, a previous biopsy site is encountered about every 15th to 20th bite.

Vascular trauma

Every so often a biopsy bite will include an intramyocardial arteriole up to 150–200 μm diameter. A record should be made of this because at a later date a biopsy with ischaemic vacuolation or sub-endocardial ischaemic fibrosis may be encountered. If no arterioles have been biopsied on previous occasions, these ischaemic changes are indicative of either acute vascular rejection or of chronic rejection, as in the case of Palmer *et al.* (1985). If, however, arterioles have been recorded in earlier biopsies, the ischaemic changes are likely to be the result of this prior vascular damage.

Occasionally, one encounters a whorled group of small myocytes with a multidirectional arrangement of the cells, the focus looking like a miniature or atrophic group of hypertrophic cardiomyopathic myocytes. Whether these are regenerating myocytes or a form of focal ischaemic atrophy is uncertain, but these foci are found adjacent to previous biopsy sites, and in some cases an arteriole was recorded in a previous biopsy. Wilcken, Shorey and Eikens (1970) showed nearly 20 years ago that regeneration can occur following experimental infarction in the dog heart.

Right coronary to right ventricular fistula has been encountered at Papworth in 5 patients (G. I. Verney, personal communication, 1985) and one of these patients has come to necropsy. In that case there was (Fig. 15.16) a sub-endocardial arteriovenous fistula with endocardial rupture. In one other patient, one biopsy bite has shown a similar vascularity and fibrosis of the endocardium at a previous biopsy site. None of these patients was symptomatic and a faint murmur was heard in only one. It is conceivable that this fistula could become the site of bacterial endocarditis, but so far this has not been encountered. Interestingly, at necropsy our patient had bacterial endocarditis on his mitral valve.

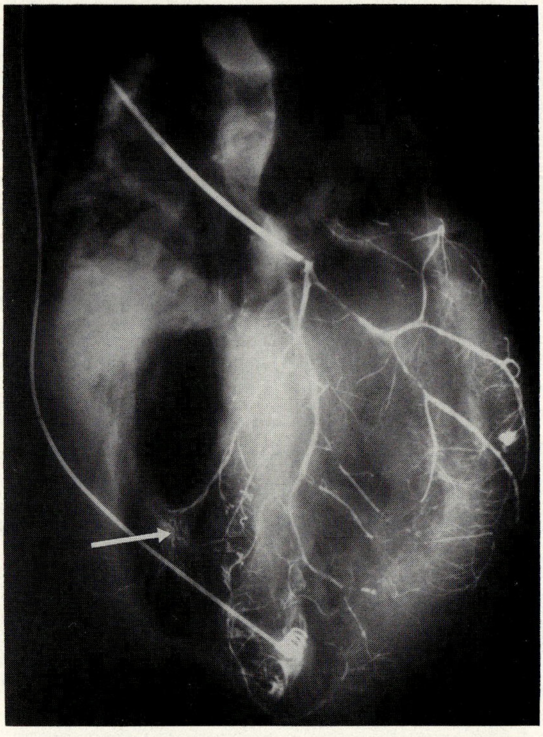

Fig. 15.16. *Left coronary–right ventricle fistula. Post-mortem angiogram. The poor filling of the coronary artery was due to the rapid flow of contrast from the fistula (arrow).*

OTHER PROBLEMS OF BIOPSIES

Donor heart preservation

In the first 7–10 days after any operation the tissues show oedema, neutrophil invasion and some haemorrhage. The transplanted heart is no exception. Caution is therefore needed in interpreting an initial biopsy as moderate or severe rejection, and it is better to rely on the intensity of the lymphocytic infiltrate. Intravascular thrombi are not normally encountered as part of the operative trauma picture, and they are indicative of serious acute vascular rejection.

The donor heart may be sub-optimally preserved or may have had some inotropic support prior to transplantation (Darracott-Cankovic *et al.*, 1987). In these circumstances, small foci of ischaemic damage are found in the myocardial biopsies. Their degree of organization is consistent with the time since the transplant operation, and by the time of the first or second myocardial biopsies any acute cellular component to the inflammatory reaction has usually largely subsided.

Inadequate donor heart preservation may also mean that repeated defibrillation was necessary at the completion of the operation. This can damage the sub-epicardial myocytes (Doherty *et al.*, 1979). Again, the grouped nature of the myocyte damage, the epicardial position and the histological age of the lesion should allow ready distinction from rejection.

An occasional finding is calcification of individual myocytes, which because of the absence of inflammatory or fibrotic response is difficult to date (McKinney, 1974; McLure *et al.*, 1981). It may possibly antedate the episode causing the brain-stem death of the donor, but is more likely to reflect some ischaemic or toxic myocyte membrane damage occurring at or about the time of the transplant. This change can develop rapidly (Hermann, Haupt and Birkhead, 1963) and may be progressive (Pardo-Mindan *et al.*, 1986).

If the donor heart is damaged or has some unsuspected disease such as myocarditis, a moderately stenotic coronary artery, anomalous coronary sinus drainage, etc., the myocardium is more oedematous than is the case with an entirely normal donor heart. Thus, when the first rejection episode occurs, with its additional oedema, the myocardial diastolic compliance will be very seriously reduced and may even lead to death, even though the rejection score has not yet achieved a moderate grade. This additive effect of two or more factors, each of which independently reduces diastolic compliance, has already been touched on in connection with Cy. It has also been seen when the donor heart has been labouring against the recipient's moderately increased pulmonary vascular resistance (Pomerance and Stovin, 1985).

Positioning of the bioptome

On most occasions the operator can judge the position of the instrument using single plane radiological screening with or without ECG monitoring. However, it does rarely happen that the biopsy bite is taken from the atrial suture line, the coronary sinus, the tricuspid chordae, or even the liver. This organ is biopsied more frequently if no radiological screening is used, but biopsies taken blindly may be necessary as an emergency procedure. None of these aberrant sites yields material that is useful for the diagnosis of rejection.

The bioptome may reach the epicardial fat on some occasions. The cellular infiltrate in the fatty tissue tends to persist longer than in the myocardium, and the fat cells damaged during the operation or by rejection appear to take a long time to recover or to be replaced by fibrous tissue. Over this period, they seem to encourage a lymphocytic reaction. The epicardium is therefore not reliable material for grading rejection.

The chief complication of endomyocardial biopsy is pneumothorax. This is not common, but it occurs when there is difficulty in finding or entering the internal jugular vein or superior vena cava. When it does occur, it is more troublesome than serious.

Cooper *et al.* (1982) have pointed out that there is a greater risk of introducing infection if a femoral site is used for inserting the bioptome than if the supraclavicular route is chosen.

Recipient compliance

Endomyocardial biopsy is an uncomfortable procedure, and for the first few times the patient is often apprehensive. The procedure is not tolerated by infants and young children unless they are anaesthetized, and even some adults refuse to undergo it. Patient compliance would not be a problem if there were non-invasive methods for detecting early changes in the myocardium, so that biopsy could be reserved for distinguishing between rejection and infection in the myocardium. Non-invasive methods which have potential for detecting rejection are reviewed in Chapter 14.

REFERENCES

Al-Rufaie, H. K., Florio, R. A. and Olsen, E. G. J. (1983). Comparison of the haematoxylin basic fuchsin picric acid method and the fluorescence of haematoxylin and eosin stained sections for the identification of early myocardial infarction. *J. Clin. Path.* **36**, 646–649.

Baandrup, U., Florio, R. A. and Olsen, E. G. J. (1982). Do endomyocardial biopsies represent the morphology of the rest of the myocardium? A quantitative light microscopic study of single v. multiple biopsies with the King's bioptome. *Eur. Heart J.* **3**, 171–178.

Barnard, C. N. (1967). A human cardiac transplant: an interim report of a successful operation performed at the Groote Schuur Hospital, Cape Town. *S. Afr. Med. J.* **41**, 1257–1274.

Bieber, C. P., Griepp, R. B., Oyer, P. E., David, L. A. and Stinson, E. B. (1977). Relationship of rabbit ATG serum clearance rate to circulating T-cell level, rejection onset, and survival in cardiac transplantation. *Transplant. Proc.* **9**, 1031–1036.

Billingham, M. E. (1979). Progress in human pathology. Some recent advances in cardiac pathology. *Hum. Path.* **10**, 367–386.

Billingham, M. E. (1981). Diagnosis of cardiac rejection by endomyocardial biopsy. *Heart Transplant.* **1**, 25–30.

Billingham, M. E. (1986). Endomyocardial biopsy detection of acute rejection in cardiac allograft recipients. *Heart Vess.* **1**, Suppl. 1, 86–90.

Brasile, L., Zerbe, T., Rabin, B., Clarke, J., Abrams, A. and Cerilli, J. (1985). Identification of the antibody to vascular endothelial cells in patients undergoing cardiac transplantation. *Transplantation* **40**, 672–675.

Caves, P. K., Stinson, E. B., Billingham, M. E., Rider, A. K. and Shumway, N. E. (1973a). Diagnosis of human cardiac allograft rejection by serial cardiac biopsy. *J. Thorac. Cardiovasc. Surg.* **66**, 461–466.

Caves, P. K., Stinson, E. B., Billingham, M. E., and Shumway, N. E. (1974). Serial transvenous biopsy of the transplanted human heart. Improved management of acute rejection episodes. *Lancet* **1**, 821–826.

Caves, P. K., Stinson, E. B., Billingham, M. E., and Shumway, N. E. (1975). Transvenous intracardiac biopsy using a new catheter forceps. *Heart Lung* **4**, 69–74.

Caves, P. K., Stinson, E. B., Graham, A. F., Billingham, M. E., Grehl, T. M. and Shumway, N. E. (1973b). Percutaneous transvenous endomyocardial biopsy. *J. Am. Med. Ass.* **225**, 288–291.

Cooper, D. K. C., Charles, R. G., Fraser, R. C., Beck, W. and Barnard, C. N. (1980). Long-term survival after orthotopic and heterotopic cardiac transplantation. *Br. Med. J.* **281**, 1093–1096.

Cooper, D. K. C., Fraser, R. C., Rose, A. G., Ayzenberg, O., Oldfield, G. S., Hassoulas, J., Novitzky, D., Uys, C. J. and Barnard, C. N. (1982). Technique, complications, and clinical value of endomyocardial biopsy in patients with heterotopic heart transplants. *Thorax* **37**, 727–731.

Darracott-Cankovic, S., English, T., Cory-Pearce, R. and Stovin, P. (1984). Quantitative birefringence measurements in cardiac transplantation. *Eur. Heart J.* **5**, 200.

Darracott-Cankovic, S., Wheeldon, D., Cory-Pearce, R., Wallwork, J. and English, T. A. H. (1987). Biopsy assessment of 50 hearts during transplantation. *J. Thorac. Cardiovasc. Surg.* **93**, 95–102.

Devineni, R., Keown, P., McKenzie, N., Stiller, C., Kostuk, W. J., Silver, M. D. and Heimbecker, R. O. (1983). Cyclosporine in cardiac transplantation: observations on immunologic monitoring, cardiac histology, and cardiac function. *Heart Transplant.* **2**, 219–223.

Doherty, P. W., McLaughlin, P. R., Billingham, M., Kernoff, R., Goris, M. L. and

Harrison, D. C. (1979). Cardiac damage produced by direct current countershock applied to the heart. *Am. J. Cardiol.* **43**, 225–232.

Duquesnoy, R. J., Zeevi, A., Fung, J. J., Kaufman, C., Zerbe, T. R., Griffith, B., Trento, A., Kormos, R. and Herdesty, R. (1987). Sequential infiltration of Class I and Class II specific alloreactive T cells in human cardiac allografts. *Transplant. Proc.* **19**, 2560–2563.

Graham, A. R. and Paplanus, S. H. (1985). Fluorescence of damaged myocardium in endomyocardial biopsy specimens for the evaluation of cardiac transplantation. *Hum. Path.* **16**, 1110–1114.

Griepp, R. B., Stinson, E. B., Bieber, C. P., Oyer, P. E., Reitz, B. A., Copeland, J. G. and Shumway, N. E. (1977). Increasing patient survival following heart transplantation. *Transplant. Proc.* **9**, 197–201.

Hakim, M., White, D. J. G., Cory-Pearce, R., English, T. A. H. and Wallwork, J. (1985a). Is cyclosporine's nephrotoxicity related to its immunosuppressive effectiveness? *Heart Transplant.* **4**, 217–219.

Hakim, M., Wreghitt, T. G., English, T. A. H., Stovin, P. G. I., Cory-Pearce, R. and Wallwork, J. (1985b). Significance of donor transmitted disease in cardiac transplantation. *Heart Transplant.* **4**, 302–305.

Hermann, G. III, Haupt, G. J. and Birkhead, N. C. (1963). Rapid myocardial calcification after cardiac surgery. *J. Am. Med. Ass.*, **186**, 260–261.

Herskowitz, A., Soule, L. M., Mellits, E. D., Traill, T. A., Achuff, S. C., Reitz, B. A., Borkon, A. M., Baumgartner, W. A. and Baughman, K. L. (1987). Histologic predictors of acute cardiac rejection in human endomyocardial biopsies: a multivariate analysis. *J. Am. Coll. Cardiol.* **9**, 802–810.

Hess, M. J., Hastillo, A., Mohanakumar, T., Cowley, M. J., Vetrovac, G., Szentpetery, S., Wolfgang, T. C. and Lower, R. R. (1983). Accelerated atherosclerosis in cardiac transplantation: role of cytotoxic B-cell antibodies and hyperlipidemia. *Circulation* **68**, Suppl. 2, 94–101.

Imakita, M., Tazelaar, H. D. and Billingham, M. E. (1986). Heart allograft rejection under varying immunosuppressive protocols as evaluated by endomyocardial biopsy. *J. Heart Transplant.* **5**, 279–285.

Joyce, L. D., Johnson, K. E., Pierce, W. S., DeVries, W. C., Semb, B. K. H., Copeland, J. G., Griffith, B. P., Cooley, D. A., Frazier, O. H., Cabrol, C., Keon, W. J., Unger, F., Bucherl, E. S. and Wolner, E. (1986). Summary of the world experience with clinical use of total artificial hearts as heart support devices. *J. Heart Transplant.* **5**, 229–235.

Karch, S. B. and Billingham, M. E. (1985). Cyclosporine induced myocardial fibrosis: a unique controlled case report. *Heart Transplant.* **4**, 210–212.

Lanza, R. P., Campbell, E. M., Cooper, D. K. C., DuToit, E. D. and Barnard, C. N. (1983). The problem of the presensitized heart transplant recipient. *Heart Transplant.* **2**, 151–154.

Matthay, R. A. and Moritz, E. D. (1981). Invasive procedures for diagnosing pulmonary infection. A critical review. *Clin. Chest Med.* **2**, 3–18.

McClure, J., Pieterse, A. S., Pounder, D. J. and Smith, P. S. (1981). Myocardial fibre calcification. *J. Clin. Path.* **34**, 1167–1174.

McGregor, C. G. A., Fleck, D. G., Nagington, J., Stovin, P. G. I., Cory-Pearce, R.

and English, T. A. H. (1984). Disseminated toxoplasmosis in cardiac transplantation. *J. Clin. Path.* **37**, 74–77.

McKinney, B. (1974). *Pathology of the Cardiomyopathies*, pp. 353–355. Butterworths, London.

Oyer, P. E., Stinson, E. B., Jamieson, S. W., Hunt, S. A., Billingham, M., Scott, W., Bieber, C. P., Reitz, B. A. and Shumway, N. E. (1983). Cyclosporin-A in cardiac allografting: a preliminary experience. *Transplant. Proc.* **15**, 1247–1252.

Palmer, D. C., Tsai, C. C., Roodman, S. T., Codd, J. E., Miller, L. W., Sarafian, J. E. and Williams, G. A. (1985). Heart graft arteriosclerosis. An ominous finding on endomyocardial biopsy. *Transplantation* **39**, 385–388.

Pardo-Mindan, F. J., Herreros, J., Marigil, M. A., Arcas, R. and Diez, J. (1986). Myocardial calcification following heart transplantation. *J. Heart Transplant.* **5**, 332–335.

Pomerance, A. and Stovin, P. G. I. (1985). Heart transplant pathology: the British experience. *J. Clin. Path.* **38**, 146–159.

Prop. J., Kuijpers, K., Petersen, A. H., Bartels, H. L., Nieuwenhuis, P. and Wildevuur, C. R. H. (1985). Why are lung allografts more vigorously rejected than hearts? *Heart Transplant.* **4**, 433–436.

Rabin, B. S. (1983). Immunologic aspects of human cardiac transplantation. *Heart Transplant.* **2**, 188–191.

Ratliff, N. B., Myles, J. L., McMahon, J. T., Golding, L., Hobbs, R., Rincon, G., Sterba, R. and Stewart, R. (1987). Myocyte injury in acute cardiac transplant rejection and in lymphocytic myocarditis is similar and reversible. *Transplant. Proc.* **19**, 2568–2572.

Reemtsma, K., Hardy, M. A., Drusin, R. E., Smith, C. R. and Rose, E. A. (1985). Cardiac transplantation. Changing patterns in evaluation and treatment. *Ann. Surg.* **202**, 418–423.

Rose, A. G., Losman, J. G. and Barnard, C. N. (1978). Evaluation of endomyocardial biopsy in the diagnosis of cardiac rejection. *Transplantation* **26**, 10–13.

Rose, A. G., Uys, C. J., Losman, J. G. and Barnard, C. N. (1978). Evaluation of endomyocardial biopsy in the diagnosis of cardiac rejection. A study using bioptome samples of formalin fixed tissue. *Transplantation* **26**, 10–13.

Rose, M. L., Gracie, J. A., Fraser, A. K., Chisholm, P. M. and Yacoub, M. H. (1984). Use of monoclonal antibodies to quantitate T lymphocyte subpopulations in human cardiac allografts. *Transplantation* **38**, 230–234.

Sibley, R. K., Olivari, M-T., Bolman, R. M. and Ring, W. S. (1986). Endomyocardial biopsy in the cardiac allograft recipient. A review of 570 biopsies. *Ann. Surg.*, **203**, 177–187.

Spiegelhalter, D. J. and Stovin, P. G. I. (1983). An analysis of repeated biopsies following cardiac transplantation. *Stats. Med.* **2**, 33–40.

Stovin, P. G. I. (1984). The morphology of myocardial rejection and transplant pathology. In *Transplantation Immunology. Clinical and Experimental* (R. Y. Calne, Ed.), pp. 78–100. Oxford University Press, Oxford.

Stovin, P. G. I. and English, T. A. H. (1987). The effect of cyclosporine on the transplanted heart. *J. Heart Transplant.* **6**, 180–185.

Stovin, P. G. I. and Hewitt, S. (1986). Conduction tissue in the transplanted human heart. *J. Path.* **149**, 183–189.

Topalidis, T., Schueler, S., Warnecke, H., Hetzer, R., Lang, W., Atay, Z. and Georgii, A. (1986). Imprint cytology of endomyocardial biopsies — diagnosis of cardiac rejection. *Transplant. Proc.* **18**, 1185–1186.

Ueda, K., Baumgartner, W. A., Beschorner, W. E., Borkon, M. A., Soule, L. M., Reitz, B. R. and Herskowitz, A. (1985). Histologic pattern of early heart allograft rejection under cyclosporine treatment. *Heart Transplant.* **3**, 296–300.

Uys, C. J. and Rose, A. G. (1983). The pathology of cardiac transplantation. In *Cardiovascular Pathology* (M. D. Silver, Ed.), pp. 1329–1352. Churchill Livingstone, New York.

Warnecke, H., Schueler, S. and Hetzer, R. (1987). Late acute rejection after cardiac transplantation: incidence and treatment. *Transplant. Proc.* **19**, 2504–2505.

Warnecke, H., Schueler, S., Schliffka, J. and Hetzer, R. (1987). Neurologic complications after heart transplantation: the influence of immunosuppression. *Transplant. Proc.* **19**, 2510–2512.

Warren, R. E. and Newsom, S. W. B. (1984). Bacterial, fungal, and protozoal infections in immunosuppressed patients. In *Transplantation Immunology. Clinical and Experimental* (R. Y. Calne, Ed.), pp. 518–566. Oxford University Press, Oxford.

Weil, R., Clarke, D. R., Iwaki, Y., Porter, K. A., Koep, L. J., Paton, B. C., Terasaki, P. I. and Starzl, T. E. (1981). Hyperacute rejection of a transplanted human heart. *Transplantation* **32**, 71–72.

Weintraub, D., Masek, M. and Billingham, M. E. (1985). The lymphocyte subpopulations in cyclosporine-treated human heart rejection. *Heart Transplant.* **4**, 213–216.

Wilcken, D. E. L., Shorey, C. D. and Eikens, E. (1970). Ultrastructural evidence for regeneration of heart-muscle cells after experimental myocardial infarction. *Lancet* **2**, 21–23.

T. G. Wreghitt and M. Hakim

16

Donor-Transmitted Disease

INTRODUCTION

In the first few months after heart transplantation, infections and rejection are the major causes of morbidity and mortality (Jamieson *et al.*, 1981; Dummer *et al.*, 1983; Ho *et al.*, 1983). Immunosuppressive agents such as cyclosporin A, azathioprine and anti-thymocyte globulin (ATG), required to subdue the recipient's cellular immune response and thus minimize graft rejection, increase susceptibility to infection with many viruses, bacteria, fungi and protozoa. The increased use of these drugs in rejection crises enhances this problem.

Infections may arise from the following:

(1) Transmission of the organism to the recipient in the donated organ(s).
(2) Transmission of the organism to the recipient in transfused blood or blood products.
(3) Increased susceptibility of the recipient to endogenous organisms, to those commonly found in the environment, and to those acquired by transmission from other persons or even animals.

After primary infection, some organisms such as cytomegalovirus (CMV) and *Toxoplasma gondii* may remain latent in the human host. In certain circumstances, such as immunosuppression, these organisms may reactivate, resulting in another episode of infection. Even so, fatal recrudescence of *T. gondii* has rarely been reported in the absence of other concurrent infections. On the contrary, in patients with some other forms of depressed immunity, as for example in the acquired immunodeficiency syndrome (AIDS), Hodgkin's disease and non-Hodgkin's lymphoma, recrudescent *T. gondii* infection is often life-threatening or fatal (Feldman, 1982; Editorial, 1984).

In addition, reactivated CMV infection may be very serious or even fatal in patients with AIDS.

While hepatitis B virus (HBV) does not usually reactivate, it has been shown that in immunosuppressed renal transplant recipients with evidence of previous HBV infection, HBsAg antigenaemia may return (Nagington, Cossart and Cohen, 1977). Furthermore, asymptomatic infection with human immunodeficiency virus (HIV) may become symptomatic in some individuals receiving immunosuppressive therapy.

In this chapter we shall consider those infections transmitted by routes (1) and (2) above, including CMV, *T. gondii*, HBV and HIV infections, with particular reference to those that have arisen in the first 160 heart and 12 heart–lung transplant recipients at Papworth Hospital, Cambridge.

TOXOPLASMA GONDII

Primary *Toxoplasma gondii* infections in non-immunocompromised patients are often asymptomatic, or manifest in glandular fever-like symptoms, perhaps with lymphadenopathy (Remington, Jacobs and Kaufman, 1960). *T. gondii* infection is usually acquired from undercooked meat containing *T. gondii* cysts, or from contact with cat faeces (Hutchinson *et al.*, 1969; Kean, Kimball and Christenson, 1969). With the exception of transplacental spread from mother to fetus, infection is not usually transmitted from man to man. The apparent transmission of *T. gondii* in leucocyte transfusions to patients with acute leukaemia has been reported (Siegel *et al.*, 1971; Roth *et al.*, 1971). Thorough studies in thalassaemia (Kimball, Kean and Kellner, 1965) and heart transplant patients (Wreghitt *et al.*, 1987) have, however, failed to show primary *T. gondii* infection acquired from blood or blood products, despite the fact that the organism may remain viable for up to 50 days in citrated blood (Talice *et al.*, 1957). In organ transplant recipients most, if not all, primary *T. gondii* infections are acquired from the organs of *T. gondii* seropositive donors.

There have been several reports of primary (or presumed primary) *T. gondii* infections in kidney, liver and heart transplant recipients (Table 16.1).

Stinson *et al.* (1971) reported a fatal case of recrudescent *T. gondii* infection in a heart transplant recipient, although the patient was also concurrently infected with *E. coli, Bacterioides, Aspergillus, Pneumocystis carinii* and CMV, which probably contributed significantly to his death.

The clinical manifestations of primary *T. gondii* infections in immunocompromised patients are highly variable (Ruskin and Remington, 1976). Table 16.2 summarizes the findings in the reported cases in heart transplant recipients, and those of the four cases in the Papworth heart, and heart and lung transplant series. As can be seen from Table 16.2, the most important

TABLE 16.1

Reports of Primary or Presumed Primary Toxoplasma gondii *Infections**

	Kidney Transplants		*Heart Transplants*		*Liver Transplants*
A	Cohen (1970)	B	Hakim *et al.* (1985)	A	Anthony (1972)
	Flament-Durand *et al.* (1967)	B	Hakim *et al.* (1986)		Ruskin and Remington (1976)
	Ghatak, Poon and Zimmerman (1970)	A	Jamieson *et al.* (1981)	A	Schroter *et al.* (1976)
A	Gleason and Hamlin (1974)	B	Luft *et al.* (1983)		Wreghitt (1987)
A	Herb *et al.* (1977)	B	McGregor *et al.* (1984)		
	Kersting and Neumann (1975)	B	Nagington and Martin (1983)		
B	Mejia *et al.* (1983)		Remington *et al.* (1972)		
B	Reynolds, Wall and Pfeiffer (1966)		Ruskin and Remington (1976)		
	Ruskin and Remington (1976)	B	Ryning *et al.* (1979)		
	Townsend *et al.* (1975)		Stinson *et al.* (1971)		
		B	Wreghitt *et al.* (1986)		

* A, presumed; B, proven.

TABLE 16.2

Clinical Details of Primary Donor-Acquired Toxoplasma gondii *Infections in Heart Transplant Recipients*

Reference	*Clinical Details*
Ryning *et al.* (1979)	35-year-old female. Raised liver enzymes 26 days after transplantation. Temperature raised to 40°C, confusion with focal neurological signs and bilateral lung consolidation. Died 30 days after transplantation; *T. gondii* seen in multiple organs in post-mortem examination
Ryning *et al.* (1979)	55-yr-old male. Reduced vision in right eye 6 months after transplantation; treated with trisulphapyrimidines and pyrimethamine. Ten months after transplantation, the patient became confused; *T. gondii* seen in material from brain abscess. Treated again but did not return to normal
McGregor *et al.* (1984)	31-yr-old male 30 days after transplantation developed peripheral oedema, intermittent fever up to 39°C with anorexia, nausea, hyponatraemia, hypoalbuminaemia, falling creatinine clearance and raised ESR. Biopsy of the right ventricle of the heart taken on day 20 after transplantation showed *T. gondii* in two muscle cells. The patient was treated with pyrimethamine (25 mg/day), sulphadiazine (1 g t.d.s.) and folinic acid. Administration of anti-thymocyte globulin (ATG) was stopped. The patient's condition deteriorated and he died 43 days after transplantation
Papworth (unpublished)	49-yr-old male, became febrile 32 days after transplantation. Three days later the patient developed diffuse bilateral shadowing in chest radiograph. Developed progressive hypoxia leading to cardiac arrest and death 36 days after transplantation. The diagnosis of disseminated toxoplasmosis was made only at post-mortem examination

TABLE 16.2 (*continued*)

Reference	*Clinical Details*
Papworth (unpublished)	43-yr-old male. Temperature of 39.5°C developed 21 days after transplantation. One week later *T. gondii* seroconversion was noted and therapy with pyrimethamine, sulphatriad and folinic acid was started on day 30. The fever resolved over the next 10 days and the patient made a full recovery
Papworth (unpublished)	20-yr-old male. On day 17 after transplantation the patient developed a dry cough and dyspnoea. On day 26, *T. gondii* cysts were seen in a routine cardiac biopsy. Focal neurological signs developed despite prompt therapy with pyrimethamine, sulphadiazine and spiramycin. Eventually the patient made a complete recovery

clinical findings in the Papworth heart transplant recipients with primary *T. gondii* infection have been fever, CNS symptoms and leucocytosis, on average 26 days after transplantation.

What has become clear in our studies on these patients and on kidney and liver transplant patients at Addenbrooke's Hospital, Cambridge, is that it is vital to document the *T. gondii* serological status of both donor and recipient, because the only situation in which primary *T. gondii* infection has been noted is when an organ from a seropositive donor has been given to a seronegative recipient.

The risk, therefore, of primary *T. gondii* infection in this group of patients depends on the incidence of previous infection (and hence the potential presence of *T. gondii* cysts) in donors and the incidence (and hence protective antibodies) in recipients. We have found 36 of 155 (23%) heart donors and 54 of 174 (31%) heart transplant recipients seropositive for *T. gondii* before transplantation. The reason for the greater incidence of seropositivity in the recipients may be explained by the fact that the average age of donors was 25 years and the average age of recipients was 40 years. This implies that approximately 0.5% of individuals acquire *T. gondii* infection per year, a figure which agrees with previous findings (Fleck, 1979). The *T. gondii* serological status of Papworth heart transplant donors and recipients in relation to age is shown in Fig. 16.1.

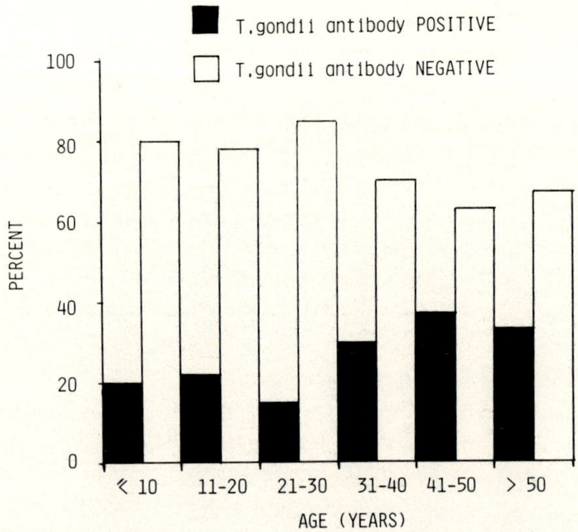

Fig. 16.1. Toxoplasma gondii *serological status and ages of Papworth heart transplant donors and recipients.*

There were 156 heart and heart–lung transplant recipients at Papworth Hospital, for whom *T. gondii* serological donor and recipient data were available. Twenty-six seronegative recipients (16.7%) received hearts from seropositive donors (i.e. mismatches) and details of the outcome in some of these patients have been published previously (Hakim *et al.*, 1985, 1986; Wreghitt *et al.*, 1986). Nine mismatched patients were not given prophylactic pyrimethamine, and of the 7 who survived for at least 1 month after transplantation, 4 (57%) acquired primary *T. gondii* infection, and 2 died (Table 16.2). The other 2 patients survived on appropriate therapy. Subsequently, mismatched patients were given pyrimethamine prophylactically (25 mg/day from day 2 or 3 after transplantation for 6 weeks). Of the 14 who survived for at least 1 month after transplantation, none has shown any clinical signs of toxoplasmosis and there is no serological evidence by latex agglutination or dye test that seroconversion has taken place. One mismatched patient, who was given prophylactic pyrimethamine, was shown to have damaged *T. gondii* cysts in the transplanted heart 55 days after transplantation. These cysts had probably been effectively destroyed by chemotherapy. The patient had neither symptoms nor antibodies attributable to *T. gondii* infection.

In a study of 54 liver transplant recipients in the Cambridge–King's College Hospital series (Wreghitt, 1987), of 5 *T. gondii* seronegative recipients who received a liver from a seropositive donor, one developed fatal primary donor-acquired *T. gondii* infection. Only one other case (Anthony, 1972) in a liver transplant recipient has been published.

More cases of fatal donor-acquired *T. gondii* infections have been reported in kidney than in heart transplant recipients. This has given a biased picture of the true situation because far more kidney transplants have been performed. In our studies of transplant recipients in Cambridge, the risk of *T. gondii* seronegative recipients acquiring primary infection from a seropositive organ donor is greater in heart (57%) than in liver (20%) transplantation. We have found no evidence of donor-transmitted *T. gondii* infection in kidney transplant recipients (G. Speirs and T. G. Wreghitt, in preparation).

T. gondii cysts are probably found more often in donated hearts than in livers or kidneys, since the organism is known to have a predilection for encysting in muscle. We have found no *T. gondii*-specific IgM in sera from donors to mismatched transplant patients, which indicates that the donors had not experienced recent primary *T. gondii* infection.

In any event, since we now know that primary *T. gondii* infection is always acquired from the donated organ, and we have shown (Hakim *et al.*, 1986; Wreghitt *et al.*, 1986) that prophylactic pyrimethamine prevents infection in mismatched patients, then provided that donors and recipients are screened at or before transplantation, and appropriate prophylactic action is taken, primary *T. gondii* infections in heart, liver and kidney patients should no longer occur.

CYTOMEGALOVIRUS

Cytomegalovirus, like *T. gondii*, is mainly transmitted to seronegative transplant recipients by the donor organ, but CMV infection may also be acquired from blood or blood products, usually given around the time of transplantation. The first report implicating blood transfusions in the transmission of CMV was in patients undergoing open heart surgery (Kaariainen *et al.*, 1966). Many workers had noted a Paul–Bunnell antibody-negative infectious mononucleosis-like syndrome which appeared 3–7 weeks after open heart surgery (Kreel *et al.*, 1960). This we now know was almost certainly caused by CMV. Some studies have shown that up to 60% of patients receiving large amounts of blood acquire CMV infection from this source (Kaariainen *et al.*, 1966; Murphy *et al.*, 1967; Embil *et al.*, 1968; Lang, Scolnick and Willerson, 1968; Paloheimo *et al.*, 1968; Henle *et al.*, 1970; Stevens *et al.*, 1970; Prince *et al.*, 1971; Lang, 1972; Kane *et al.*, 1975; Armstrong *et al.*, 1976; Evans, 1976; Ho *et al.*, 1976; Winston *et al.*, 1979; Glenn, 1981; Marker, Howard and Simmons, 1981; Pollard *et al.*, 1982; Preiksaitis *et al.*, 1985). Most investigators, however, have found the degree of transmission to be much lower than this. Henle *et al.* (1970) showed that the risk of acquiring CMV infection was related to the number of units of blood given, and was approximately 5–12% per unit. This was confirmed by Stevens *et al.* (1970) and Prince *et al.* (1971); others have found that the risk of acquiring CMV after blood transfusion is approximately 1–3% per unit (Armstrong *et al.*, 1976; Evans, 1976; Henle *et al.*, 1970; Kane *et al.*, 1975; Preiksaitis *et al.*, 1983). Much depends, of course, on the degree of CMV seropositivity in the blood donor population, since it is the latent virus in the blood of CMV seropositive donors which is responsible for transmitting the infection to seronegative recipients (Lang, 1972). Although the exact site of CMV latency is unknown, it has been suggested that the virus is latent in leucocytes (Pagano, 1975; Rinaldo, Black and Hirsch, 1977; Winston *et al.*, 1980).

Paloheimo *et al.* (1968) showed that the risk of acquiring CMV infection from blood was related to the age of the blood used. In their studies, patients given blood more than 48 h old did not acquire CMV infection, whereas 30% of patients given blood less than 48 hours old became infected. More recent studies have shown that stored citrated blood may also transmit CMV infection (Stevens *et al.*, 1970; Prince *et al.*, 1971; Monif, Dricoff and Flory, 1976). While the acquisition of primary CMV infection from blood or blood products may not be associated with symptoms in some patients (Paloheimo *et al.*, 1968; Stevens *et al.*, 1970), most infections in immunosuppressed transplant recipients are associated with significant morbidity and mortality (Winston *et al.*, 1979; Marker, Howard and Simmons, 1981; Pollard *et al.*, 1982).

Although the most severe form of CMV disease in transplant recipients relates to primary infection (Glenn, 1981), reactivation of latent CMV or reinfection may be associated with severe symptoms, particularly when patients are experiencing concurrent infections (Light and Burke, 1979). We have shown (Wreghitt *et al.*, 1986; Wreghitt *et al.*, in press) that heart transplant recipients who are CMV seropositive before transplantation are more likely to have reactivation of or reinfection with CMV if they receive a heart from a CMV seropositive rather than a seronegative donor. It seems likely that most of these infections are due to reinfection with exogenous virus rather than reactivation of latent CMV. Similar and even more striking evidence for this has been found in liver and kidney (Wreghitt, 1987; Speirs and Wreghitt, in preparation) transplant recipients in Cambridge.

In the general population, CMV is usually acquired by man-to-man transmission. In communities where people live in overcrowded conditions, CMV is usually acquired early in life (Rowe, Hartley and Cramblett, 1958; Li and Hanshaw, 1967; Haldone, Embil and Wall, 1969). Among the more affluent, infection is inclined to take place later in life, usually coinciding with the onset of sexual activity (Jordon, Rousseau and Noble, 1973; Davis, Stewart and Garvin, 1975; Stagno, Reynolds and Tsiantos, 1975). The relation of the CMV antibody status of Papworth heart transplant donors and recipients to age is shown in Fig. 16.2. A sharp increase in CMV seropositivity may be seen between patients less than 10 years of age and those aged

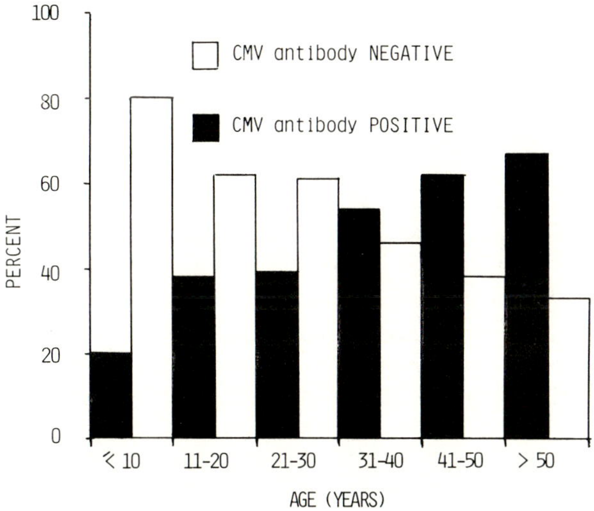

Fig. 16.2. *CMV serological status and ages of Papworth heart transplant donors and recipients.*

11–20 years. Also, only 20% under 10 years had serological evidence of previous CMV infection, whereas 67% of those aged 50 or more were seropositive.

One of the Papworth heart transplant recipients who acquired CMV infection $4\frac{1}{2}$ years after transplantation must have acquired the virus by social contact, since he had not received blood or blood products around this time.

Without doubt, the most significant route of CMV infection in organ transplant recipients is through the organ donor (Peterson *et al.*, 1980; Warrell *et al.*, 1980; Preiksaitis *et al.*, 1983; Smiley *et al.*, 1985). The risk of primary CMV infection is therefore directly related to the level of CMV seropositivity in organ donors and recipients.

In the Papworth heart transplant series, 41% of donors were CMV seropositive, as were 60% of recipients before transplantation. The reason for the difference in seropositivity is that the average age of donors was 25 years and of recipients 40 years. Of the 137 patients for whom donor and recipient CMV serological data was available, 20 seronegative recipients (14.6%) received hearts from seropositive donors (i.e. mismatches) and 17 (85%) acquired primary CMV infection (Table 16.3). Since 9 of 35 (26%) CMV seronegative patients who received a heart from a seronegative donor subsequently developed primary CMV infection, it must be presumed that this was due to blood or blood products. It is likely therefore that the same proportion of mismatched patients acquired primary CMV infection from blood. Thus, the true rate of organ donor-transmitted primary CMV disease in mismatched patients is probably in the region of 60% in our series.

TABLE 16.3
*Summary of CMV Infections in Papworth Heart Transplant Patients**

CMV Serological Status of: Donor	Recipient	*Total Number*	*No. of Patients (%) with:* Primary CMV	CMV Reactivation/ Reinfection	*Clinical Score*†
Positive	Negative	20	17(85%)	0	9.17
Negative	Negative	35	9(26%)	0	2.80
Positive	Positive	36	0	18(50%)	3.19
Negative	Positive	46	0	18(39%)	1.63
	Clinical score		7.0	2.41	

* Patients included only if they survived more than 1 month after transplantation.
† Smiley *et al.* (1985).

In an elegant study in heart transplant patients, Preiksaitis *et al.* (1983), using CMV negative blood and blood products, showed that all primary CMV infections were in CMV seronegative patients who received hearts from CMV seropositive donors. When unscreened blood was used, 1 in 5 (20%) seronegative patients who received hearts from CMV seronegative donors, acquired primary CMV infection, which agrees with our findings.

In the Papworth heart transplant series, we have found that 18 (50%) of 36 patients who were CMV seropositive and received a heart from a seropositive donor acquired CMV reactivation/reinfection after transplantation. A lower proportion (39%) of CMV seropositive recipients who received a heart from a seronegative donor acquired CMV reactivation/reinfection. Thus, in every respect, heart transplant recipients who receive a heart from a CMV seropositive donor are more likely to experience subsequent CMV infection than those who receive a heart from a seronegative donor. Furthermore, CMV disease is more severe (see clinical score, Table 16.3) in patients who received a heart from a seropositive rather than from a seronegative donor. Primary CMV infection acquired from the donor heart (clinical score 9.17) is far more serious than primary CMV transmitted by blood or blood products (clinical score 2.80). It is interesting that CMV reactivation/reinfection in seropositive recipients who receive a seropositive heart (clinical score 3.19) is more serious than primary CMV acquired from blood or blood products. This further emphasizes the point that while blood-borne CMV may cause significant morbidity, it is donor-acquired CMV infection which is more serious, even in seropositive recipients.

The first reports of donor-acquired CMV infection (Betts *et al.*, 1975; Ho *et al.*, 1975; Nankervis, 1976) involved kidney transplant recipients. Betts *et al.* (1975) showed that 78% of their CMV mismatched patients acquired primary CMV infection, but none of the CMV seronegative patients who received kidneys from CMV seronegative donors did so. Ho (1977) and

Warrell *et al.* (1980) reported similar findings. The much lower incidence of blood-borne CMV transmission in these kidney transplant patients (also found in our Cambridge series) may reflect the smaller amount of blood and blood products given to kidney than to heart transplant patients, but in a study of liver transplant patients in the Cambridge–King's College Hospital series (Wreghitt, 1987), despite their receiving a massive amount of blood perioperatively, we have been unable to find any cases of blood-borne primary CMV infection. By contrast, 3 of 8 (38%) CMV mismatched patients developed primary infection.

It is clearly beneficial to minimize the impact of CMV disease in heart (and particularly heart–lung) transplant patients. The shortage of organs for transplantation makes the strategy of not using hearts from CMV seropositive donors an impractical proposition. However, ideally, hearts (and particularly hearts and lungs) from CMV seropositive donors should not be given to CMV seronegative recipients.

For years, the relatively short ischaemic time acceptable in heart transplantation has not allowed the preoperative use of CMV antibody tests on sera from organ donors. However, a new simple quick and reliable latex agglutination test (CMV scan, Becton Dickinson) is now available. The test takes only 8 min to perform and has been found to be very reliable for donor screening (Gray *et al.*, 1987).

HUMAN IMMUNODEFICIENCY VIRUS

Human immunodeficiency virus (HIV) causes AIDS in some infected people. Infection is acquired either by sexual contact with an infected person or from blood or blood products containing HIV. It has been found recently that HIV infection can also be transmitted to transplant recipients in donated organs (L'age-Stehr *et al.*, 1985; Prompt *et al.*, 1985; Neumayer, Wagner and Kresse, 1986; J. W. Ward, personal communication). L'age-Stehr *et al.* (1985) and Neumayer, Wagner and Kresse (1986) both recorded transmission of HIV in kidneys from 3 donors with a history of intravenous drug abuse. Six kidneys were taken for transplantation but only 5 were used. All 5 recipients have developed HIV antibodies. Four patients were transplanted in Berlin and all had a similar clinical course 2–7 weeks after transplantation. Recurrent fever up to 39°C was seen between days 12 and 47 after transplantation. All 4 patients had prolonged leucopenia around day 12 which lasted until around day 55. One patient has since developed persistent generalized lymphadenopathy. Sera were not available from the donors for HIV antibody testing, but since the only other source of infection is likely to have been from blood, and the degree of HIV antibody positivity among Berlin blood donors at the time was less than 0.001%, it must be assumed that infection was acquired from the organ donors.

Two recipients of corneal grafts from one of the donors were HIV antibody negative 18 months after transplantation. Prompt *et al.* (1985) reported the transmission of HIV in donated kidneys from a haemophiliac donor. So far, however, there have not been any documented cases of transmission of HIV infection in donated organs in the USA, although it must only be a matter of time before this happens. One HIV antibody-positive person donated corneas, a kidney and heart but 6 months after transplantation none of the recipients had developed HIV antibodies nor AIDS-related symptoms (J. W. Ward, personal communication).

In June 1985, the United States Public Health Service recommended that all organ donors should be screened for HIV antibody before the organs are transplanted. Many other countries have since adopted similar measures. At present, the best way of detecting evidence of HIV infection is by antibody assay. Several tests for detecting HIV antibody are available; some are more specific than others and great care must therefore be exercised in the choice of an assay system. In Cambridge, sera from all organ and blood donors are tested by competitive enzyme-linked immunosorbent assay (ELISA, Wellcome Diagnostics). Positive sera are sent to a reference laboratory for confirmatory tests. We have found this test to be very reliable as a screening procedure. It must be stressed that while evidence of HIV antibody means that the individual is potentially infectious, and the organs should not be used, a negative HIV antibody test result may not always mean that the donor is free from infection with HIV, since it takes up to 6 weeks after HIV infection to produce an antibody response. Even so, testing for antibody is at present the best available method of screening potential organ or blood donors for evidence of HIV infection. All organ donors should be tested prospectively, since there is at present no effective therapy for HIV infection, which has an extremely poor prognosis, particularly in organ transplant recipients who are deliberately immunosuppressed.

HEPATITIS B VIRUS

Hepatitis B virus (HBV), like HIV, is usually transmitted sexually or by blood. Most developed countries have programmes designed to minimize the risk of blood-borne transmission, based on the detection of hepatitis B surface antigen (HBsAg) in blood. HBV may also be transmitted to transplant recipients in organs from HBsAg positive persons (Combined MRC and PHLS Report, 1980). It is therefore important that potential donors are screened for HBsAg before their organs are transplanted.

CONCLUSIONS

Now that the routes of CMV, *T. gondii*, HIV and HBV infection to organ transplant recipients have been elucidated, the impact of these life-threatening infections can be minimized, principally by prospective screening of potential organ donors for evidence of infection with these agents, and taking appropriate action. In particular, organs from HIV and/or HBV positive donors should not be used. Organs from CMV seropositive donors should not be given to seronegative recipients and patients should be transfused only with CMV antibody negative blood. Since, on average, there are more CMV seronegative donors than recipients, it should usually be possible to find seronegative organs for seronegative recipients. An alternative strategy would be to give CMV vaccine to seronegative potential recipients, or to give CMV mismatched patients prophylactic hyperimmune globulin against CMV so as to prevent or minimize the response to infection. Now that anti-CMV drugs (Foscarnet Astra Laboratories; B759U, Burroughs Wellcome; etc.) are available, then should primary CMV disease develop, administration of one of these drugs may modify the disease process (Klintmalm *et al.*, 1985; Ringden *et al.*, 1985; Collaborative DHPG Treatment Study Group, 1986).

Our success in eradicating primary *T. gondii* infection in heart transplant recipients at Papworth by the prophylactic use of pyrimethamine in *T. gondii* mismatched patients has proved that fatal *T. gondii* infection in organ transplant recipients should now be avoidable.

REFERENCES

Anthony, C. W. (1972). Disseminated toxoplasmosis in a liver transplant patient. *J. Am. Med. Wom. Ass.* **27**, 601–603.

Armstrong, J. A., Tarr, G. A., Youngblood, L. A., Dowling, J. N., Saslow, A. R., Lucas, J. P. and Ho, M. (1976). Cytomegalovirus infection in children undergoing open heart surgery. *Yale J. Biol. Med.* **49**, 83–91.

Betts, R. F. (1982). Cytomegalovirus infections in transplant patients. *Proc. Med. Virol.* **28**, 44–64.

Betts, R. F., Freeman, R. B., Douglas, R. G., Talley, T. E. and Rundell, B. (1975). Transmission of cytomegalovirus infection with renal allograft. *Kid. Int.* **8**, 385–394.

Cohen, S. N. (1970). Toxoplasmosis in patients receiving immunosuppressive therapy. *J. Am. Med. Ass.* **211**, 657–659.

Collaborative DHPG Treatment Study Group (1986). Treatment of serious cytomegalovirus infections with 9-(1,3-dihydroxy-2-propoxymethyl)guanine in patients with AIDS and other immunodeficiencies. *New Engl. J. Med.* **314**, 801–805.

Combined Medical Research Council and Public Health Laboratory Service Report (1980). The incidence of hepatitis B infection after accidental exposure and anti-HBs immunoglobulin prophylaxis. *Lancet* **i**, 6–9.

Davis, L. E., Stewart, J. A. and Garvin, S. (1975). Cytomegalovirus infection: a seroepidemiologic comparison of nuns and women from a venereal disease clinic. *Am. J. Epidemiol.* **102**, 327–335.

Dummer, J. S., Hardy, A., Poorsattar, A. and Ho, M. (1983). Early infections in kidney, heart and liver transplant recipients on cyclosporine. *Transplantation* **36**, 259–267.

Editorial (1984). Toxoplasmosis diagnosis and immunodeficiency. *Lancet* **i**, 605–606.

Embil, J. A., Folkins, D. F., Haldane, E. V. and Van Rooyen, C. E. (1968). Cytomegalovirus infection following extracorporeal circulation in children. *Lancet* **ii**, 1151–1155.

Evans, A. S. (Ed.) (1976). The risk factors of cytomegalovirus infection transmitted by blood transfusion. *Yale J. Biol. Med.* **49**, 3–91.

Feldman, H. A. (1982). Epidemiology of *Toxoplasma* infections. *Epidemiol. Rev.* **4**, 204–213.

Flament-Durand, J., Coers, C., Waelerbroeck, C., van Geertruyden, J. and Toussaint, G. Ch. (1967). Encephalite et myosite a toxoplasmes au cours d'un traitement immunodepresseur. *Acta Clin. Belg.* **22**, 44–49.

Fleck, D. G. (1979). Toxoplasmosis. *J. Antimic. Chemother.* **5**, Suppl. A, 87–89.

Ghatak, N. R., Poon, T. P. and Zimmerman, H. M. (1970). Toxoplasmosis of the central nervous system in the adult. *Arch. Pathol.* **89**, 337–348.

Gleason, T. H. and Hamlin, W. B. (1974). Disseminated toxoplasmosis in the compromised host. *Arch. Int. Med.* **134**, 1059–1062.

Glenn, J. (1981). Cytomegalovirus infections following renal transplantation. *Rev. Infect. Dis.* **3**, 1151–1178.

Gray, J. J., Alvey, B., Smith, D. J. and Wreghitt, T. G. (1987). Evaluation of a commercial latex agglutination test for detecting antibodies to cytomegalovirus in organ donors and transplant recipients. *J. Virol. Meth.* **15** (in press).

Grundy, J. E., Super, M. and Griffiths, P. D. (1986). Reinfection of a seropositive allograft recipient by cytomegalovirus from donor kidney. *Lancet* **i**, 159–160.

Hakim, M., Esmore, D., Wreghitt, T. G., Wallwork, J. and English, T. A. H. (1986). Toxoplasmosis in cardiac transplantation. *Br. Med. J.* **292**, 1108.

Hakim, M., Wreghitt, T. G., English, T. A. H., Stovin, P. G. I., Cory-Pearce, R. and Wallwork, J. (1985). Significance of donor-transmitted disease in cardiac transplantation. *Heart Transplant.* **IV**, 302–305.

Haldone, E. V., Embil, J. A. and Wall, A. D. (1969). A serological study of cytomegalovirus infection in the population of Easter Island. *Bull. WHO* **40**, 969–974.

Henle, W., Henle, G., Scriba, M., Joyner, C. F., Harrison, F. S., von Essen, R., Paloheimo, J. and Klemola, E. (1970). Antibody responses to Epstein–Barr virus and cytomegaloviruses after open-heart and other surgery. *New Engl. J. Med.* **282**, 1068–1074.

Herb, H. M., Jontofsohn, R., Loffler, H. D. and Heinze, V. (1977). Toxoplasmosis after renal transplantation. *Clin. Nephrol.* **8**, 529–532.

Ho, M. (1977). Virus infections after transplantation in man. *Arch. Virol.* **55**, 1–24.

Ho, M., Dowling, J. N., Armstrong, J. A., Suwansirikul, S., Wu, B., Youngblood, L. A. and Saslow, A. (1976). Factors contributing to the risk of cytomegalovirus infection in patients receiving renal transplants. *Yale J. Biol. Med.* **49**, 17–26.

Ho, M., Suwansirikul, S., Dowling, J. N., Youngblood, L. A. and Armstrong, J. A. (1975). The transplanted kidney as a source of cytomegalovirus infection. *New Engl. J. Med.* **293**, 1109–1112.

Ho, M., Wajszczuk, C. P., Hardy, A., Dummer, J. S., Starzl, T. E., Hakala, T. R. and Bahnson, H. T. (1983). Infections in kidney, heart and liver transplant recipients on cyclosporine. *Transplant. Proc.* **XV**, 2768–2772.

Hutchinson, W. M., Dunachie, J. F., Siim, J. C. and Work, K. (1969). Life cycle of *Toxoplasma gondii. Br. Med. J.* **4**, 806.

Jamieson, S. W., Oyer, P. E., Reitz, B. A., Baumgartner, W. A., Bieber, C. P., Stinson, E. B. and Shumway, N. E. (1981). Cardiac transplantation at Stanford. *Heart Transplant.* **1**, 86–91.

Jordon, M. C., Rousseau, W. E. and Noble, G. R. (1973). Association of cervical cytomegaloviruses with venereal disease. *New Engl. J. Med.* **288**, 932–939.

Kaariainen, L., Klemola, E. and Paloheimo, J. (1966). Rise of cytomegalovirus antibodies in an infectious mononucleosis-like syndrome after transfusion. *Br. Med. J.* **1**, 1270–1273.

Kaariainen, L., Paloheimo, J., Klemola, E., Makela, T. and Koivuniemi, A. (1966). Cytomegalovirus mononucleosis: isolation of the virus and demonstration of subclinical infections after fresh blood transfusion in connection with open-heart surgery. *Ann. Med. Exp. Fenn.* **44**, 297–301.

Kane, R. C., Rousseau, W. E., Noble, G. R., Tegtmeier, G. E., Wulff, H., Herndon, H. B., Chin, T. D. Y. and Bayer, W. L. (1975). Cytomegalovirus infection in a volunteer blood donor population. *Infect. Immun.* **11**, 719–723.

Kean, B. H., Kimball, A. C. and Christenson, W. N. (1969). An epidemic of acute toxoplasmosis. *J. Am. Med. Ass.* **208**, 1002–1004.

Kersting, G. and Neumann, J. (1975). Malignant lymphoma of the brain following renal transplantation. *Acta Neuropath.*, Suppl. **6**, 131–133.

Kimball, A. C., Kean, B. H. and Kellner, A. (1965). The risk of transmitting toxoplasmosis by blood transfusion. *Transfusion* **5**, 447–451.

Klintmalm, G., Lonnqvist, B., Oberg, B., Gahrton, G., Lornestedt, J., Lundgren, G., Ringden, O., Robert, K., Wahren, B. and Groth, C. (1985). Intravenous foscarnet for the treatment of severe cytomegalovirus infection in allograft recipients. *Scand. J. Infect. Dis.* **17**, 157–163.

Kreel, I., Zaroff, L. I., Canter, J. W., Krasma, I. and Baronofsky, I. D. (1960). A syndrome following total body perfusion. *Surg. Gynecol. Obstet.* **3**, 317–321.

L'age-Stehr, J., Schwartz, A., Offermann, G., Langmaack, H., Bennhold, I., Niedrig, M. and Koch, M. A. (1985). HTLV-III infection in kidney transplant recipients. *Lancet* **ii**, 1361–1362.

Lang, D. J. (1972). Cytomegalovirus infections in organ transplantation and post transfusion. *Arch. Gesamte Virus Forsch.* **37**, 365–377.

Lang, D. J., Scolnick, E. M. and Willerson, J. T. (1968). Association of cytomegalovirus infection with the post-perfusion syndrome. *New Engl. J. Med.* **278**, 1147–1149.

Li, F. and Hanshaw, J. B. (1967). Cytomegalovirus infection among migrant children. *Am. J. Epidemiol.* **86**, 137–145.

Light, J. A. and Burke, D. S. (1979). Association of cytomegalovirus (CMV) infections with increased recipient mortality following transplantation. *Transplant. Proc.* **11**, 79–82.

Luft, B. J., Naot, Y., Araujo, F. G., Stinson, E. B. and Remington, J. S. (1983). Primary and reactivated *Toxoplasma* infection in patients with cardiac transplants. Clinical spectrum and problems in diagnosis in a defined population. *Ann. Int. Med.* **99**, 27–31.

Marker, S. C., Howard, R. J. and Simmons, R. L. (1981). Cytomegalovirus infection: a quantitative prospective study of three hundred twenty consecutive renal transplants. *Surgery* **89**, 660–671.

McGregor, C. G. A., Fleck, D. G., Nagington, J., Stovin, P. G. I., Cory-Pearce, R. and English, T. A. H. (1984). Disseminated toxoplasmosis in cardiac transplantation. *J. Clin. Pathol.* **37**, 74–77.

Mejia, G., Leiderman, E., Builes, M., Henao, J., Arbelaez, M., Arango, J. L. and Borrero, J. (1983). Transmission of *Toxoplasma* by renal transplant. *Am. J. Kid. Dis.*, **11**, 615–617.

Monif, G. R. G., Diacoff, G. I. and Flory, L. F. (1976). Blood as a potential vehicle for the cytomegalovirus. *Am. J. Obstet. Gynecol.* **126**, 445–448.

Murphy, A. M., Arnold, B. J., Leogh, H. J. and Jack, I. (1967). Cytomegalovirus infection in an adult. *Med. J. Austral.* **1**, 562–563.

Nagington, J., Cossart, Y. E. and Cohen, B. J. (1977). Reactivation of hepatitis B after transplantation operations. *Lancet* **i**, 558–560.

Nagington, J. and Martin, A. L. (1983). Toxoplasmosis and heart transplantation. *Lancet* **ii**, 679.

Nankervis, G. A. (1976). Cytomegalovirus infections in the blood recipient. *Yale J. Biol. Med.* **49**, 13–15.

Neumayer, H. H., Wagner, K. and Kresse, S. (1986). HTLV-III antibodies in patients with kidney transplants or on haemodialysis. *Lancet* **i**, 497.

Orsi, E. V., Howard, J. L., Baturay, N., Ribot, S. and Eslami, H. (1978). High incidence of virus isolation from donor and recipient tissues associated with renal transplantation. *Nature* **272**, 372–373.

Pagano, J. S. (1975). Infections with cytomegalovirus in bone marrow transplantation: report of a workshop from the National Institute of Health. *J. Infect. Dis.* **132**, 114–120.

Paloheimo, J. A., Von Essen, R., Klemola, E., Kaariainen, L. and Sittanen, P. (1968). Subclinical cytomegalovirus infections and cytomegalovirus mononucleosis after open heart surgery. *Am. J. Cardiol.* **22**, 624–630.

Peterson, P. K., Balfour, H. H., Marker, S. C., Fryd, D. S., Howard, R. J. and Simmons, R. L. (1980). Cytomegalovirus disease in renal allograft recipients. A prospective study of the clinical features, risk factors and impact on renal transplantation. *Medicine* **59**, 283–300.

Pollard, R. B., Arvin, A. M., Gamberg, P., Rand, K. H., Gallagher, J. C. and Merigan, T. C. (1982). Specific cell-mediated immunity and infections with cytomegalovirus, herpes simplex virus and varicella-zoster virus in cardiac transplant recipients. *Am. J. Med.* **73**, 679–687.

Pomerance, A. and Stovin, P. G. I. (1985). Heart transplant pathology: the British experience. *J. Clin. Pathol.* **38**, 146–159.

Preiksaitis, J. K., Grumet, F. C., Smith, W. K. and Merigan, T. C. (1985). Transfusion-acquired cytomegalovirus infection in cardiac surgery patients. *J. Med. Virol.* **15**, 283–290.

Preiksaitis, J. K., Rosno, S., Grumet, C. and Merigan, T. C. (1983). Infection due to herpesviruses in cardiac transplant recipients: role of the donor heart and immunosuppressive therapy. *J. Infect. Dis.* **147**, 974–981.

Prince, A. M., Szmuness, W., Millian, S. J. and David, D. S. (1971). A serological study of cytomegalovirus infections associated with blood transfusions. *New Engl. J. Med.* **284**, 1125–1131.

Prompt, C. A., Reis, M. M., Grillo, F. M., Kopstein, J., Kraemer, E., Manfro, R. C., Maia, M. W. and Comiran, J. B. (1985). Transmission of AIDS virus in renal transplantation. *Lancet* **ii**, 672.

Remington, J. S., Gaines, J. D., Griepp, R. B. and Shumway, N. E. (1972). Further experience with infection after cardiac transplantation. *Transplant. Proc.* **IV**, 699–705.

Remington, J. S., Jacobs, L. and Kaufman, H. E. (1960). Toxoplasmosis in the adult. *New Engl. J. Med.* **262**, 180–186.

Reynolds, E. S., Walls, K. W. and Pfeiffer, R. I. (1966). Generalized toxoplasmosis following renal transplantation: report of a case. *Arch. Int. Med.* **118**, 401–405.

Rinaldo, C. R., Black, P. H. and Hirsch, M. S. (1977). Interactions of cytomegalovirus with leukocytes from patients with mononucleosis due to cytomegalovirus. *J. Infect. Dis.* **136**, 667–668.

Ringden, O., Wilcez, H., Lonnqvist, B., Gahrton, G., Wahren, B. and Lornestedt, J. O. (1985). Foscarnet for cytomegalovirus infections. *Lancet* **i**, 1503–1504.

Roth, J. A., Siegel, S. E., Levine, A. S. and Berard, C. W. (1971). Fatal recurrent toxoplasmosis in a patient initially infected via a leucocyte transfusion. *Am. J. Clin. Pathol.* **56**, 601–605.

Rowe, W. P., Hartley, J. W. and Cramblett, H. G. (1958). Detection of human salivary gland virus in mouth and urine of children. *Am. J. Hyg.* **67**, 57–63.

Ruskin, J. and Remington, J. S. (1976). Toxoplasmosis in the compromised host. *Ann. Int. Med.* **84**, 193–199.

Ryning, F. W., McLeod, R., Maddox, J. C., Hunt, S. and Remington, J. S. (1979). Probable transmission of *Toxoplasma gondii* by organ transplantation. *Ann. Int. Med.* **90**, 47–49.

Schroter, G. P. J., Hoelscher, M., Putman, C. W., Porter, K. A., Hansbrough, J. F. and Starzl, T. E. (1976). Infections complicating orthotopic liver transplantation: a study emphasizing graft-related septicemia. *Arch. Surg.* **111**, 1337–1347.

Siegel, S. E., Lunde, M. N., Gelderman, A. H., Halterman, R. H., Brown, J. A., Levine, A. S. and Graw, R. G. (1971). Transmission of toxoplasmosis by leukocyte transfusion. *Blood* **37**, 388–394.

Smiley, M. L., Wlodaver, C. G., Grossman, R. A., Barker, C. F., Perloff, L. J., Tustin, N. B., Starr, S. E., Plotkin, S. A. and Friedman, H. M. (1985). The role of pretransplant immunity in protection from cytomegalovirus disease following renal transplantation. *Transplantation* **40**, 157–161.

Speirs, G. and Wreghitt, T. G. (1988). The prevalence of organ donor-transmitted *Toxoplasma gondii* infection in heart, kidney and liver transplant recipients in Cambridge (in preparation).

Stagno, S., Reynolds, D. W. and Tsiantos, A. (1975). Comparative serial virologic and serologic studies of symptomatic and subclinical congenitally and natally acquired cytomegalovirus infections. *J. Infect. Dis.* **132**, 568–579.

Stevens, D. P., Barker, L. F., Ketcham, A. S. and Meyer, H. M. (1970). Asymptomatic cytomegalovirus infection following blood transfusion in tumor surgery. *J. Am. Med. Ass.* **211**, 1341–1344.

Stinson, E. B., Bieber, C. P., Griepp, R. B., Clark, D. A., Shumway, N. E. and Remington, J. S. (1971). Infectious complications after cardiac transplantation in man. *Ann. Int. Med.* **74**, 22–36.

Talice, R. V., Gurri, J., Royol, J. and Perez-Moreira, L. (1957). Investigations sobre la *Toxoplasma gondii* en sangue destinado a transfusao. *Fac. Medic. Montevideo* **42**, 143–147.

Townsend, J. J., Wolinsky, J. S., Baringer, J. R. and Johnson, P. C. (1975). Acquired toxoplasmosis. *Arch. Neurol.* **32**, 335–341.

Warrell, M. J., Chinn, I., Morris, P. J. and Tobin, J. O'H. (1980). The effects of viral infections on renal transplants and their recipients. *Q. J. Med.* **194** (XLIX), 219–231.

Winston, D. J., Gale, R. P., Meyer, D. V. and Young, L. S. (1979). Infectious complications of human bone marrow transplantation. *Medicine* **58**, 1–31.

Winston, D. J., Ho, W. G., Howell, C. L., Miller, C. L., Mickey, M. J., Martin, W. G., Lin, C. H. and Gale R. P. (1980). Cytomegalovirus infections associated with leukocyte transfusions. *Ann. Int. Med.* **93**, 671–675.

Wreghitt, T. G. (1987). Viral and *Toxoplasma gondii* infections. In *Liver Transplantation*, 2nd edn (R. Y. Calne, Ed.), pp. 365–384. Grune and Stratton, London.

Wreghitt, T. G., Hakim, M., Cory-Pearce, R., English, T. A. H. and Wallwork, J. (1986). The impact of donor-transmitted CMV and *Toxoplasma gondii* disease in cardiac transplantation. *Transplant. Proc.* (in press).

Wreghitt, T. G., Hakim, M., Gray, J. J., Kucia, S., Cory-Pearce, R., Wallwork, J. and English, T. A. H. (1988). A detailed study of CMV infections in the first 160 heart and heart/lung transplant recipients at Papworth Hospital, Cambridge, England. *Transplant. Proc.* (in press).

Sharon A. Hunt and
Edward B. Stinson

17

Accelerated Atherosclerosis in the Cardiac Allograft

INTRODUCTION

A variety of complications limits the long-term survival of cardiac transplant recipients. The most common, allograft rejection and opportunistic infection, are expected consequences of the current imperfect regimens of immunosuppression for all solid organ grafting. Others, such as renal dysfunction and arterial hypertension, are related to particular agents in the immunosuppressive regimen, such as cyclosporin. A very diffuse and often rapidly progressive type of occlusive epicardial coronary artery disease, termed accelerated graft atherosclerosis (AGAS), has been found to affect a substantial number of cardiac allograft recipients in the late postoperative period. This accelerated form of atherosclerosis is not a process which would have been predicted, and does not seem to be related to any individual immunosuppressive agent. It may be analogous to the chronic vascular injury, termed chronic rejection, seen in renal allografts.

As survival after transplantation improves, because of increasingly successful management of allograft rejection and infectious complications, the development of AGAS may well become the major limitation to long-term survival in cardiac allograft recipients. The study of this devastating disease in order to define high-risk subgroups of patients, and eventually to institute measures to modify its course, will be a major area of research in cardiac transplantation in coming years.

INCIDENCE

The incidence of AGAS by angiographic criteria was first reported by the Stanford group (Bieber *et al.*, 1981) to be approximately 40% (21 of 55 patients) 5 years after transplantation. Of these 21 patients, the findings in 10 were incidental in routine annual coronary arteriograms, and had not then led to myocardial infarction or graft failure. More recent data from the same group (Zusman *et al.*, 1985) suggest that the incidence of AGAS has not changed since the introduction of cyclosporin-based immunosuppression in 1980. Although the follow-up period is not as long with the cyclosporin cohort, it appears that in this group also a 30–40% incidence of AGAS can be predicted by 5 years post-transplant.

Since the disease is diffuse and affects vessels in a concentric fashion, as will be detailed below, it is possible that standard angiographic criteria used in the past have underestimated the incidence of the disease. By studying the annual coronary arteriograms, starting with a 'baseline' investigation, a month or two after the operation, and measuring changes in coronary artery diameter with a calibrated catheter, it is hoped that a more accurate assessment can be made. Only by such accurate measurement will it be possible to assess the effects of any intervention aimed at changing the incidence or course of this disease.

MORPHOLOGY

At the microscopic level, the lesions of AGAS were first described (Kosek, Hurley and Lower, 1968) in cardiac transplants in dogs treated with immunosuppressive agents. There was a time-related occurrence of coronary intimal thickening, not correlated with acute myocardial rejection, in almost all of the large coronary arteries in 2 dogs surviving longer than 1 year. Five of their dogs who died earlier had recent myocardial infarction at necropsy, and similar lesions in the arteries. This process was then termed chronic rejection, although its relation to immunological processes was deduced rather than proved. Other investigators have demonstrated the induction of occlusive allograft coronary arterial disease in rat (Lurie *et al.*, 1981) and rabbit (Alonso, Starek and Minick, 1977) models.

The histology of AGAS in human cardiac allograft recipients (Fig. 17.1) was first described by Bieber *et al.* (1970). At necropsy they found circumferential and longitudinal increase in intimal fibrous tissue and myo-intimal cells, limited to coronary arteries with muscular media, and not present in arterioles or veins in 12 patients. The thickness of the intima was roughly proportional to the age of the graft, some thickening developing as early as 9 days; in 6 of 7 allografts from patients surviving more than 1 month,

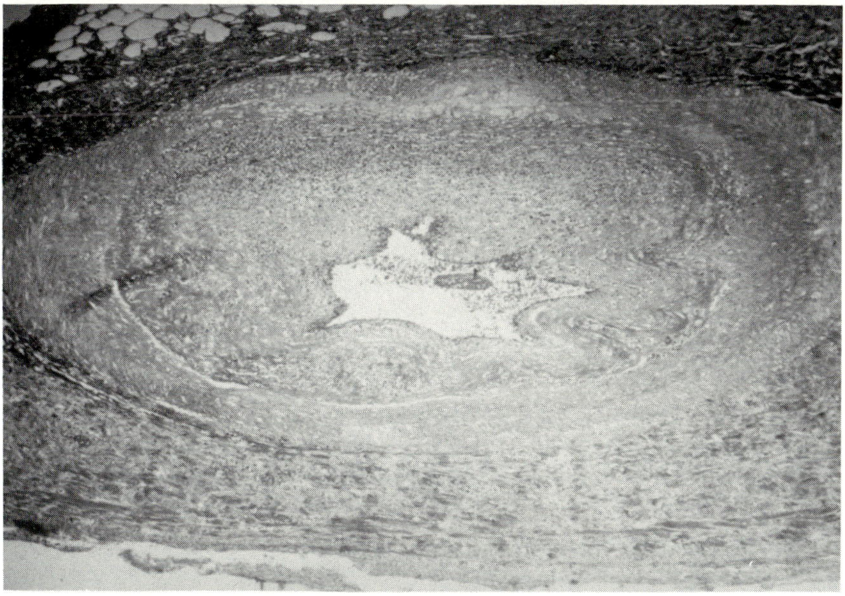

Fig. 17.1. *Histological section: cross-section of left anterior descending artery from heart explanted at time of re-transplantation 2 years after initial transplant. Heart was from 18-year-old donor.*

thickening was present. Purely proliferative intimal lesions were seen in early grafts, and large numbers of lipophages and lipid droplets appeared only in later grafts. None of these patients, however, died of ischaemic heart disease or had clinical signs of myocardial ischaemia. The histopathology of the major coronary arteries in patients who die from AGAS is quite similar to that of native atherosclerosis except for its diffuseness. These findings gave rise to the assumption that initial proliferative intimal lesions eventually become infiltrated with lipid, and the subsequent fibrous scarring leads to ordinary atherosclerotic disease by the time the process is clinically advanced enough to result in death.

The most distinctive morphological characteristic of AGAS relevant to its clinical recognition is its diffuseness and the lack of development of collateral vessels (Gao *et al.*, 1988). When first detected angiographically, it is almost always a concentric process diffusely affecting all the major epicardial coronary vessels and their branches. The focal proximal stenoses of ordinary atherosclerotic disease are uncommon. Moreover, the rate of progression can be quite rapid in comparison with the expected rate of progression of ordinary coronary disease. Rapid rates of progression of lesions over a 3-month interval are not unusual (Fig. 17.2). As mentioned above, the very diffuseness of the process can lead to angiographic under-estimation of its severity.

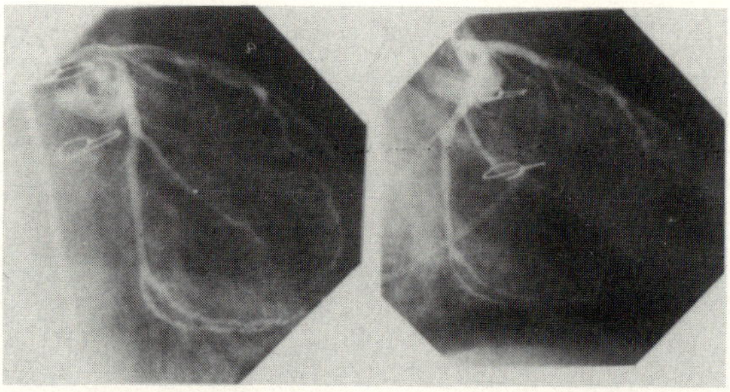

Fig. 17.2. *Serial coronary arteriograms (left coronary injection, RAO position) in heart transplant recipient 303, 13 months postoperatively on left panel and 15 months postoperatively on right panel. Note diffuse narrowing and distal 'pruning' of all vessels.*

Without careful comparison of serial angiograms, the observer can easily fail to identify a diffuse decrease in calibre of coronary vessels or the uniform shortening or 'pruning' of all the branches characteristic of AGAS.

There have been occasional reports (Mason and Strefling, 1979; Billingham, 1983; Palmer *et al.*, 1985) and anecdotal discussions describing a much rarer form of arterial disease of the cardiac allograft affecting the small intramyocardial arterioles only. Right ventricular biopsies of these patients are generally normal unless they happen to contain a section of arteriole (Palmer *et al.*, 1985). Coronary arteriograms can also be quite normal, but the patients die of complications of ischaemic heart disease. We have seen one such patient at Stanford in 18 years and are aware of the existence of several others.

AETIOLOGY

It seems clear that the occurrence of AGAS is not related to the risk factors for the occurrence of 'ordinary' coronary artery disease (Gao *et al.*, 1987). AGAS occurs as frequently in patients whose underlying cardiac disease was cardiomyopathy as in those who originally had arteriosclerotic vascular disease. The cause of AGAS has been postulated to be a process involving initial immune injury of the coronary endothelium, exposing a thrombogenic surface, with subsequent platelet aggregation, lipid infiltration and fibrous tissue accumulation, leading to intimal thickening and occlusive arterial lesions. This assumption is attractive because of the solid experimental evidence suggesting that arterial intimal injury of a variety of types is followed by local reactive changes which favour lipid deposition and lead to atherosclerosis (Hardin, Minick and Murphy, 1973; Minick, Stemerman and Insull, 1979). Indeed, in experimental rabbit (Alonso, Starek and Minick,

1977) and rat (Lurie *et al.*, 1981) models, morphologically similar lesions have been produced in cardiac allografts. These lesions are more prominent in cholesterol-fed rabbits. The relevance of these animal models to human disease is not clear, since vessel disease occurred in virtually all of the experimental animals at risk within a matter of days to months. However, the disease is evident, even at necropsy, in only a minority of patients over the intermediate term (1–5 years). Differences in the quality of immunosuppressive control or incompleteness of clinical data may account for this discrepancy.

In the rat model, there was no apparent correlation between the degree of vessel disease and the severity of graft rejection, a discordance which on the surface seems inconsistent with the theory of underlying immune injury causing the vessel disease. This discrepancy is also seen at the clinical level, as reflected in the general experience that a patient's rejection history is not a reliable predictor of his probability of developing AGAS. The Stanford group (Zusman *et al.*, 1985) reported a weak correlation between the number of rejection episodes and the probability of AGAS in cyclosporin-treated patients, but such a correlation has never been demonstrated in azathioprine-treated patients. Multivariate analysis has identified only mismatches at the HLA-A2 locus and elevated serum triglyceride (but not cholesterol) levels to be associated with the development of AGAS (Pennock *et al.*, 1982); the significance of these findings is not well understood.

There has been some speculation that antibody-mediated immune injury, independent of the usual clinically diagnosed cell-mediated graft rejection, might play a role in initiating the coronary endothelial injury leading to AGAS. Evidence in favour of this theory is so far limited to the observation of cytotoxic B-cell antibodies in 6 of a group of 14 cardiac transplant patients, all of whom developed AGAS less than $2\frac{1}{2}$ years after transplantation (Hess *et al.*, 1983). Why these antibodies should be injurious to the arterial wall, and why they should be elaborated apparently independently of the cell-mediated immune response, remains to be explained.

Thus, while the theory of immune injury to the coronary intima leading to AGAS is the most attractive and intuitively acceptable explanation of its aetiology, its mechanism remains unexplained and the relevance of current animal models is not clear.

CLINICAL CONSEQUENCES

Although the mechanisms leading to AGAS are not well understood, its consequences have become well appreciated. It follows a similar clinical pattern to ordinary occlusive coronary disease. Myocardial infarction, congestive heart failure and ventricular arrhythmias are all seen; sudden death is perhaps the most common clinical presentation. Angina pectoris is notably absent in these patients, presumably because of the lack of afferent re-innervation of the allograft. Myocardial infarctions are frequently 'silent', detected only by virtue of changes on routine serial electrocardiograms or of the onset of congestive heart failure or ventricular ectopic activity. The lack of the usual warning symptom of angina has led to the policy in most centres of performing annual coronary arteriograms on cardiac transplant recipients in an effort to detect AGAS before it leads to ischaemic graft injury. No reliable non-invasive method for detecting this form of coronary disease has emerged. Specifically, treadmill testing may be negative even with advanced disease, although the specificity and sensitivity of this or other non-invasive techniques for detecting AGAS have yet to be clarified.

AGAS currently ranks third, behind rejection and infection, as a cause of death in cardiac transplant recipients and is clearly emerging as a leading cause of death after the second postoperative year.

TREATMENT

The diffuseness of the occlusive disease seen in AGAS has precluded standard forms of therapy such as coronary bypass grafting or percutaneous transluminal coronary angioplasty (PTCA), which are designed to re-establish perfusion beyond discrete proximal arterial stenoses. Several unpublished attempts at PTCA in patients with AGAS have led to the expected disappointing results. In one attempt at Stanford, a discrete proximal lesion was easily dilated, but an angiogram 2 months later revealed re-stenosis and diffuse advance of the disease in all vessels. The patient died of congestive heart failure.

The only definitive therapy currently available is re-transplantation. Patients in the Stanford programme are offered the option of elective re-transplantation when the severity or rate of progression of asymptomatic AGAS is judged to be life-threatening, or when ischaemic complications have supervened. Figure 17.3 shows separate patient and graft actuarial survival curves from the Stanford programme; the difference of 4% at 5 years represents the small but definite impact of re-transplantation. Twenty-five of the 46 second transplants in the Stanford programme have been carried out because of AGAS in the original allograft, and the remainder because of intractable rejection. Survival rates after a second transplant are 60% at 3 months and 36% at 1 year.

Whether factors leading to the occurrence of AGAS in a first allograft will lead to its recurrence in an antigenically different second graft is not settled, in part because of the small number of patients available for analysis. In the Stanford series, 2 of 25 patients with second grafts implanted because of

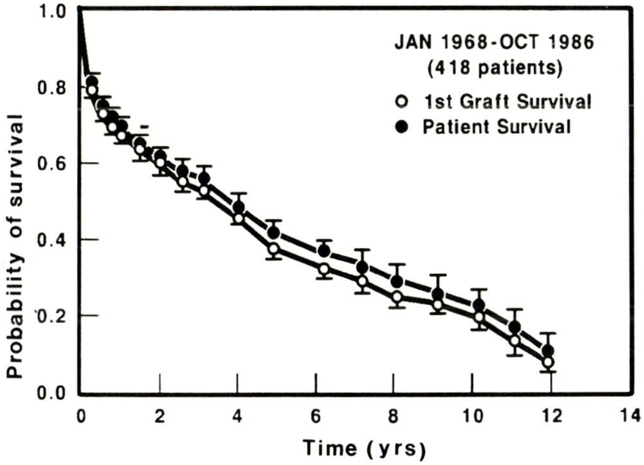

Fig. 17.3. *Patient survival vs. first graft survival (Stanford cardiac transplantation programme).*

AGAS rapidly developed AGAS; the rest have not. The ability to identify subgroups at high risk for recurrence would be most useful in terms of allocating scarce donor resources.

Prevention of AGAS is perhaps an even more important subject for investigation. Although some early reports suggested that prophylactic regimens employing systemic anticoagulation, the anti-platelet agent dipyridamole, and a low cholesterol, low saturated fat diet were effective in reducing AGAS (Griepp *et al.*, 1977), later analysis showed that the systemic anticoagulation could be omitted without changing the incidence of AGAS. In addition, analysis has not demonstrated any correlation between serum cholesterol measurement or hypertension and the incidence of AGAS. One of the animal experimental models (Lurie *et al.*, 1981) did demonstrate a strong protective effect of dipyridamole against the development of arteriolar lesions in rat cardiac allografts. Anti-platelet agents, including dipyridamole and aspirin, have been used routinely in most clinical programmes, largely because of their lack of adverse side effects, but no controlled clinical trial has demonstrated their efficacy, if any, in reducing AGAS. Thus, while the control of risk factors for ordinary coronary artery disease, and the routine use of antiplatelet agents, are strongly advocated by clinicians caring for cardiac transplant recipients, it remains unclear whether even the most meticulous adherence to such advice influences the probability of developing AGAS. The rational design of other interventions must await a clearer understanding of the basic causes of the disease.

Thus, even after 20 years of clinical work in cardiac transplantation, the often clinically silent but eventually lethal disease which we term AGAS remains a well-described but poorly understood phenomenon. As noted above, its other appellation, chronic rejection, is based on intuition rather than any solid evidence. Any logical attempts to prevent or modify this disease need to be based on some better understanding of its pathogenesis. Such understanding becomes most crucial as the occurrence of AGAS emerges as the main factor limiting long-term survival after what is otherwise the only successful treatment for end-stage heart disease.

REFERENCES

Alonso, D. R., Starek, P. K. and Minick, R. (1977). Studies on the pathogenesis of atheroarteriosclerosis induced in rabbit cardiac allografts by the synergy of graft rejection and hypercholesterolemia. *Am. J. Pathol.* **87**, 415–435.

Bieber, C. P., Hunt, S. A., Schwinn, D. A., Jamieson, S. A., Reitz, B. A., Oyer, P. E., Shumway, N. E. and Stinson, E. B. (1981). Complications in long-term survivors of cardiac transplantation. *Transplant. Proc.* **13**, 207–211.

Bieber, C. P., Stinson, E. B., Shumway, N. E., Payne, R. and Kosek, J. (1970). Cardiac transplantation in man: cardiac allograft pathology. *Circulation* **41**, 753–772.

Billingham, M. E. (1983). Diseases of the transplanted heart. In *Specific Heart Muscle Disease* (C. Symons, T. Evans and A. G. Mitchell, Eds), pp. 130–139. Wright, Bristol.

Gao, S. Z., Alderman, E. L. *et al.* (1988). Accelerated coronary vascular disease in the heart transplanted patient: coronary arteriographic findings. *J.A.C.C.* **12**.

Gao, S. Z., Schroeder, J. S., Alderman, E. L., Hunt, S. A., Silverman, J. F., Wiederhold, V. and Stinson, E. B. (1987). Clinical and laboratory correlates of accelerated coronary artery disease in the cardiac transplant patient. *Circulation* **76** (Suppl. V), V56–61.

Griepp, R. B., Stinson, E. B., Bieber, C. P., Reitz, B. A., Copeland, J. G., Oyer, P. E. and Shumway, N. E. (1977). Control of graft arterio-sclerosis in human heart transplant recipients. *Surgery* **81**, 262–269.

Hardin, N. J., Minick, R. and Murphy, G. E. (1973). Experimental induction of atheroarterio-sclerosis by the synergy of allergic injury to arteries and lipid-rich diet. *Am. J. Pathol.* **73**, 301–321.

Hess, M. L., Hastillo, A., Mohanakumar, T., Cowley, M. J., Vetrovac, G., Szentpetery, S., Wolfgang, T. C. and Lower, R. R. (1983). Accelerated atherosclerosis in cardiac transplantation: role of cytotoxic B-cell antibodies and hyperlipidemia. *Circulation* **68**(II), 94–101.

Kosek, J. C., Hurley, E. J. and Lower, R. R. (1968). Histopathology of orthotopic canine cardiac homografts. *Lab. Invest.* **19**, 97–112.

Lurie, K. G., Billingham, M. E., Jamieson, S. W., Harrison, D. C. and Reitz, B. A. (1981). Pathogenesis and prevention of graft arteriosclerosis in an experimental heart transplant model. *Transplantation* **31**, 41–47.

Mason, J. W. and Strefling, A. (1979). Small vessel disease of the heart resulting in myocardial necrosis and death despite angiographically normal coronary arteries. *Am. J. Cardiol.* **44**, 171–176.

Minick, C. R., Stemerman, M. B. and Insull, W. (1979). Role of endothelium and hypercholesterolemia in intimal thickening and lipid accumulation. *Am. J. Pathol.* **95**, 131–151.

Palmer, D. C., Tsai, C. C., Roodman, S. T., Codd, J. E., Miller, L. W., Sarafian, J. E. and Williams, G. A. (1985). Heart graft arteriosclerosis: an ominous finding on endomyocardial biopsy. *Transplantation* **39**, 385–388.

Pennock, J. L., Oyer, P. E., Reitz, B. A., Jamieson, S. W., Bieber, C. P., Wallwork, J., Stinson, E. B. and Shumway, N. E. (1982). Cardiac transplantation in perspective for the future: survival, complications, rehabilitation, and cost. *J. Thorac. Cardiovasc. Surg.* **83**, 168–177.

Zusman, D. R., Stinson, E. B., Oyer, P. E., Baldwin, J. C., Jamieson, S. W., McGregor, C. G., Hunt, S. A., Schroeder, J. S. and Shumway, N. E. (1985). Determinants of accelerated graft atherosclerosis (AGAS) in conventional and cyclosporine treated heart transplant recipients (Abstract). *J. Heart Transplant.* **4**, 587.

M. J. Buxton

18

Resource Implications of Heart Transplantation

INTRODUCTION

Heart transplantation shares at least one major characteristic with most other modern developments in medicine: its transition from an experimental technique to an accepted patient therapy has raised important questions about its resource implications. On the one hand, proponents have found it necessary to argue for additional direct funding for the programmes, or for specific insurance coverage for transplant patients, basing their arguments on the new 'lease of life' that transplantation offers. On the other hand, external critics (and clinical colleagues competing for resources for other patient groups) have argued against heart transplantation, suggesting that it is unduly expensive and diverts resources from more valuable health care uses.

Such was the nature of the debate in the early 1980s in the UK and USA — a debate which served only to highlight the paucity of systematic information on the costs and benefits of the procedure. Although for many comparable procedures, including for example liver transplantation, the lack of relevant economic data has persisted, heart transplantation has been the subject of at least two major economic studies involving the collection of primary data (one in the UK and one in the USA), and similar studies are under way in other countries such as the Netherlands. Thus heart transplantation is unusual (perhaps unique in terms of non-capital-intensive technologies) in that its diffusion has been influenced by evaluation at an early stage.

This chapter focuses on the resource use and cost data generated in the UK study of the costs and benefits of heart transplantation — UK HTS

(Buxton *et al.*, 1985). It compares these with data from the USA, principally from the US National Heart Transplantation Study — US NHTS (Evans *et al.*, 1984). It then discusses some of the issues involved in using these data to compare the cost-effectiveness of heart transplantation with that of different procedures. Finally, it considers how the various cost parameters have changed, and are still changing, and what factors are likely to influence future resource requirements.

COSTS OF HEART TRANSPLANTATION: UK EVIDENCE

The UK HTS was funded by the Department of Health and Social Security and was carried out between 1982 and 1984. It involved the collection of detailed patient-specific data on resource usage for heart transplant patients at Harefield and Papworth hospitals. In the National Health Service, where patient-based costing is exceptional because of the fixed budget nature of hospital funding, this required the introduction of very detailed data collection procedures.

The simplest indicator of resource usage, however, is length of stay at different stages in the programme. This is shown in Table 18.1. At Papworth, a standardized assessment procedure occurs, organized so that assessment normally takes place over 3 days. It relies on the patients having had various tests performed in advance at their local hospital or referring centre. Thus, the mean length of stay at assessment during the period of study (1 January 1982–30 September 1984) was 3.1 days, a figure that reflected a slight increase in the length of stay in each of the three years 1982–84.

At Harefield, the mean length of stay for assessment fell dramatically from a figure of 17.3 days in 1982 to 8.2 days in 1984, although this figure was still considerably greater than that for Papworth. This reflected, among other factors, much less reliance than at Papworth on the performance of tests elsewhere in advance of admission. The length of stay at Harefield for assessment has continued to fall to 5.0 days in 1986.

The figures for postoperative lengths of stay are rather different. At both centres the length of stay fell initially, but at the end of the formal study there remained a substantial difference between the two centres for the lengths of in-patient (IP) stay for patients discharged alive. The figures for 1984 for this postoperative period as IPs were 15.0 days at Harefield and 42.4 days at Papworth. Some of this difference was explained by the use of the 'transplant flats' provided in Harefield village by the Harefield Heart Transplant Trust. These provide a 'halfway house' for many patients between their discharge as an IP and their actual return home, if that home is some distance away from the centre. During the period in the flats, they

TABLE 18.1

Numbers of Transplants and Average Lengths of Stay 1982–86 (UK Heart Transplant Study Centres)

Study Centre	*1982*	*1983*	*1984*	*1985*	*1986*
HAREFIELD					
No. of heart transplants	20	34	75*	83†	80‡
Length of stay (days):					
assessment	17.3	9.9	8.2	6.4	5.0
transplant to discharge	30.3	18.0	15.0	19.8	20.0
post-discharge stay in flats	20.5	13.7	§	§	§
transplant to death (prior to discharge)	20.6	22.5	18.9	10.7	10.4
PAPWORTH					
No. of heart transplants	16	19	39	44	52
Length of stay (days):					
assessment	2.7	3.2	3.4	3.3	3.3
transplant to discharge	51.9	46.1	42.4	32.2	27.1
post-discharge stay in flats	0.0	0.3	0.8	5.8	10.1
transplant to death (prior to discharge)	17.4	21.0	17.0	31.3	12.0

* Plus 2 transplants performed elsewhere but transferred and followed up as part of the Harefield programme.

† Plus 6 transplants performed elsewhere but transferred and followed up as part of the Harefield programme.

‡ Plus 31 transplants performed elsewhere but transferred and followed up as part of the Harefield programme.

§ Detailed figures not available but routinely a stay of about 2 weeks.

Source: UK Heart Transplant Study data (Tables 3.1 and 3.3 updated to end of 1986).

attend Harefield Hospital regularly (initially daily) as outpatients (OPs). An equivalent arrangement for Papworth patients did not become a regular feature until 1985. Since then, length of IP stay at Papworth has continued to fall, whereas at Harefield it has risen again from the 1984 low. Thus, in 1986, the length of IP stay after transplantation was 20.0 days at Harefield and 27.1 at Papworth, plus routinely a 2-week stay in the flats at Harefield and 10.1 days at Papworth.

In the UK HTS, detailed analysis of costs was conducted for the main stages of treatment during the period 1 July 1983–30 June 1984. This cost analysis included direct attribution of nursing costs, drugs and blood products, costs relating to the operation, and all diagnostic tests. It included by apportionment ward/ICU consumables and all general hospital services. However, these patient-specific figures *exclude* capital costs, and the main inputs of the surgical staff teams responsible for the programmes. The latter

TABLE 18.2

Average Lengths of Stay and Cost per Patient; Assessment, July 1983–June 1984 (UK Heart Transplant Study Centres)

	Harefield (n = 65)	*Papworth (n = 49)*
	(1983–84 prices)	
	£	£
Nursing	390	83
Consumables	39	8
Drugs	33	7
Respiratory physiology	25	2
Radiography, etc.	64	12
Pathology, etc.	181	120
Electrocardiography	20	1
Other	11	27
Sub-total	762	260
General services	418	169
Grand total	1180	429
Length of stay (days)	9.7	3.6

Source: UK Heart Transplant Study (Table 6.1 and unpublished data).

were treated as overhead costs, in that they could not be allocated to specific patients, but only to the programme as a whole.

Table 18.2 presents a breakdown of costs for assessment at each of the centres; these costs closely reflect the differences in length of stay for these patients — and imply a very similar 'cost per day of assessment' at each hospital.

Table 18.3 similarly presents costs for the period of transplant to discharge for patients discharged alive, and (in summary) for patients who died in hospital. In the case of Harefield, the intermediate discharge was to the Harefield flats, from where transplant recipients could be treated as OPs. Unlike assessment costs, the differences between centres in costs from transplant to discharge might be expected to reflect not simply differences in total length of stay, but also the 'one-off' costs of the operation and the higher costs of the period of ICU care.

Subsequent to the Report of the UK HTS, further analysis of these patient-specific cost data has focused on the variability within the averages cited and possible explanatory factors. It emphasizes the wide variations within each centre in treatment costs for patients, particularly for drug,

TABLE 18.3

Average Length of Stay and Cost per Patient; Transplant Operation to Discharge, July 1983–June 1984 (UK Heart Transplant Study Centres)

	Harefield (*1983–84 prices*)		*Papworth*
	Hospital	*Flats*	
PATIENTS DISCHARGED ALIVE	($n = 47$)		($n = 21$)
	£	£	£
Nursing	1490	—	2735
Consumables	149	—	273
Drugs	767	452	1445
Recipient operation	934	—	1711
Respiratory physiology	47	—	—
Radiography, etc.	170	68	584
Pathology, etc.	642	153	1656
Blood products	377	—	465
Electrocardiography	66	17	76
Physiotherapy	26	—	110
Sub-total	4668	691	9055
General services	615	207	2103
Grand total	5283	898	11 158
Length of stay total (days)	14.2	12.2	44.3
Length of stay in ICU (days)	11.4	—	15.4
DIED IN HOSPITAL PRIOR TO DISCHARGE:	($n = 4$)		($n = 3$)
Grand total cost	10 071		8187
Length of stay, total (days)	19.0		12.7
Length of stay, ICU (days)	17.2		12.7

Source: UK Heart Transplant Study (Tables 6.3 and 6.4 and unpublished data).

pathology and radiography costs. An analysis by Bell (1987) found that these variations in costs could not generally be explained in terms of differences in basic patient characteristics (age, sex, diagnosis, previous surgery or period on the waiting list), nor of donor characteristics (age, sex or ischaemic time).

Transplant type was significant — heterotopic transplants were found to employ a significantly higher level of resources. In addition, this analysis re-confirmed that there was a highly significant time trend in costs — with nearly all elements of resource usage declining over time.

Nevertheless, the remarkable finding from the further analysis of the data relating to 66 transplant patients discharged alive from the two hospitals was that 89% of the variation in transplant to discharge costs for each patient could be explained by a single simple linear regression of length of stay.

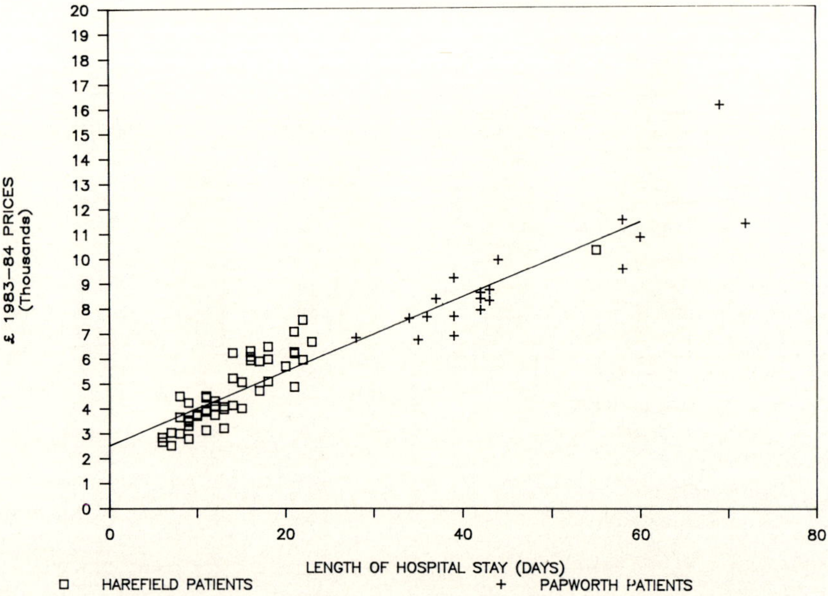

Fig. 18.1. *Lengths of stay and costs: transplant to discharge (UK HTS Centres).*

Figure 18.1 illustrates this with a scattergram of length of stay and costs and the regression line.

However, costs continue beyond discharge and, as has already been indicated, the point of discharge may itself be influenced by whether or not

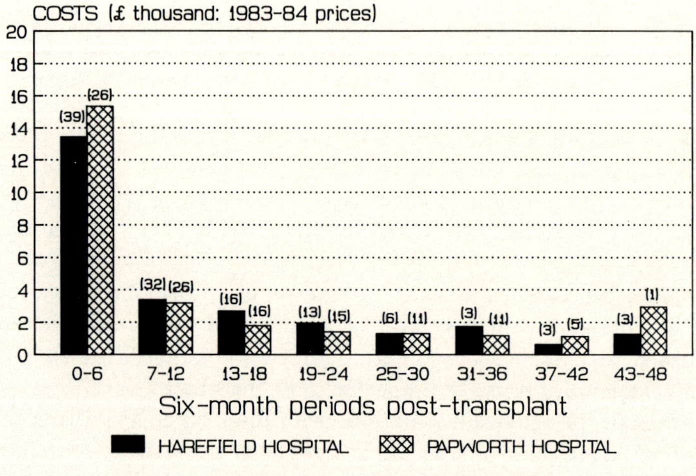

Fig. 18.2. *Average 6-monthly costs per patient (UK HTS Centres). Numbers of observations in parentheses. (Source: Reanalysis of UK Heart Transplant Study data)*

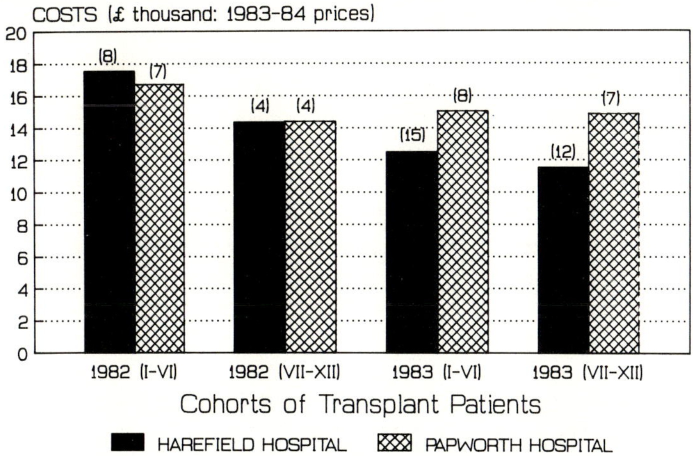

Fig. 18.3. *Average cost per patient: transplant to discharge (UK HTS Centres). Numbers of observations in parentheses. (Source: Reanalysis of UK Heart Transplant Study data)*

convenient arrangements can be made for the patient to be seen regularly as an OP following early discharge. For this reason, the UK study costed patients on a basis of 6-month periods from transplant, so enabling a time profile of costs to be built up. Figure 18.2 presents an analysis of costs in this way. The major element in the cost of ongoing therapy is that of the immunosuppressive drug regimen. In addition, there are the costs of OP visits, and both routine and unscheduled readmissions. The data in Fig. 18.2 are estimates of all these costs including OP attendances at the patient's local hospital.

Within the limits of the period for which detailed cost data was collected, the study also examined change in costs over time. Figure 18.3 shows how costs for the first 6-month period from transplant (including costs of donor operation and the immediate postoperative period) changed for 4 consecutive cohorts of transplanted patients. It shows a steady reduction in costs at Harefield, whereas at Papworth costs levelled out after an initial reduction.

COSTS OF HEART TRANSPLANTATION: US EVIDENCE

US Heart Transplantation Study

The main source of cost analysis for the USA is the National Heart Transplantation Study (US NHTS) from Evans *et al.* (1984). This study obtained information on patients from six centres (University of Arizona; Presbyterian Hospital, Columbia; Medical College of Virginia; University of

Minnesota; University of Pittsburgh; and University Medical Centre, Stanford) for the period 1 January 1978–30 June 1983.

Table 18.4 shows data for assessment (or evaluation as it is referred to in the USA). These figures show considerable variation in average cost between centres, and even greater variation within centres. A mean charge of $8.3 thousand dollars, reflecting 8.9 days of hospitalization at this period, was estimated. However, the modal period for the actual evaluation was only 4.0 days. The data suggest that although a routine assessment pattern of 4.0 days existed in most centres, for a number of patients evaluation took place over a much more extended period.

Table 18.5 shows the US NHTS data on a similar basis for transplant hospitalization (equivalent to the UK transplant–discharge data), for patients discharged alive and separately for those who died prior to discharge. It indicates lengths of stay in the ICU and in general wards, and hospital *charges*. The 'total charge' figures represent actual billing data. The 'Medicare costs' are estimates of what would have been the charge to Medicare (before allowing for patient cost-sharing) on the basis of the then ruling Medicare cost reimbursement system. Evans *et al.* (1984) suggest that these estimates may be the better indicator of resource costs. Like the UK figures (although for different pragmatic reasons), all these charges exclude the main fees for physician services which were estimated to be in the order of an additional $10 000. The lengths of stay and charges again show considerable variation in means between centres, and the standard deviations indicate a broad range of costs within centres. The total lengths of stay (and stay in the ICU) are higher than for the UK.

Evans and his colleagues also estimated the ongoing cost of care for transplant patients, including further hospitalization at the transplant centre or at other hospitals, OP costs and drug costs. However, unlike the UK data these are calculated in terms of one-year *post-discharge*, and are not published for each centre or for different time periods. Figure 18.4 shows the annual pattern of costs for survivors (including transplant costs into the first year's costs) to give a broadly comparable figure to that from the 6-monthly UK data in Fig. 18.2. These figures are estimated from the US NHTS Report and are only approximate.

National Health Services and Practice Patterns Survey data

More recently in the USA, the National Health Services and Practice Patterns Survey (NHSPPS) on heart transplantation has been published by the Medical Technology and Practice Patterns Institute (1986). This is based on cost data from 11 centres (Barnes Hospital, St. Louis; Foster G. McGaw Hospital, University of Chicago; Hartford Hospital, Hartford; Methodist

TABLE 18.4

Average Lengths of Stay and Costs per Patient: Evaluation for Transplant (US Heart Transplant Study Centres)

	Arizona (*n* = 23)	*Columbia* (*n* = 18)	*MCV* (*n* = 29)	*Minnesota* (*n* = 19)	*Pittsburgh* (*n* = 47)	*Stanford* (*n* = 93)	*Weighted Mean*
Mean Length of Hospital Stay (days)							
ICU/CCU	4.4	2.8	2.1	4.3	1.6	3.8	
Ward	3.3	10.3	7.1	7.9	4.2	4.2	
Total	7.7	13.1	9.2	12.2	5.7	8.1	8.9
Total Length of Evaluation Period (days)							
Mean	8.5	13.7	12.1	11.5	12.6	9.5	10.8
(Standard deviation)	(11.5)	(25.0)	(28.8)	(10.8)	(36.4)	(20.8)	
Mode	3.0	4.0	4.0	4.0	4.0	4.0	4.0
				(US$ thousand; 1983 prices)			
Total charge	4.5	8.9	5.8	12.1	6.7	11.1	8.3
(Standard deviation)	(5.0)	(5.6)	(4.0)	(8.2)	(7.1)	(21.5)	

Source: Evans *et al.* (1984) (based on Table 28.4).

TABLE 18.5

Costs per Patient and Average Lengths of Stay: Transplant Hospitalization (US Heart Transplant Study Centres)

	Arizona	*Columbia*	*MCV*	*Minnesota*	*Pittsburgh*	*Stanford*	*Weighted Mean*
PATIENTS DISCHARGED ALIVE:	($n = 31$)	($n = 12$)	($n = 17$)	($n = 12$)	($n = 37$)	($n = 99$)	
Total charge (US$ thousand; 1983 prices)	63.8	103.7	63.1	55.3	67.7	89.3	
(Standard deviation)	(25.0)	(48.1)	(23.4)	(26.6)	(22.7)	(39.4)	
'Medicare cost' (US$ thousand; 1983 prices)	51.9	72.8	53.5	54.4	47.5	74.1	61.7
Length of stay (days):							
ICU/CCU	31.3	23.3	11.5	27.9	6.3	30.9	
ward	25.1	40.7	66.4	8.0	45.5	19.8	
Total	56.4	64.0	77.9	35.9	51.8	50.7	55.9
PATIENTS WHO DIED BEFORE DISCHARGE:	($n = 8$)	($n = 10$)	($n = 8$)	($n = 8$)	($n = 12$)	($n = 20$)	
Total charge (US$ thousand; 1983 prices)	56.5	77.0	42.0	55.9	52.9	161.6	
(Standard deviation)	(42.1)	(44.5)	(46.5)	(44.4)	(38.0)	(103.6)	
'Medicare cost' (US$ thousand; 1983 prices)	33.8	43.4	36.9	47.8	39.0	133.8	66.8
Length of stay (days):							
ICU/CCU	12.5	17.0	15.3	14.3	9.0	64.2	
ward	5.5	9.1	9.6	3.1	13.8	13.2	
Total	18.0	26.1	24.9	17.4	22.8	77.5	38.3

Source: Evans *et al.* (1984) (based on Tables 28.7 and 28.8).

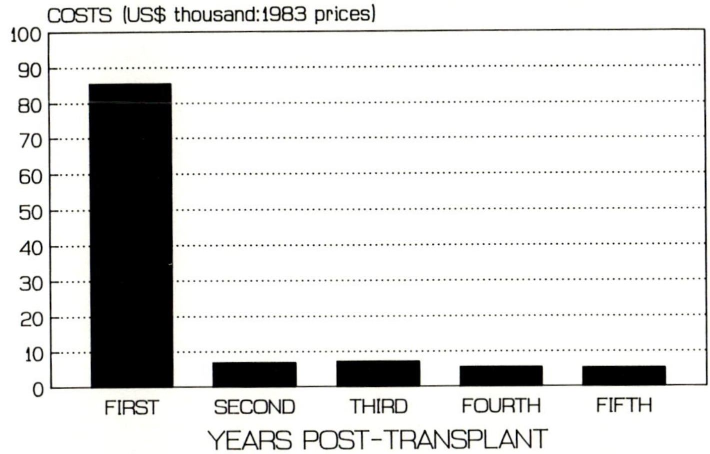

Fig. 18.4. *Average annual costs per patient (US Heart Transplant Study Centres). (Source: Based on US Heart Transplant Study data)*

Hospital of Indiana, Indianapolis; Presbyterian University Hospital, Pittsburgh; Sharp Memorial Hospital, San Diego; St. Luke's Episcopal Hospital, Houston; St. Luke's Hospital, St. Louis; Tallahasse Memorial Regional Medical Center, Tallahassee; Temple University Hospital, Philadelphia; University of Utah Health Sciences Center, Salt Lake City). Of these, only the University of Pittsburgh was included in the Evans study. It is claimed that this sample of 11 hospitals was 'representative of the universe of heart transplant centers, both established and emerging' in the USA. The study used data on costs and resource requirements for all heart transplant procedure cases at these centres from the beginning of 1985 through to mid-1986 — a total of 237 discharges. Their analysis included the small subset of patients who died in hospital. The average length of stay from transplant to discharge for these patients was 41 days — a lower figure than that observed in the earlier US NHTS. Table 18.6 shows that *costs* also appear similarly to have fallen when compared with the nearest equivalent US NHTS data (revalued to 1987 prices). This table also shows the difference in costs between Medicare and non-Medicare patients: the NHSPSS study suggests that the 'Medicare-eligible patients are likely to represent a patient population with greater severity of illness, long-standing conditions and presence of co-existing disease'.

COMPARING COSTS AND BENEFITS

Information on the costs of heart transplantation, or the resources it uses, is really only helpful when put into the context of the benefits gained from

TABLE 18.6

Costs per Patient for Hospitalization to Discharge (Comparison of US Data Sources)

		US$ thousand (1987 prices)
MTPPI Data		
Non-Medicare discharges	$n = 178$	59.3
Medicare discharges	$n = 59$	66.8
All discharges	$n = 238$	63.7
*UK HTS Data**		
Survivors	$n = 208$	72.1
Decedents	$n = 66$	78.2
Case-weighted combination	$n = 274$	73.6

* 'Medicare cost' estimates (see Table 18.5), inflated from 1983 prices to 1987 prices (by 1.17 price inflation factor).

Source: MTPPI (1986) (calculated from Table 6).

heart transplantation and from other competing claims on health care resources. Costs then become a shorthand linkage to benefits forgone elsewhere.

The UK and US studies both emphasize the need for this perspective, and both include important data on survival and on patients' quality of life. The US NHTS study explores one of the main analytical routes to making comparisons between alternative uses of the resources, by integrating the cost information with benefit data (on survival and quality of life), and presents estimates of cost per 'quality-adjusted life year' or (QALY).

The idea of using 'cost per QALY' as a cross-programme indicator of the cost-effectiveness of health care interventions has been advocated both in the USA and in the UK. Weinstein and Stason (1977), from the Harvard School of Public Health, have presented the conceptual approach. Since about that time it has been applied extensively in North America, particularly by Torrance and colleagues at McMaster University — for a review see Torrance (1986). In the UK, its use has been championed particularly by Williams (1985), and is now beginning to be seen in official reports; for example, the 'Forrest Report' on breast cancer screening (UK Department of Health and Social Security, 1986b).

Applied to heart transplantation, the cost per QALY concept could be represented as in Fig. 18.5. It would involve the estimation of the average costs (including assessment costs, donor organ operation, transplant to discharge, and post-discharge costs) of a transplant (at time T) associated with an average expected survival experience to ST years, and a quality of life

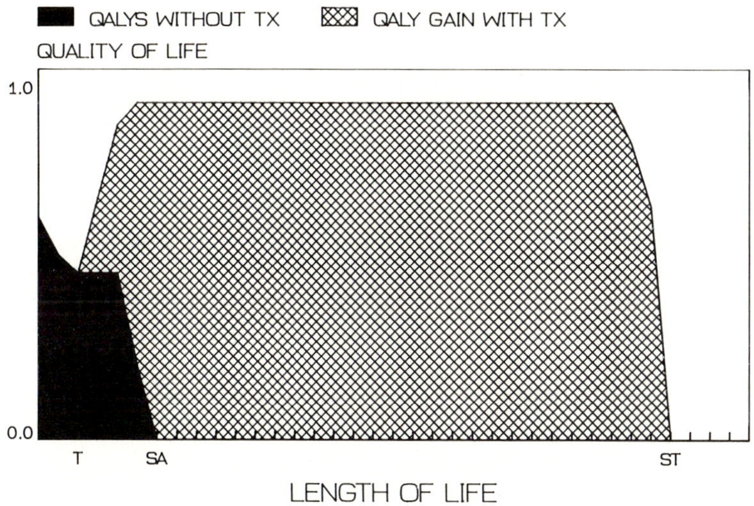

Fig. 18.5. *QUALYs gained from transplantation.*

profile as shown by the upper curve. From these would be deducted the alternative costs of 'routine' medical management (if the patient were not transplanted) associated with the alternative average survival to *SA* years, and the lower quality of life profile. These net costs would be the costs of achieving the net gain in QALYs: the hatched area.

The US NHTS study calculates a 'base case' estimate of $23.5 thousand per life-year gained, within a range of $14.0–$30.0 thousand. This range reflects 'various plausible assumptions about discount rates and the costs of alternative treatment (i.e. not receiving a transplant)'. These figures do not include any quality-adjustment of the life-years gained and are based on a mean estimated post-transplant survival of 6.5 years — a figure derived from a hypothetical survival probability model that, rather than being mathematically derived from actual data, was 'rough, subjective estimates, balancing apparent trends intuitively' — Chapter 29.18 in Evans *et al.* (1984).

However crude or sophisticated in detail, the QALY approach involves extrapolating future long-term survival. The UK study had reasonably firm data for survival for only 3 years, and the authors took the view that any calculation of cost per QALY at that stage would involve too many subjective assumptions that could not be substantiated or justified by the empirical data.

More recently, UK survival data for 287 patients (up to 30 April, 1985) was used to illustrate the effect on estimated net survival of alternative estimation procedures (O'Brien, Buxton and Ferguson, 1987). A simple linear extrapolation (as in the US study) of the observed survival probabilities was compared with two parametric survival projections (a simple exponential model and the Weibull model). Although all three models related well to the short period of observed data, at 20 years' projection the degree of uncertainty is considerable. In addition, the paper attempted to make the best estimate of survival without transplantation calculated from mean survival time from *acceptance* (based on all pre-transplant experience). This suggested an alternative average survival of about 10 months. Subtracting this from the alternative 20-year survival projections gives us a wide range of estimates of life-years gained of from 2.6 to 9.3 years. Given such uncertainty, the niceties of quality adjustment, etc., seem rather theoretical, particularly since (as is indicated in Chapter 19) post-transplant quality of life has been found to be very close to normal 'full' health.

However, the 'cost per QALY' framework is worth exploring further. The costs of heart transplantation can usefully be seen in terms of three elements — the 'screening' costs of identifying, selecting and assessing potential transplant recipients; the 'investment' costs of the surgery, and immediate post-operative period; and the ongoing 'maintenance' costs of drug therapy, monitoring, etc.

As survival increases, so the 'screening' costs and the surgical 'investment' are amortized over a greater number of life-years gained, and the cost per life-year gained approaches the annual maintenance cost which sets a lower bound for the cost per life-year. This annual cost is heavily dependent on the immunosuppressive regimen. The US NHTS figures included an estimated $810 per year for immunosuppressive drugs, but the report notes that this 'mean for immunosuppressive drugs is well below the $10 000–$11 000 per year that might possibly be charged if cyclosporin is the drug of choice' — Chapter 28.42 in Evans *et al.* (1984). The UK study suggested that the then current cyclosporin-based drug therapy had an average cost of approximately £3000 per patient per year. A more recent US estimate suggests annual cyclosporin costs of $4–5 thousand per patient (Evans, 1986). In 1994, the 20-year UK patent for Cyclosporine will expire and lower price generic substitutes may appear; however, it appears likely that by then a new generation of (expensive?) immunosuppressants will be available.

The 'investment' costs of the surgery and immediate postoperative period have generally been falling, but there seems to be only limited scope in the UK for further substantial falls in these costs (resulting from reductions in length of stay) when in 1986 postoperative lengths of hospital IP stay averaged only 20 days at Harefield and 27 days at Papworth. Furthermore, the 'screening' costs per patient screened are unlikely to fall much further, although the cost per subsequent *transplant* may be reduced by two factors: first, careful pre-selection of patients at referral, so that very few patients are rejected after the assessment (evaluation) work-up, and secondly by careful management of the programme, so that patients are assessed only if there is a high probability of a donor heart being available sufficiently soon — so minimizing deaths among assessed patients.

If current data on observed costs and observed survival experience are extrapolated to estimate 'costs per QALY' for heart transplantation, it is neither as expensive as its critics would infer, nor as cheap as its proponents would wish. Evans (1986) concludes that, in the US context, 'the annual per-case cost of heart transplantation compares well with that of the other forms of long-term life-saving therapy such as kidney dialysis, management of the cancer patient and total parenteral nutrition'. He suggests that 'if we decide we cannot or do not want to afford a new technology, such as heart transplantation, then it is only fair that we reconsider other "accepted" therapies that have lesser or equal benefits'.

In the UK, Williams, in advocating a 'cost per QALY' approach to prioritizing health care expenditures, has frequently cited heart transplantation (quoting not implausible estimates of 'cost per QALY' of £5000 (Williams, 1985) and more recently £8000 (Williams, 1987). At first sight, the implication of his figures and argument must be that resources should not be devoted to heart transplantation in the UK until a number of other services have been expanded that are more beneficial in cost per QALY terms. However, he recognizes that uncompromising rigidity in allocating all resources according to cost per QALY might stifle medical progress in that 'many of the interventions which are now commonplace (and cost-effective) started off being very expensive in relation to the rather uncertain benefits they initially generated during the experimental stage' (Williams, 1987). He suggests that any intervention that is too costly in relation to its benefits to be worth funding out of the therapeutic budget of the health service should compete for research funding, which would be provided *only if* there is a reasonable prospect that its results will improve or costs fall significantly and *if* it is funded as a research activity subject to formal protocols, independent evaluation and full disclosure of data.

The UK and US studies indicate that the exact position of heart transplantation in the cost per QALY league table of therapeutic interventions depends upon uncertain extrapolations of survival data and estimates of future cost changes. However, heart transplantation undoubtedly qualifies for support in Williams' 'research' category. Indeed, it is clear that even pessimistic estimates of cost per QALY for heart transplantation are lower than for several of the routinely accepted therapeutic interventions (such as haemodialysis) for which data are available (Hurst, 1987). How it compares with the all too many interventions that as yet have been subjected to absolutely no economic evaluation will only emerge when these too are subject to rigorous analysis (Buxton, 1987a).

COSTS AND BENEFITS: THE FUTURE

If heart transplantation were a fully developed technology in a stable state the problems of costing and evaluation would be much reduced. But, as has been stressed, the available data show considerable evidence of change in costs and benefits over the past few years, and this changing basis makes extrapolation of future benefits and costs exceedingly difficult (Buxton, 1987b).

In terms of costs, a number of important changes are still taking place:

(1) *Changes in patient management in the transplant–discharge period.* The reduction in length of stay has been an important feature, and may continue to be so at centres where it is still longer than others. With changes in total length of stay may come further reductions in the expensive period in ICU/CCU. At Papworth, the average stay for transplant patients in ICU/CCU in 1984 was 15.4 days; by 1986 this had fallen to 5.6 days. At the end of the hospital stay, arrangements for patients temporarily to live locally may allow further substitution of OP for IP care. At Papworth, the UK HTS data include the cost of a pacemaker for all patients. At present at Papworth, pacemaker leads are inserted during all heart transplant operations, but the need for the pacemakers is assessed before discharge home and in 1986 only in 1 in 4 patients was it necessary to fit a pacemaker.

(2) *Changes in long-term management.* The most important element in long-term costs is the immunosuppressive regimen. Cyclosporin increased costs (but also increased cost-effectiveness through improved survival). The long-term side effects of cyclosporin may, however, be a negative factor. Future changes in this area are uncertain but potentially very important.

(3) *Changes in technology related to the 'replacement' heart.* Two separate developments in this field have rather different implications. Techniques for increasing the 'safe' ischaemic time may be important in reducing some of the costs of donor procurement and of the recipient operation by relaxing time constraints and so permitting rather more routine management of the transplant episode. More dramatically, the use of an artificial heart as a bridging device — or a temporary holding state more comparable with renal dialysis — appears to offer a major technical advance. However, it may simply reduce cost-effectiveness by increasing costs while not improving the survival from the programme as a whole. Certainly, if the supply of donor hearts is the limiting factor, or indeed if the shortage of resources constrains the number of transplant operations, then the temporary artificial heart will merely change the allocation of donor hearts among the excess demand from potential

recipients. Improvements in programme survival would only arise if the survival prognosis of a patient transplanted after being maintained with an artificial heart is better than the survival prognosis of the patient (the same patient without the intervening assist period, or another patient) who would otherwise have received the donor organ.

(4) *Changes in patient selection.* Running counter to the various tendencies to reduce costs may be the trend to relax exclusion criteria in patient selection. For example, diabetes is no longer considered a contraindicator. *If* newly included categories of patients have greater costs associated with them due to their age or concomitant disease or have poorer survival/quality of life prospects, then 'cost per QALY' will increase.

Each of these factors has potential for changing costs and benefits and so changing the cost-effectiveness of the procedure. Heart transplantation has been unusual in the intensity and extensiveness of early economic evaluation. However, evaluation is not a one-off single point-of-time process. A continuing process of monitoring is required to identify and formally consider the economic (i.e. cost *and* benefit) implications of changes in the available technology, of changes in patient selection, etc. This monitoring, particularly if it involves comparative analysis of the performance of different centres, can indicate positive changes that can be made to reduce the costs while at the same time improving results. The UK evidence shows that clinicians have been willing to respond to such information produced as a by-product of the UK HTS to increase their cost-effectiveness. Such a process needs to be maintained in the context of an ongoing monitoring system.

ECONOMICS AND POLICY DECISIONS

In both the UK and USA explicit policy decisions have been made that appear to be broadly consistent with the economic picture described above.

For a number of years in the UK, after the two heart transplant programmes had been set up with mainly charitable funding, specific *ad hoc* grants were centrally allocated by the Department of Health and Social Security (Buxton, 1988). However, in 1985, following receipt of the UK HTS Report, the Secretary of State sought the advice of the Supra-Regional Services Advisory Group regarding the most appropriate way to develop the heart transplant programme. The Advisory Group recommended that heart transplantation should be recognized as a supra-regional speciality, and designated the existing units at Papworth and Harefield Hospitals, and a new centre at the Freeman Hospital in Newcastle-upon-Tyne. In allocating funds for 1986–87, the original two centres were expected to maintain their levels of activity while the new unit expanded to approximately the same level (UK Department of Health and Social Security, 1986b).

In their allocations for 1987–88, the Advisory Group announced that a programme of heart transplants for children would be added (as a joint venture between the Hospital for Sick Children, Great Ormond Street, London and Papworth) and suggested that funds for a fourth adult centre would be approved for the subsequent financial year.

Thus, the policy is one of cautious expansion of a limited number of centres. It is not as tight a *research* environment as Williams would require, not is it an unrestrained adoption of the technology as routine. Typically for the NHS, costs are constrained through programme budgets; the procedure is available to those who can be treated within those official budgets, supplemented by whatever charitable support the centres can obtain.

In the USA, the major step by the Federal Government was taken in June 1986, when it announced that Medicare (the programme of health care benefits, available to those 65 or over and the disabled, administered by the Health Care Financing Administration) would provide coverage for heart transplantation, provided the transplants were carried out in facilities that met certain eligibility criteria aimed at identifying necessary experience and expertise (US Department of Health and Human Services, 1986). The US Department of Health and Human Services estimated that up to 10 transplant centres would qualify to perform heart transplants for Medicare and that up to 65 transplants would be covered in the first year. This imposition of eligibility criteria is particularly significant, when in the USA 94 different hospitals performed heart transplants during 1986 (Office of Health Technology Assessment, 1987). They carried out 1368 heart transplants. Although this decision directly affects Medicare patients only, it may be significant in encouraging private insurers to adopt similar criteria.

However, in the USA the major resource constraint is not now finance but donor availability. The critical resource is the donor hearts (Evans *et al.*, 1986). Various efforts have been made to increase the supply of donors, including the required request legislation now adopted in many states, and the changes permitting procurement agencies primarily established to supply kidneys for transplantation to charge for the procurement of other organs. The US 'Task Force on Organ Transplantation' (1986) made a large number of specific recommendations to help further increase the supply of donor organs. However, while a shortage of donor hearts clearly exists in the USA, and to a lesser extent is arising in the UK, it then becomes essential that programmes are managed not only to maximize cost-effectiveness but also to maximize the benefit from this vital constrained resource. This in itself may require specific policies as regards allocation of organs within and between centres (O'Brien, 1987). It will require careful consideration as to the real implications of the use of artificial hearts as a temporary measure. It may also hasten the development of totally implantable assist devices.

Heart transplantation has been subjected to unusually rigorous economic scrutiny, and the initial indicators of cost-effectiveness are not unfavourable. The various changes outlined above, and other smaller technological changes, will continue to occur and will affect costs and benefits. These changes will need monitoring and active management, if heart transplantation is to become firmly and incontrovertibly accepted as a cost-effective routine therapy.

REFERENCES

Bell, R. (1987). *Modelling the costs of heart transplants by patient characteristics: a perspective on DRGs*. HERG Discussion Paper no. 5. Health Economics Research Group, Brunel University, Uxbridge.

Buxton, M. J. (1987a). Problems in the economic appraisal of new health technology: the evaluation of heart transplants in the UK. In *Economic Appraisal of Health Technology in the European Community* (M. F. Drummond, Ed.), pp. 103–118. Oxford University Press, Oxford.

Buxton, M. J. (1987b). The economic evaluation of high technology medicine: the case of heart transplants. In *Health and Economics* (A. Williams, Ed.). Macmillan, London.

Buxton, M. J. (1988). Heart transplantation in the U.K.: the decision making context of an economic evaluation. In *European Regulatory Mechanisms for Technology Assessment* (B. Stocking, Ed.), pp. 36–48. Oxford University Press, Oxford.

Buxton, M., Acheson, R., Caine, N., Gibson, S. and O'Brien, B. (1985). *Costs and benefits of the heart transplant programmes at Harefield and Papworth Hospitals*. DHSS Research Report no. 12. Her Majesty's Stationery Office, London.

Evans, R. W. (1986). The heart transplant dilemma. *Iss. Sci. Technol.* Spring, 91–101.

Evans, R. W., Manninen, D. L., Garrison, L. P. and Maier, A. M. (1986). Donor availability as the primary determinant of the future of heart transplantation. *J. Am. Med. Ass.* **255**(14), 1892–1898.

Evans, R. W., Manninen, D. L., Overcast, T. D., Garrison, L. P., Yagi, J., Merrikin, K., Jonsen, A. R. *et al.* (1984). *The National Heart Transplantation Study: final report*. Battelle Human Affairs Research Centers, Seattle, Washington, D.C.

Hurst, J. W. (1987). New attitudes in assessing benefits. In *Costs and Benefits of Pharmaceutical Research* (G. Teeling Smith, Ed.), pp. 18–24. Office of Health Economics, London.

Medical Technology and Practice Patterns Institute (1986). *National health services and practices patterns survey: report on heart transplantation procedure operating costs, Medicare payments and utilization rates*. MTPPI, Washington, D.C.

O'Brien, B. J. (1987). A game—theoretic approach to donor kidney sharing. *Social Science and Medicine* (in press).

O'Brien, B. J., Buxton, M. J. and Ferguson, B. A. (1987). Measuring the effectiveness of heart transplant programmes: quality of life data and their relationship to survival analysis. *J. Chron. Dis.*, **40**, Suppl. 1, 1375–1535.

Office of Health Technology Assessment (1987). *Transplant activity summary: December 1986* (mimeo). OHTA, Rockville, MD.

Task Force on Organ Transplantation (1986). *Organ transplantation: issues and recommendations.* US Department of Health and Human Services, Washington, D.C.

Torrance, G. W. (1986). Measurement of health state utilities for economic appraisal. *J. Health Econ.* **5**, 1–30.

US Department of Health and Human Services (1986). *Press release*, 27 June. DHHS, Washington, D.C.

UK Department of Health and Social Security (1986a). *Breast cancer screening: report by a working group chaired by Professor Sir Patrick Forrest.* Her Majesty's Stationery Office, London.

UK Department of Health and Social Security (1986b). *On the state of the public health for the year 1985.* Her Majesty's Stationery Office, London.

Weinstein, M. C. and Stason, W. (1977). Foundations of cost-effectiveness for health and medical practices. *New Engl. J. Med.* **296**, 716–721.

Williams, A. (1985). Economics of coronary artery bypass grafting. *Br. Med. J.*, **291**, 326–329.

Williams, A. (1987). The importance of quality of life in policy decisions. In *Quality of Life: Assessment and Application* (S. R. Walker, Ed.). MTP Press, London.

Noreen Caine and Virginia O'Brien

19

Quality of Life and Psychological Aspects of Heart Transplantation

INTRODUCTION

The analysis of quality of life components and their measurement have gained momentum over the past 10 years. There are two main reasons for this development — the high cost of modern medicine in a resource conscious health service, and a long overdue recognition of the patient's right and ability to form an opinion on the effectiveness of a course of treatment which the doctor has judged to be for the best. Clinicians involved in costly or invasive forms of therapy are experiencing an unprecedented scrutiny of their traditional clinical freedom and their natural pioneering instincts. They are finding also that it is no longer sufficient to demonstrate good survival rates; quality is running parallel to quantity in the valuation stakes. Heart transplantation is both costly and invasive and in addition it has had a highly emotive and political impact. It is not surprising therefore that in the UK and in the USA there has been simultaneous support for detailed cost and benefit studies (Evans *et al.*, 1984; Buxton *et al.*, 1985).

Many treatment justification studies have concentrated on describing objective indicators of quality of life which have been relatively simple to measure, such as return to work after surgery. The incisive critique by Najman and Levine (1981) of 23 studies of the outcome of various medical interventions effectively demonstrates the need for including both objective and subjective indicators of quality of life, particularly if changes due to medical interventions are to be appreciated. These authors also assert that more attention should be given to study design if the results are to be worth while. Too many projects have looked at too few patients, have ignored control or comparison groups or have failed to appreciate the importance of paired comparisons before and after intervention. Of course, some compromise in study design is often required, as with heart transplantation in the

1980s, since it is not always possible ethically to advocate a randomized control trial.

Any study of the quality of life in patients who have undergone a major medical intervention must include the individual's circumstances both before and after treatment. This necessitates a prospective framework of study in which the structure allows for the relative importance, to the individual patient, of some aspects of life quality as opposed to others. In his thought-provoking reflections on a theory of life quality, based on the patient's capacity to realize his own 'life plan', Cohen (1982) demonstrates the importance of an understanding of the distinction between general and individualized quality of life components when investigating treatment outcome. For example, return to an occupation undertaken prior to illness, whether it is work, study or being a housewife, is vitally important to most people and would be one of the generally agreed components of a successful outcome. Yet for some individuals, return to work is a more direct function of the need for income than the actual impact of treatment on the patient's state of health. Where financial circumstances permit, full or partial retirement after surgery, not returning to a former occupation and finding alternative, more fulfilling activity may best enhance life quality. Generalized features of life enhancement are important, but Cohen suggests that we also take account of the individual's life plan by asking patients before treatment what their expectations of a good outcome are, and what changes in their lives they hope to effect. Then, in follow-up studies, we can determine whether individual goals have been realized and, if not, whether this is because of some limitation which the treatment has not improved or because the life plan has changed. Such an approach will give a more reliable measurement of the effects of a specific treatment, and a better understanding of the impact of that intervention, on quality of life.

The study design adopted in the UK research into the costs and benefits of heart transplantation attempted to incorporate the principles outlined by Najman and Cohen, relying almost exclusively on prospectively collected data. Unfortunately, from the point of view of the evaluation, a randomized control structure was not possible and so every attempt was made to ensure the inclusion of as much relevant comparative information as possible from the various patient groups accessible to the researchers. The aim was to identify the extra costs and benefits resulting from the existence of the cardiac transplant programmes compared with those of conventional medical and surgical therapy. It was recognized of course that no other treatments provided true alternative forms of management for patients requiring a heart transplant; rather, they provided contextual comparisons useful in the understanding of extra costs and benefits, and demonstrated the feasibility of applying the same evaluation methods to various forms of intervention.

The research team decided on a dual approach to the study of quality of life. In order to measure changes in the general health status of patients at intervals before and after operation, the Nottingham Health Profile (NHP) was chosen (Hunt, McKenna and McEwen, 1981). The NHP's 38 statements in Part I, covering aspects of physical, social and emotional functioning, had been well tested in other studies and had been widely used with normal populations, thus providing comparisons for the heart transplant patient results before and after surgery. The second, more exploratory and informal element was a series of interviews carried out before transplantation, and six months, 1 year and 2 years after transplantation. The seven areas of life most affected by health, as identified in Part II of the NHP, were used as a basis for the interview, to which aspects more specific to the transplantation were added.

At the end of 1984 the research team prepared its final report to the DHSS and the study was terminated. However, at Papworth it was decided to continue to monitor patients' quality of life, with three specific objectives:

(1) To study more patients and thereby increase the data available for the analysis of NHP scores, in particular paired comparisons before and after surgery.
(2) To study the longer term health status of patients after transplantation.
(3) To develop a questionnaire from the experience gained in the many interviews undertaken with transplant patients, which would be used alongside the NHP, thus forming a routine 'package' of quality of life questionnaires which would be acceptable to patients for use at regular intervals before and after surgery.

In the quality of life sections below, some early results from the continued study are combined with the interview material and NHP data from the formal research study.

The psychological problems encountered by patients during all stages of the transplant experience were touched on in the quality of life studies both in the NHP, which has an 'emotional reactions' dimension, and in the interviews during discussions regarding changes in quality of life experienced during illness and after transplantation, but no specific study was made of psychological effects.

The psychological problems for those involved in the trauma of terminal illness, major surgical intervention and its outcome, and the understanding of the psychological strengths needed to cope with this experience, provide a fascinating area of observation. At Papworth, the same social worker has been working as a member of the transplant team since 1981 and has been closely involved with the patient experience during all aspects of treatment and recovery. She has identified (O'Brien, 1985) five stages during this process, each with its unique problems. These are: diagnosis and referral, assessment for transplantation, the waiting period, the operation and early recovery (in-patient) period, and discharge from hospital. McAleer *et al.* (1985), using a series of 12 tests, identified six stages of psychological adjustment which follow the major crisis points after admission to hospital. These two frameworks, independently defined, are remarkably similar, their differences being more of title than content.

The patient

The patients fall into three main disease categories, namely ischaemic heart disease, cardiomyopathy and valvular/congenital heart disease. The 'typical' cardiomyopathy patient is a young man or woman who has been quite suddenly overtaken by illness, and who deteriorates rapidly from a fit and healthy state to a severely restricted existence and certainty of imminent death without transplantation. It is possible for all this to happen within a matter of months. Other cardiomyopathy patients will have had the disease from childhood. By contrast, the 'typical' ischaemic patient is male, has been ill for several years, and may have experienced more than one heart attack and had coronary artery bypass surgery, intensive medical therapy or both. Occasionally, however, the ischaemic patient can progress rapidly from onset of illness to transplantation. The difference in length of history between individual patients is very important for those dealing directly with the psychological support of the patient and family and to the researcher approaching the task of assessing changes in quality of life before and after transplantation.

STAGE I: DIAGNOSIS AND REFERRAL

Patients and their partners often make very good historians not just about the progression of the disease, which can either be slow and debilitating or rapid and frightening, but also about the effects of the illness and its emotional impact. The initial reaction to being told about the seriousness of the illness is often one of disbelief and despair. The impact leaves them quite defenceless and their reaction may be to try to push the reality away. Initial periods of depression are not uncommon and anger and bitterness sometimes follow as slow adjustments are made. It is surprising how often what is happening is seen as a punishment. But for what? Why does it happen to me? A detailed examination of one's personality and its shortcomings is a painful and often destructive process, but it is undertaken in an effort to find an answer. Many people feel that they could accept the situation if cause and effect could be clearly seen, but they are left mystified with the recognition that their life history so far does not justify such an outcome.

Fortunately, few personalities remain frozen at this particular stage of development and they move on in an effort to deal with the situation. Gradually they come to terms with the reality and find their own level of acceptance. Some patients have expressed astonishment at the discovery of an inner strength, the existence and depth of which they have been previously unaware. Others say that their illness has meant a period of reflection, resulting in a greater appreciation of everything in their lives which had previously been taken for granted. Most people have a strong hold on life and do not view its loss with equilibrium. For the majority of patients, their marriage and family, their work and their way of life are too precious to be relinquished without a fight. It is this 'life force' which allows them to move on to consider the alternative, which offers the possibility of holding on to relationships and retrieving their previous quality of life.

The patients with sudden onset of illness who are often in the younger age groups are denied this gradual process of adjustment. They and their families are still reeling from the first impact of the disease, the effects of which are in such marked contrast to the healthy life of a few short weeks ago. Patients are often so desperately ill that they do not realize the proximity of death, and those families who know this intellectually still find it hard to accept emotionally.

It is against such a background that patients are referred for assessment for transplantation. How they and their families are coping, with the illness and its consequences, will often provide an indication of how they will cope with future traumatic events. The turbulence of feelings at this point can be likened to a psychological strait-jacket from whose fetters the patient and his family need to be freed in order to confront the taxing demands of the next stage.

STAGE II: ASSESSMENT FOR TRANSPLANTATION

The patient is accompanied by his or her spouse, or a friend or relative, who will be closely involved in all discussions and interviews. The objectives of the assessment period are threefold: to determine the patient's clinical and psychological suitability for transplantation, to inform the patient and companion about what to expect during all stages of transplantation and to provide the appropriate support for each individual.

The assessment process is difficult to define. Crucial to the surgeon's decision is his judgement as to the patient's prognosis in terms of length of survival without transplantation. Apart from the purely medical criteria, however, the surgeon needs to assess the patient's suitability as regards personality and ability to achieve successful rehabilitation. He needs to consider the patient's motivation, coping skills, comprehension and understanding of what heart transplantation entails, and the strength of family support available. It is not enough that patients accept the prospect of transplantation because they do not want to die; they must also have a strong desire to live. To quote one patient: 'Life may be finished with me but I am not finished with life.' While exposure to a long period of stress and uncertainty in the general population has its incidence of psychiatric disorder, the fact that after transplantation none of our own patients has required treatment for such disorder would seem to reflect the efficacy of the assessment process.

At Papworth Hospital, Cambridge, UK, the social worker coordinates the assessment. On admission, she gives the patient an initial summary of the assessment process and over the next few days coordinates the input of those wards and departments involved in transplant patient care. She answers patients' questions and satisfies herself that they understand the full implications of transplantation.

The assessment period is probably the most important time available to work with patients and their partners. It is essential that they become active participants, not passive recipients. At no other time are they in this same psychological state or so receptive to advice and influence. The object is to help them to achieve a balanced view of the process, providing adequate factual information while allowing the expression of natural feelings of fear and uncertainty. This balance is important. To be too pessimistic merely increases anxiety and causes undue distress, whereas to be too optimistic can lead to long-term problems. Patients are given a clear understanding of the risks involved in this type of surgery, with a full explanation of the survival statistics. They need to be made fully aware of the postoperative regimen, with its discipline and constraints as well as the demands of the drug therapy and its possible side effects. The resulting strain and tension and the effects these may have at the difficult stages of postoperative care must be clearly understood and must not be underestimated. Patients also need encouragement to look at their own strengths, motivation and self-discipline.

On admission for assessment, anxiety is the dominant emotional symptom often expressed by those patients who are able to do so. They are anxious about what is going to happen to them during the assessment and what is expected of them, but their greatest anxiety is centred on the momentous decision to be made. By the time they arrive most patients have already decided to accept transplantation if it is offered. The interval between referral and admission has given time for reflection on the stark options, namely to stay as they are and face early death or to have an operation with its chance of not simply continuing to live, but a return to normal life. For these patients the possibility of being refused an operation is their greatest fear because they know there is nowhere else to go.

This very natural anxiety for acceptance can often mask the real issues surrounding the actual operation. Many lessen the reality of what will be involved, both the risks and dangers for them and the difficulties for their families. In wanting to put the past behind them and in their anticipation of a better future, they can, and often do, disregard the present. Perhaps for the first time since the severity of their illness was fully understood they can contemplate a future and this can have the effect of obliterating any obstacle. This is a difficult and sensitive time when patients need the assistance of those closely involved in this process to help them disregard the fantasies they may have and to make the necessary adjustments to reality.

Some patients have thought deeply about the issues involved and will have come to terms with them: the need to accept an organ from another human being, the inevitable loss of a life which makes transplantation a reality, the sense that for them to gain, others will have suffered loss. Many people will already feel comfortable about the religious, philosophical and ethical issues involved. For those who have not progressed as far, it is necessary to bring them to contemplation of these issues at this stage.

Perhaps one of the most significant meetings the patients and their partners have is with other transplant patients and their families. For most patients this will be the first time they have met someone who has had the operation and it can prove to be the most rewarding experience of the assessment. It is an opportunity to share for a few brief days other patients' experiences, and the advice and help gained can prove very beneficial to their own future progress. The mutual support between transplant patients at all stages of treatment can bring much comfort to all concerned.

The assessment procedure is undertaken in the clear knowledge that it is impossible for the potential recipients and their families to retain all the facts they are given. All those who work with them during this admission know that discussing theoretical future events is not always commensurate with their ability to assimilate full understanding at a time when their anxiety levels are at their highest. However, if good foundations are laid at this time they can be built upon and reinforced subsequently, particularly during the next very difficult stage.

STAGE III: THE WAITING PERIOD

Patients who have been accepted for transplantation return home to their families with a new-found sense of hope and optimism for the future. From their frank discussions with staff and patients they feel relieved, reassured, better informed and most of all hopeful for the future. They see transplantation as a 'chance for life', the only alternative to 'waiting to die'. At the same time, however, they are facing perhaps one of the most difficult periods in their lives. The initial euphoria lessens all warnings of the difficulties of the waiting period. Having emerged from the assessment admission with the answer they wanted, most are now impatient for action. They feel psychologically ready for the operation and yet have to adjust to waiting. Emotion can play havoc with people's logic. Doubts and uncertainties about what really happened during the assessment are raised. The very real fear that they will die before a donor becomes available can become paramount. Guilt feelings may emerge if they dwell on the fact that for their lives to continue, others must die.

The original state of dependence upon the family, with all its inherent frustrations and anger, is now increased by a state of dependence upon the transplant centre. For those lacking the physical and mental strength to fight it, deep depression often follows. Much of this is understood by the patients and their families, but the ability to continue as before can become severely impaired and the resulting stress is felt by all the family members. During this difficult time contact may be maintained with the transplant hospital as a means of keeping in touch with events and seeking support. At Papworth Hospital such support is given freely and requests are met in a constructive and sympathetic way without giving false reassurance. For many patients the assessment had provided them with a tantalizing promise for a future. Feelings of frustration can be great when they feel that the transplant centre is impotent at the time they need help the most. During this period patients have to draw heavily upon their own inner resources and those of their family. It is a time of reflection and reappraisal of the present situation and its certain outcome if a donor does not become available in time, of coming to terms with death and all its emotional and practical elements. It is a time when the whole family may enter into a period of anticipatory grieving for the patient and make plans for coping with such an eventuality. It is a time for many to experience a resurgence of deeper religious and philosophical beliefs; for some this will be a normal part of their lives and one which has helped them greatly during previous difficult times; for others it may be an entirely new experience, but one which can bring them much comfort.

About a quarter of all patients on the waiting list die before a donor organ becomes available, and a great many grieving families have seen their hopes for the future, once felt to be within their grasp, snatched away from them. Many families express bitterness at being denied the chance of surgery and feel that they could have coped with the death of the patient so much better if it had followed an unsuccessful operation.

STAGE IV: THE OPERATION AND IN-PATIENT PERIOD

The practical arrangements and the speed of the journey to hospital conspire to keep reality at bay, and it is usually during the last quiet hour or so before surgery that the impact of what is imminent is absorbed fully. Of all the possible life-threatening events which may lie ahead, it is the operation itself which is regarded as the greatest risk by most patients and their partners and they are often afraid, even though it is rare (< 1.0%) for a patient to die during the operation.

The patient

Patients often feel ashamed of their fear and few recognize their remarkable bravery and strength of character. Coupled with this fear is a sense of relief and excitement — relief that the long wait is over, excitement at the prospect of being made to feel well again. Those patients who have been very ill for a long time are at peace at this moment, having decided that death would be preferable to their intolerable symptoms. For others who are undergoing the operation at a stage when they are relatively symptom-free, there is often a feeling of conflict in having the operation at that particular time. A few patients have said that they would have turned back at this point if they had felt that the decision was theirs alone or that they were accepting transplantation for themselves alone, but that love of their families, their commitment to them and perhaps also to the medical staff, left them with no alternative but to proceed.

For most patients the immediate postoperative period is relatively uncomplicated medically. Many are surprised at how well they feel on recovery from the anaesthetic. Often the more immobilized the patient was before surgery, the greater the sense of well-being immediately afterwards, particularly for those patients who had been affected previously by severe breathlessness. For others, these benefits may be masked by adverse reactions to the trauma of surgery, the anaesthetic or the drug regimen, sometimes causing confusion, aggression or depression. For almost all patients and their partners, however, this period is an intensely emotional one.

There are few patients who do not experience overwhelming feelings of gratitude towards the donor family and a great desire to let that family know what their generosity of spirit has meant to them. The feeling of having received the ultimate gift, of life itself, holds true for each patient undergoing cardiac transplantation; at a later stage, it can lead to a whole complex area of personal sense of responsibility and indebtedness. In the first flush of these feelings many patients feel they would like to make contact with the donor family, even though there may be an underlying sense of unease about such a course of action. Patients are advised to let their initial feelings settle, and to consider the effect this may have upon the donor family as well as their own; most, later, are relieved that they refrained from such action. Whatever feelings they may have had at different stages of their illness, for most patients the heart ceases to have a conscious meaning in relation to another human being and becomes an organ capable of effecting a return to a normal way of life.

With few exceptions patients, in the early days following surgery, experience a period of almost total dependence upon the medical and nursing staff. Feelings connected with earlier states of dependence, which often involved deep resentment, anger and frustration, are not apparent, as this stage is viewed as a short but necessary transitory state leading to eventual independence. At Papworth Hospital, the first few days spent in the intensive care unit lead swiftly to a move to a surgical ward where patients can begin to have some control over their everyday lives within the constraints of normal ward management. Being able to visit other patients, go to physiotherapy or walk in the grounds, all enhance the patient's well-being. Although there are the normal anxieties that something may suddenly go wrong, most patients are well motivated to contribute to their own recovery, becoming knowledgeable about their daily regimen and medical therapy and learning a considerable amount about the fundamentals of transplantation.

Patients will have been well prepared for the possibility of rejection and infection and most view the first episode of rejection with reasonable equilibrium. We do not highlight it as being a significant stage of psychological adjustment. An understanding of the delicate balance between body, donor organ and immunosuppression drugs leads patients to expect rejection at some stage. They know it could be serious, but they often continue to feel well and this helps them to view it as an inevitable routine occurrence. Minor episodes of infection are dealt with similarly, but when they are more severe they can cause renewed alarm, as patients often feel unwell.

Patients exhibit great bravery in their ability to strike out for the future when they know their progress may come to a sudden end. A difficulty sometimes expressed by patients is their attitude to physical exercise. What would once have been a life-threatening and forbidden activity is now encouraged by the medical staff. Feelings of uncertainty can sometimes immobilize the patient until he can gain sufficient confidence.

For those patients who have suffered a sudden onset illness, the post-operative period can be a time of some difficulty. They have had no time of preparation and adjustment. On recovering, they first have to come to terms with what has happened to them and this can cause much emotional turbulence. Uncooperative behaviour and feelings of depression can interfere with progress. Episodes of rejection and infection are viewed as more threatening than they sometimes are, by both patient and relatives. Over-protective relatives can cause intense anger and frustration in a patient, especially when some conflict already existed before illness. Parents for instance may fail to understand that transplantation does not give their child instant maturity and can be disappointed in what they view as inappropriate responses from the patient. Having adjusted to his survival, many parents have time to consider their child's future and the uncertainty this holds in view of the anticipated life span of transplant patients.

Most patients, however, appear to bask in the fulness and richness of these early days following the operation which are in such marked contrast to their immediate preoperative experience. Even with the limitations of ward routine, the paramount feeling is one of celebration of life, shared between the patient and his family and other transplant patients and their families. A strong bond is established between patients and a feeling of specialness emerges. Sometimes the unlikeliest friendships are formed that would probably never have occurred prior to transplantation. Strong feelings of gratitude towards surgeons and affection towards staff often run parallel to the desire to help others in repayment for what they have received. Their willingness to support and help patients admitted for assessment is often very touching. Their almost evangelical attitude in celebration of good health is often expressed in their plans for the future. Some consider a new career in the caring professions. They have for so long felt receivers that they want to put all their energies into giving. This not unnatural overreaction will hopefully in time settle to a normal level. It should be neither unrealistically encouraged nor severely discouraged. The passage of time, the return home and the gradual resumption of normal activity usually brings stability, although most patients continue to gain great satisfaction from their efforts to help other patients at difficult stages of transplantation. Their feelings towards the transplant hospital remain strong and are often expressed in fund-raising activities and general promotion of transplantation.

The partner

During the operation the partners suffer the 3–5 hours of waiting. At this time and in the early days after the operation they may need the opportunity to re-explore their sometimes ambivalent feelings. Anticipating an unsuccessful outcome, some feel guilty about the active part they have played in encouraging the idea of transplantation, perhaps at a time when the patient was unsure about proceeding. If postoperative problems arise, the possibility of what the partner may feel to be unnecessary prolonged suffering for the patient causes great distress, resulting sometimes in a desire to terminate further medical therapy before the surgeon is prepared to do so. Occasionally partners express the fear that the patient will die in hospital leaving them alone, a long way from home and uncertain of how to cope. In response to this reaction it is necessary to discuss these fears with the partner in some detail. It has been found beneficial to help them to separate two possible outcomes: first survival, an understanding of the importance of their role and the enhancement of their coping skills, and secondly, death and all the practical issues which would be involved. It is often only when these aspects can be separated and discussed that the relative is able to cope, sometimes putting an end to sleepless nights, nightmares and the fear of a temporary breakdown of personality. While the patient is surrounded by a world of high-tech surgery and intensive care, the partner needs to be surrounded by support, comfort and guidance.

While the patient's energy increases, the partner's may decrease, leading to physical and emotional exhaustion. This is often a good time for the partner to return home for a break. Other relatives may come to stay nearby or perhaps the patient is quite happy to be supported by other patients and staff. This short break away from the hospital is often very therapeutic both to the partner and to the patient.

Intermediate discharge

Discharge home, direct from the closely supervised routine of ward life, can be a traumatic experience. Many patients have reported their distress when discovering that the excitement of going home was shattered, perhaps just a few miles from the hospital, by feelings of fear which in some cases completely immobilized them. They felt cut off, not just from medical help but also from the personal support offered by other patients and the staff.

The policy of providing accommodation close to the hospital, helping to bridge the gap between hospital and home, was started in the UK at Harefield Hospital and was adopted by Papworth in 1985. Its beneficial effects have been obvious. Patients who are doing well, 2–3 weeks after operation, no longer need to be in hospital, but they still require physiotherapy and regular surveillance by the nursing and medical staff. This 'halfway house' policy and the counselling provided by all the staff involved help to ease patients and their families into a more confident independence.

For many couples this is a particularly important time of readjustment. They feel the need to regroup and reassemble themselves as a partnership before taking on the whole family and friends. Their time and privacy will soon be invaded and most report this period just before returning home as a very special time together. They begin to absorb the full impact of their recent experiences and in particular patients will begin to realize what their time in hospital has been like for their partners. Previously preoccupied with their own recovery, there has been some consciousness of the role of the partner but not necessarily a full appreciation of what has been involved. Partners during this time begin the often difficult task of 'letting go' of the strong hold as carer. The village house provides a setting 'like home' and is greatly appreciated. However, they all long for the day when they may return home.

STAGE V: DISCHARGE FROM HOSPITAL

The stated aim of all transplant patients is to be made well again and to return to a 'normal' way of life, and little which happens to them during the process changes this goal. However, normality is not easy to reach after such an extraordinary experience. Perhaps what many patients mean by normality is in fact a previous state of 'unawareness', a 'taking for granted' of their everyday lives. This state can never be returned to completely. They are not the same people as they were before their illness. Many will have grown significantly in their emotional lives and they often express the belief that it is impossible for them to have been so close to death without strong feelings of the 'specialness' of life. For them each day becomes a celebration of life, with a freshness and richness of quality not felt by people who have not shared similar experiences. Patients may become impatient with those around them who do not view the world as they do and this makes them feel 'different'.

Some patients feel that with their new life come new responsibilities. This feeling has several origins; the donor family's gesture of giving is one, the skill and commitment of the surgeons is another and the care and love of the nursing and paramedical staff is yet another. Many patients emerge with a deeper respect for their own bodies and become committed to keeping themselves fit, not only to help them survive but because they feel they 'owe it to others'. Most patients feel they have become ambassadors of their transplant centre and that they have a responsibility to do what is 'right'.

Almost all patients describe feelings of overwhelming joy on returning home, of rediscovering the pleasure of undertaking the most mundane domestic tasks which had previously been denied them and of sharing this simple pleasure with their families. There are of course adjustments to be made, some more painful than others.

A recurring problem is one of reassessment of the reversal of traditional roles in the family which may have been necessary because of the patient's illness. Some wives who have become used to going out to work and organizing the finances, as well as running the home and taking full responsibility for their children's upbringing, find themselves easily relinquishing their extra responsibilities and returning to a life at home without complaint, particularly if their partner resumes his occupation. Other women find it difficult or even impossible to give up a job they have enjoyed. Some patients have problems in returning to work for one reason or another, and they may find satisfaction in running the home, particularly if they have their own interests and hobbies or are active in voluntary work. Other men find it very difficult to come to terms with unemployment or alternative work and this can cause stress in family relationships. The frustration of feeling well and yet being unable to find employment can cause bitterness and resentment, especially when the consequence is to remain dependent upon state aid and/or a partner's income and to be denied the opportunity of becoming the 'breadwinner' again. About 75% of patients do return to work, and often this is possible very soon, perhaps 3–4 months after their operation. Some are well supported by employers, receiving a full salary during their illness and returning to their previous occupation. For them there is a gradual and very natural return to their former lifestyle.

Not uncommonly the patient's partner becomes 'depressed' some 2–3 months after the patient's return home. It may be that for these people the prolonged period of daily stress since the patient first became ill has to take its toll. As their partners become healthier and fitter they can allow themselves the luxury of becoming 'ill'. Often they are at a loss to understand what is happening. They know they should 'feel happy' because everything is going well and the whole family is settling back into a routine way of life, but instead they feel sad, depressed and unhappy. Sometimes this can be ascribed to the strain of having to cope with an uncertain future. Sometimes it may be attributed to the inability to 'let go', a sense of disbelief that the patient is really well; such behaviour is observed by patients with obvious irritation, as they cannot understand why their partners are still treating them as though they were ill. Perhaps it is unreasonable to expect people who have been through so much, who have experienced every emotion leading to the brink of a loved one's death, to resolve the resultant emotional difficulties in a short space of time.

All patients and families have to learn to live with the uncertainties of the future. No one knows how long each patient will live. The effect of transplantation is that death can be postponed, but for an unknown length of time. Many patients realize this and speak of 'borrowed time'. Some older patients feel guilty that this 'bonus' has been given to them and not to someone younger who they feel may have 'done more' with it. This is based presumably upon the assumption that life is somehow sweeter and more precious for younger people. It is more difficult for younger transplant patients to come to terms with these uncertainties, but eventually they have to consider what their future can hold within the predicted length of survival, particularly in terms of relationships, marriage and children. Perhaps an expression of faith in that future can be seen from the several young married patients who have decided to start a family.

All these underlying problems and adjustments are part of the transplant patient survivor's life and, for most, life after transplantation cannot be lived at a constant emotional peak, with daily speculation of their special circumstances. It is impossible for patients not to look back and contemplate the events of their illness and their close proximity to death, but the natural life force inherent in most people causes them to enjoy today and to look forward to however many days they have before them. They return home from hospital to their families, their work, their interests and social life and a future of which the most often quoted comment is: 'If I should die tomorrow it has all been worth while.'

QUALITY OF LIFE BEFORE AND AFTER TRANSPLANTATION

During a series of interviews with patients the effects of illness and transplantation on quality of life were recorded. When the series was completed in 1984 a questionnaire was developed from the interview experience, which is now used routinely at Papworth Hospital together with the NHP. From this routine questionnaire there were data available from 75 assessment patients and 21 patients at 3 months after transplantation, at the time of writing. In addition, in September 1986, a sample of 76 surviving transplant patients completed questionnaires aimed at updating our information on their work status, their symptoms and overall condition. In this section we will look at the combined impressions gained from both the interview and questionnaire data, with particular consideration given to the symptoms suffered by patients and the effects of, first, illness and then transplantation on working life, daily activities, social life and home relationships.

In general discussions about quality of life during interviews with patients before transplantation, it was loss of independence which was most keenly felt, leading to intense feelings of frustration. This theme recurred constantly. The particular element of independence most missed varied between patients. For many, of course, it was their work. For some, often the younger patients, it was an active sporting and social life, whereas for others it was the enjoyment of activities in the home and with the family. Some of the following comments from patients describing their quality of life were typical: 'I'm existing, not living'; 'I'm clinging on to life but nothing is left really'. Quality of life was 'non-existent', 'very poor' or 'nil'. A patient who was to die a few days after his assessment and interview said: 'Recently I haven't been able to do anything. I have felt ill and have been walking a few yards when absolutely necessary. I feel I am getting worse.'

The main symptoms experienced by patients waiting for a transplant were breathlessness, pain on exertion, tiredness, loss of appetite, coughing and swelling of limbs due to fluid retention. Constant physical discomfort and the resulting restrictions dominated everything in their lives, even making sleeping or lying down in bed very difficult. The degree of mobility varied. Some were bed-bound, others house-bound, while some were still capable of walking several hundred yards on a good day.

In a sample of 75 patients who completed a questionnnaire at the time of assessment, 94.7% said they suffered from breathlessness, 42.8% said they

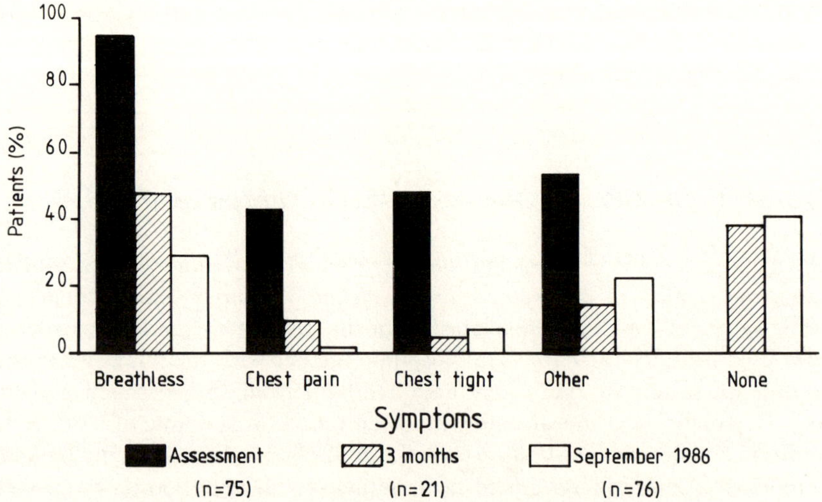

Fig. 19.1. *Transplant patients' symptoms, before and after surgery.*

suffered from chest pain, 48.0% from tightness in the chest, and 53.4% from other types of symptoms, specified as mainly tiredness and fluid retention (Fig. 19.1). In Fig. 19.2 an indication is given of the level of exertion at which these symptoms were experienced. This shows that for 92% of

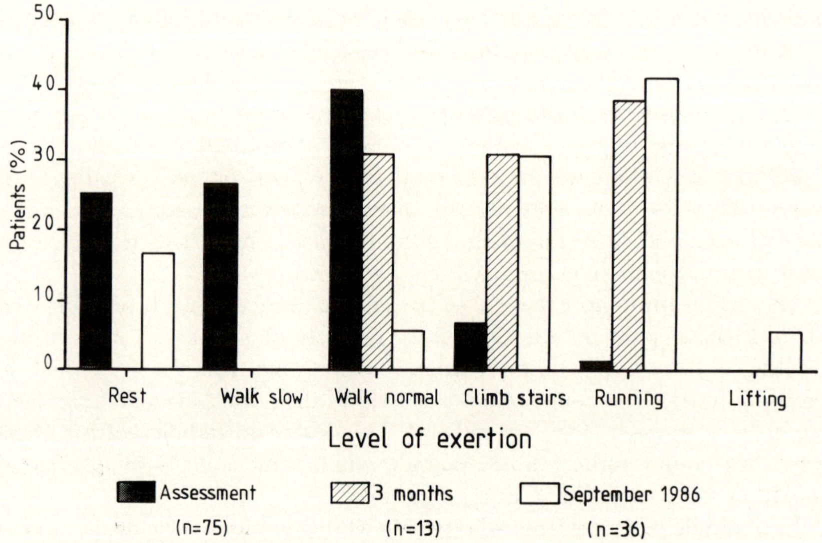

Fig. 19.2. *Level of exertion producing symptoms, before and after transplant.*

patients a very low level of exertion, i.e. being at rest or walking at a slow or normal pace, could produce symptoms.

At interviews held with patients at 6 months, 1 year and 2 years after surgery the aspects of quality of life discussed followed closely the format of the pre-surgery investigations. In discussing quality of life in general terms, the accent was on the contrast to life shortly before the operation. The lack of restrictions, especially at the interview 1 year after operation, was to these patients remarkable after the confinement of a serious illness. Most people said they were completely back to normal and were leading full, active lives. Some patients said that it was not until their health was restored that they could appreciate how ill they had been. Regained independence in looking after the home, in driving and walking, in simple daily activities, was very satisfying. Freedom from unpleasant symptoms, like breathlessness, chest pain, tiredness and oedema, added greatly to the quality of life. Those patients who had been ill for several years, some of them for most of their lives, particularly appreciated the difference. They spoke of how minor health problems, usually side effects of the drugs they were taking, were a small price to pay for being returned to an essentially normal way of life. Temporary difficulties in the months immediately following operation included muscle weakness in arms and legs, hand cramps, slight oedema or breathlessness and some pain in the re-uniting sternum. At 3 months after transplantation, 47.6% of 21 patients were still experiencing some breathlessness, whereas 38.1% of patients were symptom-free. Breathlessness persisted in about 30% of the 76 patients completing questionnnaires in September 1986, although for 8 out of 10 of these cases it occurred as a result of exertion like climbing stairs, running or heavy lifting (Figs 19.1 and 19.2). Persisting complications, some of which were related to the immunosuppressive drug therapy, were extra hair growth, Cushingoid features, and various skin rashes, but the only depressing feature was weight gain and the inability to lose weight even when diets were strictly followed.

Of the 21 patients completing questionnaires at 3 months after transplantation, 38.1% said they were completely better and 61.9% said their condition was definitely improved. In questionnaires completed in September 1986, 65.8% of the 76 respondents said they were completely better and 31.6% said they were definitely improved compared with immediately before their transplant (Fig. 19.3).

On a quality of life scale from 0 to 10 (low to high), 66.6% of the 21 patients completing questionnnaires at 3 months after their transplant produced a high score, 28.6% a medium and only 4.8% a low rating (Fig. 19.4). This compares with the ratings given at assessment by the sample of 75 patients, when only 8.0% gave their quality of life a high score.

Away from the strictly physical problems, some patients would talk about needing to be accepted as 'normal', particularly in the job market, and of the uncertainty of length of survival, which could affect their plans for the

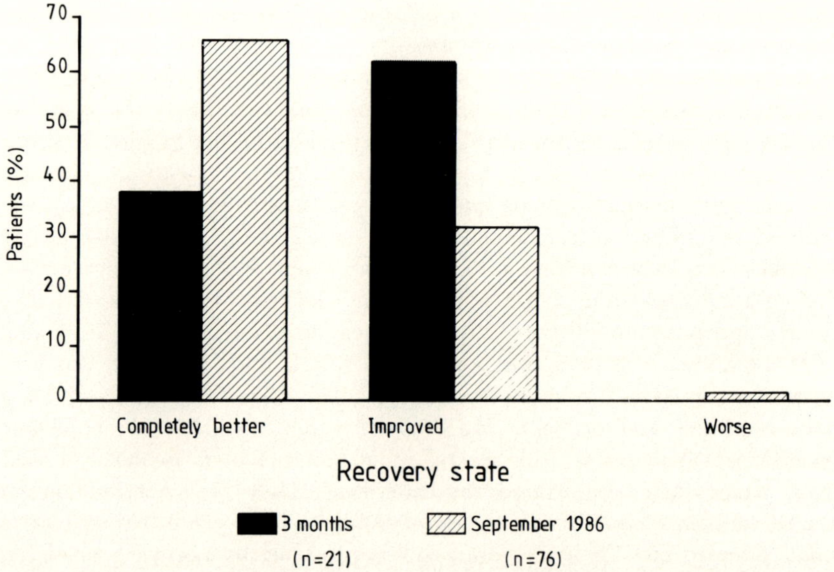

Fig. 19.3. *Recovery state after transplantation.*

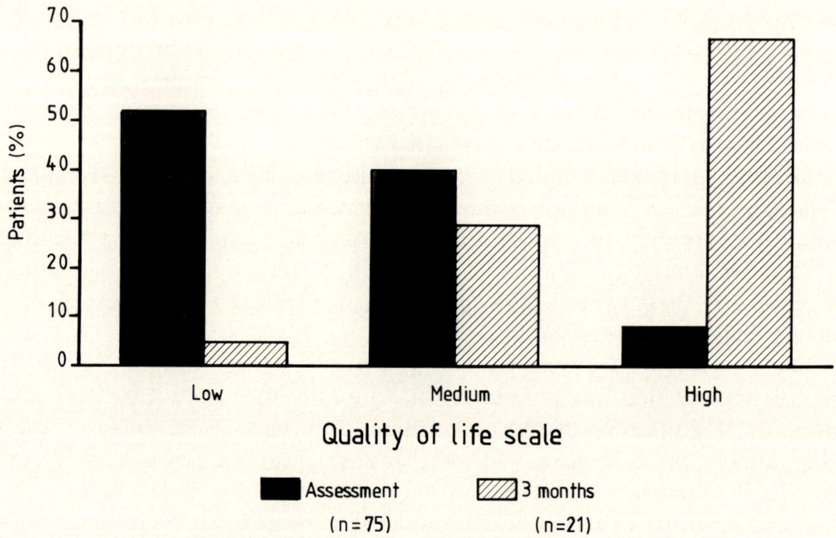

Fig. 19.4. *Quality of life scale, before and after transplant.*

long-term future. However, when asked whether the transplant had been worth while, all patients interviewed said that it had, even those who had experienced a very difficult recovery period in hospital or still had infection or rejection episodes several months or years afterwards. Every one of the 21 patients who completed questionnaires 3 months after operation said that if they had to make the same choice again they would decide to have the transplant. Many patients said they would recommend transplant surgery to anyone who found themselves in the same desperately ill state, because it was like being given a second chance at life, like being 're-born'.

Working life

Of the 75 patients who completed a questionnaire at assessment, 96.0% were not working at the time and in most cases (89.3%) this was due directly to their illness. For 41.3% of these patients, their job was being held open for them. Many patients had undergone changes in their working lives because of their illness; 29.3% of patients had changed to lighter work within their employment, 18.7% worked fewer hours, and 14.7% underwent a change of employment.

During the interviews patients were encouraged to talk in a general way about their working lives since they became ill and about their attitudes to any changes that had proved necessary. Many patients commented on the frustration and anguish caused by their inability to work. Most of them had enjoyed their jobs very much and missed the work and the social contact it brought, but most important of all they felt they had been denied their rightful function in life, and hated to see their families suffering, financially and emotionally. For many, the alternative to work was confinement to the house or perhaps to a hospital bed. The loss of a job and subsequent loss of earnings brought important changes to the family. Wives who had never worked, or perhaps had worked part time, became full-time breadwinners. Gradual changes in the traditional roles within the household resulted in psychological and emotional difficulties prior to any subsequent adjustment. The few patients who said that they had adjusted reasonably well to not working usually enjoyed interests which helped to keep their minds active. Some men had taken over the housekeeping role while their wives went out to work and found fulfilment in doing something useful.

The resilience and adaptability of some of the patients with regard to their working lives since their illness began were very striking. Several had changed to a physically less demanding occupation in an effort to keep working despite their illness. A change of job could mean a loss of self-esteem, a lack of job satisfaction and perhaps loss of earnings. Sometimes resentment at employers' attitudes was expressed. One man commented that in the 9 years of his illness his main worry had been holding down a job: 'If heart disease is mentioned to employers,' he commented, 'they don't want to know.' Several patients were particularly distressed at the loss of their businesses, while some found it difficult to sit back while others ran them. One man who was still working at the time of the interview said that he felt he was not being promoted as quickly as would have been possible if he had not been suffering from heart disease.

The financial aspects of changes in working status could be devastating. Only 21.3% of the 75 patients completing the questionnaire said that they were still receiving a full salary; another 30.7% were receiving a pension; 74.7% were receiving some kind of state benefit because of their illness; and 69.3% judged themselves to be financially worse off since the onset of their illness. The detrimental psychological effects, however, could prove more difficult to cope with than the financial constraints. People entering, perhaps for the first time, the apparently hostile world of state aid with its charitable associations found themselves in a new climate of economic dependence which was often in marked contrast to their previous economic status. Being in this position for any length of time could leave them with a keen sense of humiliation, poor self-esteem and feelings of inadequacy. The different roles of 'husband', 'father' and 'breadwinner' are considered by many men and women as interdependent; if one is affected, they are all affected.

In interviews following transplantation, a few patients felt that their quality of life would not be completely restored until they could return to work. This was especially true for the men who had been trying to find employment for a long time, sometimes years. Buxton *et al.* (1985) reported that 6 out of 10 patients were able to resume employment or to fulfil their role as housewife and mother. In recent figures taken from questionnaires completed in September 1986, this rate was confirmed in the population of all respondents, but was 75.0% for those patients who had been transplanted at least 2 years.

Those patients who had returned to work felt quite capable of holding down full-time and sometimes physically demanding jobs. When questioned about changing to lighter work or shorter hours, surprisingly few felt this was necessary. Those who did had often been employed in heavy industry and for these patients the road back to full employment was a difficult one, perhaps entailing rehabilitation courses and many applications and interviews. Not being able to obtain employment was often distressing, annoying and frustrating, especially when patients felt perfectly capable of doing a full-time job. Sometimes patients were resentful about prospective employers' attitudes. They commented that it could be difficult to convince employers that a heart transplant patient could do a normal day's work. Persuading employers to make allowances for the time away from work for check-ups was another major hurdle, as were the complicated problems of insurance and pension schemes. Some patients, however, believed that the level of unemployment was the main obstacle to their getting work, especially in the industrial sector. On the whole, the patients who found it easiest to return to work were those whose jobs had been kept open and who were lucky enough to have understanding employers.

Daily activities

The areas of daily life other than working life discussed at interview and in the questionnaires were: looking after the home, interests and hobbies and social life. In the questionnaires, patients were asked to list their usual activities under these three headings and say to what degree each activity had been affected first by illness and then by transplantation. They were given four choices: was the activity undertaken more often, less often, not at all, or had there been no change? The results in this section are expressed in terms of the percentage of patients who specified these activities as part of their daily living experience. For example, some patients did not complete the section on 'looking after the home' because this was not an area of activity in which they normally participated.

Looking after the home

In most cases, the usual activities around the home had been affected in some way by illness. For the men, it was most often the gardening, decorating and general repairs. Although many of the men were spending a great deal of time at home, they could usually only manage very light chores. Sometimes, even jobs like washing up and making tea were found to be too much of an effort. Several men commented on how much they resented having to ask a friend or relative to do repair jobs around the house, while they looked on helplessly. For the women, especially the housewives, this was the area of daily activity which was most affected by their illness. If they could manage any jobs around the house, it was usually only very light duties. For them, the inability to look after the home and family was both frustrating and distressing. From the questionnaires completed at assessment, it was found that 56.4% of 39 patients were performing very light duties around the home less often, while another 28.2% had given them up completely. For heavier chores, 38.2% of 68 patients said that their ability was limited and for a further 58.8% these had become impossible (Fig. 19.5).

Most of the men interviewed after surgery were able to do the usual jobs around the house that had been neglected during their illness; repair work, decorating, gardening and general chores were all mentioned. Some patients commented that the only restriction they felt in the early months was in those chores requiring heavy lifting. Some male patients who were not working had taken on the housekeeping role while their wives went out to work. For those patients whose main hobby was taking care of the family

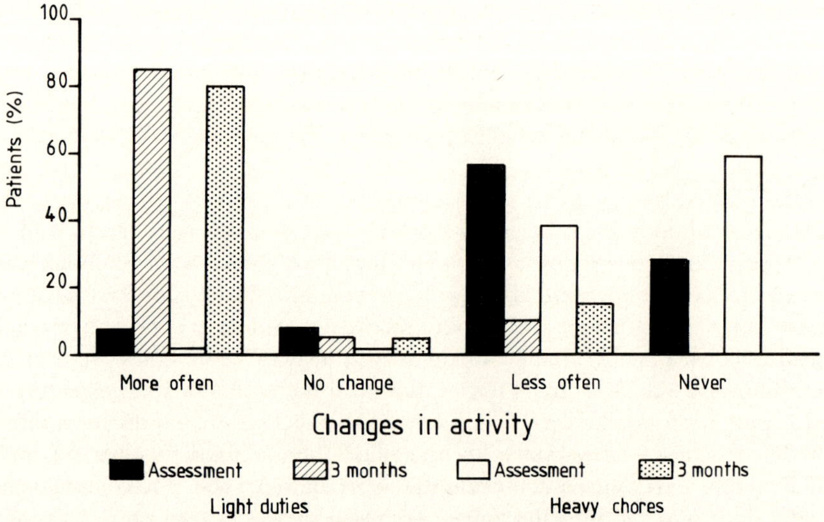

Fig. 19.5. *Daily life activities — looking after the home.*

home, being able to do jobs around the house was one of the most rewarding aspects of feeling well again. Of the 21 patients completing questionnaires 3 months after surgery, 80.0% of 20 reported being able to undertake heavy chores around the house more often than before their surgery (Fig. 19.5).

Both housewives and working female patients spoke of the pleasure and relief experienced in being able to look after the home and family once more. Sometimes they would comment that they were still working at a slower pace than normal or that heavier chores like cleaning windows were still difficult, but they could feel themselves improving and doing more every day.

Interests and hobbies

At the interviews with patients being assessed for transplantation, the activities under this heading fell into four main categories. The first was sporting interests, both playing and watching. A wide variety of sports were mentioned at interview, ranging from squash, badminton, cycling, tennis, football and cricket to fishing, darts and snooker. Sometimes, playing sport had been replaced by attending games, but for many this activity was reduced to viewing sport on television. The second main category was family activity; this included walking, boating, caravanning, country drives or just playing with the children. For many people, most of their interests apart from work revolved around outings with the family, and these were sorely missed. A third category could be labelled community activities and these ranged from

From the results of the assessment questionnaires it was apparent that of the 66 patients who specified social activities as part of their lives before their illness, 95% said that these were undertaken less often or not at all (Fig. 19.7).

The withdrawal from working and family activities, sports, hobbies and normal social interaction could result in total isolation, the patient becoming trapped by illness within his own mind. He feels very vulnerable and it becomes increasingly difficult for him to view the world in general, his own world and his participation in it, with a balance which, together with good health, is essential to a well-adjusted ego.

Very soon after leaving hospital following transplantation most patients found few restrictions in their social life, although some avoided large gatherings, preferring to mix with close friends who understood something of their recent experience. Patients' ability to cope with larger social gatherings seemed to improve over time. Of those 20 patients reporting on social activities in the questionnaires completed 3 months after surgery, 35% felt that there was no improvement in their ability or inclination to participate in social events, ranging from visiting the pub or cinema to attending football matches and rock concerts (Fig. 19.7). Some commented, however, that this restriction had more to do with finances than their state of health.

Family relationships

The strain of a serious illness and the frustration and anger it generates can and do affect personal relationships, within marriage, with children and the wider family. Many families spoke of the gradual and painful adjustments which have to be made as they come to terms with the patient's condition and learn to accept, with a certain sense of helplessness, what is happening to them. There is often an initial difficulty in adjusting to the new circumstance of having a formerly active member of the family gradually or, worse perhaps, very suddenly becoming a mere invalid. Tension mounts and not infrequently erupts, leaving patient and family regretful of things said in the heat of the moment. Perhaps some equilibrium could be found if this were known to be a permanent but stable state of ill health which would not deteriorate, but the conflict for family members is in trying to balance their attitude to the patient against the knowledge that his is a progressive disease with a poor prognosis. As a result, a type of 'queen bee' syndrome may develop, with the entire family having to subjugate their own needs to those of the patient, at the same time leaving him suffering the effects of overprotectiveness. It is not uncommon for patients to go through a phase of feeling a burden to their wives and families.

Families who have undergone several years of anxiety because of the illness of one of their members have different problems from those for whom

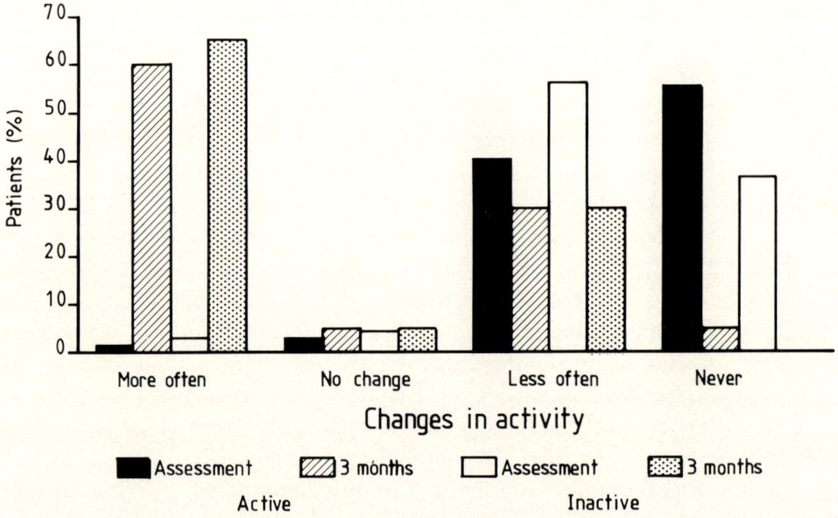

Fig. 19.7. *Daily life activities — social life.*

the process has been very sudden. The latter are often teenagers or young adults who have been bright, alert, high achievers enjoying a varied field of activity in which perhaps their relatives have played an interested, participatory and encouraging role. For such families the dramatic and sudden transformation to the helpless state of having to face the death of a member is a trauma of great intensity.

Usually, the spouse was considered to be extremely understanding when it came to making allowances for bad temper and irritability, but patients often expressed concern about the effect of their illness on relationships with children. Children could take a while to adjust to the new situation at home and to accept Dad's new crankiness, and even when they did they would often try simply to avoid the situation, perhaps becoming less boisterous and argumentative, less natural, and even subdued.

Nevertheless, for many families there is no doubt that the effects of the illness have been directly responsible for the strengthening of relationships. It is a time to 'take out and examine' the quality of relationships, most of which have been previously taken for granted. The most frequent comment was how the crisis had drawn the patient and family together. For about a third of the patients interviewed, the strain of the illness had caused actual problems, but even among these cases a better understanding and a closer relationship was often the final result.

When asked in the questionnaire whether their sex life had deteriorated because of their illness, 90.7% of 75 patients replied that it had, 5.3% said that it had not and 4% of patients did not answer the question. After transplantation, 14.3% of the 21 patients at 3 months said their sex life had deteriorated since their transplant, for 28.6% it had improved, the same number said it had not changed and the remaining 28.5% did not answer the question.

NOTTINGHAM HEALTH PROFILE DATA

The NHP was adopted by the DHSS research team as the formal instrument for measuring the health status of patients before and after transplant surgery during the study of the costs and benefits of the heart transplant programmes at Harefield and Papworth hospitals from 1982 to 1984. At the end of the study period it was agreed to continue using the NHP, with the intention of increasing the data available for analysis of changes before and at intervals after surgery, particularly longer term follow-up. Results are presented from those Profiles completed by Papworth patients up to the end of 1986.

The NHP was devised by a team from the Department of Community Medicine at the Nottingham University School of Medicine, together with the then Social Science Research Council. It is divided into two parts. Part I consists of 38 statements which all relate to limitations of activity or aspects of distress in six dimensions: physical mobility, pain, sleep, energy, social isolation and emotional reactions. Patients are required to indicate by a 'yes' or 'no' which of the problems they are experiencing at the time of completing the questionnaire. The weight applied to each statement allows a score ranging from 0 to 100 to be calculated for each dimension of Part I of the Profile. The higher the score, the more the respondent is suffering limitations in activity or distressing social and emotional problems. The process by which these statements were derived and the calculation of the weighting system have been reported (McKenna, Hunt and McEwen, 1981; McEwen, 1983). Part II of the Profile lists the seven areas of 'task performance' most affected by health status: occupation, ability to perform jobs around the house, home relationships, sex life, social life, hobbies and holidays. Again patients are asked to answer 'yes' or 'no' to indicate which areas are being affected by their state of health. The number of affirmative responses is used as a summary statistic.

The NHP is brief, easily understood and acceptable as a routine task over a long period of time. Patients are required to complete the Profile at 3-month intervals from their acceptance on the waiting list for operation, 3 months and 6 months after operation and at 6-month intervals thereafter. By the end of 1986, 111 Papworth transplant patients had completed NHPs before operation, 51 at 3 months, 42 at 1 year and 38 at 2 years. In Fig. 19.8, the mean scores from Part I of the Profile give a general picture

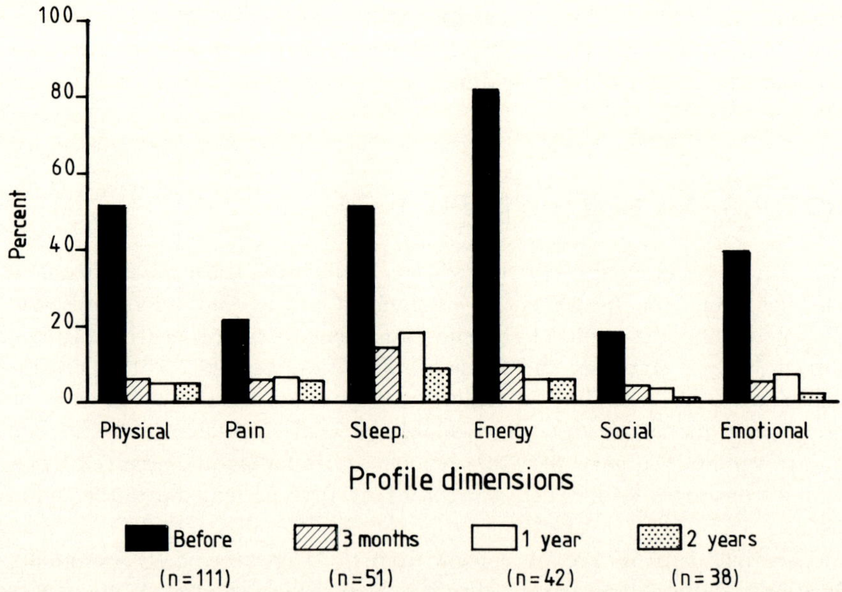

Fig. 19.8. *Nottingham Health Profile, Part I — mean scores before and after transplant.*

of the 'before' and 'after' experience for these patients, indicating an overall improvement in health at an early stage. From the analysis of the Profiles completed by 48 pairs of patients before and 3 months after operation, there was a significant improvement ($p < 0.001$) in all six dimensions of Part I. There is no evidence, however, of change in the health status of patients between 3 months after transplantation and later intervals.

One of the reasons the NHP was selected by the DHSS research team as the formal instrument for the subjective measurement of these patients' health status was that it had been used widely in the UK, not only in studies measuring change after a variety of medical or surgical interventions, but also in general population studies. In Table 19.1, the mean scores from the Profiles completed by transplant patients 1 and 2 years after operation can be compared with those from a 'normal' male population. The similarity in scores in all six dimensions is evidence of the extent to which these patients are restored to a level of health which would have been the expected experience for their age group if they had not suffered heart disease and undergone transplantation. The one area in which some patients were still experiencing problems a year after surgery was in sleeping, and this ranged from just waking up early in the morning, which patients often commented was a long-term habit, to sleeping badly or lying awake at night. There is some evidence that this was less of a problem for these patients 2 years after operation (Fig. 19.8).

TABLE 19.1

*Nottingham Health Profile Part I: Mean Scores for Transplant Patients at 3 months and 1 year After Surgery Compared With Scores From a Normal Population Sample**

	Transplant Patients		*Normal Population*	
	1 year ($n = 42$)	*2 years* ($n = 38$)	*35–39 years*	*40–44 years*
Physical mobility	5.12	5.11	1.2	3.2
Pain	6.29	5.84	2.6	5.8
Sleep	18.18	8.90	5.7	11.9
Energy	5.81	5.79	5.0	10.1
Social isolation	3.40	0.95	2.7	5.0
Emotional reactions	6.86	1.95	10.3	10.4

* Sample of 2173 men randomly drawn from a general practice.

For the analysis of the data from Part II of the Profiles completed by the 48 pairs of patients before and 3 months after operation, the McNemar test for paired comparisons was used. The results show a significant ($p < 0.01$) difference in all seven areas, indicating that most patients found a decreasing number of activities affected by their health just 3 months after operation. The areas in which the greatest number of patients expressed a marked improvement were in their home and social activities: 94% experienced problems before and only 20% 3 months after surgery. The aspect of life least affected by health problems before operation was home relationships, less than 50% of patients expressing difficulties, yet even here there was significant improvement (Table 19.2).

DISCUSSION

A comparison of observations and results from other quality of life studies with the UK experience highlights many similarities in method and conclusions.

Christopherson, Griepp and Stinson (1976) reviewed 56 Stanford patients who had heart transplantations between 1968 and 1975 and who had survived more than 6 months. They found that 91% of these patients were able to resume active lives which included 'tasks identical to or perceived as equivalent to those in which they had engaged prior to the onset of severe cardiac disease'. Being able to return to tasks perceived by the patients as their usual or normal experience is an important element of successful

TABLE 19.2

*Nottingham Health Profile Part II: Percentage of Patients Indicating Problems Caused by State of Health Before and After Transplant (n = 48)**

	Pre-transplant (%)	*3 months After Transplant* (%)
Job of work	84.1	50.0
Looking after the home	93.5	19.6
Social life	93.5	19.6
Home life (relationships)	45.7	15.2
Sex life	84.4	28.9
Interests and hobbies	93.5	26.1
Holidays	91.3	26.1

*$p < 0.01$.

rehabilitation. In the UK studies, a similar question was included in interviews and is used currently in the routine Papworth questionnaires; however, it has been adapted to include comparisons of activity before and after the onset of illness, before transplantation.

Christopherson showed that 75% (38) of the 51 patients achieving successful rehabilitation had returned either to school, employment or homemaking (67.9% of the 56). Twelve returned to jobs previously held, 9 to self-employment and 5 found new employment. For these five, in each instance the salary and fringe benefits of their new job were inferior to those enjoyed preoperatively. Christopherson comments that the 'hiring discrimination often experienced by cancer patients and kidney transplant recipients appeared to be expressed even more strongly against cardiac recipients', a view which some of the Papworth patients would endorse. Thirteen of the 51 chose active retirement. Important factors contributing to this decision included a sufficient income without working, a conviction shared by the patient and family that the extra time gained by transplantation would be better spent in pursuits other than competitive employment, and a pre-illness history of avocational interests or involvement in community or civic groups.

In another report from Stanford, Pennock *et al.* (1982) looked at the rehabilitation of 106 heart transplant patients who had survived more than 1 year. They found that 82% had achieved active rehabilitation, 'defined simply as restoration of overall functional capacity sufficient to provide the patient with an unrestricted option to return to active employment or an activity of choice'. In the same year, English, Cory-Pearce and McGregor (1982) reported on the quality of life of the 14 survivors who had been discharged from Papworth Hospital, commenting that most of the heart recipients were delighted with the degree of rehabilitation they had attained.

Samuelsson, Hunt and Schroeder (1984) reported on results from 38 patients aged less than 30 who were transplanted during the period from 1974 to 1981. Twenty-three of the 24 survivors completed a questionnaire relating to rehabilitation and quality of life. Whether working or not, no patient considered himself completely unable to work and only 4 patients had not returned either to work or school, although 8 recognized some restriction in work activity. When questioned about physical mobility, 20 patients described themselves as 'completely free to come and go as they please'. In response to the question, 'If you had to make the same decision again, whether to accept a heart transplantation, would you make the same choice?', 22 answered yes and 1 patient was undecided. In the Papworth questionnaires, all 21 patients said they would make the same choice again. In the study by Lough *et al.* (1985) a similar question was asked, with a 95% positive response.

Lough and her colleagues sent questionnaires to 100 Stanford heart transplant recipients, all of whom were over the age of 18 and had survived 6 months from surgery. Replies were received from 75 patients. Their ages ranged from 19 to 60 years, with a mean of 42, and time from transplant ranged from 7 months to 14 years, with a mean of 3.7 years. The quality of life of 89% of patients was rated by them as good to excellent on the Likert scale and 82% expressed themselves highly satisfied with their current quality of life. Using a life-change scale, Lough found that positive changes had occurred in health status, physical condition, sense of achievement, future outlook and feelings of independence. Less change had occurred in close relationships, but where this was reported it was positive. These findings are very similar to the impressions gained in interviews with Papworth patients and data from the NHP. The factors showing negative changes for most of this Stanford group were financial situation and physical appearance ($p < 0.001$), the latter being true for both immunosuppressive therapy groups, azathioprine–prednisolone (Aza-Pred) and cyclosporin–low dose prednisolone (Cy-Pred). Changes for the worse in sexual function did not reach statistical significance, although of the 41% reporting a negative change, this was described as severe by 71% of that group. This compares with 28.9% of 48 Papworth patients who indicated problems in their sex lives because of their state of health at 3 months after surgery, the figure for the same individuals before transplantation being 84.4% ($p < 0.001$) (Table 19.2).

One of the most interesting aspects of Lough's data, however, relates to the results concerning symptom frequency and symptom distress. Recipients were asked to report the frequency of 27 symptoms related to immunosuppressive drug side effects and the degree of distress caused by them. Of the recipients receiving Aza-Pred therapy, 60% reported bruises and fragile skin. In the Cy-Pred group, excessive hair growth was the most frequently experienced symptom. It was impotence, however, occurring in 28% of the men in the Aza-Pred group and 11% of the Cy-Pred group, which was the most distressing symptom. However, a negative association was found between quality of life and both symptom frequency ($p < 0.001$) and symptom distress ($p < 0.009$). The conclusion was that symptoms and distress associated with them had little impact upon recipients' subjective evaluation of their overall quality of life. These data help to explain an apparent anomaly in the Papworth questionnaire results when a number of patients who were experiencing symptoms said, at the same time, that they were 'completely better'.

In the National Heart Transplantation Study (NHTS) of Evans *et al.* (1984), patients from six major transplant centres in the USA were studied after transplantation, using a variety of quality of life indicators. The Indices of Psychological Affect and Life Satisfaction, with scores ranging from 1 to 7, together with the Index of Well-Being, which is calculated by combining the first two, resulting in a score ranging from 2.1 to 14.7, were used in a survey of 152 patients. The higher the score, the more positive the psychological effect, the level of life satisfaction or feeling of well-being. The heart transplant recipients' mean scores were 5.49, 5.11 and 11.11, respectively. The Karnofsky Index was used as an indicator of patients' physical functional status, as judged by medical staff, the scores ranging from 1 (normal) to 10 (moribund). The heart transplant recipients' mean score was 1.47. The Sickness Impact Profile (SIP) measured patient perceived health status, with an overall score ranging from 0 to 100. In this case, the higher the score the poorer the health status, rather like the NHP, except that with the SIP it is possible to calculate a total mean score; for the heart transplant recipients it was 9.60.

The return to work figures in the NHTS were perhaps a little disappointing when compared with other studies. Only 58% of patients judged themselves able to work and fewer than 4 out of 10 patients had actually returned to full or part-time employment, school or looking after the home.

In a survey of psychological problems related to heart transplantation, reported by McAleer *et al.* (1985), in Arizona, data were collected by transplant coordinators from 595 recipients in 11 US transplant centres, as well as from the Arizona programme's own patients. All centres reported problems during the initial hospitalization, including depression and mood alterations in patients and an increase in family and marital stress. After discharge from hospital, family-related stress was the most common problem, non-compliance increased, depression and mood changes were still apparent and some patients had problems with impotence, personality changes or chronic pain. As these data are presented as the number of centres reporting problems, rather than numbers of patients, it is difficult to determine just how widespread the problems were; although in the Arizona programme in 1983, all 28 patients who had survived more than 3 months were noted to have psychological problems. Psychiatric services had been utilized in the initial evaluation of patients for potential recipient selection since 1980, and in 1983 support groups for heart transplant patients' families were instituted, 75% of members responding favourably. Although none of the other centres studied had started support groups at the time of reporting, these were being planned in several centres, and at one the transplant patients had formed a subgroup of a support group started for coronary artery bypass patients.

For the future, the Arizona programme was planning to start a support group for patients, hoping that other centres would follow this example so that a patient could attend the group closest to his home. We would agree with the authors, however, when they comment that further study is required to identify how patients perceive their own problems and how these evolve during prolonged survival.

To provide patients and their families with appropriate support before and after transplantation is a responsibility which should be recognized and pursued. However, caution is needed in treating these patients as a special group. Such an approach could even incur the risk of denying them what they most want and need, i.e. to feel normal and be accepted as such by society.

The overwhelming evidence from studies around the world is that heart transplantation, despite all the physical and psychological problems which may be involved, is to the vast majority of patients well worth while. Greater understanding of the problems still encountered is one of the main concerns now, especially identifying those which could be alleviated, thus reducing morbidity and mortality and thereby helping to decrease patients' anxieties with regard to the future. These include learning more about immunosuppression, thus reducing the incidence of rejection and infection, and side effects; developing techniques for the earlier and perhaps less invasive detection of rejection; and better preservation of organs and greater understanding of graft atheroma in the transplanted patient. Apart from the purely physical problems, better education of the general public and prospective employers may help more patients to return to work, and better counselling of patients and families regarding problems which may be encountered after surgery will give them the best possible preparation and help to reduce crisis disruption in their lives. This is a possible role for psychology support/therapy groups. Continuing to monitor levels of efficiency, financial management and outcome measures in terms of morbidity, survival and quality of life, i.e. remaining open to the evaluative process, will encourage governments to increase support and allow the expansion of an essentially successful form of treatment for end-stage cardiac disease.

REFERENCES

Buxton, M., Acheson, R. M., Caine, N., Gibson, S. and O'Brien, B. (1985). *Costs and Benefits of the Heart Transplant Programmes at Harefield and Papworth Hospitals: Final Report.* HMSO, London.

Christopherson, L. K., Griepp, R. B. and Stinson, B. (1976). Rehabilitation after cardiac transplantation. *J. Am. Med. Ass.* **236**(18), 2082–2084.

Cohen, C. (1982). On the quality of life: some philosophical reflections. *Circulation* **66** (suppl. III), 29–33.

English, T. A. H., Cory-Pearce, R. and McGregor, C. (1982). Heart transplantation at Papworth Hospital. *Heart Transplant.* **1**(2), 110–111.

Evans, R. W., Manninen, D. L., Overcast, T. D., Garrison, L. P., Yagi, J., Merrikin, K., Jonsen, A. R. *et al.* (1984). *The National Heart Transplantation Study: Final Report.* Battelle Human Affairs Research Centers, Seattle.

Hunt, S. M., McKenna, S. P. and McEwen, J. (1981). *The Nottingham Health Profile: Manual* (mimeo, unpublished).

Lough, M. E., Lindsey, A. M., Shinn, J. A. and Stotts, N. A. (1985). Life satisfaction following heart transplantation. *Heart Transplant.* **IV**(4), 446–449.

McAleer, M. J., Copeland, J., Fuller, J. and Copeland, J. G. (1985). Psychological aspects of heart transplantation. *Heart Transplant.* **IV**(2), 232–233.

McEwen, J. (1983). *The Nottingham Health Profile: A Measure of Perceived Health in 'Measuring the Social Benefits of Medicine'*, pp. 75–84. Office of Health Economics, London.

McKenna, S. P., Hunt, S. M. and McEwen, J. (1981). Weighting the seriousness of perceived health problems using Thurstone's method of paired comparisons. *Int. J. Epidemiol.* **10**(1), 93–97.

Najman, J. M. and Levine, S. (1981). Evaluating the impact of medical care and technologies on the quality of life: a review and critique. *Soc. Sci. Med.* **15F**, 107–115.

O'Brien, V. (1985). Some psychological and social aspects of heart transplantation. *Heart Transplant.* **IV**(2), 229–231.

Pennock, J. L., Oyer, P. E., Reitz, B. A., Jamieson, S. W., Bieber, C. P., Wallwork, J., Stinson, E. B. and Shumway, N. E. (1982). Cardiac transplantation in perspective for the future: survival, complications, rehabilitation and cost. *J. Thorac. Cardiovasc. Surg.* **83**, 168–177.

Samuelsson, R. G., Hunt, S. A. and Schroeder, J. S. (1984). Functional and social rehabilitation of heart transplant recipients under age thirty. *Scand. J. Thorac. Cardiovasc. Surg.* **18**, 97–103.

Michael P. Kaye

20

Results — The International Register*

It is now apparent that heart transplantation is no longer an experimental procedure, but rather a highly effective therapy for the treatment of end-stage heart disease. As a consequence of the demonstrated efficacy of this procedure, 3623 heart transplant procedures have been performed and reported to the Registry of the International Society for Heart Transplantation during the past 5 years. Although the increase in numbers of procedures performed from 1982 to 1983 was only 111, the increase from 1983 to 1984 was 360, and in the subsequent 2 years it was 358 and 478 per year. These data are graphically depicted in Fig. 20.1.

The data presented in this report were obtained from 78 centres in the USA and 37 centres from other sites around the world. At the end of the calendar year 1986, all the centres were sent a list of their patients and asked to provide the Registry with an updated statement of current patient status. It is from this updated list that the data presented are derived. It should be noted that some of the reporting centres have chosen to report for consortia, and hence the actual number of hospitals with the necessary staff to perform transplants is somewhat greater than the number of reporting centres.

The database of the Registry now consists of greater than 4600 patients. The average age for patients undergoing heart transplantation is 41.68 years, with a range in ages from newborn to 66 years. The majority of patients in the heart transplant group were male, only 15% of heart transplant patients being female. For the heart–lung transplant patients, the age range is not dissimilar, being 0.7–51 years (mean 32.54 years). However, the sex distribution of heart–lung patients is almost equal, 48% male and 52% female.

* First published in *The Journal of Heart Transplantation*, **6**(2), 1987, reproduced by permission.

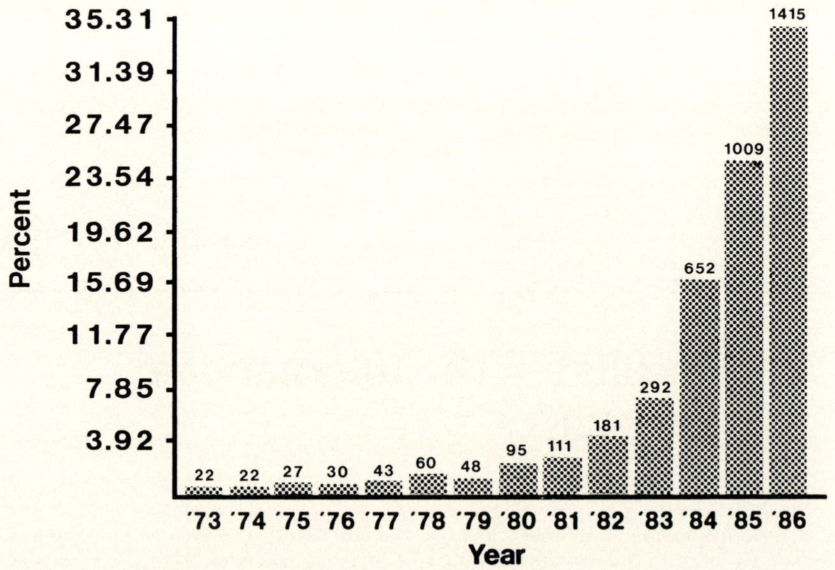

Fig. 20.1. *Number of heart transplant procedures per year.*

As progress has been made in increasing the survival after heart transplantation, the limitation of candidates to an age range of 15–50 years has been broadened. Table 20.1 details the distribution of patients undergoing heart transplantation by age, grouped in 5-year intervals. It is apparent from this table that the majority of patients undergoing transplantation fall into the 40–55-year age range. For the patients undergoing heart–lung transplantation, the age distribution table (Table 20.2) indicates that these patients tend to be somewhat younger than those subjected to heart transplantation, with most of the patients being between ages 35 and 40 years. Figure 20.2 shows the number of heart–lung transplants that have been reported to the Registry up until 1986. We are aware that these data are incomplete because of lack of data from one major centre, but we believe that they represent the trend for an increasing number of heart–lung transplants being performed throughout the world.

The most common indications for heart–lung transplantation continue to be primary pulmonary hypertension and the Eisenmenger's complex. For patients undergoing heart transplantation, cardiomyopathy and coronary artery disease continue to be the prime indications for surgery. These data are shown in Table 20.3, as well as the 30-day mortality in these groups of patients. Although there appears to be no difference in the 30-day mortality in the two primary groups, this mortality is increased in those patients

TABLE 20.1
Heart Transplant Patients by Age Group

Age Range	*Patient Count*
0–4	22
5–9	13
10–14	76
15–19	147
20–24	215
25–29	224
30–34	275
35–39	472
40–44	641
45–49	781
50–54	711
55–59	392
60–64	85
65–69	6
≥70	0
Total	4060

TABLE 20.2
Heart–Lung Transplant Patients by Age Group

Age Range	*Patient Count*
0–4	1
5–9	2
10–14	1
15–19	6
20–24	17
25–29	29
30–34	27
35–39	31
40–44	19
45–49	11
50–54	3
55–59	0
60–64	0
65–69	0
Total	147

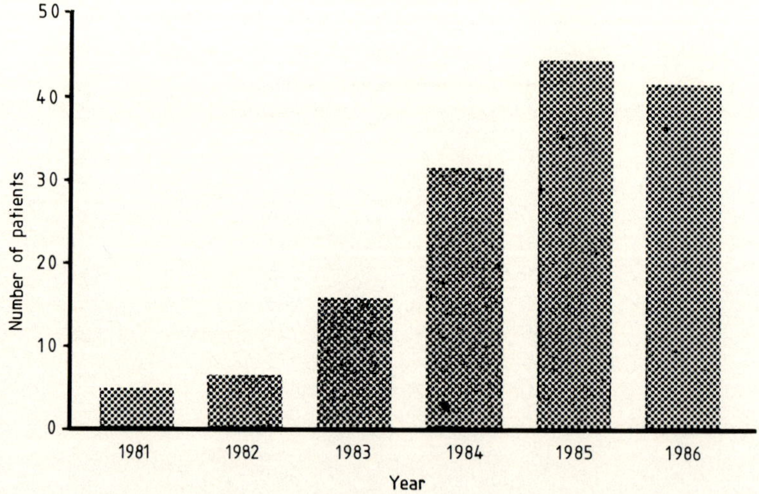

Fig. 20.2. *Number of heart–lung transplants per year.*

undergoing surgery for congenital and valvular heart disease and for graft rejection.

Table 20.4 details the 30-day mortality by age, grouped in 5-year increments for all heart transplant patients. Although there is no significant difference between any of the groups, it is of interest to note the relatively low 30-day mortality for those patients in the 55–65-year age range.

The 30-day mortality seems to indicate that the results of heart transplantation are continuing to improve with experience. Table 20.5 details the 30-day mortality for the years 1980–86, demonstrating a significant improvement in survival. This decrease in mortality has occurred as the number of heart transplant procedures increased from 652 in 1984, to 1010 in 1985, and to 1488 in 1986.

TABLE 20.3
Indications for Heart Transplantation, 1967–86

Indication	*Patient No.*	*Mortality (%)*
Cardiomyopathy	2325	12.26
Coronary artery disease	1481	12.42
Congenital disease	76	27.63
Graft rejection	46	28.26
Valvular disease	80	17.50

TABLE 20.4
Thirty-Day Mortality by Age

Age Range	*Patient Count*	*Mortality Count*	*Mortality (%)*
0–4	22	4	18.18
5–9	13	0	0.00
10–14	76	10	13.16
15–19	147	24	16.33
20–24	215	36	16.74
25–29	224	26	11.61
30–34	275	38	13.82
35–39	472	60	12.71
40–44	641	62	9.67
45–49	781	82	10.50
50–54	711	90	12.66
55–59	392	39	9.95
60–64	85	8	9.41
⩾65	6	1	16.67
Total	4060	480	11.82

Overall survival as calculated from actuarial tables continues to improve. Figure 20.3 compares 5-year actuarial survival for all patients undergoing orthotopic or heterotopic heart transplantation from 1967 to 1986, with those patients treated with cyclosporin during the same time period. Complete data are available in the Registry on 4095 patients, 3393 of whom have been treated with cyclosporin. As can be seen in Fig. 20.3, the 1-year actuarial survival in the entire group is 76%, and the 5-year survival is 71.3%. For those patients treated with cyclosporin, the 1-year actuarial survival is

TABLE 20.5
Thirty-Day Mortality

Year	*Mortality (%)*
1980	16.84
1981	15.32
1982	18.23
1983	16.10
1984	14.57
1985	12.21
1986	7.40
1967–86	12.14
1980–86	11.94

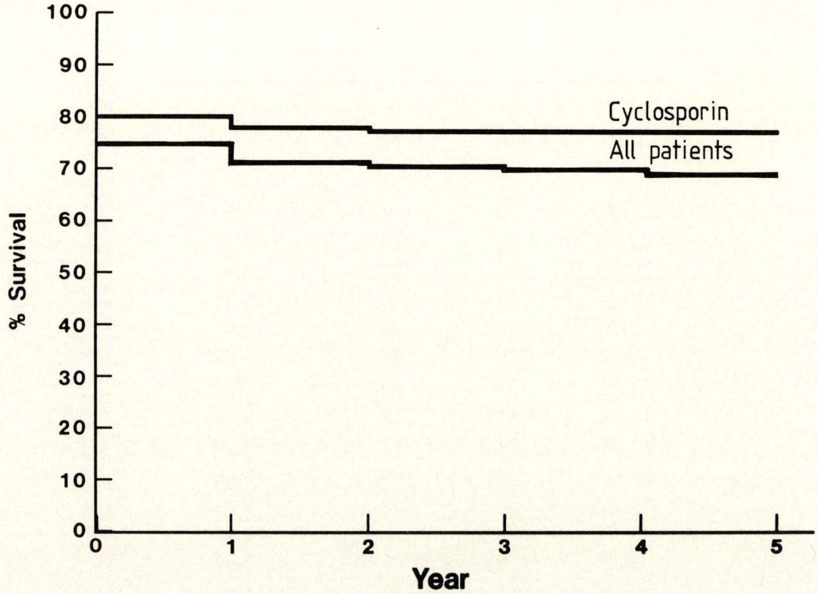

Fig. 20.3. *Heart actuarial survival.*

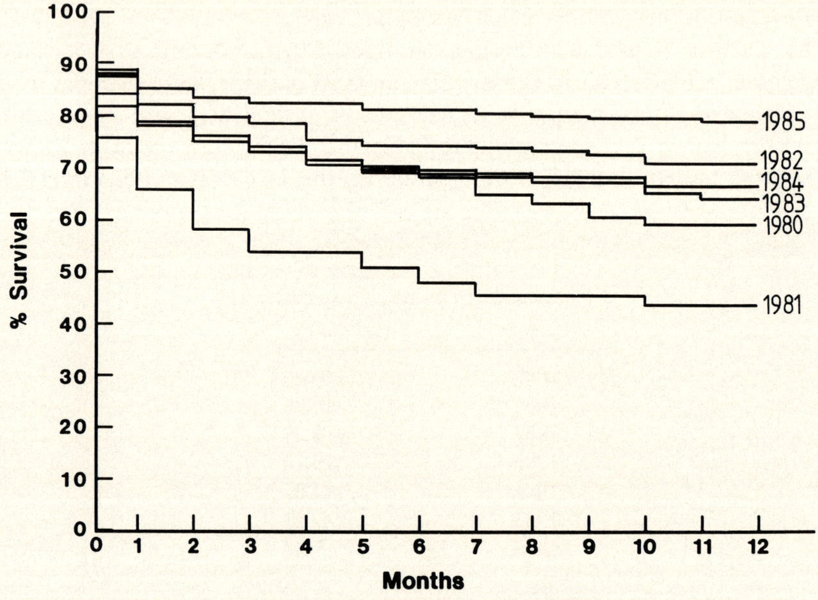

Fig. 20.4. *Kaplan–Meier survival graph.*

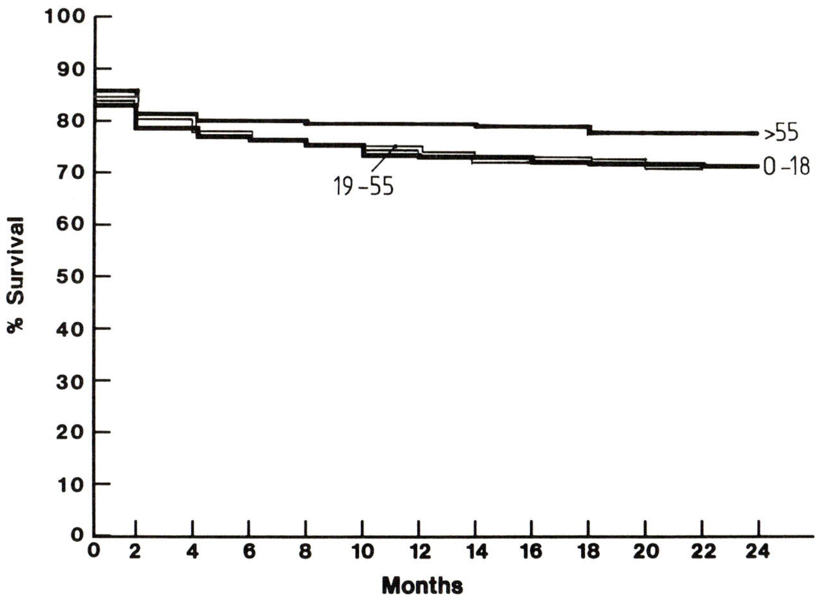

Fig. 20.5. *Actuarial survival according to age group.*

increased to 80.6%, and the 5-year actuarial survival rate is increased to 78.3%.

Figure 20.4 depicts the 1-year actuarial survival curves of the individual years 1980–85. Although the data from 1983 and 1984 appear almost to overlap, it is apparent that a marked upward shift occurred in 1985, with the 1-year actuarial survival at approximately 80%. On the basis of this trend and the 30-day mortality cited earlier, we would anticipate that the 1-year actuarial survival rate for 1986 will be even better than that for 1985.

As was mentioned previously, the limits of age have been extended in recent years to encompass patients from the newborn period until well into the sixth decade. Figure 20.5 depicts 2-year actuarial survival curves for three groups of patients according to age: 0–18 years, 19–55 years and >55 years. As can be seen, there is no apparent difference in the 2-year survival rates of patients aged 0–18 and 19–55 years. Remarkably, there is an increased survival of the patients in the 55 years and over age range. Because the number of patients is still somewhat small, this apparent enhanced survival is not statistically significant at this time.

There appears to be an increasing trend for many of the institutions that have staff members who are able to perform transplantation to use combinations of immunosuppressive drugs, with the most common combination being cyclosporin, azathioprine and steroids, in different dosages and for

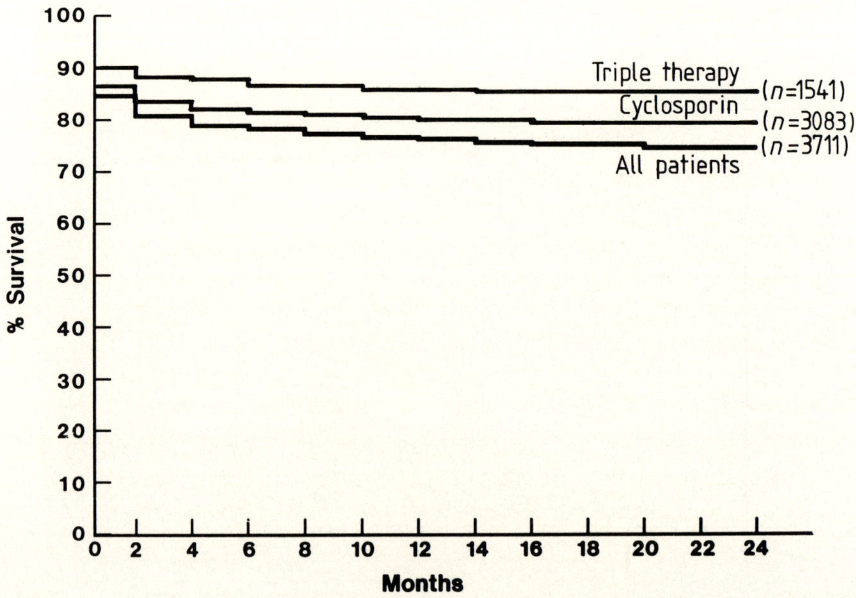

Fig. 20.6. *Actuarial survival, 1980–86, vs. immunosuppressive therapy.*

various periods of time. Because there is a great inter-institutional variability in dosage levels and administration schedules, we have simply categorized the use of these drugs as triple therapy. Figure 20.6 depicts 2-year actuarial survival curves for patients undergoing heart transplantation during the years 1980–86. Three groups of patients are compared: a group made up of all patients who had transplants in those years ($n = 3711$), a group who received cyclosporin with or without any other therapy ($n = 3083$), and a group who received triple therapy as described above ($n = 1541$). Two-year actuarial survival in the first group was 74.8%. In those patients receiving cyclosporin, survival at 2 years was increased to 79.2%, whereas in the group receiving triple therapy, the 2-year actuarial survival was 85.2%. It thus appears that alterations in immunosuppressive therapy can indeed enhance survival after heart transplantation.

The results presented thus far represent the combined data from those patients undergoing either orthotopic or heterotopic heart transplantation. Figure 20.7 demonstrates the number of heterotopic heart transplants reported to the Registry for the years 1973–86. In reviewing the indications for transplantation in these patients, there is no apparent reason for the increased numbers of heterotopic transplants performed in 1986. Survival data on these patients are unlike those from orthotopic heart transplant patients, with a 1-year actuarial survival of 61.4% and a 2-year actuarial survival of 56%.

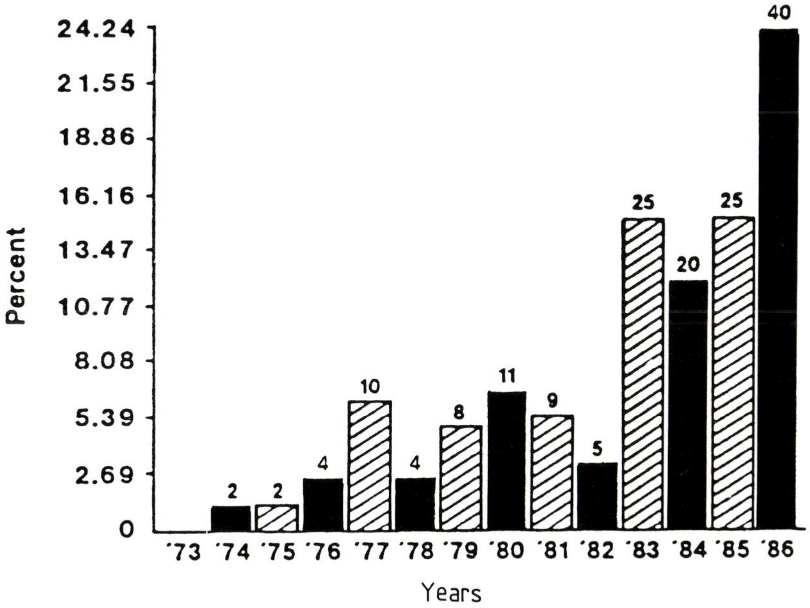

Fig. 20.7. *Number of heterotopic heart transplants, 1973–86.*

Of the data submitted to the Registry on heart-lung transplantation, information adequate to permit actuarial analysis is available on 126 patients as of March 1987. These data are presented in graphic form in Fig. 20.8 and indicate a 1-year actuarial survival of 55.4% and a 2-year rate of 51.9%.

Despite the increased survival in the transplanted patients and the apparent improvements in immunosuppression therapy, infection still remains the major cause of death after heart transplantation. Table 20.6 lists the causes of death in these patients. Although infection and rejection continue to be the primary causes of death, the number of patients dying of cardiac causes

TABLE 20.6
Causes of Death, 1967–86

Cause of Death	%
Infection	39
Acute rejection	26
Chronic rejection	9
Cardiac causes	21
Other causes	5

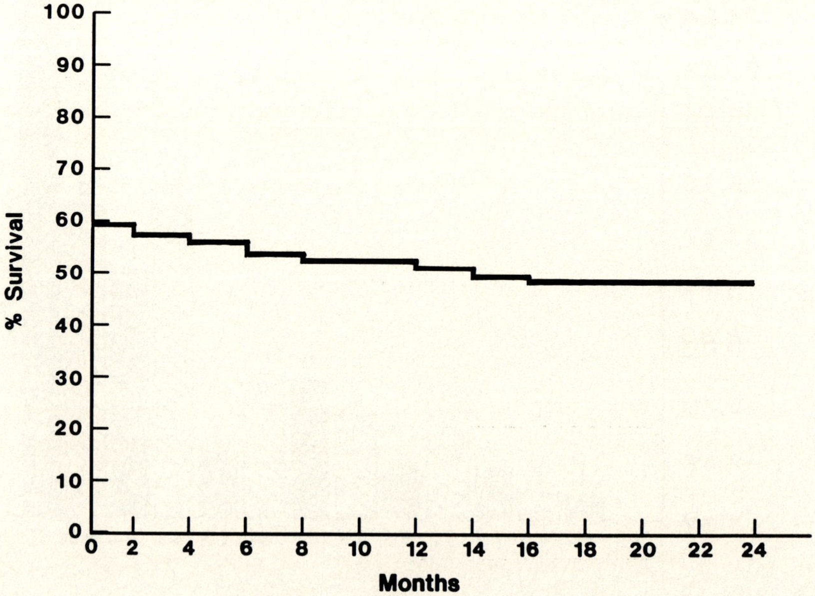

Fig. 20.8. *Heart–lung actuarial survival.*

TABLE 20.7
*Donor Age Distribution**

Age	*Number*	*30-Day Mortality (%)*
0–3	8	25.00
4–7	2	0.00
8–11	13	15.40
12–15	73	5.50
16–19	233	7.30
20–23	212	10.40
24–27	154	7.89
28–31	136	7.41
32–35	86	14.12
36–39	71	10.00
40–43	32	3.13
44–47	14	7.14
48–51	4	25.00

* Range 0.1–51 years; mean 24.8 years.

TABLE 20.8
Ischaemic Time

Ischaemic Time (h)	*Donors*
⩾1	76
1–2	211
2–3	269
3–4	142
4–5	23
5–6	2

appears high. Data are not available to permit conclusions, but we might speculate that deaths from cardiac causes may be related to the donor hearts and that improvements in techniques for harvesting and transportation of the donor hearts might decrease the number of deaths resulting from cardiac-related causes.

During the past year we have expanded the reporting form and have begun to accumulate data on heart and heart–lung donors. To date, data on 1085 donors have been filed with the Registry. These data indicate that 684 of the 1085 donor organs were procured from distant hospitals, whereas only 175 of the 1085 were from in-house donors. The age range for donors was from 0.1 to 51 years, with a mean of 24.8 years. Table 20.7 depicts the distribution of donors by age groups and as expected demonstrates that the donor population comes primarily from the 16–30-year age groups. This may well be related to the fact that the most common cause of death in the donor population continues to be motor vehicle accidents. Table 20.8 demonstrates the range of ischaemic times in the heart transplant donors. In Table 20.9, the donor ischaemic time is related to the 30-day mortality after transplantation. It appears from this table that there is a relationship between the ischaemic time and the 30-day mortality. The accumulation of more data will clearly define this relationship.

TABLE 20.9
Mortality Within 30 Days by Ischaemic Time

Time (h)	*Patients*	*Mortality (%)*
Up to 1	82	4.88
1–2	255	6.27
2–3	314	11.46
3–4	166	15.66
4–5	28	28.57
Total	845	10.65

Part II

Heart–Lung Transplantation

B. A. Reitz

21

Development of Heart–Lung Transplantation

Achievement of success in clinical heart–lung transplantation is an excellent example of evolutionary progress in cardiac surgery. All the general factors necessary for successful cardiopulmonary bypass and the management of acutely ill patients were a requirement, together with a specific understanding of the technique of heart–lung transplantation, the control of breathing after denervation, and the ability to diagnose and effectively suppress allograft rejection.

The beginnings of cardiac surgery and the transplantation of vascularized organs can be traced to the pioneering work of Alexis Carrel (Carrel and Guthrie, 1905; Carrel, 1907). In a series of elegant experiments, he demonstrated the feasibility of arterial and venous anastomoses, and their application to the transplantation of numerous organs. In a description of early experimental transplantation of a puppy's heart into the neck of an adult dog, Carrel describes another experiment, in which he transplanted the lungs together with the heart:

> Both lungs, the heart, the aorta, and vena cava of a cat one week old were extirpated and put into the neck of a large adult cat. The aorta was anastomosed to the peripheral end of the carotid, and the vena cavae to the peripheral end of the jugular vein. The coronary circulation was immediately re-established and the auricles began to beat. The lungs became red and after a few minutes, effective pulsations of the ventricles appeared. But the lungs soon became edematous, and distention of the right part of the heart occurred. This accident seems difficult of prevention. A phlegmon of the neck terminated this observation two days later.

Although this experiment met little success, it and numerous other observations by Carrel predicted the eventual utility of the transplantation of organs. It was many years before numerous advances in anti-coagulation, blood typing and artificial oxygenators made possible modern open heart surgery.

In the meantime, other also quite dramatic experiments were performed in the late 1940s by a Russian surgeon, V.P. Demikhov. These were reported in the West in 1962, with the publication of his book (Demikhov, 1962). He developed a technique using a working heart–lung preparation which allowed him to transplant the organs. By removing the heart–lung bloc at normothermia, and by maintaining a heart beat, he was able to transfer the heart and both lungs, or the heart and one lung into recipient dogs. One of many variations of this experiment is shown in Fig. 21.1. With his methods, neither cardiopulmonary bypass nor hypothermia were required, since the heart–lung preparation from the donor continued to function normally as it was being sutured into the recipient. This was accomplished by alternating one of two venous inflow anastomoses (either the superior or inferior vena cava) with one of two outflow anastomoses (either the brachiocephalic artery or the transverse aortic arch just distal to the brachiocephalic artery) and then the trachea. Thus, he replaced the heart and lungs of the recipient animal while both the donor and recipient heart and lungs continued to function.

In the first experiment, the dog in which the heart and lungs had been totally replaced survived for about 2 h with the donor organs. In May 1948, on the fourteenth attempt, the experiment resulted in a dog which survived for 7 h after the complete replacement of the heart and lungs. In the fifteenth experiment, they were at last able to complete the operation and take the dog alive from the operating table. The notes from this experiment recorded that after the chest was closed, 'spontaneous respiration was resumed, but respirations were infrequent and deep, 7 per minute. Later, respiration ceased, and the animal died shortly thereafter'. Other experiments confirmed that the respiratory pattern was very deep and the animals used the muscles of the abdominal wall and neck, with their mouths open. These changes in respiratory pattern were later associated with complete cardiopulmonary denervation in the dog.

In all, Demikhov subjected 67 dogs to replacement of the heart and lungs together. Twenty-three died on the operating table, 30 survived less than 24 h after the operation, 6 less than 48 h, 6 less than 4 days, 1 less than 5 days, and 1 less than 6 days. His experiments showed beyond doubt that from the point of view of surgical technique, the operation was feasible. The longest surviving animal (dog 'Damka') lived for 6 days and is shown in Fig. 21.2. In a prophetic statement, Demikhov noted: 'In the surgery of the future, when the causes of the complications and failures attending these operations have been studied and overcome, the transplantation of the heart, together with the lungs, will find its application in irreversible forms of cardiopulmonary insufficiency.'

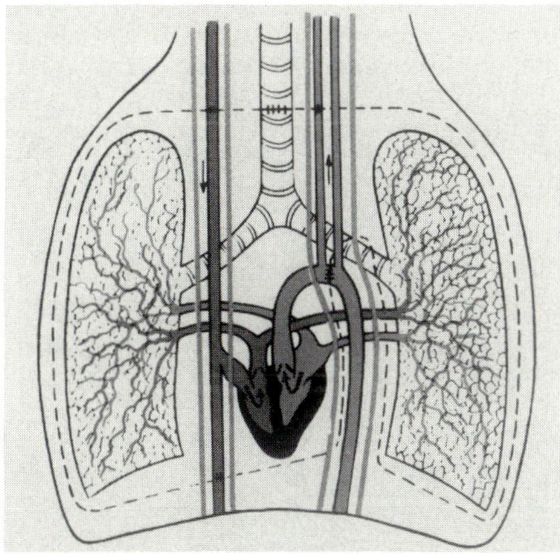

Fig. 21.1. *Experiment by V. P. Demikhov, showing the transection and anastomoses of the vena cava, transverse arch and brachiocephalic artery, and the trachea.*

The next reports of experiments on heart and lung replacement appeared in two papers which are consecutive in the volume of the *Archives of Surgery* for 1953. The first of these is by Neptune and associates, from Hahneman Medical College in Philadelphia (Neptune *et al.*, 1953). They reported what they felt was the first successful replacement of the heart and both lungs using the technique of hypothermia and circulatory arrest. They performed three experiments, and one animal survived as long as 6 h, maintaining a satisfactory blood pressure, spontaneous respiration and return of reflexes.

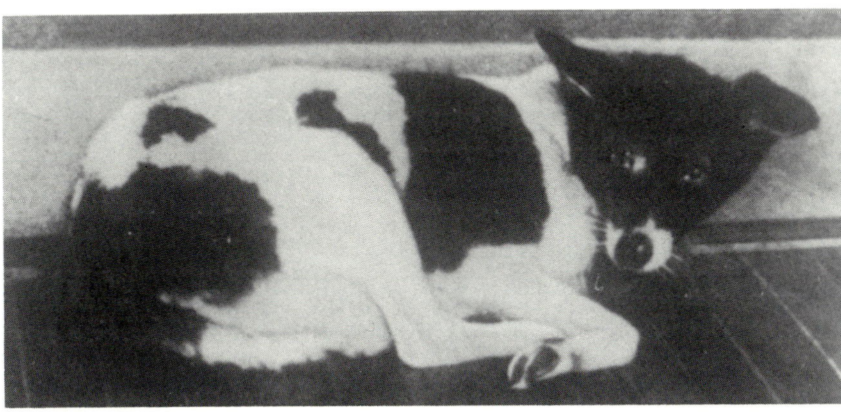

Fig. 21.2. *'Damka', the longest survivor after heart–lung transplantation performed by V. P. Demikhov in 1948. The dog lived until the sixth postoperative day, dying of pulmonary failure.*

They concluded that this preparation is an 'ideal way of obtaining a completely denervated heart, as well as lungs, for physiologic study'.

The following paper in the same journal is entitled 'Homologous heart grafts' and is written by Marcus and associates from the Chicago Medical School (Marcus, Wong and Luisada, 1953). Their experiments describe heterotopic heart–lung transplantation to the intra-abdominal aorta and vena cava of a recipient animal. In 8 animals, they sutured the superior and inferior venae cavae of the donor heart and lung to the distal inferior vena cava of the recipient, the brachiocephalic artery of the donor to the proximal abdominal aorta, and the transverse aortic arch to the distal abdominal aorta. The trachea was then exteriorized and mechanically ventilated. Nitrogen was given to the recipient's own trachea, and circulation was maintained by administering oxygen to the trachea of the donor animal. The experimental preparation is demonstrated in Fig. 21.3. They were able to maintain the recipient for approximately 75 min after the heart of the host animal had died.

Marcus described a second ingenious experiment. While the heart and lung preparation was working in the abdominal position, the chest of the host was entered and the main pulmonary artery was temporarily occluded to empty the left side of the heart. The host heart was then opened with an incision in the left atrial appendage, and manipulations of the mitral valve were made under direct vision. After 7 min of intracardiac exposure, the atrium was closed, and the heart was allowed to beat again. Thus, the authors had ingeniously devised a method for open intracardiac surgery using a donor heart and lungs as the pump oxygenator. The authors note in their discussion that 'a transplanted heart or heart–lung preparation might be used for replacement of a diseased organ'.

Many significant advances in cardiac surgery then followed, including the use of hypothermia and circulatory arrest for successful closure of an atrial septal defect by Lewis and his colleagues (Lewis and Taufic, 1953) and the demonstration by Gibbon that an artificial pump and oxygenator could be used to perform open intracardiac surgery (Gibbon, 1954).

These procedures initiated the era of modern open heart surgery. The surgeon then had the technical tools to routinely transplant intrathoracic organs. In 1957, the use of a pump oxygenator to perform heart–lung transplantation in dogs was reported (Webb and Howard, 1957). These authors found it was possible to restore the heart to relatively normal function, and the animals lived from 75 min to 22 h. Their experiments anticipated the technical difficulties of later surgeons; they noted continued bleeding from the extensive raw surfaces developed during the dissection, and none of their animals returned to spontaneous normal respiration. They also reported four attempts at autotransplantation of the heart and lung, but noted that in several of their animals cardiac function was sufficient but the animals were

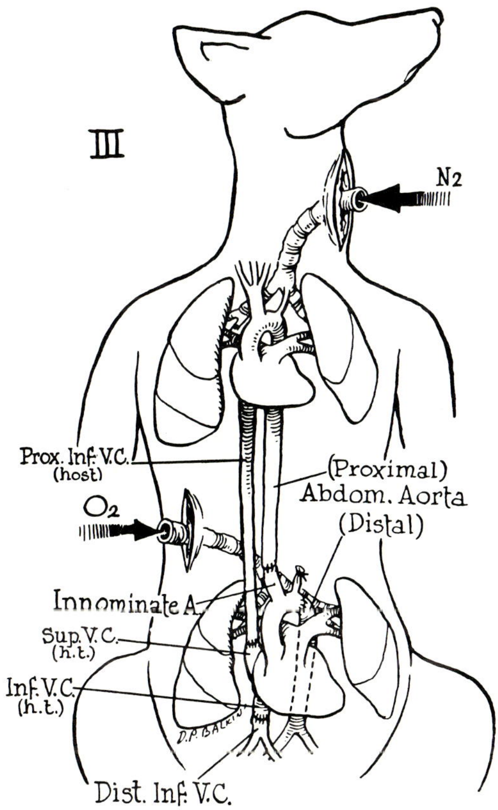

Fig. 21.3. *Heterotopic, working heart–lung transplantation in the dog. Support of the circulation was demonstrated by ventilating the host with nitrogen gas (From Marcus, Wong and Luisada (1953), reproduced by permission. Copyright 1953, American Medical Association).*

unable to breathe spontaneously. This was in contradistinction to other experiments they performed, in which heart transplantation alone was done. In those instances, there was an immediate return to spontaneous respiration. This again suggested that cardiopulmonary denervation was not well tolerated by dogs. They concluded that transplantation of the heart and both lungs was not practical, due to respiratory paralysis. They suggested that transplantation of the heart with one lung be considered, since respiratory paralysis would be prevented by retaining one innervated lung.

In 1958, Blanco and associates reported eight attempts at orthotopic heart and lung replacement, maintaining the recipient on a pump oxygenator (Blanco *et al.*, 1958). In two of their animals spontaneous respirations appeared after the respirator was disconnected, but no animal survived more than 5 h.

The next encouraging report was from Lower *et al.* (1961). This group had previously reported the first significant survival after orthotopic heart transplantation in the dog (Lower and Shumway, 1960). They now turned their efforts to complete heart–lung replacement, and 6 animals resumed spontaneous respiration. They pointed out the need for preservation of the recipient's phrenic and vagus nerves, and careful ligation of bronchial vessels. The donor organs were immersed in cold saline solution at 4°C for topical hypothermia, and anastomoses were performed at the aorta, trachea and both venae cavae. In those dogs that resumed spontaneous respirations, the respiratory pattern was altered with increased tidal volume and slow respiratory rate. This now familiar pattern is typical of a dog with cardiopulmonary denervation. Despite this, 2 of the animals survived for as long as 4 days postoperatively. Lower and his colleagues believed the study demonstrated that the lung could survive without a bronchial arterial supply, but the question of prolonged survival after pulmonary denervation remained unanswered.

Sen and colleagues from India reported experiments in cardiopulmonary transplantation (Sen *et al.*, 1965). Survival of 5–12 h was obtained, but haemorrhage was a significant problem. Another report using similar techniques was presented by DeBono (1966). In a study of the heart–lung working preparation to examine heart viability after storage, Robicsek *et al.* (1967) repeated Demikhov's method with up to 37 h survival. Again, respiratory difficulties prevented long-term survival.

In an extensive study of heart–lung transplantation in dogs, Longmore *et al.* (1969) introduced the concept of a single inflow anastomosis at the right atrium. There was 1 survivor for 25 h. A co-author, D. K. C. Cooper, wrote a historical review as part of the study (Cooper, 1969). Clearly, although surgical technique was up to the task of heart–lung transplantation, cardiopulmonary denervation had to be overcome.

Insight into the breathing difficulties after denervation came from the excellent experiments of Nakae *et al.* (1967), who performed different types of cardiopulmonary autotransplantation in several species of animals. First, they divided the great vessels, venae cavae and trachea, and divided all other tissue connecting the heart and lungs with the surrounding structures. In dogs who had this type of denervation, the breathing pattern was extremely slow and abnormal, as in all of the dogs who had heart–lung transplantation. When mediastinal denervation was complete, but without transection of the great vessels, the breathing pattern was also abnormal. In a third group, complete mediastinal denervation without tracheal transection was also accompanied by an abnormal breathing pattern, and the animals died of respiratory failure. A final group of dogs underwent division of the major vessels only without pulmonary denervation, and these all resumed spontaneous respirations with a normal respiratory pattern. Then, they repeated the procedure in cats with the same results. Finally, when the same experiments were performed in monkeys, there was the resumption of a relatively normal respiratory pattern despite mediastinal denervation. Deaths in this group were due to technical factors such as bleeding or air leakage and not to respiratory insufficiency. These experiments confirmed the suggestion from earlier work by Haglin *et al.* (1963) that denervation of both lungs did not prevent a return of adequate spontaneous respiration in primates as it did in dogs.

Proof of these physiology experiments came with a report by Castaneda *et al.* (1972a). In trying to avoid respiratory difficulties they operated on primates, and avoided allograft rejection by performing autotransplants. In a series of 40 baboons, 6 animals survived for more than 1 month, several surviving for several years. In addition to technical success, they examined the pulmonary ventilation and perfusion and circulatory haemodynamics in these baboons (Castaneda *et al.*, 1972b). In all respects they were found to be normal, and the authors predicted that heart–lung transplantation would be successful in patients.

Additional primate studies were begun in 1978 by Reitz and colleagues at Stanford University, California (Reitz *et al.*, 1980). The initial experiments in small cynomolgus monkeys were with autotransplants. First, hypothermia and circulatory arrest was the technique, and later, cardiopulmonary bypass was found to give better success (Reitz, Pennock and Shumway, 1981). A method for right atrial cannulation and anastomosis was developed, as illustrated in Fig. 21.4. Again, autotransplanted animals had normal cardiopulmonary function and long-term survival.

In the late 1970s, cyclosporin was being studied in several laboratories, and it was suggested that this new immunosuppressive drug could prevent allograft rejection very effectively (Kostakis, White and Calne, 1977). A small amount of the material was available for study in the Stanford laboratory and it was used for the treatment of monkeys after heart–lung allotransplantation. It soon became apparent that this drug was able to prevent allograft rejection without obvious toxicity, and several animals survived for periods of greater than 1 year after heart–lung allotransplantation (Reitz *et al.*, 1980). Several of these animals lived for well over 5 years after allotransplantation (Harjula *et al.*, 1987). The early results in these monkeys suggested that the degree of rejection in the heart and lung was similar, and that the clinically useful endomyocardial biopsy might be sufficient for following the rejection post-transplant. Later, clinical experience proved that pulmonary rejection could occur without cardiac rejection. The survival of these animals gave encouragement for a new clinical trial.

Before the clinical trials of 1981, there were three earlier heart–lung transplants performed during the initial period of enthusiasm over heart transplantation in the late 1960s. The first of these was in September 1968 by

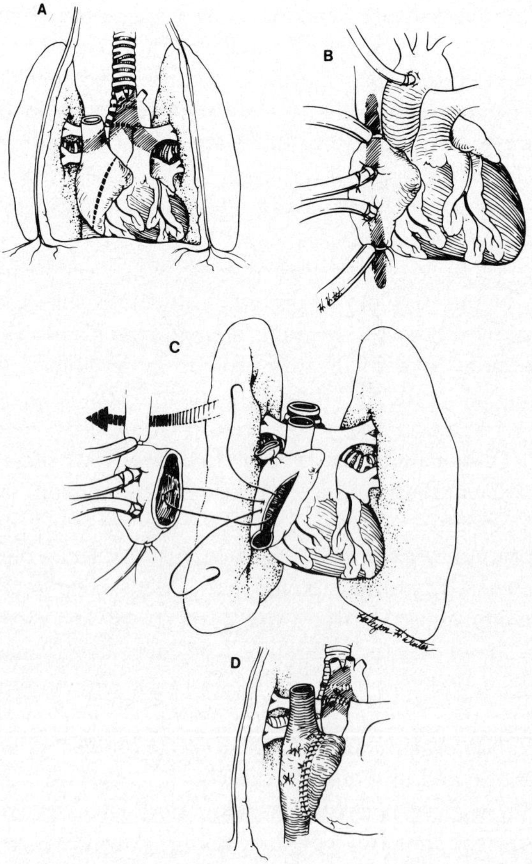

Fig. 21.4. *Cannulation, transection, and re-anastomosis for heart–lung transplantation in primates. This method was suggested for clinical procedure by Reitz, Pennock and Shumway (1981).*

Cooley and associates. The recipient was a $2\frac{1}{2}$-month-old child with atrioventricular canal defect and pulmonary hypertension. She died from pulmonary insufficiency with evidence of pulmonary consolidation 14 h postoperatively (Cooley *et al.*, 1969). In December 1969, Lillehei and colleagues transplanted the heart and lungs of a 50-year-old woman into a 43-year-old man with terminal emphysema. He was extubated on the first postoperative day and was ambulatory for several days before becoming ill with severe bronchopneumonia. He died 8 days following transplantation (Lillehei, 1970). A third human heart–lung transplantation was performed by Barnard in 1971; this patient developed a tracheobronchial fistula and intractable pneumonia, but survived for 23 days (Losman *et al.*, 1982). These

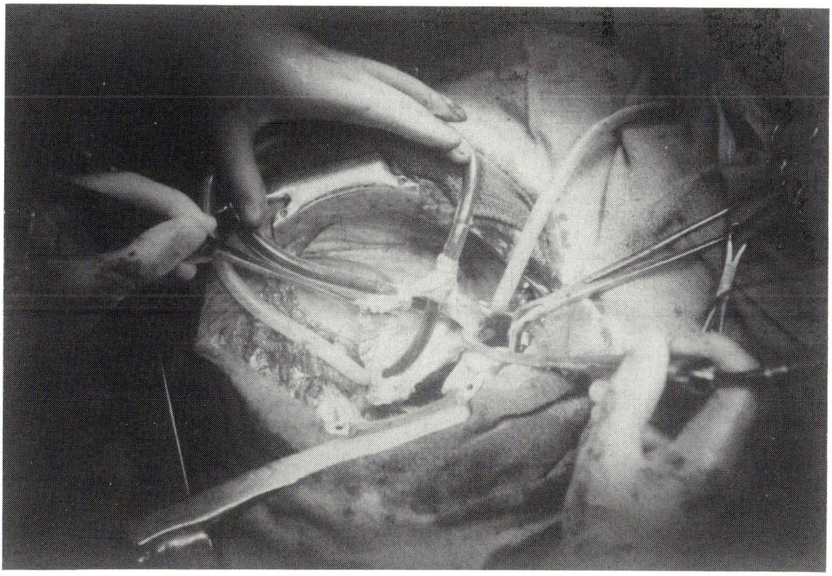

Fig. 21.5. *Empty thorax, after heart–lung removal, of a 45-year-old patient with primary pulmonary hypertension. The right atrial cuff with venous cannula, and the transected aorta with cross-clamp, are both shown. This patient had excellent long-term survival.*

results were similar to those of isolated lung transplants performed at that time, and the ability of both Lillehei's and Barnard's patients to breathe spontaneously was helpful evidence that heart–lung denervation would not preclude patient survival, as it had in the canine experiments.

With the laboratory success of cyclosporin in small primate heart–lung transplants, a new clinical trial began in March 1981 at Stanford. The protocol for these operations was approved by an institutional review board, and cyclosporin A for clinical use gained Federal approval as an investigational new drug. The first patient was a 45-year-old woman with end-stage primary pulmonary hypertension. The donor for the procedure was brought to the transplant centre in order to minimize the ischaemic time, and the heart–lung transplant was performed with the method previously described (Reitz, Pennock and Shumway, 1981). The patient's thorax with heart and lungs removed is shown in Fig. 21.5. She was treated with a combination of cyclosporin and azathioprine for 14 days, and then azathioprine was discontinued and prednisone was added. An acute rejection episode at 10 days post-transplant required intubation and ventilatory assistance, but ultimately she was discharged from the hospital in good condition and subsequently did very well for more than 5 years after transplantation. The chest radiograph 1 year post-transplant is shown in Fig. 21.6. A second patient,

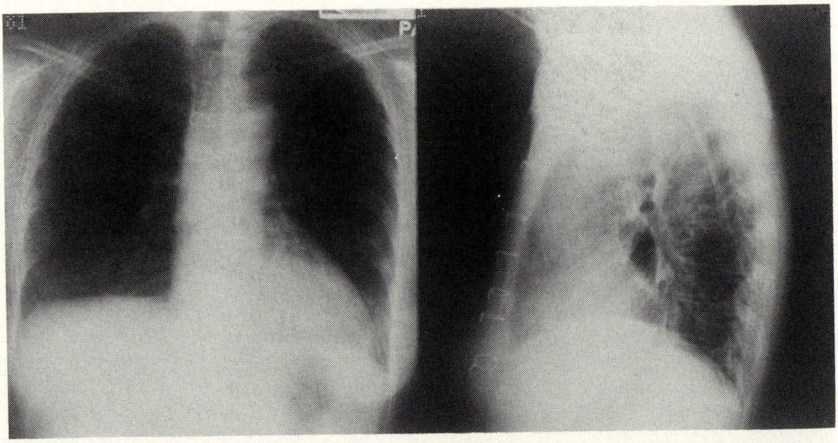

Fig. 21.6. *Chest radiograph of the first long-term survivor after heart–lung transplantation, 1 year postoperatively. This patient had excellent cardiopulmonary function for 5 years. She died of complications of trauma.*

with Eisenmenger's syndrome caused by a large membranous ventricular septal defect, had heart–lung transplantation several months later, and also had a remarkable recovery with long-term success (Reitz *et al.*, 1982).

The advent of clinically successful heart–lung transplantation sparked interest in the procedure in a number of centres. Further experimental studies were directed at methods for the preservation of lung tissue in order to extend the allowable ischaemic time of the donor organs. Studies were performed to examine the relationship between heart and lung rejection, the vascularity of the tracheal anastomosis, and the effects of pulmonary denervation, among others. These later experiments are too numerous to review adequately in this chapter.

As clinical heart–lung transplantation expanded, various additional problems were identified, including bronchiolitis obliterans and a lack of donors to meet the need. The record of the development of this procedure has shown that when advances have occurred, they have been preceded by experimental laboratory investigation. Such studies will continue to lead the way as the testing ground for techniques and treatments which will improve the results of all transplant procedures.

REFERENCES

Blanco, G., Adam, A., Rodriguez-Perez, D. and Fernandez, A. (1958). Complete homotransplantation of canine heart and lungs. *Arch. Surg.* **76**, 20.

Carrel, A. (1907). The surgery of blood vessels, etc. *Bull. Johns Hopkins Hosp.* **18**, 18–28.

Carrel, A. and Guthrie, C. C. (1905). The transplantation of veins and organs. *Am. Med.* **10**, 1101–1102.

Castaneda, A. R., Arnar, O., Schmidt-Hableman, P., Moller, J. H. and Zamora, R. (1972a). Cardiopulmonary autotransplantation in primates. *J. Cardiovasc. Surg.* **37**, 523.

Castaneda, A. R., Zamora, R., Schmidt-Habelmann, P., Hornung, J., Murphy, W., Ponto, D. and Moller, J. H. (1972b). Cardiopulmonary autotransplantation in primates (baboons). Late functional results. *Surgery* **72**, 1064.

Cooley, D. A., Bloodwell, R. D., Hallman, G. L., Nora, J. J., Harrison, G. M. and Leachman, R. D. (1969). Organ transplantation for advanced cardiopulmonary disease. *Ann. Thorac. Surg.* **8**, 300.

Cooper, D. K. C. (1969). Transplantation of the heart and both lungs, I. Historical review. *Thorax* **24**, 383–390.

DeBono, A. H. (1966). La transplantation cardiopulmonaire totale. *Ann. Chir. Thorac. Cardiovasc.* **5**, 243.

Demikhov, V. P. (1962). *Experimental Transplantation of Vital Organs.* Consultants' Bureau, New York.

Gibbon, J. H. (1954). Application of a mechanical heart and lung apparatus to cardiac surgery. *Minn. Med.* **37**, 171.

Haglin, J., Telander, R. L., Muzzall, R. E., Kiser, J. C. and Strobel, C. J. (1963). Comparison of lung autotransplantation in the primate and dog. *Surg. Forum* **14**, 196–198.

Harjula, A., Baldwin, J., Henry, D., Tazelaar, H., Jamieson, S., Reitz, B. and Shumway, N. (1987). Minimal lung pathology in long-term primate survivors of heart–lung transplantation. *Transplantation* **44**, 852–854.

Kostakis, A. J., White, D. J. G. and Calne, R. Y. (1977). Prolongation of rat allograft survival by cyclosporin A. *IRSC Med. Sci.* **5**, 280.

Lewis, F. and Taufic, M. (1953). Closure of atrial septal defects with the aid of hypothermia; experimental accomplishments and the report of one successful case. *Surgery* **33**, 52–59.

Lillehei, C. W. (1970). Discussion of Wildevuur, C. R. H., Benfield, J. R. A review of 23 human lung transplantations by 20 surgeons. *Ann. Thorac. Surg.* **9**, 489.

Losman, J. G., Campbell, C. D., Replogle, R. L. and Barnard, C. N. (1982). Joint transplantation of the heart and lungs. Past experience and present potentials. *J. Cardiovasc. Surg.* **23**, 440.

Longmore, D. B., Cooper, D. K. C., Hall, R. W., Sekabunga, J. and Welch, W. (1969). Transplantation of the heart and both lungs. II. Experimental cardiopulmonary transplantation. *Thorax* **24**, 391–398.

Lower, R. R. and Shumway, N. E. (1960). Studies on orthotopic homotransplantation of the canine heart. *Surg. Forum* **11**, 18.

Lower, R. R., Stofer, R. C., Hurley, E. J. and Shumway, N. E. (1961). Complete homograft replacement of the heart and both lungs. *Surgery* **50**, 842.

Marcus, E., Wong, S. N. T. and Luisada, A. A. (1953). Homologous heart grafts. *Arch. Surg.* **66**, 179–191.

Nakae, S., Webb, W. R., Theodorides, T. and Sugg, W. L. (1967). Respiratory function following cardiopulmonary denervation in dog, cat, and monkey. *Surg. Gynecol. Obstet.* **125**, 1285.

Neptune, W. B., Cookson, B. A., Bailey, C. P., Appler, R. and Rajkowski, F. (1953). Complete homologous heart transplantation. *Arch. Surg.* **66**, 174–178.

Reitz, B. A., Burton, N. A., Jamieson, S. W., Bieber, C. P., Pennock, J. L., Stinson, E. B. and Shumway, N. E. (1980). Heart and lung transplantation, autotransplantation and allotransplantation in primates with extended survival. *J. Thorac. Cardiovasc. Surg.* **80**, 360.

Reitz, B. A., Pennock, J. L. and Shumway, N. E. (1981). Simplified operative method for heart and lung transplantation. *J. Surg. Res.* **31**, 1–5.

Reitz, B. A., Wallwork, J., Hunt, S. A., Pennock, J. L., Billingham, M. E., Oyer, P. E., Stinson, E. B. and Shumway, N. E. (1982). Heart–lung transplantation: successful therapy for patients with pulmonary vascular disease. *New Engl. J. Med.* **306**, 557–564.

Robicsek, F., Lesage, A., Sanger, P. W., Daugherty, H. K., Gallucci, V. and Bagby, E. (1967). Transplantation of 'live' hearts. *Am. J. Cardiol.* **20**, 803.

Sen, P. K., Parulkar, G. B., Panday, S. R. and Kinare, S. G. (1965). Homologous canine heart transplantation: a preliminary report of 100 experiments. *Ind. J. Med. Res.* **53**, 674.

Webb, W. R. and Howard, H. S. (1957). Cardiopulmonary transplantation. *Surg. Forum* **8**, 313.

John Wallwork

22

Indications for Operation, Patient Selection and Assessment

Heart–lung transplantation has followed other organ transplant procedures by rapidly going through an early period of development since the first successful operation in 1982 (Reitz *et al.*, 1982). The indication for that first operation was primary pulmonary hypertension. Since then the disease processes which can be treated by heart–lung transplantation have become more numerous and diverse than at first thought (Penketh *et al.*, 1987; Scott *et al.*, 1988b; Hutter *et al.*, 1988a). Furthermore, the criteria for acceptance of individuals from these groups and the timing of intervention continue to change. This evolution and expansion of the scope of heart–lung transplantation will continue as more knowledge is gained of the short, mid- and long-term results (Copeland, 1987). Criteria regarded as contraindications to surgery 5 years ago (Burke *et al.*, 1986), are now not so regarded. For example, some patients with previous cardiac or thoracic surgery are now accepted and a major group of patients, those with cystic fibrosis (Jones, Higenbottam and Wallwork, 1987a; Scott *et al.*, 1988b), are now acceptable as potential recipients; they may indeed be one of the largest groups to benefit.

The demand for heart–lung transplantation is already greater than current activity can meet (Higenbottam, Caine and Wallwork, 1988). As the procedure becomes more established and successful, the demand will rise further. The ultimate determinant of heart–lung transplant activity will be donor organ supply. Even if 'required request' or similar legislation and guidelines (Oh and Uniewski, 1986; DHSS, 1987) were widely accepted, and thus donor organ availability increased, there would still be limits on

TABLE 22.1
Conditions Potentially Suitable For Heart-Lung Transplantation

Eisenmenger's syndrome
Primary pulmonary hypertension
Cystic fibrosis
Fibrosing alveolitis
Emphysema
Sarcoidosis
Bronchiectasis
Histiocytosis X
Pulmonary fibrosis

heart–lung transplantation because of lack of resources. Careful selection of potential recipients and evaluation of results will determine how best to use this scarce resource.

This chapter describes the current indications for and assessment of patients for heart–lung transplantation, illustrated by the Papworth Hospital, Cambridge, programme experience. It will also assess the potential need as far as can be determined from mortality data of the major disease categories currently acceptable for heart–lung transplantation.

INDICATIONS FOR SURGERY

The conditions potentially suitable for heart–lung transplantation are outlined in Table 22.1. They are basically divided into two major groups: those patients with primary lung disease, including primary pulmonary hypertension, and those patients with secondary pulmonary hypertension due to cardiac disease. The largest group among these latter patients comprises those with congenital heart disease who may or may not have had previous surgery, but for whom there is now no anatomical or physiological chance of correction. It is among this group of patients that the majority of future expansion will take place in the development of heart–lung transplantation for infants and children. The list of potential diseases given in Table 22.1 is not exhaustive. There will be many individuals with a variety of disorders which lead to chronic cardiorespiratory failure who will be suitable for heart–lung transplantation. The three major diagnostic groups are patients with Eisenmenger's syndrome, primary pulmonary hypertension and cystic fibrosis. Patients with other forms of lung disease make up a further sizable heterogeneous group of potential patients.

Some patients, particularly those with fibrosing lung disease, will be suitable for single lung transplantation (Cooper *et al.*, 1987) and some patients without cardiac involvement may be suitable for double lung transplantation (Patterson *et al.*, 1988). These parallel developments are described in Chapter 25. All patients with Eisenmenger's syndrome, however, will need both heart and lung transplantation. It is too early in the development of these procedures to give definitive guidelines which will determine the particular procedure most suitable for those potential recipients for whom there is a possible choice of operation.

It used to be thought, for example, that one of the advantages of combined heart–lung transplantation was the ability to monitor rejection of the heart–lung bloc by way of endomyocardial biopsy (Reitz *et al.*, 1983). We now know that this is not the case, as the lungs tend to reject prior to and without cardiac rejection (Scott, Hoverick and Billingham, 1984; McGregor *et al.*, 1985; Prop *et al.*, 1985). Indeed, at Papworth we have, like several other centres, abandoned routine cardiac biopsy in heart–lung transplant recipients (Hutter *et al.*, 1988b).

There is still concern about the mid- and long-term problems of stenosis of the bronchial/tracheal anastomosis in isolated lung transplants. In heart–lung transplantation, a systemic bronchial blood supply from coronary collaterals is retained, which is not the case in isolated lung transplantation. Although satisfactory healing can be achieved, the lack of a native bronchial blood supply may be responsible for these problems.

Double lung transplantation for primary lung disease has been advocated in order to maximize donor organ supply, enabling the heart to be given to a second recipient (Cooper *et al.*, 1987). However, Reitz and Yacoub have introduced independently the concept of the heart of a heart–lung transplant recipient, if it is suitable, being donated to a heart transplant patient as an alternative to maximize organ usage. This procedure still maintains the benefits of transplanting the heart–lung bloc intact. The future of this development again awaits full evaluation before definite statements can be made about the most appropriate operation for the individual recipient.

NEED FOR HEART–LUNG TRANSPLANTATION

The true potential need for heart–lung transplantation can only be estimated. As acceptance criteria change, the size of the recipient pool will alter accordingly. No morbidity data are available to assess the size of the recipient population, but a *minimum* estimated need can be derived from the *mortality* data for the major disease groups in the appropriate age ranges (Higenbottam, Caine and Wallwork, 1988).

An analysis of the Department of Health and Social Security mortality figures for England and Wales for 1984 has been used to make this estimate (HMSO, 1984). Ages in the ranges 10–49 and 5–9 years have been analysed separately, to help in the assessment of need in younger children.

The number of deaths per year was considered for each of the following major disease groups: Eisenmenger's syndrome, pulmonary hypertension, cystic fibrosis and other parenchymatous lung diseases which include cryptogenic fibrosing alveolitis and granulomatous diseases such as sarcoidosis. The annual death rates for a population of approximately 30 million people are shown in Table 22.2 for both age groups. Miscellaneous diseases of the lung account for the majority of the deaths, and the largest single disease group is patients with cystic fibrosis. This is also true of the younger age group, although Eisenmenger's syndrome is also important.

The deaths per year per million population of patients who could be potential heart–lung transplant recipients are 5.8 in the 5–9 year olds and 11.3 in the 10–49 age group. It must be stressed that the potential recipient population is probably much greater than this figure when the large pool of chronically disabled patients not immediately at risk of death is taken into account. Not all of these patients would prove to be acceptable, however, because of other contraindications to surgery. At Papworth during the past 2 years, 26% of patients assessed have been excluded because of factors such as previous pleurectomy or high-dose steroid therapy.

The need for heart–lung transplantation undoubtedly exceeds our capacity to transplant all these patients. Some selection of patients will continue to be imposed to maximize the benefit of heart–lung transplantation to the population and minimize the risks to the individual.

SELECTION CRITERIA

In any restricted form of medical or surgical therapy, selection criteria have to be considered to make the most appropriate use of resources available. The most important criteria for selection are shown in Table 22.3. One of the major difficulties in selection of patients for heart–lung transplantation compared with heart transplantation is prediction of prognosis. This is of particular importance in patients with Eisenmenger's syndrome and chronic lung disease where progressive deterioration may temporarily cease, leaving patients in a state of severe disability without immediate risk of death for many years.

Acceptance of a patient as a potential recipient depends therefore on a constellation of features. For patients without contraindications the decision

TABLE 22.2
Potential Population For Heart–Lung Transplantation in England and Wales

Disease Group	Mortality Rates Per Million Population (England and Wales, 1984) Age Groups 5–9	10–49
Eisenmenger's syndrome	1.0	1.8
Primary pulmonary hypertension	0.7	1.2
Cystic fibrosis	4.1	3.3
Other lung disease	—	5.0
Total	5.8	11.3

is easy. For example, patients who have progressed to a wheelchair existence or who are in need of regular oxygen therapy are obvious candidates for transplantation. For others, this decision is more difficult. One of the most important features to be considered is the life-threatening condition of the patient. Syncope at rest, frequent haemoptysis and severe hypoxaemic angina are all important.

The rate of progress of disease in any particular patient is relevant. Deterioration from a chronic stable state towards inability to work, becoming house-bound, the occurrence of more frequent hospital admissions and the appearance of new clinical features over a short period of a few months or years may warrant acceptance.

For those patients in whom there has been some doubt as to the level and rate of change in disability, we have found a standardized 12-minute walk (McGavin, Gupta and McHardy, 1976) to be a good objective measurement which can be repeated to show changes over time. We regard a distance of

TABLE 22.3
Recipient Criteria and Potential Contraindications for Heart–Lung Transplantation

Recipient Criteria	*Potential Contraindications*
End-stage pulmonary vascular or parenchymal disease	Other non-reversible organ dysfunction or disease
Positive attitude and good family support	Major thoracotomy, e.g. pleurectomy or lung resection
Age <50 years	High-dose steroid therapy
	Insulin-dependent diabetes

less than 200 metres over a 12-minute period to be a good indicator of disability severe enough to warrant transplantation.

Of great importance is the patient's attitude towards the prospect of heart–lung transplantation. A passive ambivalence will be a relative contraindication for surgery, however acceptable the patient might otherwise be. If a patient has one of the diseases amenable to heart–lung transplantation but has become stable at a reasonable level of disability, or there is some doubt as to whether he has deteriorated significantly, then no definite decision is needed. Patients will be reviewed by their referring physicians as well as by the transplant centre and at the appropriate time accepted onto a definite waiting list.

Because of the increasing demand for heart–lung transplantation and the unpredictable supply of donor organs, there are inevitable delays between acceptance and surgery. This gives us time to consider and reflect on each case. It is always better to see patients early in the disease process, sometimes before heart–lung transplantation is necessary, and then to keep them under review. Such a referral pattern is far better than one in which moribound patients are referred for resurrection heart–lung transplantation.

At the inception of clinical heart–lung transplantation an arbitrary upper age limit for potential transplant recipients was set at 45 years. At Papworth Hospital we have raised the limit to 50 years. More centres are now performing heart–lung transplantation on younger children, a trend which will continue as more is learned about the long-term outcome of transplantation and methods of avoiding some of the potential long-term problems.

Patients are excluded as potential recipients if they have other systemic illness or conditions that are considered non-reversible and likely to inhibit mid- and long-term survival. However, conditions such as cystic fibrosis and alpha-1 antitrypsin deficiency are not now regarded as contraindications to surgery, nor are fibrosed lungs from sarcoidosis. Insulin-dependent diabetes has changed from being an absolute to a relative contraindication for heart transplantation, but again this decision may change with time. A tumour not absolutely confined to the lungs would remain a contraindication to surgery. Previous intrathoracic surgery was regarded as an absolute contraindication for heart–lung transplantation at its inception. The risk of major bleeding from the extensive dissection of adhesions during surgery was the main concern. Patients with a previous median sternotomy are, however, now accepted for heart–lung transplantation. A previous thoracotomy, for lung biopsy or for shunt procedures, is also acceptable, but a previous thoracotomy involving a pleurectomy or major lung resection remains a contraindication for surgery because of the increased risk of life-threatening perioperative haemorrhage.

Many patients, particularly those with chronic parenchymatous lung disorders, are on steroid therapy, which will inhibit wound healing, that of the

TABLE 22.4
Referral Pattern For Heart–Lung Transplantation (November 1982–December 1987), Papworth Hospital

Category	*Male*	*Female*	*Total*
Referrals	159	174	333
Assessments	51	78	129
To be assessed	24	15	39

trachea being of particular concern (Penketh *et al.*, 1987). All patients, therefore, except those on very low-dose steroids, have to be reviewed carefully. Many patients with non-active end-stage lung disease have been maintained on steroid therapy long after it has ceased to be effective. Often they can be weaned from steroids with little effect, thus making them acceptable candidates for heart–lung transplantation.

REFERRAL PATTERNS

The potential demand for heart–lung transplantation can be illustrated by the referral pattern at Papworth Hospital (Table 22.4). Between November 1982 and December 1987 a total of 333 patients were referred as potential heart–lung transplant recipients. At the beginning of the programme, many referrals were totally unacceptable; patients were often in the terminal stages of acute or chronic respiratory illness, being ventilated, in renal failure or infected. As the criteria for acceptance for heart–lung transplantation have become more widely known and the beneficial results seen, the patterns of referral have become more realistic.

The most striking contrast with heart transplantation referral is that approximately 50% of potential patients for heart–lung transplantation are female and they are younger, with a mean age of 30.

TABLE 22.5
Waiting Times For Heart–Lung Transplantation, Papworth Hospital

	Mean	*Range*
Assessment ($n = 86$)	6 months	1–18 months
Transplant ($n = 34$)	8 months	1 week–25 months

TABLE 22.6
Results of Assessments for Heart–Lung Transplantation (November 1982–December 1987), Papworth Hospital

Assessments	129
accepted	77
provisional	28
waiting	26
died waiting	17
transplanted	34

Excluding totally unsuitable patients and those above the age of 50 or with major contraindications, 129 patients have been admitted for assessment for transplantation. There is a growing list of patients waiting to be assessed: 39 patients at the end of 1987 (Table 22.4). At our institution we currently see 1 or 2 patients per week and there is a considerable delay between referral and assessment for surgery (Table 22.5).

Of those assessed (129), 77 have been definitely accepted as recipients (Table 22.6). A further 28 have been accepted provisionally, including those

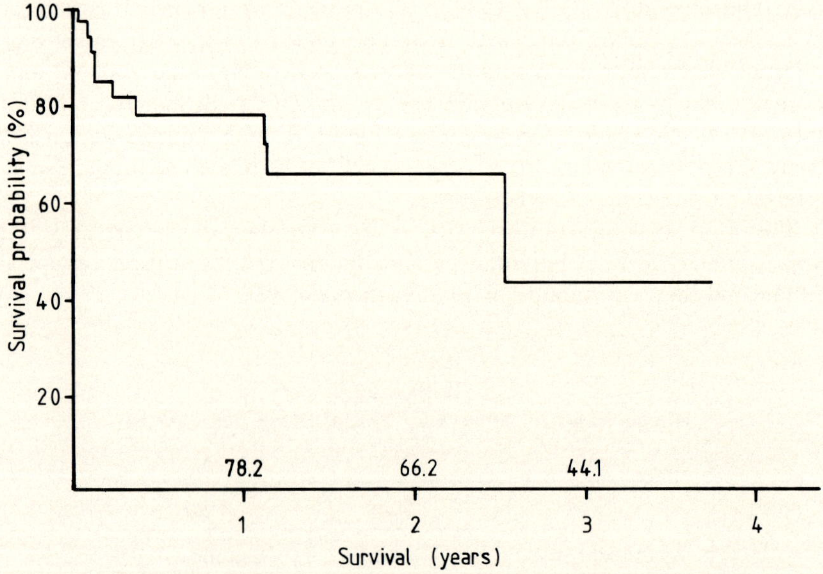

Fig. 22.2. *Heart–lung transplant patient survival at Papworth Hospital (December 1987).*

TABLE 22.7
Diagnoses of Patients Accepted For Heart–Lung Transplantation (November 1982–December 1987), Papworth Hospital

Accepted for transplant	77
Eisenmenger's syndrome	26
primary pulmonary hypertension	13
thrombo-embolic pulmonary hypertension	2
fibrosing alveolitis	7
cystic fibrosis	13
emphysema	5
sarcoidosis	3
histiocytosis X	1
α_1-antitrypsin deficiency	2
bronchiectasis	1
systemic lupus erythematosus + pulmonary hypertension	1
cardiomyopathy and pulmonary hypertension	1
pulmonary fibrosis	1
primary biliary cirrhosis + pulmonary hypertension	1

patients, discussed above, who were relatively well at the time of assessment but because of their diagnosis will eventually need heart–lung transplantation. The provisional list also includes a group described below, those with primary pulmonary hypertension, where alternative novel therapies have been instituted as a temporary measure to improve their quality of life prior to transplantation.

Twenty-two per cent of the patients accepted have died before they could be transplanted and at the end of 1987, 26 patients were on the waiting list for heart–lung transplantation. Since 1981 we have performed 34 heart–lung transplants and it is intended that our activity will rise to approximately 25 heart–lung transplants per year from 1988. This number is still obviously inadequate to meet the demand. However, with careful patient selection as part of an overall strategy of care for heart–lung transplant recipients, an actuarial survival at 1 year of 78% has been achieved (Fig. 22.1).

The diagnoses of those patients accepted for transplantation are shown in Table 22.7. The three largest groups are Eisenmenger's syndrome, primary pulmonary hypertension and cystic fibrosis.

ASSESSMENT PROCEDURE

We believe that it is important that the period of assessment be as comprehensive as possible. The 3–4-day admission allows time for the patients and their families to adjust to the concept of heart–lung transplantation and to gain as much knowledge as they can to enable them to take part in the decision-making process. They are seen by key members of the medical, nursing and support staff and have an opportunity to visit the various areas of the hospital with which they will come into contact following transplantation. They also have an opportunity to see patients who have received a heart or heart–lung transplant. A full and frank discussion of their medical condition occurs and the prospects and problems surrounding heart–lung transplantation are described.

Many of the patients have been fully and appropriately investigated prior to admission by the referring physician. A list of investigations routinely performed at the transplant centre is shown in Table 22.8. Although many of these will previously have been performed at the referral centre, they are repeated to provide baseline data. Some procedures, such as right heart catheterization, may only be needed on selected patients.

The majority of patients with Eisenmenger's syndrome will have had a cardiac catheterization to confirm the diagnosis and its underlying anatomical abnormalities at some stage. For many there is no need to repeat this. Echocardiography, in combination with previous investigation, is necessary to confirm the anatomy of the systemic venous drainage prior to acceptance for transplantation. Whatever the complexity of the intracardiac lesions, heart–lung transplantation is possible provided there is situs solitus with or without a left superior vena cava, and an aorta to which an anastomosis can be made. The remainder of any abnormal anatomy is irrelevant to heart–lung transplantation. Single atrium, for example, can be simply dealt with by over-sewing of the pulmonary veins following removal of the right lung, using this single chamber as a new right atrium.

For those patients who are not wheelchair-bound or bedridden and who can exercise, we have found a standard 12-minute walk (McGavin, Gupta and McHardy, 1976; Lipkin *et al.*, 1986) a useful way of assessing their exercise tolerance. This simple test, which measures the total distance a patient can walk on the flat over a period of 12 minutes, including as many rests as they require, can be repeated to show any changes if reassessment is needed. We regard less than 200 metres in 12 minutes as showing severe restriction. Aterial desaturation on exercise measured by a pulse oximeter is also a good prognostic indicator of severe problems, particularly in parenchymatous lung disease or primary pulmonary hypertension.

Virology screening is important for heart–lung transplant recipients, particularly to avoid cytomegalovirus (CMV) mismatches between the donor and the recipient. By avoiding transmission of CMV in the donor organs to CMV-negative recipients, severe and usually fatal primary CMV infection in a heart–lung transplant recipient can be eliminated (Gray *et al.*, 1987).

Open lung biopsy may be necessary to establish a final diagnosis in some patients, particularly those with parenchymatous lung diseases, to ensure that all avenues of conventional therapy have been explored.

TABLE 22.8
Investigations at Assessment For Heart–Lung Transplantation, Papworth Hospital

Routine
haematology
biochemistry
bacteriology
Coagulation screen
Blood gases
Preformed antibody screen
Tissue-typing (for retrospective analysis)
Virology titres
CMV
toxoplasma
EBV
HIV
Right heart cardiac catheter
Echocardiography
Pulmonary function tests
12-minute walk
Open lung biopsy

Right heart cardiac catheterization is performed in the main for patients with primary pulmonary hypertension who may go on to long-term prostacyclin infusion therapy. We have found that self-administered continuous 24-hour infusion of prostacyclin has considerably improved the quality of life of many of these patients, has avoided pre-terminal syncope and has 'bought time' for some patients who would otherwise die before receiving a transplant (Jones, Higenbottam and Wallwork, 1987b). For this therapy we have selected patients who have failed to improve on conventional vasodilator therapy and whose mixed venous oxygenation has been less than 63%. These patients have a 17% 3-year survival untreated (Fuster *et al.*, 1984). We have been able to improve their exercise tolerance and prevent dangerous syncopal episodes. Many of these patients been improved sufficiently to allow their transfer from the provisional waiting list. The progress of primary pulmonary hypertension is not reversed, however, and ultimately they either die or require heart–lung transplantation. Nevertheless this therapy has improved the 1-year survival from 37% to 68% (Scott *et al.*, 1988a). Long-term prostacyclin therapy is an expensive form of treatment and is reserved for those who have failed to improve on conventional vasodilator drugs. It provides only a temporary respite in the progressive deterioration towards death.

At the end of the assessment period, suitable patients are accepted onto the heart–lung waiting list. If further information is required, or they are regarded as being too well for definite acceptance, they are placed in a provisional group. The latter group is subsequently reviewed and patients are placed on the definite waiting list once they have deteriorated. A few patients are not accepted for transplantation; this number is kept to a minimum by screening patients for definite contraindications at referral. Once the patients have been assessed, they are discharged back to the care of their referring physician and the majority wait at home for a suitable donor to become available.

Inevitably deaths occur on the waiting list before transplantation. Twenty-two per cent of our patients have died on the waiting list for heart–lung transplantation. The waiting times on average between referral and assessment and acceptance and transplantation are shown in Table 22.5. They reflect the discrepancy between supply and demand of heart–lung transplantation in a unit which had the second or third highest heart–lung transplant activity worldwide in 1987.

WHO TO TRANSPLANT?

The waiting period between assessment and surgery can be a difficult time for the patients and their families. Some of the psychological factors involved are discussed in Chapter 19.

When a donor becomes available, the decision-making process for the selection of a particular patient from the list to be transplanted goes through an orderly sequence. In addition, the recipient has to be matched for blood group and size. If there is more than one suitable candidate having regard to these criteria, the patient considered to be the most seriously ill is chosen. If no such distinction is possible, the patient who has been waiting longest on the list is selected. Occasionally time and distance constraints affect the choice of recipient, but these are secondary considerations. No consideration is given to tissue-typing, as this is impractical currently for heart–lung transplantation. A direct cross-match is only performed if the patients demonstrate a significant (>10%) number of preformed antibodies against a random pool of lymphocyte donors from the assessment investigations.

CONCLUSIONS

Such is the current state. The ground is shifting, and the indications and acceptance of individual patients will change as heart–lung transplantation continues to develop. Demand will rise from both the medical profession and the public. As the results improve, more recipients will receive a heart–lung transplant in centres with established heart transplant programmes. Crucial to this expansion will be the appropriate dispersion of experience and access to all possible donor organs. Donor care and donor organ preservation will need to be enhanced to allow long-distance procurement to become the normal method of organ retrieval.

The successful development of heart–lung transplantation has already made possible a 1-year survival rate >75%, thus negating the argument that heart–lung transplantation wastes hearts that could be used for heart transplant recipients. The current developments of the so-called 'domino' operation will provide more organs to the heart donor pool and in particular offer some hearts for patients with marginally raised pulmonary vascular resistance, for whom a conventional donor would not be suitable. However, heart–lung transplantation will never be an open-ended service. With resources restricted either because of fiscal constraints or lack of donors, it will be important to maximize the benefits to the large potential recipient pool. Because of the waiting times already involved, it is probably inappropriate to consider emergency heart–lung transplantation for moribund patients without their being fully assessed, except under very exceptional circumstances. Doing so would lessen the chances for transplantation of those chronically disabled but fully assessed, by further limiting resources. Choices will still have to be made in selecting patients, and continuing audit, both in terms of survival and quality of life, still needs to be performed in order for us to make the best use of this developing service.

REFERENCES

Burke, C. M., Theodore, J., Baldwin, J. C., Tazelaar, H. D., Morris, A. J., McGregor, C., Shumway, N. E., Robin, E. D. and Jamieson, S. W. (1986). Twenty-eight cases of human heart–lung transplantation. *Lancet*, **i**, 517–519.

Cooper, J. D., Pearson, F. G., Patterson, G. A., Todd, T. R., Ginsberg, R. J., Goldberg, M. and DeMajo, W. A. P. (1987). Technique of successful lung transplantation in humans. *J. Thorac. Cardiovasc. Surg.* **93**, 173–181.

Copeland, J. G. (1987). Heart–lung transplantation: current status. *Ann. Thorac. Surg.* **43**, 2–3.

DHSS (1987). Conference of Medical Royal Colleges and their faculties in the U.K. Report of the Working Party on the Supply of Donor Organs for Transplantation. Department of Health and Social Security, London.

Fuster, V., Steele, P. M., Edwards, W. D., Gersh, B. J., McGoon, M. D. and Frye, R. L. (1984). Primary pulmonary hypertension: natural history and the importance of thrombosis. *Circulation* **70**, 580–587.

Gray, J. J., Alvey, B., Smith, D. J. and Wreghitt, T. G. (1987). Evaluation of a commercial latex agglutination test for detecting antibodies to cytomegalovirus in organ donors and transplant recipients. *J. Virol. Meth.* **16**, 13–19.

Higenbottam, T. W., Caine, N. and Wallwork, J. (1988). Heart–lung transplantation: the size of the problem estimated from mortality data in England and Wales. *Lancet* (submitted).

HMSO (1984). *OPCS Mortality Statistics: Causes.* Her Majesty's Stationery Office, London.

Hutter, J., Despins, P., Higenbottam, T. W., Stewart, S. and Wallwork, J. (1988a). Heart–lung transplantation: the Papworth experience. *Am. J. Med.* (in press).

Hutter, J. A., Higenbottam, T. W., Stewart, S. and Wallwork, J. (1988b). Routine endomyocardial biopsy is redundant in heart–lung recipients. *J. Heart Transplant.* (in press).

Jones, D. K., Higenbottam, T. W. and Wallwork, J. (1987a). Long-term survival after heart–lung transplantation in cystic fibrosis. *Chest* (in press).

Jones, D. K., Higenbottam, T. W. and Wallwork, J. (1987b). Long-term treatment of primary pulmonary hypertension with prostacyclin. *Br. Heart J.* **57**, 270–278.

Lipkin, D. P., Scriven, A. J., Crake, T. and Poole-Wilson, P. A. (1986). Six minute walking test for assessing exercise capacity in chronic heart failure. *Br. Med. J.* **292**, 653–655.

McGavin, C. R., Gupta, S. P. and McHardy, G. J. R. (1976). Twelve minute walking test for assessing disability in chronic bronchitis. *Br. Med. J.* **1**, 822–824.

McGregor, C. G. A., Baldwin, J. C., Jamieson, S. W., Billingham, M. E., Yousem, S. A., Burke, C. M., Oyer, P. E., Stinson, E. B. and Shumway, N. E. (1985). Isolated pulmonary rejection after combined heart–lung transplantation. *J. Thorac. Cardiovasc. Surg.* **90**, 623–626.

Oh, H. K. and Uniewski, M. H. (1986). Enhancing organ recovery by initiation of required request within a major medical centre. *Transplant. Proc.* **18**, 426.

Patterson, G. A., Cooper, J. D., Goldman, B., Weisel, R. D., Pearson, F. G., Waters, P. F., Todd, T. R., Scully, H., Goldberg, M. and Ginsberg, R. J. (1988) Technique of successful double lung transplantation. *Ann. Thorac. Surg.* (in press).

Penketh, A., Higenbottam, T. W., Hakim, M. and Wallwork, J. (1987). Heart and lung transplantation in patients with end-stage lung disease. *Br. Med. J.* **295**, 311–314.

Prop, J., Kuijpers, K., Pereson, A. H., Bartels, H. L., Nieuwenhuis, P. and Wildevuur, C. R. H. (1985). Why are lung allografts more vigorously rejected than hearts? *J. Heart Transplant.* **4**, 433–436.

Reitz, B. A., Gaudiani, V. A., Hunt, S. A., Wallwork, J., Billingham, M. E., Oyer, P. E., Baumgartner, W. A., Jamieson, S. W., Stinson, E. B. and Shumway, N. E. (1983). Diagnosis and treatment of allograft rejection in heart–lung transplant recipients. *J. Thorac. Cardiovasc. Surg.* **85**, 354–361.

Reitz, B. A., Wallwork, J., Hunt, S. A., Pennock, J. L., Billingham, M. E., Oyer, P. E., Stinson, E. B. and Shumway, N. E. (1982). Heart–lung transplantation: successful therapy for patients with pulmonary vascular disease. *New Engl. J. Med.* **306**, 557–564.

Scott, J., Higenbottam, T. W., Caine, N., Wallwork, J. and Jones, K. (1988a). The long-term use of prostacyclin in the management of primary pulmonary hypertension. *Chest* (submitted).

Scott, J., Higenbottam, T. W., Hutter, J., Hodson, M. and Wallwork, J. (1988b). Heart–lung transplantation for cystic fibrosis. *Br. Med. J.* (in press).

Scott, W. C., Hoverick, A. and Billingham, M. E. (1984). Lethal rejection of the lung without significant rejection in primate heart–lung allografts. *J. Heart Transplant.* **4**, 33–39.

J. A. Hutter, N. Cavarocchi
and John Wallwork

23

Donor Selection and Preservation of Donor Lungs

SELECTION OF DONORS

The criteria for selection of donors for heart–lung transplantation (HLTx) are necessarily more stringent than for isolated cardiac transplantation. It was estimated by Reitz (1982) that 25% of donors suitable for heart transplantation may be suitable for HLTx, although more recent estimates (Harjula *et al.*, 1987) suggest a figure of only 10–15%. Not only must the donor have a stable circulation, but the lungs must be normal in terms of compliance and gas exchange in the absence of trauma or infection. The lungs must also be of a comparable volume to those of the intended recipient. A significant mortality and morbidity has occurred from primary cytomegalovirus infection (CMV) (Dummer *et al.*, 1985; Burke *et al.*, 1986; Hutter *et al.*, 1988b); therefore, a CMV-negative recipient should only receive organs from a CMV-negative donor. As with other organ transplantation, donor and recipient are matched for ABO blood group and occasionally for lymphocyte compatibility. It is not practicable to perform prospective HLA matching. Table 23.1 lists the criteria for the selection of heart–lung donors, while Table 23.2 gives the criteria used at Papworth Hospital, Cambridge, for donor–recipient compatibility.

Age

The upper age limit for heart–lung donors was initially arbitrarily set at 35 years. This age limit has been maintained by some units, but the scarcity of suitable donors within this age limit has led other units to extend the

TABLE 23.1
Criteria For Heart–Lung Donors

Age <45 years
No major thoracic trauma
No past history of pulmonary disease, including asthma
A short period of ventilation
No systemic or pulmonary infections
Normal chest radiograph
Normal lung compliance with a peak inspiratory pressure below 20 mmHg, tidal volume of less than 15 ml/kg and respiratory rate of between 10 and 14 per min.
Normal gas exchange (Pa_{O_2} > 15 with FI_{O_2} of 30%).
Inotropic requirement of less than 10 μg/kg per min of dopamine or dobutamine
Normal ECG

maximum acceptable age to 45 years (Hutter *et al.*, 1988a). Inspection of the organs in older donors has not revealed more unrecognized cardiac or pulmonary pathology. Although more extensive investigation of potential donors with echocardiography, coronary angiography or computed tomography scanning could exclude such disease, these investigations are expensive and if routinely requested may deter centres from participating in organ donation.

Past medical history

Donors with a history of cardiac or pulmonary disease are excluded, but a previous spontaneous pneumothorax or mild hypertension may be acceptable. A history of asthma is a definite contraindication, but light cigarette smoking in the donor would not lead to exclusion.

TABLE 23.2
Criteria For Donor–Recipient Compatibility, Papworth Hospital

Size	Comparable measurements taken from chest radiograph
Blood group	ABO group compatible
Cytomegalovirus (CMV)	Antibody-negative recipient should receive organs only from antibody-negative donor

Cause of death

Initially it was considered likely that donors for HLTx would be cases of fatal spontaneous intracranial haemorrhage or primary brain tumours (Hakim *et al.*, 1988). However, in our experience trauma resulting in brain death but without significant pulmonary injury occurred in 16 of 31 donors. Fourteen donors resulted from a spontaneous subarachnoid haemorrhage and in only a single case was death due to a primary brain tumour (Hutter *et al.*, 1988a). In the Stanford experience (Harjula *et al.*, 1987), 68% of donors resulted from road traffic accidents, 15% from intracranial haemorrhage, and 17% from gunshot wounds to the head. In a consecutive series of 44 paediatric donors (aged 2–16 years) referred to Addenbrooke's Hospital, Cambridge, for liver transplantation, the heart and lungs were also transplanted in 15. Thirteen of these donors died following a head injury; epiglottitis and spontaneous intracranial haemorrhage each led to a single case.

Duration of ventilation

A short period of ventilation of the heart–lung donor is desirable, as areas of atelectasis and subsequent infection become increasingly likely with prolonged periods of ventilation (Ruiz, 1987), although physiotherapy and regular endotracheal suction may minimize this occurrence. The period of ventilation has varied in reported series, with an average period of 58 h (range 15–140 h) in the Stanford experience (Harjula *et al.*, 1987) and between 10 h and 95 h, mean 34 h, in the Papworth experience (Hutter *et al.*, 1988a).

Neurogenic pulmonary oedema

Brain stem death is commonly associated with pulmonary oedema, although the pathogenesis is unclear. Novitzky *et al.* (1987) have demonstrated in the Chacma baboon that brain death, induced by acute intracerebral hypertension, results in a marked increase in circulating catecholamines and a rise in the systemic vascular resistance (SVR). The rise in SVR may be as great as 537% to a peak value of 800 Wood units (Novitzky *et al.*, 1987). This resulted in acute left ventricular failure, leading to pulmonary oedema in 4 of 11 animals. The agonal period during which the left atrial pressure rose above the pulmonary artery pressure was only of short duration, but disruption of capillaries during this period may result in high protein content pulmonary oedema. A period of severely elevated systemic vascular resistance and an elevated LVEDP may also result in subendocardial infarction of the heart (Griepp *et al.*, 1971; McLeod *et al.*, 1982). The vascular changes may be transient and although a history of a pulmonary oedema does not necessarily preclude use of the organs for HLTx, extreme caution is advised in selecting donors with this history. In our experience, 2 of 31 donors had a history of neurogenic pulmonary oedema and although all parameters of lung function were normal when the organs were removed, the immediate post-implant period suggested that some damage had occurred. The eventual outcome, however, was good in both cases.

DONOR MANAGEMENT

Prior to confirmation of brain stem death, the clinical management of the donor will have been directed towards minimizing cerebral oedema. In many cases a diuresis will have been induced with mannitol and diuretics. Inotropes may have been required to maintain a satisfactory circulation in the presence of hypovolaemia. Diabetes insipidus is common following brain stem death and may contribute to fluid depletion. When tests have established the absence of brain stem function the clinical management should be directed towards maintaining the organs for transplantation in optimal condition.

It is well established in cardiac transplant recipients that initial cardiac function is related to the requirement for inotropes in the donor prior to removal of the organs. Restoration of the circulatory volume with fluid will usually decrease the requirement for inotropes, but great care is required in the heart–lung donor to ensure that excessive administration of fluid does not result in oedematous lungs. It is therefore essential that the central venous pressure is accurately monitored by insertion of a central venous cannula. For HLTx this cannula should be inserted in the right internal jugular vein or right subclavian vein, as the innominate vein is divided early during the procurement procedure. Infusions of large volumes of crystalloid solutions are more likely to result in oedematous lungs; blood, plasma, or a plasma substitute such as Haemaccel are recommended. In some instances a volume of 4–5 litres has been required to optimize the haemodynamic state and has allowed a reduction in the inotrope requirement without producing oedematous lungs. Ventilation with a positive end expiratory pressure (PEEP) will minimize areas of atelectasis and also reduce the tendency to pulmonary oedema. If the urine volume exceeds 3 ml/kg body weight per hour, DDAVP (Pitressin) should be given (10 units over 4 h).

Recent studies (Novitzky, Cooper and Reichart, 1987) have shown that a variety of other hormonal and metabolic abnormalities occur following brain death. In one study, a metabolic acidosis due to high lactic acid levels, and low blood glucose and thyroxine (T3) levels were seen in potential organ donors. Initial attempts to correct these low T3 levels have not been effective. It is suggested that these abnormalities may explain why some cardiac donors show cellular damage, measured by birefringence (Darracott-Carnkovic *et al.*, 1987), in cardiac biopsies and why further deterioration occurs during the preservation period.

CRITERIA FOR ORGAN FUNCTION

The following criteria have been suggested by the Papworth group (Hakim *et al.*, 1988) for assessment of satisfactory organ function, but as each potential donor is considered individually the criteria should act only as guidelines.

Chest radiograph

The chest radiograph should not show any abnormality suggestive of infection, contusion, pulmonary oedema or atelectasis. Complete radiographic resolution of neurogenic pulmonary oedema is essential.

Pulmonary function

Lung compliance assessed by the peak inspiratory pressure should be below 20 mmHg, with a tidal volume of 15 ml/kg and a respiratory rate of between 10 and 14 breaths/min. An inspired oxygen concentration of 30% should produce a minimum arterial oxygen concentration (Pa_{O_2}) of 15 kPa.

Cardiac function

The haemodynamic state of the donor must be stable, and the inotropic requirements of dopamine or dobutamine below 10 mg/kg per min. The electrocardiogram should be normal.

Bacteriology

A Gram stain of the tracheal aspirate should not demonstrate any pathogenic organisms, but normal commensal organisms are acceptable.

The importance of the bacteriology in the donor has recently been emphasized by the Stanford group (Harjula *et al.*, 1987). In a series of 40 heart–lung donors Gram stains of the donor tracheal aspirate revealed Gram-positive bacteria in 80% and Gram-negative bacteria in 35%. Yeasts were seen on smear in 25%. When the Gram stains demonstrated a heavy concentration of bacteria, the hospital mortality of the recipients was 83%. A heavy concentration of polymorphonuclear lymphocytes on Gram stains was associated with a hospital mortality of 50% (3 of 6). The hospital mortality associated with fungus on Gram stains was 40% (4 of 10). The overall hospital mortality for this group was 27.5% (11 of 40), demonstrating that these findings were a major risk factor for the recipient.

In the Papworth experience (Hutter *et al.*, 1988a), the Gram stain of the donor trachea was negative for pathogenic bacteria and fungi in 34 of 35 cases. The recipient of organs with pathogenic bacteria was the only patient to die in the early postoperative period with a bacterial infection.

DONOR–RECIPIENT COMPATIBILITY

Having established that a donor is suitable for HLTx, a recipient must be selected by matching for size, blood group and cytomegalovirus (CMV) antibody status.

Size matching

Transplantation of lungs with a greater volume than the volume of the recipient's chest cavity will result in areas of atelectasis (Burke *et al.*, 1986) and subsequent infection. Significant cardiac tamponade may also occur when the sternum is closed. Conversely, if the transplanted lungs are too small to fill the recipient's chest cavity, hyperinflation of the lungs may be encouraged by applying a negative pressure to the intercostal drainage tube. As the lungs become hyperinflated, air leaks are common and require prolonged intercostal suction. If the pneumonthorax is allowed to remain, pleural effusions develop and may result in an empyema. However, if the recipient's chest is hyperinflated as a result of cystic fibrosis, emphysema or other chronic lung diseases, then the chest volume may be expected to decrease after transplantation. Under these circumstances, transplantation with slightly smaller lungs may be appropriate.

Two techniques are currently used to obtain a suitable size match. The external measurements of the donor's chest may be compared with similar measurements of the recipient, but we have preferred to compare measurements made from chest radiographs taken at a standard focal length (Hakim *et al.*, 1988). The distance between the first and both the tenth and twelfth thoracic vertebrae and the transverse diameter of the chest at the junction of the second and third ribs and the lower border of the tenth rib are compared (Fig. 23.1). We believe that these measurements more accurately reflect the intrathoracic volume of the donor and recipient and are not influenced by muscle and fatty tissue external to the rib cage.

Ideally the donor should be about 10% smaller than the recipient (Hutter *et al.*, 1988a). Whenever possible the donor's chest radiograph is brought to Papworth Hospital and directly compared to chest radiographs of various

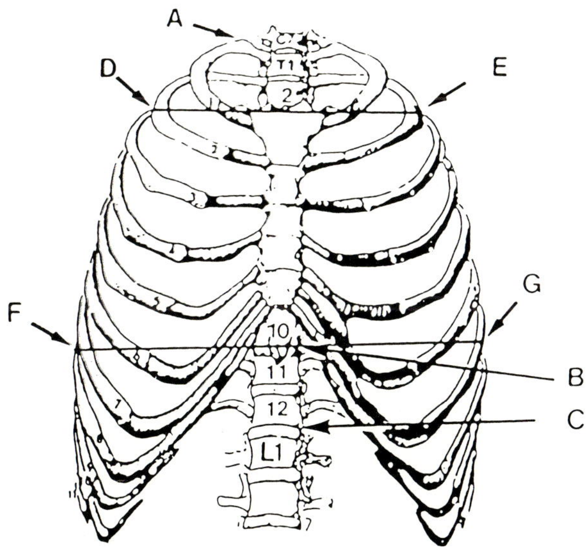

Fig. 23.1. *Four dimensions used for radiological assessment of chest size: A–B, neck of 1st rib to lower border of 10th thoracic vertebra; A–C, neck of 1st rib to lower border of 12th thoracic vertebra; D–E transverse diameter at level 2nd and 3rd ribs cross; F–G, transverse diameter at lower border of 10th thoracic vertebra.*

potential recipients; the best match is then chosen. If a direct comparison of radiographs is not possible before selecting a recipient, the chest radiograph of the recipient chosen on the basis of the measurements is taken to the donor hospital for a final assessment of size compatibility.

Serological matching

Donor and recipient should be matched for ABO blood group. A lymphocytotoxic crossmatch to exclude the presence of preformed antibodies to the donor's lymphocytes is required if the percentage of reactive antibodies to a panel of lymphocytes is greater than 15%.

The importance of organ-transmitted disease including cytomegalovirus (Hakim *et al.*, 1985; Dummer *et al.*, 1985; Burke *et al.*, 1986; Hutter *et al.*, 1988b) has been previously reported in cardiac and heart–lung recipients. We have demonstrated that significant mortality and morbidity results from transplantation of heart and lungs from a CMV-positive donor to a CMV-negative recipient (Hutter *et al.*, 1988b). In our experience, 8 of 18 patients (aged 26 $\pm$ 10 years) who were CMV antibody negative prior to transplantation received organs from CMV antibody positive donors. All but one developed primary CMV, with a fatal pneumonitis in 3 cases. Three recipients recovered after severe CMV disease. When CMV antibody negative recipients received organs from CMV antibody negative donors only mild symptoms of CMV occurred in 3 patients. As a rapid latex agglutination test (Gray *et al.*, 1987; Hakim *et al.*, 1988) to assess CMV status is now available, we recommend that CMV-negative recipients receive organs only from CMV-negative donors.

Because the length of time required to carry out HLA-Dr tests is greater than the acceptable ischaemic period for the donor lungs, tissue-typing is not performed prospectively. Retrospective analysis of HLA-DR matching may be shown to be a factor in determining the outcome of HLTx (Harjula *et al.*, 1987), but the numbers of patients for analysis are too small to allow definite conclusions.

PRESERVATION TECHNIQUES FOR HEART–LUNG TRANSPLANTATION

These stringent criteria make suitable donors scarce. Initially, donors for HLTx were transported to the transplant centre so that donor and recipient procedures could be performed in adjoining theatres, minimizing the ischaemic period for the organs. This procedure is logistically complex and is excessively distressing for the bereaved relatives. Fortunately, organ-preservation techniques are now available to allow ischaemic periods of sufficient duration for distant procurement. Two approaches to organ preservation have been developed and used clinically. The organs may be transported in a warm, ventilated, autoperfused heart–lung preparation (Hardesty and Griffith, 1987); alternatively hypothermia may be induced by extracorporeal circulation (Khaghani, 1986) or by a cold perfusion technique (McLeod *et al.*, 1982; Jones *et al.*, 1985; Hakim *et al.*, 1988).

Autoperfusion technique

In 1969, Robicsek and colleagues developed an experimental model and demonstrated that it was possible to keep the heart 'alive' and functioning outside the body for prolonged periods (Robicsek *et al.*, 1968, 1985). A similar system was first used clinically in 1984 (Ladowski *et al.*, 1985). Both coronary and pulmonary arterial blood flow are maintained to preserve the heart and lungs in a modified Starling preparation. The heart pumps fresh heparinized, normothermic whole blood into a reservoir suspended at 100 cm to maintain a pressure of 75 mmHg within a closed segment of aorta, which in turn perfuses the coronary arteries. Venous return to the right atrium from the reservoir and through the coronary sinus determines right ventricular preload, and therefore pulmonary arterial flow. The preparation is enclosed in a sterile bag, allowing hand ventilation of the lungs. Hypothermia must be avoided at all stages; during procurement all infusions are warmed and when liver procurement is required only a preliminary dissection of the porta hepatis is allowed prior to removal of the heart–lung block. During transport the requirement for heaters necessitates that the ambulance and aircraft are equipped with a suitable power source.

Recently, the results for 30 procurements using this technique were reported from Pittsburgh (Hardesty and Griffith, 1987). Technical failures occurred in 6 procurements, 4 from hypothermia and ventricular fibrillation, 1 from haemorrhage and 1 from distension of the left ventricle. These failures may be attributed to the complexity of the technique, which limits its clinical application. Adequate preservation of the heart and lungs was achieved in 14 of 20 recipients (Hardesty and Griffith, 1987). Early pulmonary function was determined by calculation of the alveolar–arterial (A–a) oxygen gradient. This gradient was initially elevated but rapidly returned to a normal value (130 ± 11 torr) during the week after transplantation. In one case the donor lung was considered to have been poorly preserved, as evidenced by an A–a oxygen gradient greater than in those whose preservation was good. This patient died of pulmonary insufficiency and hypoxia after 72 h. In this case, however, the A–a gradient during transport had also been high. In one case the donor cardiac preservation was poor and the recipient died of cardiac failure 24 h postoperatively.

The technique is also complicated by the need to cooperate with other transplant surgeons to permit multi-organ harvesting. Most of the supradiaphragmatic vena cava is required for the autoperfusing heart–lung; this may not be acceptable to many liver transplant surgeons.

Although this technique has achieved clinical success, its complexity and the requirement for constant attention with the possibility of unsuspected failure limits its clinical application.

Experimental work in dogs (Miyamoto *et al.*, 1987) has also suggested that with this technique prolongation of the preservation period will be difficult to achieve. These workers found that the Pa_{O_2} during 100% oxygen ventilation decreased significantly after 6 h. Pulmonary vascular resistance increased transiently after harvest; thereafter it normalized and remained constant for several hours, but again increased markedly after 8 h. Pulmonary compliance also decreased after 7 hours. They concluded that the autoperfused heart–lung preparation showed good viability up to 5 h, but then deterioration was multifactorial including complement activation, trapping of leucocytes and platelet aggregation. It is suggested that to prolong the viability of the autoperfused heart–lung preparation, inhibition of complement activation (Wonders *et al.*, 1983), removal of leucocytes (Breda *et al.*, 1985) or prevention of platelet aggregation (Utsunomia *et al.*, 1980) by administration of prostaglandins should be considered.

Core-cooling by extracorporeal circulation

This approach to graft preservation was introduced by Hardesty and Griffith in 1985 and used with clinical success when the organs were implanted immediately (Hardesty and Griffith, 1987). Yacoub has successfully developed the technique to allow distant procurement (Khaghani, 1986).

Cardiopulmonary bypass is instituted with venous drainage from the right atrium and return to the aorta. Cooling is continued to a core temperature of 10°C. Depending on the size of the donor, this takes between 15 and 45 min (Khaghani, 1986). When ventricular fibrillation occurs a vent is inserted into the left ventricle to avoid distension. The organs are then removed and immersed in cold blood for transport.

Changes in alveolar capillary endothelial permeability, resulting in a significantly increased amount of serum protein within the alveolar space, have been shown to occur (Wells, 1985) in animals subjected to cardiopulmonary bypass. In some animals there was also an increase in alveolar epithelial permeability, measured by the clearance rate of ^{99m}Tc–DTPA, and a significant correlation with other parameters of pulmonary change such as erythrocyte and leucocyte infiltration and septal and peribronchovascular oedema. These changes may not only explain the haphazard frequency of non-cardiogenic, high-protein pulmonary oedema following cardiopulmonary bypass, but also predispose to poor organ function following HLTx.

Hypothermia by pulmonary artery flush

This simple technique is comparable to the well-established techniques for preservation of the liver (Calne, 1981), kidneys (Collins, Bravo-Shugarman and Terasaki, 1969), and heart (Watson *et al.*, 1979) for transplantation.

After mobilization of the major vessels and trachea, the aorta is clamped and cardioplegia solution at 4°C infused into the aortic root. When cardiac arrest occurs a hypothermic pulmonary preservation fluid is perfused into the pulmonary artery. Prior to removal of the organs, the lungs are inflated and the trachea clamped. The organs are placed in a cold storage box for transport.

The importance of hypothermia in preservation of the heart and lungs was described by Joseph and Morton (1971). Improved preservation of primate lungs was found after storage at 10°C, compared with normothermic storage.

Veith *et al.* (1971) have investigated the importance of maintaining the lungs inflated during preservation. In studies on dogs, Veith found that a deflated lung preserved for more than 1 h at normothermia could not support life. However, lungs inflated and kept at 38°C remained functional after 2 h or 3 h of ischaemia (6 of 10 survivors), but not after 4 h (0 of 4 survivors). In baboons, slightly better survival was achieved after auto-lung transplantation of ventilated, rather than inflated, lungs kept ischaemic and normothermic for 4–6 h (Joseph and Morton, 1971). As a result of these studies in clinical practice, both inflation of the lungs and hypothermia are considered to be essential for successful preservation. At Papworth Hospital the pulmonary preservation fluid is passed through a simple heat exchanger and infused into the pulmonary artery at 4°C. The fluid should not be infused at a pressure of more than 60 cmH_2O, as changes in the delicate structure of the alveolar capillaries may occur.

Composition of the pulmonary preservation fluid

The composition of fluids used for pulmonary preservation was comprehensively reviewed by Haverich, Scott and Jamieson (1985). The fluids may be characterized as the intracellular type, the extracellular type or the blood type. No solution has found universal acceptance and a variety of solutions of all types has been used clinically with varying success.

Experimental background

Experimentally, both non-colloid (Veith *et al.*, 1976) and colloid (Castagne, Shors and Benfield, 1972) extracellular solutions have been shown to be harmful for lung preservation. Similar results were obtained for preservation with serum or plasma fractions of blood (Garzon *et al.*, 1968). Successful preservation has been achieved experimentally with intracellular type (low sodium, high potassium concentration) fluids, with the addition of phosphate buffers as developed for kidney (Collins, Bravo-Shugarman and Terasaki, 1969; Sachs, Petritsch and Kaufman, 1973) transplantation. Using one such fluid, the Collins solution with added glucose, Grosjean *et al.* (1972) reported the first consistent survival after unilateral lung transplantation in dogs, following 24 h storage. However, dogs with functional contralateral lungs were the only long-term survivors. Using the Sachs solution (Sachs, Petritsch and Kaufman, 1973), which has approximately the same intracellular ionic composition as the Collins solution but contains mannitol instead of dextrose and has a higher osmolarity (430 mosmol/litre), bilateral lung transplantation experiments resulted in good function after 3 h of normothermic ischaemia and after 5 h of ischaemia at 4°C (Kondo, Turner and Cockrell, 1974).

Modry *et al.* (1983) reported the use of cold blood, an 'interstitial' solution (tissue culture medium) and a Collins-type solution in 24 h preservation, followed by unilateral lung transplantation. The 'interstitial' solution did not preserve the lung any better than the Collins solution, neither one protecting the lung sufficiently to ensure survival of the animal.

In this study, cold blood preservation resulted in far better lung function after transplantation, as assessed by serial arterial Po_2 measurements.

Clinical experience

In the clinical setting, ischaemic periods of 3–4 h will allow distant procurement of organs, although future developments may achieve adequate preservation after 24 h.

At Papworth Hospital, distant procurement was introduced in 1985 (Jones *et al.*, 1985) using an extracellular-type fluid. The composition of the fluid (Table 23.3) was derived from considerations of a variety of evidence relating to pulmonary preservation and also as a result of the clinical experience gained in the treatment of primary pulmonary hypertension with prostacyclin (Jones, Higenbottam and Wallwork, 1987). The often extremely heterogeneous histological findings within preserved lungs (Garzon *et al.*, 1968), with areas of severe reperfusion injury next to normal lung, suggested uneven distribution of the pulmonary preservation fluid. It was anticipated that prostacyclin, which is known to be a potent pulmonary vasodilator, would ensure more even pulmonary preservation. Prostacyclin may also

TABLE 23.3
Constituents of the Papworth Pulmonary Preservation Solution

Constituent	*Quantity* (ml)
Ringer's solution	700
20% Albumin	200
20% Mannitol	100
Citrate–phosphate–dextrose	63
Donor blood	400
Heparin (1000 iu/ml)	10
Total	1473

prevent leucocyte sequestration (Moncada, 1982), platelet aggregation (Moncada *et al.*, 1977) and damage to the pulmonary vascular endothelium by complement activation (Moncada, 1982). A cytoprotective property for prostacyclin (Mundy *et al.*, 1980) has also been reported, and infusion of prostacyclin has protected transplanted kidneys from hyperimmune rejection in dogs (Mundy *et al.*, 1980). The high osmolarity of the flushing solution, due to the addition of mannitol and albumin, may reduce the degree of

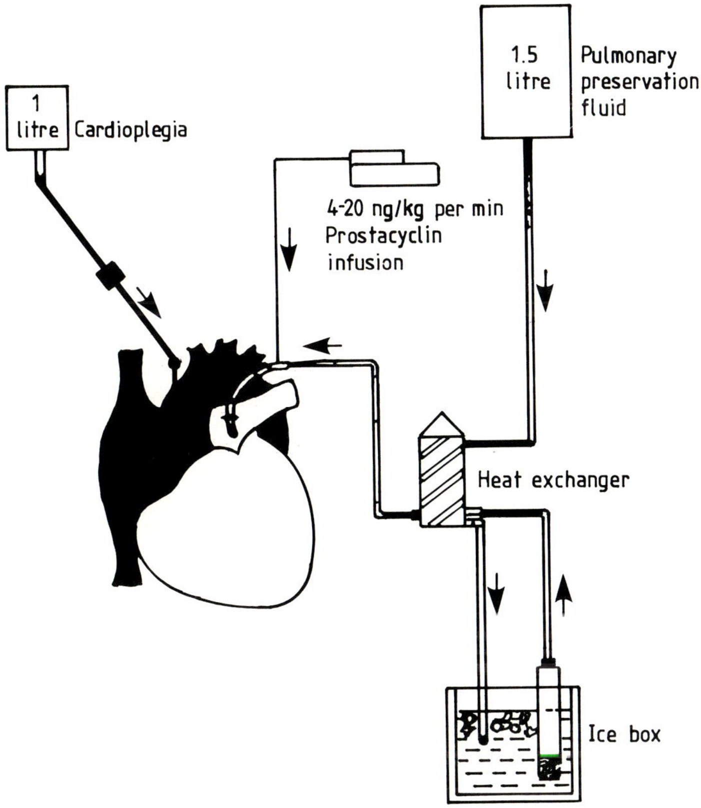

Fig. 23.2. *Circuit used for infusion of prostacyclin and preservation solution for organ preservation.*

pulmonary oedema. Mannitol can also act as a free oxygen radical scavenger (Magovern *et al.*, 1984) and may inhibit complement activation. The addition of blood increases the buffering capacity and may help to maintain a certain degree of cellular metabolism due to the oxygen content.

We consider that the infusion of prostacyclin prior to the preservation fluid is an essential part of the preservation technique (Fig. 23.2). When the great vessels and trachea have been mobilized, a cannula is inserted into the pulmonary artery and a prostacyclin infusion is started at 4 ng/kg per min. The rate of infusion is increased to 20 ng/kg per min, provided there is no significant systemic hypotension or tachycardia. The aorta is then clamped and cardioplegic solution infused into the ascending aorta. When cardiac activity ceases, the pulmonary preservation fluid is infused through the same cannula as the prostacyclin, which results in a bolus of prostacyclin preceding the preservation fluid. The organs are then removed and stored.

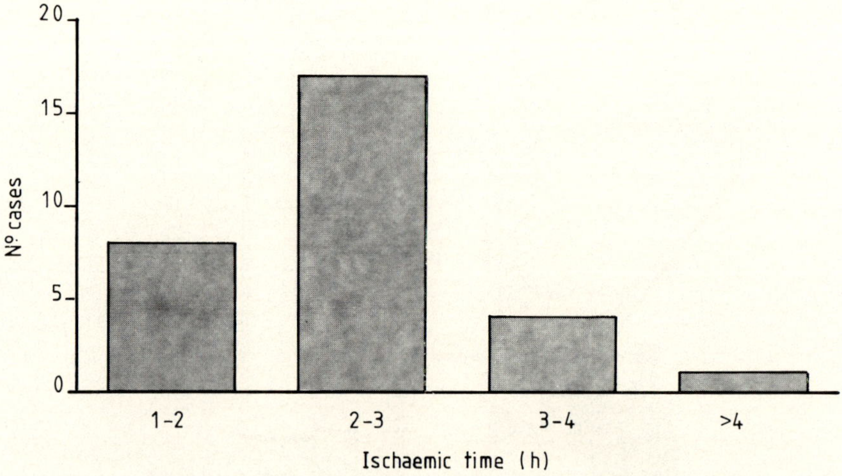

Fig. 23.3. *Heart–lung transplantation: ischaemic time distribution* ($n = 30$).

This technique has been used successfully for HLTx in 30 patients at this institute (Hakim *et al.*, 1988; Hutter *et al.*, 1988a). Ischaemic periods (Fig. 23.3) have varied between 70 min and 249 min, with a mean period of 150 ± 41 min (mean ± s.d.). In this group of patients immediate lung function has been good in all cases, so that cardiopulmonary bypass was readily discontinued on 50% or less inspired oxygen concentration. Twenty-four patients were extubated within 48 h and 21 were able to maintain a normal arterial Po_2 without an oxygen mask by the end of the first postoperative week. Although the A–a oxygen difference was high immediately after implantation, it had returned to normal by the end of the first postoperative week in all but one case.

Experimental comparison of preservation techniques

Various attempts have been made to compare the techniques available for lung preservation using a variety of animal models. Wahlers *et al.* (1986) compared preservation by the single flush technique using modified Euro-Collins solution with core-cooling by extracorporeal circulation in mongrel dogs after heterotopic heart and left lung transplantation, leaving the right lung of the recipient in place. The organs were transplanted after 6 h ischaemia at 4°C. Pulmonary vascular resistance was lower in the group preserved by extracorporeal circulation, possibly reflecting superior lung preservation. Impaired oxygenation was, however, seen in all cases, suggesting inadequacies in both techniques. The authors comment that impaired oxygenation under these circumstances is related to oedema and thickening of the alveolar capillary membrane.

A different animal model and different criteria for assessing preservation were used by Adachi *et al.* (1987) to compare preservation by core-cooling with preservation by the autoperfusing heart–lung preparation. Eighteen dairy cows received HLTx after 4 h preservation. Pulmonary function was assessed 6 h after implantation, by measuring the arterial oxygen concentration when the animal was ventilated with 100% oxygen. The animal was then killed and the lungs assessed by measurement of extravascular lung water and according to a histological lung injury score. No significant differences were seen between the groups. The authors conclude that either method provides adequate preservation, but comment that hypothermic preservation is simpler and more stable than autoperfusion.

Further studies are undoubtedly required to compare the various preservation techniques and investigate the mechanisms leading to cell damage. The beneficial constituents of pulmonary preservation fluid must be identified and their mode of action determined.

The ideal animal model, however, for these studies is not available. Long-term survival in animals following HLTx is very difficult to achieve and studies have only investigated the immediate results achieved with various preservation techniques. Long-term survival has been achieved in animals after single lung transplantation, but in these models the bronchial collateral circulation is interrupted so that relevance to the clinical situation is difficult to assess.

CONCLUSIONS

Successful HLTx is undoubtedly dependent upon selection of good donor organs. The scarcity of donors must not be allowed to precipitate acceptance of unsuitable donors. Careful matching of the recipient and donor with respect to size and serology is required. Good preservation of the heart and lungs is essential, clinical experience suggesting that this may be achieved by either a core-cooling technique using cardiopulmonary bypass or by a pulmonary artery flush technique. The composition of the preservation fluid is critical and must be emphasized when comparisons between techniques are made. Prostacyclin appears to be essential for the success of the flush technique, although the mechanism of its action is not yet known. Although the autoperfusion technique has also provided good organ preservation in clinical practice, it is too complex to gain wide acceptance.

A fuller understanding of pulmonary preservation is required before further advances can be made, but unfortunately the ideal animal model is not available as long-term survival has rarely been achieved. However, the results of HLTx are encouraging and we hope that the increasing awareness of the potential of transplantation will allow an increased number of patients to benefit.

REFERENCES

Adachi, H., Fraser, C. D., Kontas, G. J., Borton, A. M., Hutchins, G. M., Galloway, E., Brawn, J., Reitz, B. A. and Baumgartner, W. A. (1987) Autoperfused working: heart–lung preparation versus hypothermic cardiopulmonary preservation for transplantation. *J. Heart. Transplant.* **6**, 253–260.

Breda, M. A., Hall, H. S., Stuart, R. S. *et al.* (1985). Twenty-four hour lung preservation by hypothermia and leukocyte depletion. *J. Heart Transplant.* **4**, 325–329.

Burke, C. M., Glanville, A. R., Macoviek, J. A., O'Connel, B. M., Tazalaar, H. D., Baldwin, J. C., Jamieson, S. W. and Theodor, J. (1986). The spectrum of cytomegalovirus infection following human heart–lung transplantation. *J. Heart Transplant.* **5**, 267–272.

Calne, R. Y. (1981). In: *Liver Preservation of Organs for Transplantation* (A. M. Karrow and D. E. Pegg, Eds) Marcel Dekker, New York, pp. 617–624.

Castagne, J. T., Shors, E. and Benfield, J. R. (1972). The role of perfusion in lung preservation. *J. Thorac. Cardiovasc. Surg.* **63**, 521–526.

Collins, G. M., Bravo-Shugarman, M. B. and Terasaki, P. I. (1969). Kidney preservation for transplantation: 3. Initial perfusion and 30-hour ice storage. *Lancet* **2**, 1219–1222.

Darracott-Carnkovic, S., Wheeldon, D., Cory-Pearce, R., Wallwork, J. and English, T. A. H. (1987). Biopsy assessment of 50 hearts during transplantation. *J. Thorac. Cardiovasc. Surg.* **93**, 95–102.

Dummer, J. S., White, L. T., Monto, H. O., Griffiths, B. P., Hardesty, R. L., and Bahnson, H. T. (1985). Morbidity of cytomegalovirus infection in recipients of heart or heart–lung transplants who received cyclosporine. *J. Inf. Dis.* **152**, 1182–1191.

Garzon, A. A., Cheng, C., Pangan, J. and Karlson, K. E. (1968). Hypothermic hyperbaric lung preservation for twenty-four hours with reimplantation. *J. Thorac. Cardiovasc. Surg.* **55**, 546–554.

Gray, J. J., Alvey, B., Smith, D. J. and Wreghitt, T. G. (1987). Evaluation of a commercial latex agglutination test for detecting antibodies to cytomegalovirus in organ donors and transplant recipients. *J. Virol. Meth.* **16**, 13–19.

Griepp, R. B., Stinson, E. B., Clark, D. A., Dong, E. and Shumway, N. E. (1971). The cardiac donor. *Surg., Gynecol. Obstet.* **133**, 792–798.

Grosjean, O., Noirclerc, M., Duvinage, J. F., Sudan, N., Tedeschi, J., Coutant, P. and Lejeune, G. (1972). Pulmonary transplantation with immediate return of function after twenty-four hours of preservation. *Acta Chir. Belg.* **71**, 321–333.

Hakim, M., Higenbottam, T., Bethune, D., Cory-Pearce, R., English, T. A. H., Kneeshaw, J. D., Wells, F. C. and Wallwork, J. (1988). Selection and procurement of combined heart and lung grafts for transplantation. *J. Thorac. Cardiovasc. Surg.* (in press).

Hakim, M., Wreghitt, T. G., English, T. A. H., Stovin, P. G. I., Cory-Pearce, R. and Wallwork, J. (1985). Significance of donor-transmitted disease in cardiac transplantation. *Heart Transplant.* **4**, 302–306.

Hardesty, R. L. and Griffith, B. P. (1987). Autoperfusion of the heart and lungs for preservation during distant procurement. *J. Thorac. Cardiovasc. Surg.* **93**, 11–18.

Harjula, A., Baldwin, J. C., Starnes, V. A., Stinson, E. B., Oyer, P. E., Jamieson, S. W. and Shumway, N. E. (1987). Proper donor selection for heart–lung transplantation: the Stanford experience. *J. Thorac. Cardiovasc. Surg.* **94**, 874–880.

Haverich, A., Scott, W. C. and Jamieson, S. W. (1985). Twenty years of lung preservation — a review. *Heart Transplant.* **4**, 234–240.

Hutter, J. A., Higenbottam, T., Stewart, S. and Wallwork, J. (1988a). Heart–lung transplantation: the Papworth experience. *Am. J. Med.* (in press).

Hutter J. A., Wreghitt, T., Scott, J. P., Higenbottam, T. and Wallwork, J. (1988b). The importance of cytomegalovirus in heart–lung transplantation. *Chest* (in preparation).

Jones, K. D., Cavarocchi, N., Hakim, M. and Wallwork, J. (1985). A single flush technique for successful distant organ procurement in heart–lung transplantation. *J. Heart Transplant.* **4**, 614.

Jones, P. K., Higenbottam, T. and Wallwork, J. (1987). Treatment of primary pulmonary hypertension with intravenous epoprostenol (prostacycline). *Br. Heart J.* **57**, 270–279.

Joseph, W. L. and Morton, D. L. (1971). Influence of ischaemia and hypothermia on the ability of the transplanted primate lung to provide immediate and total respiratory support. *J. Thorac. Cardiovasc. Surg.* **62**, 752–761.

Khaghani, A. (1986). Discussion of Wahlers *et al.* (1986) — see below.

Kondo, Y., Turner, M. D. and Cockrell, J. U. (1974). Ischaemic tolerance of the canine autotransplanted lung. *Surgery* **76**, 447–453.

Ladowski, J. S., Kapelanski, D. P., Teodori, M. F., Stevenson, W. C., Hardesty, R. L. and Griffith, B. P. (1985). Use of autoperfusion for distant procurement of heart–lung allografts. *J. Heart Transplant.* **4**, 330–333.

McLeod, A., Dwyer, G., Meyer, G., Richardson, P., Crinkshank, J. and Bartlett, J. (1982). Cardiac sequelae of acute head injury. *Br. Heart J.* **47**, 221–226.

Magovern, G. J., Bolling, S. F., Casall, A. S., Bulkley, B. H. and Gardner, T. J. (1984). The mechanism of mannitol in reducing ischaemic injury; hyperosmolarity or hydroxyl scavenger? Circulation **70**, 191–195.

Miyamoto, Y., Lajos, T. Z., Bhayana, J. N., Bergsland, J. and Celik, C. F. (1987). Physiologic constraints in autoperfused heart–lung preservation. *J. Heart Transplant.* **6**, 261–266.

Modry, D. L., Walpoth, B. W., Cohen, R. G., Seifert, F. C. and Bleese, N. M. (1983). Heart–lung preservation in the dog followed by lung transplantation: a new model for assessment of lung preservation. *Heart Transplant.* **2**, 287–298.

Moncada, S. (1982). Biology and therapeutic potential of prostacycline. *Stroke* **14**, 157–168.

Moncada, S., Herman, A. G., Higgs, E. A. and Vane, J. R. (1977). Differential formation of prostacycline (PGX or PGIs) by layers of the arterial wall. An explanation for anti-thrombotic properties of vascular endothelium. *Thromb. Res.* **11**, 323–344.

Mundy, A. R., Bewick, M., Moncada, S. and Vane, J. R. (1980). Short term suppression of hyperacute renal allograft rejection in presensitized dogs with prostacycline. *Prostaglandins* **19**, 595–603.

Novitzky, D., Cooper, D. K. C. and Reichart, B. (1987). The value of hormonal therapy in improving organ viability in the transplant donor. *Transplant. Proc.* **19**, 2937–2938.

Novitzky, D., Wicomb, W. N., Rose, A. G., Cooper, D. K. C. and Reichart, B. (1987). Pathophysiology of pulmonary edema following experimental brain death in the Chacma baboon. *Ann. Thorac. Surg.* **43**, 288–294.

Reitz, E. A. (1982). Heart–lung transplantation — a review. *Heart Transplant.* **4**, 291–297.

Robicsek, F., Master, T. N., Duncan, G. D., Denyer, M. H., Rise, H. E. and Etchison, M. (1985). An autoperfused heart–lung preparation: metabolism and function. *J. Heart Transplant.* **4**, 334–338.

Robicsek, F., Pruitt, J. R., Sanger, P. W., Daugherty, H. K., Moore, M. and Bagby, E. (1968). The maintenance of function of the donor heart in the extracorporeal stage and during transplantation. *Ann. Thorac. Surg.* **6**, 330–342.

Ruiz, S. (1987). ICU pneumonias. *Crit. Care Med.* **15**, 930.

Sachs, S. A., Petritsch, P. H. and Kaufman, J. J. (1973). Canine kidney preservation using a new perfusate. *Lancet* **1**, 1024–1028.

Utsunomia, T., Krause, M. M., Valeri, C. R., Shepro, D. and Hechtman, H. B. (1980). Treatment of pulmonary embolism with prostacycline. *Surgery* **88**, 25–30.

Veith, F. J., Crane, R., Torres, M., Colon, I., Hagstrom, J. W. C., Pinsker, K. and Koerner, S. K. (1976). Effective preservation and transportation of lung transplants. *J. Thorac. Cardiovasc. Surg.* **72**, 97–105.

Veith, F. J., Sinha, S. B. P., Graves, J. S., Boley, S. J. and Dougherty, J. C. (1971). Ischaemic tolerance of the lung: effect of ventilation and inflation. *J. Thorac. Cardiovasc. Surg.* **61**, 804–810.

Wahlers, T., Hauerich, A., Fieguth, H. G., Schafers, H.-J., Takayama, T. and Borst, H. G. (1986). Flush perfusion using EuroCollins solution vs. cooling by means of extracorporeal circulation in heart–lung preservation. *J. Heart Transplant.* **5**, 89–98.

Watson, D. C., Reitz, B. A., Baumgartner, W. B., Oyer, P. E., Stinson, E. B. and Shumway, N. E. (1979). Distant heart procurement for transplantation. *Surgery* **86**, 56–59.

Wells, F. C. (1985). The effects of cardiopulmonary bypass on alveolar pathway barrier function, with particular emphasis on alveolar epithelial permeability. *M.S. thesis*, University of London.

Wonders, T., Huttermeier, P., Berry, D., Schuette, A., Kong, D., Watkins, W. D. and Zapol, W. M. (1983). Complement depletion prevents pulmonary hypertension and leukopenia in sheep extracorporeal membrane oxygenation. *Trans. Am. Soc. Artif. Intern. Org.* **29**, 210–213.

Stuart W. Jamieson and Michael P. Kaye

24

Operative Procedure and Postoperative Management

INTRODUCTION

Preceding chapters have dealt with the history of heart–lung transplantation, recipient and donor selection and the preservation of donor lungs. The ultimate fate of the recipient will obviously depend heavily on the condition of the donor as well as the recipient prior to and during the donor harvest and recipient implantation.

The obtaining of donors for combined heart and lung transplantation remains one of the most significant obstacles to the wide application of this procedure. Although these aspects have been discussed in Chapter 23, their importance warrants summarizing the technique at our centre (the Minnesota Heart and Lung Institute).

Donors must, of course, meet the criteria of brain death, and be without cardiac or pulmonary impairment by history or physical examination. It is important that donors are free of excessive inotropic support, systemic infection or malignancy. Pulmonary function must provide a pO_2 >100 torr with an FiO_2 of 40%, peak inflation pressures of <30 torr on physiological tidal volumes, and there should be no grossly infected secretions. The chest radiograph must be clear.

The donor operation is timed to co-ordinate with that of the recipient so as to minimize ischaemic time. Timing is more difficult than for heart transplantation, since the recipient operation may be prolonged if extensive adhesions are present. Almost all practising centres now make use of distant procurement techniques (see Chapter 23). Although other methods have been used, the accepted techniques for preservation of the heart and lung block hinge upon cooling. Cooling may be through hypothermia on bypass or flush perfusion of the pulmonary artery. Good results have been obtained with both these techniques. If flush perfusion is to be used, it is important to use sufficient perfusate to ensure adequate cooling (at least 60 ml/kg per min for 4 min) and to use an intracellular rather than extracellular type of fluid.

The donor operation is co-ordinated with other organ procurement teams, and it is important that they all have an understanding of each other's needs so as to maximize the viability of each organ. Generally, the heart and lungs are inspected early in the operation, and preliminary communication is made with the recipient team. Other organs are then fully mobilized. Towards the end of this time, after the heart has been exposed, both pleural cavities are opened, care being taken to avoid injury to, or undue manipulation of, the lungs. The phrenic nerves are sacrificed. The absence of adhesions of the lungs to the chest wall is confirmed.

The aorta is mobilized, and retracted to the left in order to expose the trachea. An infusion line is placed in the main pulmonary artery (a size 14 pulmonary artery vent catheter is convenient for this). After administration of heparin, the superior vena cava is tied and divided well above the right atrium to avoid damage to the sinus node. The inferior vena cava is mobilized and clamped at the level of the diaphragm, then divided above the clamp. This prevents excessive spillage of inferior vena caval blood into the chest cavity during the remainder of the dissection. Occasionally, the liver procurement team will request that the inferior vena cava is not clamped, so that a longer length of inferior vena cava can be left attached to the liver. This does not cause any great difficulty.

A cardioplegic infusion catheter is placed in the ascending aorta, and after the heart has emptied the aorta is clamped above the catheter and 500 ml of cardioplegic solution is infused into the aortic root. Simultaneously 4 litres of modified cold Collins' solution is infused into the main pulmonary artery. As soon as infusion of these solutions is established, the tip of the left atrial appendage is excised, to allow free drainage of the infusate after it has passed through the lungs. The left ventricle is examined periodically to ensure that it is not distending. During infusion of the cold solutions, the heart and lungs are bathed in cold Ringer's solution.

Ventilation may be continued using unheated room air. High levels of inspired oxygen must be avoided at all times. After completion of the infusions, the aorta is divided as high as is convenient, usually at the level of the take-off of the innominate artery. If the recipient has Eisenmenger's syndrome with a single arterial trunk, the donor's aortic arch is also removed. When widely opened it provides a large area for subsequent implantation to the recipient arterial trunk.

The trachea is identified to the right of, and posterior to, the divided aorta, and it is clamped as high as possible, with the lungs 50% inflated.

Using the clamp as a retractor, the trachea is pulled forward out of the wound, and the lungs progressively freed on both sides using electrocautery to divide the posterior reflections of the pleura in the plane anterior to the oesophagus. The vagus nerves are usually cut during this process.

Finally, the pulmonary ligaments are divided on both sides, and the heart and lungs lifted out of the chest. They are then transferred to a bowl containing cold Ringer's solution. If the organs are to be transported to another hospital they are placed in a plastic bag containing cold Ringer's solution, which is then sealed in a similar sterile plastic bag also containing cold solution. The whole is now transferred to a sealed container containing cold (4°C) saline, which is packed in ice. Using this method a total ischaemic time of 4 h is readily tolerated.

THE RECIPIENT OPERATION

The patient is placed on the operating table in the standard position for a median sternotomy incision. A roll is placed beneath the shoulders so as to elevate the chest. A median sternotomy incision is made and the pleura incised on both sides. Each lung is then gently palpated for adhesions. The major operative complication in heart–lung transplantation is bleeding from adhesions within the chest. The maintenance of haemostasis is an absolute prerequisite, but the visualization of peripheral, and especially apical, adhesions from a median sternotomy incision can be most difficult. If adhesions are present, they should if possible be divided at this stage, prior to heparinization, although the usual cardiomegaly may prohibit this in some cases.

The pericardium is now incised longitudinally and attached to the wound edges. The thymic fat pad is removed, care being taken to prevent injury to the phrenic nerves as they course anteriorly cephalad. Heparin (300 units/kg) is administered. The ascending aorta is cannulated as high as possible for the arterial return, and two caval cannulae are placed low in the atrium for venous drainage. After initiation of bypass, the superior and inferior venae cavae are snared. The aorta is cross-clamped and the heart fibrillated.

The heart is excised first. The incision follows the atrioventricular groove, but the atrial appendage is also removed. The incision is carried into the atrial septum either superiorly or inferiorly, the septum incised, and the incision carried around the left atrium, again at the atrioventricular groove, although excluding the appendage.

The ascending aorta is now transected as high as possible. It is important not to cut this vessel obliquely. The pulmonary artery is transected at its midpoint. The heart is lifted out of the chest.

The pericardial edge on the left side is grasped with two clamps and retracted anteriorly and to the left. An incision is made in the pericardium

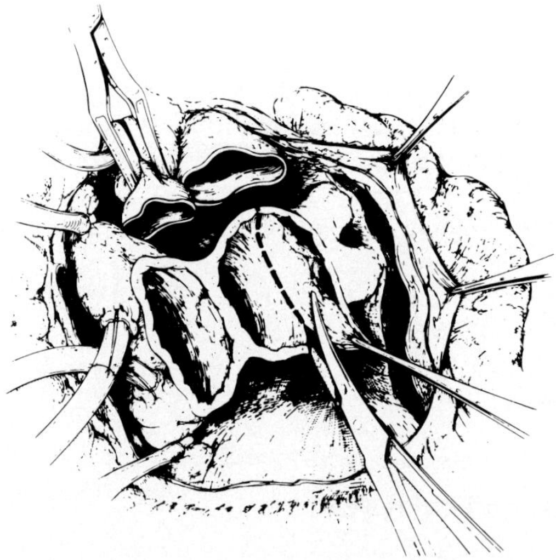

Fig. 24.1. *The recipient heart has been removed. The left atrium is now incised across the oblique sinus, so as to separate right and left pulmonary veins. An incision is made beneath the left phrenic nerve. (From Jamieson, 1986, reproduced by permission.)*

immediately anterior to the pulmonary veins. This incision is carried inferiorly as far as the diaphragm, care being taken to stay well behind the course of the phrenic nerve. Superiorly, the incision should be discontinued when the level of the left pulmonary artery is reached. Further cephalad there is a risk of injury to the vagus and the phrenic nerves which approach each other here.

A vertical incision which divides the left atrium in two is now made through the oblique sinus of the remnant of the left atrium (Fig. 24.1). This has the effect of separating the right and left pulmonary veins. The left atrial remnant on the left side, together with the left pulmonary veins, are retracted anteriorly and electrocautery used to separate these structures from the posterior pericardium and posterior mediastinum (Fig. 24.2). Important structures posteriorly are the oesophagus and the left vagus nerve.

The pulmonary ligament on the left side is now ligated and cut. The left lung remains attached only by the pulmonary artery and the bronchus, and the posterior pleural reflection. The whole left lung is now drawn out of the wound anteriorly and towards the right side, and electrocautery used to separate the remaining pleura posteriorly so that the hilum comes free. The left pulmonary artery is now divided. The left main bronchus is then progressively dissected with electrocautery, during which several bronchial arteries are encountered. These arteries, which of course are considerably enlarged in Eisenmenger's syndrome, should be secured individually (Fig.

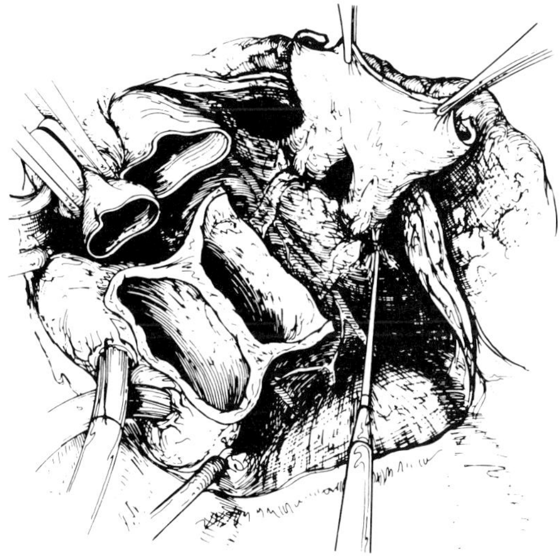

Fig. 24.2. *The remnants of the left atrium together with the left pulmonary veins are removed from the posterior pericardium. Posterior relations here are the left vagus nerve and the oesophagus. When the pulmonary veins have been fully freed, the veins with the left atrial remnant are passed beneath the phrenic nerve pedicle into the left chest. (From Jamieson, 1986, reproduced by permission.)*

24.3). The left lung is now attached only by the left main bronchus, which is closed with a TA 30 stapler using 35 mm staples. The bronchus is cut distal to the staples, and the left lung removed. Because of the potential for contamination from the cut bronchus, the instruments and lung should be considered unsterile and handled accordingly.

The heart and the left lung having been removed, attention is turned to the right lung. The phrenic nerve lies much closer to the hilum on the right than the left, and when the pleura is incised posteriorly care must be taken to avoid injury to the nerve. The pleura is incised widely, downwards from the hilum to the diaphragm, and upwards to the level of the right pulmonary artery. This provides an adequate opening for the subsequent passage of the donor right lung. The ribbon of pericardium containing the phrenic nerve is gently retracted, and an incision made in the roof of the remaining left atrial remnant on the right side, as for a mitral valve replacement. Inferiorly, this incision passes below the inferior vena cava into an open space; superiorly, the incision continues across the roof of the atrium to sever all the remaining attachments of the pulmonary veins to the left atrium. Care should be taken not to injure the atrial septum which will serve as the posterior wall of the new right atrium.

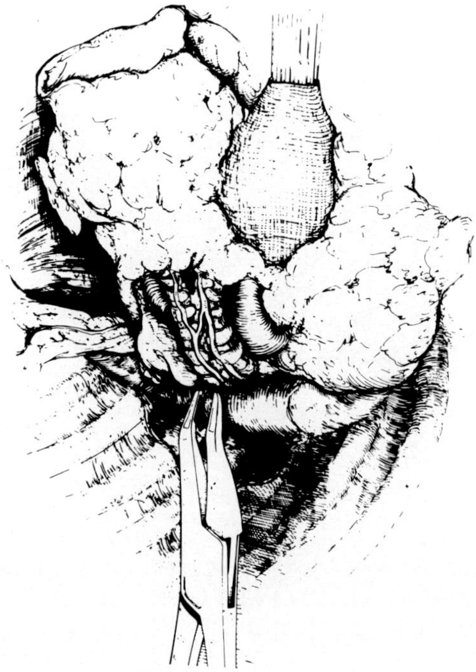

Fig. 24.3. *The left lung is now retracted medially. The bronchial arteries are individually secured with clips. (From Jamieson, 1986, reproduced by permission.)*

The right pulmonary ligament is divided. The right lung is retracted anteriorly and towards the left, and the pulmonary veins and the bronchus are freed from the posterior pleura with electrocautery. The bronchial arteries should be individually clipped as they come into view. The vagus nerve lying immediately posterior to the hilum can be tented upwards when the lung is retracted anteriorly, and care must be taken to avoid injury to it. The right pulmonary artery is divided at the level of the hilum and the right bronchus fully exposed.

The lung is retracted to the right and the bronchus stapled. The remnants of the pulmonary artery are excised, although a small disc of pulmonary artery is left around the ductus ligament to avoid damaging the left recurrent laryngeal nerve.

The ascending aorta is retracted to the left. An incision is made directly posterior and to the right of it, to expose the trachea. The stapled stump of the left main bronchus is identified and grasped with a clamp. It is drawn anteriorly and to the right, and dissected proximally, using electrocautery. The carina is reached, and the right main bronchus also freed (Fig. 24.4). The remnant here is shorter than that on the left side. The trachea is

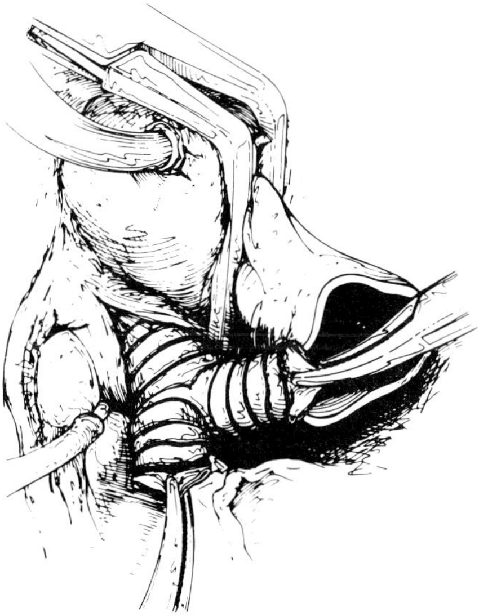

Fig. 24.4. *The heart and both lungs are now removed. Dissection to the right of the aorta posteriorly exposes the trachea and the two freed main bronchi. (From Jamieson, 1986, reproduced by permission.)*

exposed at the carina, but care is taken not to clear it excessively of its surrounding tissue, in order to preserve its blood supply. Meticulous haemostasis is now obtained throughout the chest cavity. Many of the posterior structures cannot be seen after the implantation of the new heart and lungs, which makes subsequent haemostasis difficult.

When the donor heart and lungs are received, the donor trachea is trimmed with a scalpel immediately above the carina. Cultures are taken from the donor trachea, the lumen of which is then thoroughly but gently cleaned with a small sucker. The main bronchi are gently irrigated with saline.

The donor right lung is passed beneath the right atrium and both venae cavae, and the left lung beneath the left phrenic nerve and its associated pedicle (Fig. 24.5). The recipient trachea is trimmed immediately above the carina. Cultures are taken. All that now remains to complete the operation is the anastomosis of the trachea, aorta and right atrium.

The tracheal anastomosis is performed with continuous 000 polypropylene (Fig. 24.6). The cold irrigating solution is aspirated at the level of the anastomosis so that it does not run into the trachea.

The atrial anastomosis is performed. The donor right atrium is opened as for cardiac transplantation, with a curvilinear incision that avoids the sinus node. The anastomosis is performed with a continuous suture of poly-

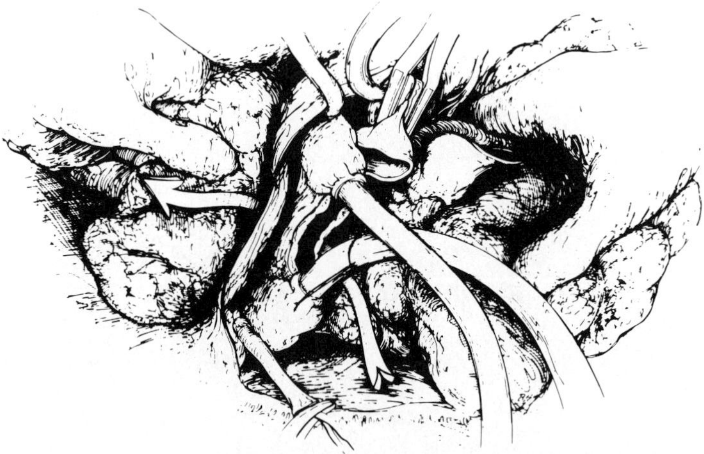

Fig. 24.5. *The donor heart and lungs are put in place. The right lung is passed beneath the right atrium and right phrenic nerve pedicle. (From Jamieson, 1986, reproduced by permission.)*

propylene including, on the posterior side, all remnants of the left atrium and the intra-atrial groove.

Finally, the aortic anastomosis is performed (Fig. 24.7). Air is removed from the heart and the aortic cross-clamp removed. The lungs are inflated gently with 5 ml of PEEP using 40% oxygen. Completion of the procedure is

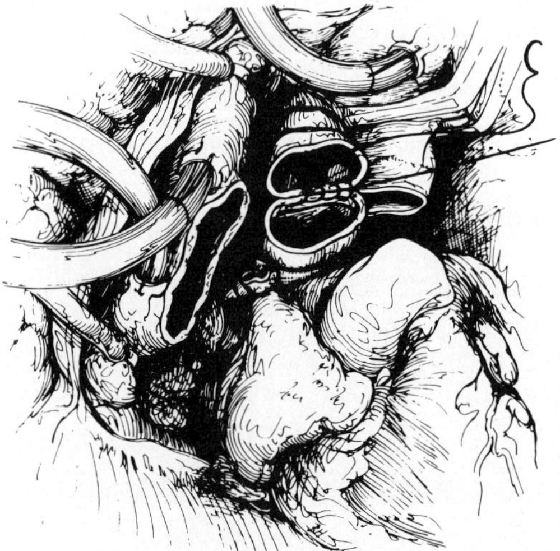

Fig. 24.6. *The tracheal anastomosis is performed first, with a continuous running suture of polypropylene. (From Jamieson, 1986, reproduced by permission.)*

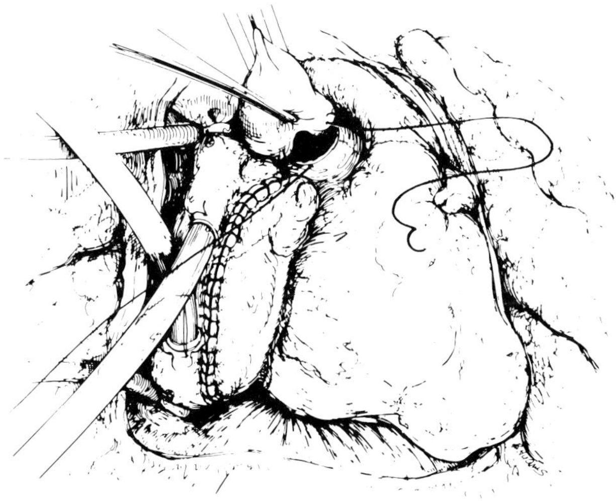

Fig. 24.7. *After the right atrial anastomosis is performed, the operation is completed by suturing the aorta. (From Jamieson, 1986, reproduced by permission.)*

now carried out in a standard fashion. Generally, we have initiated an isoprenaline infusion at the discontinuation of bypass, the infusion titrated to maintain the heart rate at about 110 beats/min. Fluid balance is critical, and we prefer not to reinfuse the pump contents unless urine output is substantial. It is often useful to ultrafiltrate the perfusate during the period of bypass to eliminate excess water.

POSTOPERATIVE CARE

Postoperative care is mainly concerned with careful fluid balance and the administration of immunosuppressive agents. The chest tubes are generally left *in situ* for at least 48 h because of the increased drainage associated with the large posterior dissection. An aggressive diuresis is instituted, with the aim of returning the patient to preoperative weight by 24 h after operation.

Immunosuppression

When clinical heart–lung transplantation was begun in 1981, our experience with cyclosporin after heart transplantation was limited to its use with steroids and anti-thymocyte globulin (ATG). It was felt important to avoid the use of steroids for the combined operation, at least initially, because of the risk of impaired tracheal healing with subsequent dehiscence. Cyclosporin was therefore administered with azathioprine and a short course of

ATG, converting this to cyclosporin and steroids (oral prednisone) after 2 weeks.

Further experience has modified this protocol. We still avoid steroid therapy for the first 10 days, but now do not use ATG, which in our experience has been associated with a high risk of infection. Immunosuppression begins with cyclosporin given orally at a dose of 6 mg/kg immediately before the operation, together with intravenous azathioprine 2 mg/kg after induction of anaesthesia. Immediately after operation, methylprednisolone 500 mg is given intravenously, followed by 125 mg intravenously every 8 h for 3 doses. No further steroids are given for 10 days.

Cyclosporin is given at 6 mg/kg daily in 2 divided doses. The administration of this drug is governed by the levels of cyclosporin, which are maintained at 200 μg/kg serum trough level for the first month, and at 100 μg/kg thereafter. After 10 days, prednisone, 0.2 mg/kg daily, is begun. Treatment with azathioprine, which is given orally from the time of the operation at the highest dose compatible with an adequate white count (usually 2 mg/kg), is continued indefinitely.

As for transplantation of the heart, strict sterile technique is of utmost importance in the immediate postoperative period in these immunosuppressed patients. Patients are usually extubated within the first 24–48 h, and vigorous pulmonary toilet is instituted. Because clearing pulmonary secretions is more difficult than normal in these patients, since they have no afferent nervous pathways from the lung, vigorous postural percussion physiotherapy is given frequently during the first 2 weeks.

Of utmost importance in this immediate postoperative period is the effort directed to the maintenance and preservation of normal lung function. Because of the frequency of compromised renal function preoperatively in these patients, and the nephrotoxity of cyclosporin, careful monitoring of fluid and electrolyte balance is essential. Hydration is minimized and a vigorous diuresis is initiated and maintained.

REFERENCE

Stuart W. Jamieson (1986). Transplantation. In *Operative Surgery* (*Cardiac Surgery*), 4th edn (S. W. Jamieson and N. E. Shumway, Eds), pp. 584–605. Butterworths, London.

J. D. Cooper and G. A. Patterson

25

Lung Transplantation

HISTORICAL INTRODUCTION

Surgical interest in organ transplantation developed in the 1950s, the decade following establishment of the immunological basis of allograft rejection by Medawar (1944). Metras (1950), in France, and Hardin and Kittle (1954), in the USA, demonstrated the feasibility of lung transplantation in dogs. In 1963, Dr James Hardy and co-workers reported the first human lung transplant (Hardy *et al.*, 1963). The recipient survived for 18 days, demonstrating the technical feasibility of lung transplantation and the capability of the transplanted lung to function. This success, although limited, was sufficient to stimulate worldwide interest in lung transplantation.

The next two decades saw rapid developments in organ transplantation, and the demonstration of repeated long-term clinical success with transplantation of the kidney, heart and liver. However, success with lung transplantation was more elusive. In the 20 years following Hardy's initial attempt, there were approximately 40 lung or lobe transplants performed around the world, but unfortunately no patient was restored to normal health for any significant period of time. Only one recipient survived long enough to be discharged from hospital, a 23-year-old patient of Derom *et al.* (1971) who underwent right lung transplantation for advanced silicosis. The patient was discharged from hospital 8 months after transplantation and died a short while later with chronic rejection, sepsis and bronchial stenosis. Most recipients succumbed within 2 weeks of transplantation, usually from primary organ failure, sepsis and rejection. Of the first 38 transplants, only 9 patients survived more than 2 weeks and 6 of these died in the first month of bronchial anastomotic disruption. This was the outcome of our initial attempt at lung transplantation — a right lung transplant performed in 1978 for a ventilator-dependent victim of inhalation burns (Nelems, 1980).

After this experience, we undertook a laboratory programme to evaluate factors affecting bronchial anastomotic healing following lung transplantation. The initial experiments involved canine lung autotransplantation, half of the animals receiving no immunosuppression and the other half receiving standard immunosuppression with azathioprine and prednisone. The results of these experiments demonstrated significant bronchial complications in the treated animals, including ischaemia, necrosis and disruption of the bronchial anastomosis, similar to complications previously reported following human lung transplantation (Lima *et al.*, 1981). Subsequent experiments demonstrated that the adverse effect on bronchial healing in these experiments was entirely due to the prednisone and that the use of azathioprine did not prejudice satisfactory healing of the bronchial anastomosis. When cyclosporin was substituted for the prednisone in these experiments, bronchial anastomotic healing in the animals treated with cyclosporin and azathioprine did not differ from that in untreated animals (Goldberg *et al.*, 1983).

In order to buttress the bronchial anastomosis, and rapidly restore bronchial artery circulation, we employed a pedicle of omentum brought up into the chest to wrap around the bronchial anastomosis at the time of lung transplantation in dogs. These studies resulted in further improvements in bronchial anastomotic healing, and demonstrated rapid restoration of bronchial circulation via collateral vessels from the omentum (Morgan *et al.*, 1983; Dubois, Choiniere and Cooper, 1984).

CLINICAL LUNG TRANSPLANTATION

Following this laboratory success, we embarked on a limited programme of clinical lung transplantation. Our initial attempt was in a victim of paraquat poisoning with hepatic and renal failure, who was on a ventilator as well as on extracorporeal membrane oxygenator support for respiratory failure. A right lung transplant initially functioned well, but then sustained damage from high levels of residual circulating paraquat. Subsequent left lung transplantation was performed with restoration of satisfactory pulmonary gas exchange, but the patient died 10 weeks following initial lung transplantation never having recovered renal function (Saunders, Alpert and Cooper, 1985).

SELECTION OF RECIPIENTS

On reviewing the world experience of lung transplantation we concluded that poor recipient selection significantly contributed to the unfavourable outcome, as with our paraquat victim. We decided to employ, at least initially, very strict criteria for recipient selection, in the hope of improving the outcome. Patients with bilateral pulmonary sepsis, either acute or chronic, seemed ill-suited for unilateral lung transplantation as the remaining, infected lung would not only contaminate the transplanted lung, but would serve as a focus for systemic infection following institution of immunosuppression. In patients with emphysema, unilateral lung transplantation might result in hyper-expansion of the contralateral native lung with mediastinal shift and crowding of the transplanted lung. We also excluded ventilator-dependent patients, as such individuals may have airway sepsis, multi-system failure, and in general insufficient stamina to permit rapid recovery and cessation of ventilatory assistance early in the postoperative period. We decided that patients with end-stage fibrotic lung disease represented ideal candidates. In such individuals, the restrictive nature of the lung defect would lead to preferential ventilation of the transplanted lung. The increased vascular resistance in the native lung would similarly create a diversion of the majority of the cardiac output to the transplanted lung, thus avoiding a ventilation–perfusion imbalance, or any significant degree of wasted ventilation.

Patients with end-stage pulmonary fibrosis are frequently treated with high-dose prednisone in an attempt to retard the progression of the disease. Because of the animal experimentation indicating the adverse effects of prednisone in the early postoperative period, we require that all transplant recipients be weaned entirely from prednisone for at least 1 month prior to transplantation. In patients with end-stage pulmonary fibrosis requiring transplantation, we are usually dealing with 'burned-out' fibrotic lungs with little, if any, active inflammation. Thus steroid administration at this stage is usually of no benefit, and for this reason such patients can be weaned entirely from their steroids without adverse effect in anticipation of a transplant.

We have attempted to identify as candidates patients who are likely to die of their disease within 12–18 months. Such candidates are patients who are oxygen-dependent, who have demonstrated progressive deterioration in pulmonary function, and an increasing requirement for oxygen administration over the previous 12 months. Even while receiving supplemental O_2, such patients generally demonstrated a prompt fall in oxygen saturation upon exercise.

Patients with end-stage pulmonary fibrosis generally have excellent respiratory muscle strength due to the chronic workload of ventilating the poorly compliant, fibrotic lungs. These patients have some degree of pulmonary hypertension, but this is usually moderate so that cor pulmonale is not present. Right ventricular function is evaluated non-invasively using echocardiography, and gated nuclear angiography to compute the first pass right ventricular ejection fraction.

Prospective recipients are thoroughly evaluated and any having significant psychosocial problems are excluded because of the considerable stress which the preoperative assessment, long waiting period and postoperative recovery impose. Furthermore, the need for strict patient compliance and cooperation is essential to ensure a satisfactory long-term result.

DONOR SELECTION

The lack of suitable donors is currently the major obstacle to more widespread application of lung transplantation. Only a fraction of organ donors have lungs which remain suitable for transplantation. We require that the donor chest radiograph be entirely clear and that the arterial oxygen tension exceed 300 mmHg when 100% oxygen is administered with 5 cm of positive end-expiratory pressure. We also require that bronchoscopy reveal no purulent secretions.

In order to minimize ischaemic injury to the lung, we initially utilized only donors whose families would permit transfer of the donor to our hospital, so that the removal of the lung, and its subsequent transplantation, were carried out in adjacent operating rooms. With increasing experience we have abandoned this policy, and at the present time the majority of donor lungs are excised elsewhere and transported to our hospital for implantation.

LUNG PRESERVATION

Our method of lung preservation is simple. After excision from the heparinized donor, the lung graft is immersed in EuroCollins solution at 4°C. Using this simple technique, we have had satisfactory results with ischaemic periods up to 4 h. To date, we have not used the technique of flushing with cold electrolyte solution as has been routinely utilized for heart–lung transplants. We anticipate that flush techniques in the future will be developed which are superior to simple immersion and which will extend the period of safe ischaemia up to 12 h or longer. Limited success with such a technique in animals has been previously reported from several centres (Haverich, Scott and Jamieson, 1985; Todd *et al.*, 1988; DeMajo, Zulys and Cooper, personal communication).

SIZE MATCHING

For purposes of size matching, the vertical and transverse radiological dimensions of the chest are used. The transverse diameter is measured at the level of the apex of the diaphragm, and the vertical measurement on each side from the apex of the chest to the apex of the diaphragm. Unfortunately, donor lateral films are not usually available so we must rely on portable anteroposterior films in most cases. Therefore, exact comparison with the intended recipient is often difficult. Body weight, height and chest circumference are also utilized in an attempt to assess the suitability of the match. Initially we sought a donor lung of approximately the same size as the recipient chest. With experience, however, we realized that a donor lung which was considerably oversized was not only suitable, but desirable. With pulmonary fibrosis, the recipient's chest is contracted because of the nature of the disease process, and insertion of a larger lung will allow for chest expansion back toward normal and provide better lung function. The accommodation of the recipient chest to the larger donor lung is facilitated if the left side is used for transplantation, since the left diaphragm descends more readily than the right, and the mediastinum easily shifts toward the right. This is illustrated in Fig. 25.1.

CHOICE OF SIDE

We have performed lung transplantation on either side, but in general we prefer the left side for several technical reasons:

(1) It is easier to clamp the left atrium proximal to the pulmonary veins on the left side, because on the right side the pulmonary veins enter the left atrium near the inter-atrial groove.
(2) For this same reason, separate extraction of the donor heart for cardiac transplantation is easier if the donor's left lung is to be used for a lung transplant, since on the left, larger atrial cuffs can be preserved on the heart and lung grafts.
(3) The recipient bronchus is longer on the left, making the bronchial anastomosis somewhat easier.
(4) For reasons noted above, an oversized donor lung may be more easily accommodated on the left than on the right.

If the recipient has had a major thoracotomy on the left side, we would favour a right lung transplant.

DONOR PREPARATION

At the present time, most donor lungs are extracted in conjunction with separate cardiac extraction. To facilitate such coordination, and to minimize delay of the cardiac team, the heart is removed initially leaving a small cuff of left atrium attached to the donor lung. Immediately following inflow occlusion and cardioplegic arrest, the cardiac extraction is performed *in situ*.

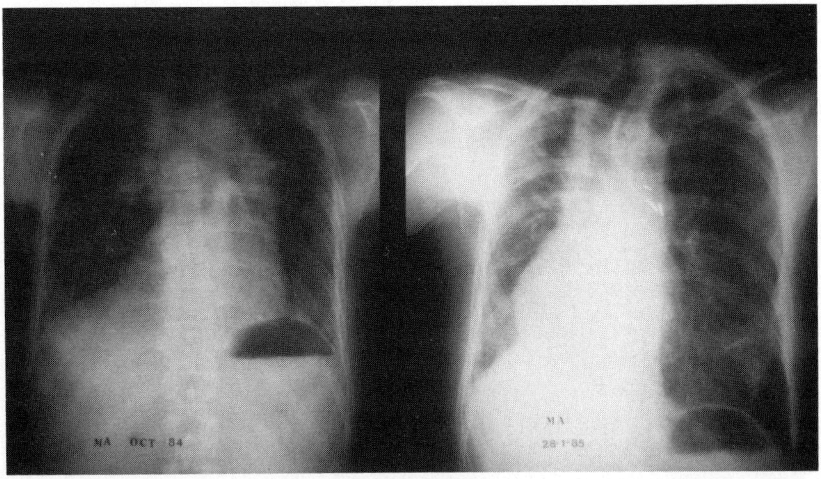

Fig. 25.1. *Preoperative and postoperative chest radiographs from a patient who has undergone left lung transplantation. Note the enormous discrepancy in the recipient and donor left lung. The postoperative film on the right shows a marked mediastinal shift and inferior displacement of the diaphragm to accommodate the oversized left lung.*

The superior and inferior venae cavae, and the ascending aorta are divided as is the common pulmonary artery just proximal to the bifurcation. This leaves the base of the heart attached only by the left atrium. Meticulous division of the left atrium is then carried out under direct vision, enabling the surgeon to leave an adequate left atrial cuff on the heart and lung side. Separate excision of the heart requires only a few minutes more than is required when there is no concern for a lung graft. Following cardiac extraction, the trachea is severed at its mid-point, with stapling of the distal end. The lungs are extracted *en bloc*, and immersed in a bag containing Collins' solution at 4°C. This bag is then placed on ice for transportation of the lungs to our hospital. Just prior to implantation, the donor lung is trimmed from the specimen, dividing the donor bronchus two rings proximal to the upper lobe take-off and the ipsilateral pulmonary artery at its origin. The atrial cuff is fashioned at the time of cardiac extraction. We leave large flaps of pericardium attached to the hilum of the donor lung as a route for systemic revascularization of the bronchi.

ANAESTHESIA

Prior to induction of anaesthesia, a Swan–Ganz thermal dilution catheter is inserted into the recipient and positioned in the pulmonary artery of the lung opposite the one to be transplanted. This position is verified by chest radiograph. An arterial line permits continuous blood pressure monitoring and frequent arterial blood gas analysis. Pulse oximetry and continuous end tidal CO_2 monitoring are also employed. Femoro-femoral veno-arterial extracorporeal bypass with a micro-porous membrane oxygenator is always on standby, although not usually required. It has been utilized only if adequate gas exchange or haemodynamic stability could not be achieved with ventilation and perfusion of the contralateral native lung. Bypass has been utilized in 4 of 15 cases to date. To minimize bleeding, bypass is instituted only after the recipient lung has been entirely mobilized, so that no anticoagulation is utilized during dissection of the scarred lung from the chest wall and diaphragm.

For patients undergoing a left lung transplant, a left bronchial blocker (Fogarty no. 14 French venous occlusion catheter — Model no. 62-080-8, American Hospital Supply), is inserted into the distal trachea, after which a standard single lumen endotracheal tube is inserted. A flexible bronchoscope is then inserted through the endotracheal tube and under direct vision the bronchial blocker is positioned in the proximal left main bronchus about 2 cm distal to the carina. The balloon is inflated with 5–7 cc of air to verify complete occlusion of the left main bronchus, after which the balloon is deflated and the bronchoscope is removed.

For patients undergoing a right lung transplant, a left double-lumen endotracheal tube is inserted and the appropriate position verified by clinical assessment and fibre-optic bronchoscopy.

OPERATIVE PROCEDURE

After anaesthetic induction, and intubation, the patient is placed supine. The abdomen and groin on the side of the proposed transplant are prepared and draped. A small upper midline incision is made and the greater omentum is withdrawn through the wound. It is usually necessary to dissect the omentum from the transverse colon in order to provide an adequate length. Additional omental length can be obtained if necessary by division of the right or left vascular arcade. A tunnel is made immediately behind the xiphisternum by means of blunt dissection with the index finger. This tunnel is enlarged to several finger breadths and the apex of the omentum is placed in it prior to closing the abdominal incision.

The abdominal procedure requires 15–20 min. During this time the anaesthetist performs a thorough assessment of haemodynamics and gas exchange while ventilating both lungs. The lung to be transplanted is then collapsed and the measurements repeated after 15 min. At this point, a preliminary decision is made as to whether the patient can possibly be managed without the use of cardiopulmonary bypass during extraction of the lung. If bypass is thought likely, the femoral vessels on the side of the proposed thoracotomy are exposed and prepared. Otherwise no groin dissection is done, but the groin area is always draped in the field when preparing for the thoracotomy, should the need for intraoperative extracorporeal support arise.

Once the abdomen has been closed, the patient is turned to the thoracotomy position and the chest, abdomen and ipsilateral groin area are prepared and draped. The chest is entered through the bed of the excised 5th rib and adhesions between the lung and the chest wall or diaphragm are carefully dissected free, using cautery as much as possible. The pulmonary veins are isolated extrapericardially and the proximal pulmonary artery is circled intrapericardially. On the left side, the ligamentum arteriosum is divided to facilitate subsequent proximal clamping of the pulmonary artery. On the right side, exposure is facilitated by division of the azygus vein and intrapericardial dissection of the right pulmonary artery posterior to the superior vena cava.

During this mobilization, the lung has been collapsed, if the patient can tolerate it, in order to facilitate dissection. After isolation of the pulmonary veins and pulmonary artery, the bronchus is minimally mobilized just proximal to the upper lobe takeoff, special care being taken not to dissect tissue from around the recipient bronchus proximal to the point of proposed division.

If a previous temporary occlusion of the pulmonary artery was well tolerated, a vascular clamp is once again placed on the proximal pulmonary artery and the first branch to the upper lobe is isolated and divided between ligatures. The pulmonary artery will be subsequently divided just distal to this point, providing additional length as well as a somewhat smaller calibre in order to reduce the usual discrepancy between a large recipient pulmonary artery and a normal size donor pulmonary artery.

The two pulmonary veins are ligated extrapericardially and the veins are divided peripheral to these ligatures. The pulmonary artery is divided transversely just beyond the ligated first branch, and the bronchus is divided transversely proximal to the upper lobe bronchus. After removal of the recipient lung, the pericardium is opened circumferentially around the stumps of the pulmonary veins and a Satinsky clamp is placed as centrally as possible on the left atrium without impinging on the contralateral pulmonary veins. On the right side, it may be necessary to dissect into the intra-atrial groove, in order to mobilize enough left atrium to allow satisfactory proximal placement of the Satinsky clamp. After the atrium has been clamped, the previously placed ligatures on the pulmonary venous stumps are removed and the bridge between the pulmonary veins is divided to create a suitable atrial cuff. This cuff is then fashioned to match the size of the donor atrial cuff.

Lung implantation

The pleural cavity is inspected carefully to ensure that haemostasis has been accomplished. The previously prepared, deflated donor lung is then positioned posteriorly in the chest. The atrial anastomosis is the first to be performed. The back wall of the anastomosis is sutured from the front using continuous 3–0 polypropylene. The front wall of the atrial anastomosis is similarly performed without the need to reposition the lung. The donor and recipient pulmonary arteries are then trimmed if necessary and proper orientation is determined. The previously ligated first branch of the recipient pulmonary artery, and the first branch of the donor pulmonary artery, can be lined up to ensure that no rotation of the donor pulmonary artery occurs. The posterior wall of the pulmonary anastomosis is then sutured with continuous 5–0 polypropylene. The anterior wall of the pulmonary anastomosis is then constructed, but the running suture is not tied at this point, so as to allow subsequent flushing and back-bleeding through the anastomosis.

The bronchial anastomosis is performed with interrupted 4–0 Vicryl sutures with knots placed exterior as far as possible. Following completion of the bronchial anastomosis, the left atrial clamp is gradually released. Back-bleeding through the untied pulmonary artery suture line should occur within several minutes. Gentle inflation of the lung at this point may facilitate back-bleeding. After back-bleeding has been observed, or after 3–5 min if it has not, the pulmonary artery clamp is momentarily released to flush the pulmonary artery. When the pulmonary artery suture line has been tightened, the pulmonary artery clamp is removed.

The mediastinal pleura is then opened just above the diaphragm anteriorly, adjacent to the pericardium, and the omentum is withdrawn from its retrosternal position. If for some reason an adequate length of omentum is not easily withdrawn into the chest, the previously closed abdominal wound, which has been prepared and draped, could be reopened for further abdominal mobilization. The omentum is brought inferior and then posterior to the hilum of the lung. Its apex is passed medial to the bronchial anastomosis around the bronchus and back to itself, creating a broad blanket of omentum completely encircling the bronchus and separating it from the pulmonary artery suture line. The omentum is tacked to itself to avoid subsequent displacement.

The lung is retracted posteriorly, and the free edge of the donor pericardium is loosely attached to the omentum with several interrupted sutures. Collateral circulation from the omentum rapidly restores circulation in the

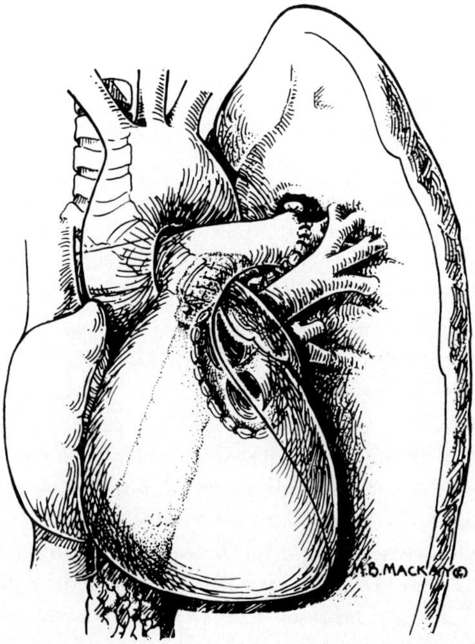

Fig. 25.2. *A completed left lung transplantation depicting the large left atrial anastomosis which on the donor side contains the confluence of both pulmonary veins. The pulmonary arterial anastomosis is shown constructed immediately distal to the first branch of the recipient pulmonary artery. The bronchial anastomosis is illustrated wrapped securely in the pedicled flap of omentum.*

pericardial vessels which are in continuity with the bronchial circulation at the hilum of the lung.

Two chest tubes are placed and the chest is closed in standard fashion. The bronchial anastomosis is assessed bronchoscopically prior to termination of the procedure. The average blood requirement for this procedure has been one unit. This technique of single lung transplantation has been previously reported (Cooper *et al.*, 1987). The completed implantation is shown in Fig. 25.2.

Use of extracorporeal bypass

If contralateral ventilation or temporary clamping of the proximal pulmonary artery before excision of the diseased lung indicates the need for extracorporeal support, partial veno-arterial bypass is instituted through the femoral vessels. This is begun after the lung has been completely mobilized and continues until circulation is restored to the transplanted lung.

IMMUNOSUPPRESSION

Cyclosporin A, 5 mg/kg (oral), and azathioprine, 2 mg/kg (intravenous), are given to the recipient immediately preoperatively. Postoperatively, oral cyclosporin (5 mg/kg) is administered twice daily, with a dose adjusted to produce a plasma trough level of 200 ng/ml, as measured by radioimmunoassay. Azathioprine, 1.5 mg/kg per day, is administered as a single intravenous dose for the first week and thereafter orally. Minnesota antilymphoblast globulin, 10–20 mg/kg per day, is administered by continuous intravenous infusion for the first 7–14 days until satisfactory plasma cyclosporin levels are achieved. Suspected rejection episodes are treated with intravenous bolus doses of methylprednisolone sodium succinate (solumedrol), 500 mg to 1 g intravenously, for 3 successive days. Routine use of prednisone is avoided for the initial 2–3 weeks. At that time, if the thoracotomy wound is healing well and if bronchoscopy reveals normal bronchial healing, oral prednisone is begun in a dose of 0.5 mg/kg per day. Our immunosuppressive protocol has been evolving with time, and currently long-term maintenance is with azathioprine, cyclosporin and alternate-day prednisone.

DIAGNOSIS OF REJECTION

The diagnosis of rejection remains imprecise and is based on a combination of one or more of the following features: deterioration in Pa_{O_2}, modest pyrexia, development of a radiological diffuse infiltrate or hilar flare, decreased oximetry saturation with exercise, increased fatiguability or dyspnoea. The single most useful diagnostic tool is the response to a pulse dose of 500 mg to 1 g of intravenous methylprednisolone. Improvement in arterial oxygenation and reduction in temperature occur within hours, improvement in the chest radiograph occurring over a somewhat longer period of time. We have found sequential quantitative lung perfusion scans to be of diagnostic value. A decline in perfusion to the transplanted lung, with corresponding increased perfusion to the native lung, has frequently been observed in association with rejection episodes. This shift in perfusion promptly reverses after administration of intravenous methylprednisolone.

Most recipients have undergone two or three significant rejection episodes in the first 3 weeks. The first episode most commonly occurs at about day 5, but may occur as early as 48 h after transplantation.

The vast majority of rejection episodes occur within the first 6 weeks and we have not recognized acute rejection episodes beyond this time. Two patients, however, have developed chronic rejection, proven on open lung biopsy. This has led to the death of one patient and to reduced pulmonary function in the second. We have not recognized the development of obliterative bronchiolitis in any case, contrary to the significant incidence of this condition following combined heart–lung transplant.

RESULTS

Fifteen patients with end-stage pulmonary fibrosis have undergone lung transplantation at our centre, 2 right lung and 13 left lung transplants. There have been 4 postoperative deaths, 2 related to poor donor selection, 1 due to viral pneumonia, and 1 due to accidental venous air embolism on the 10th postoperative day. Of the 11 survivors, 2 have subsequently died, 1 from chronic rejection at 6 months, and 1 from B-cell lymphoma at 8 months. Seven patients have survived more than 1 year, the longest being alive and well more than 4 years after transplantation.

Bronchial healing

No patient has died as a result of complications of bronchial anastomotic healing. Of the 11 long-term survivors, 9 had normal bronchial healing. Two patients developed partial necrosis of the donor bronchus just distal to the anastomosis. In both instances, repeated pulse doses of steroids had been required in the early postoperative period for rejection episodes. Neither individual developed a bronchovascular or bronchopleural fistula, presumably because of the protection afforded by the encircling omental wrap (Fig. 25.3). Both individuals required repeated bronchial dilatation and were ultimately treated by endoscopic insertion of a short silicone rubber stent into the left main bronchus. This has remained in place for 6 months in once case and $2\frac{1}{2}$ years in the other, without further difficulty.

Rehabilitation

The oxygen dependency and prompt desaturation with exercise exhibited by these patients preoperatively, leads to marked limitation in their activity resulting in generalized muscular weakness and loss of stamina. We require all candidates to participate preoperatively in a structured rehabilitation programme involving treadmill walking, cycling, and strengthening exercises, using weights. We have been able to demonstrate improvement in the exercise capacity of many of these end-stage patients prior to transplantation and feel that this procedure improves the chances for prompt postoperative recovery. Most transplant recipients are able to resume rehabilitation exercises 3–4 weeks after operation. Such rehabilitation is maintained on an outpatient basis for a minimum of 3 months, for at least 3 days per week. Improvement in overall performance continues for 6–12 months, although

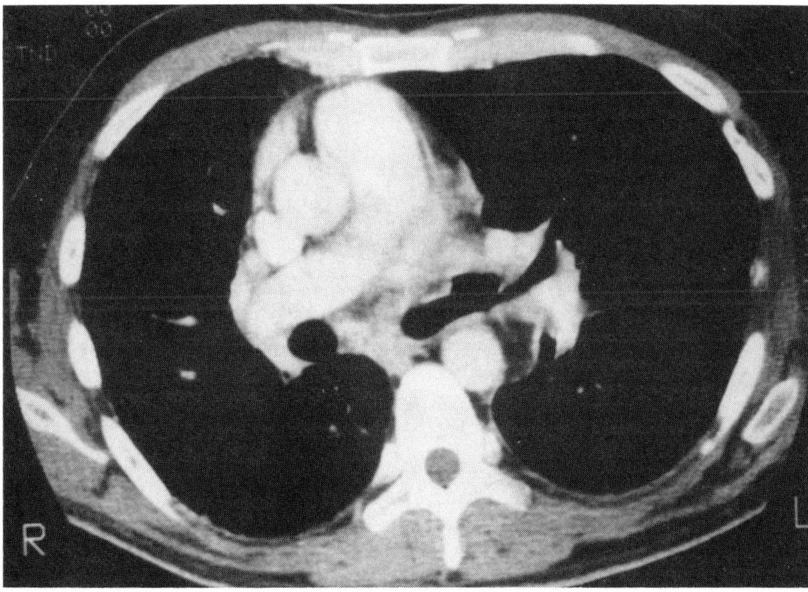

Fig. 25.3. *A computerized axial tomographic cut in a patient with a postoperative bronchial anastomotic dehiscence. The dehiscence and mediastinal cavity can be seen immediately anterior to the left main bronchus. The large bulk of omentum wrapped around the bronchial anastomosis can be best seen as a fatty density lying immediately posterior to the bronchus and lateral to the descending thoracic aorta.*

patients are able to resume normal activity and usually return to full employment within 3–6 months.

DOUBLE-LUNG TRANSPLANTATION

For patients with chronic bilateral pulmonary sepsis, such as cystic fibrosis or bronchiectasis, or patients with emphysema, we have not to date considered single lung transplantation for the reasons previously noted. We were impressed by the early results obtained with combined heart–lung transplantation at Stanford for patients with pulmonary hypertension and cor pulmonale (Reitz *et al.*, 1982) and sought to apply this form of transplantation to patients with end-stage pulmonary disease deemed unsuitable for single lung transplantation. We soon recognized that this type of transplant was not ideal for recipients with adequate or recoverable right ventricular function. The recipient must give up his own heart unnecessarily. The recipient is required to accept transplantation of two major organ systems, each of which is associated with its own problems, including rejection of one independent of the other. Advanced coronary sclerosis has been reported after several years in recipients of heart or heart–lung transplants. The donor heart would best be used in an individual requiring heart transplantation, without prejudicing the use of the lungs for the recipient with pulmonary disease. By separately extracting the heart for cardiac transplantation and the lungs for bilateral pulmonary transplantation, many more donor lungs are available, especially considering the proliferation of centres for cardiac transplantation.

The concept of simultaneous *en bloc* bilateral pulmonary transplantation is not a new one and was demonstrated in dogs by Vanderhoeft *et al.* (1972). We developed, in dogs and monkeys, a technique for *en bloc* double-lung transplantation with three anastomoses, namely the trachea, the common pulmonary artery, and a cuff of donor left atrium containing the pulmonary veins (Dark *et al.*, 1986). We subsequently described the application of this technique for human double-lung transplantation (Patterson *et al.*, 1988). Our initial double-lung transplant was performed in November 1986, and to date 7 such transplants have been performed: 1 for primary pulmonary hypertension and 6 for obstructive lung disease (4 emphysema, 1 bronchiolitis obliterans, 1 eosinophilic granuloma). Six patients remain alive and well up to 14 months. The completed double-lung implantation is illustrated in Fig. 25.4.

We have utilized the omental wrap for the tracheal anastomosis in the double-lung transplant. Nevertheless, ischaemic tracheal complications have been more frequent than with single-lung transplant, undoubtedly a reflection of the long donor airway of the double-lung graft. One patient died as a result of ischaemic necrosis of the donor trachea and main bronchi. Prolonged postoperative hypotension is thought to have contributed to this complication. A second recipient, also with prolonged postoperative hypotension, developed late ischaemic necrosis of the membranous tracheal wall without adverse clinical effect. At 5 months, the distal tracheal lumen is narrowed with granulation tissue which may require repeated dilatation and/or insertion of a silicone stent. A third recipient developed an ischaemic stricture of the proximal left main bronchus, requiring initial dilation followed by transbronchoscopic insertion of a silicone stent. Four recipients had completely normal healing of the airway. The 6 surviving recipients, ranging from 4 to 14 months postoperatively, all have excellent lung function and have resumed a normal life. Thus, in spite of an increased rate of airway complications, overall results to date have been very encouraging. We plan to explore the possibility of direct restoration of the bronchial circulation in order to further reduce the incidence of ischaemic airway damage with this procedure.

At the present time, we recommend unilateral lung transplantation for patients with end-stage pulmonary fibrosis, double-lung transplantation for patients with obstructive lung disease or bilateral pulmonary sepsis, and

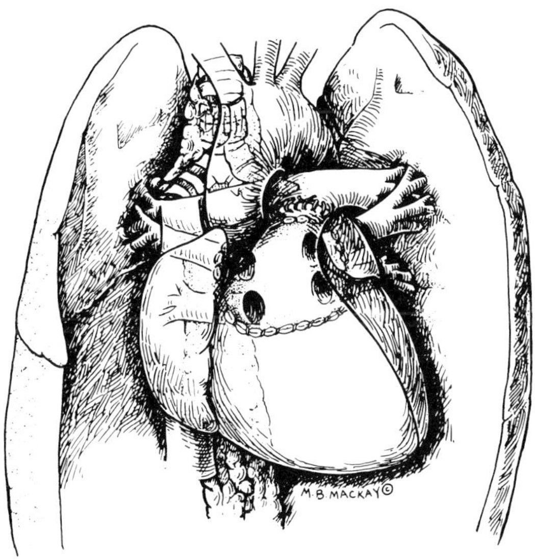

Fig. 25.4. *A completed double-lung graft. The tracheal anastomosis performed immediately proximal to the carina is wrapped securely in omentum. The left atrial anastomosis is illustrated with the donor cuff containing the orifice of all four pulmonary veins. The pulmonary artery anastomosis connects the donor and recipient main pulmonary artery, just distal to the pulmonic valve.*

combined heart–lung transplantation for patients with the combination of irreversible cardiac and pulmonary disease. Clinical and experimental evidence suggests that the adverse effects of pulmonary hypertension on the right ventricle may be reversible in many cases, following restoration of normal pulmonary vascular resistance. For patients with primary pulmonary hypertension, therefore, the application of single- or double-lung transplantation seems promising. Further clinical experience with all three forms of transplantation will be required before a final evaluation as to the role, benefits and long-term results of each is established. It seems apparent at the present time, however, that transplantation for end-stage lung disease can produce the degree of success already achieved with renal, cardiac and hepatic transplantation.

REFERENCES

Cooper, J. D., Pearson, F. G., Patterson, G. A., Todd, T. R., Ginsberg, R. J., Goldberg, M. and DeMajo, W. A. P. (1987). Technique of successful lung transplantation in humans. *J. Thorac. Cardiovasc. Surg.* **93**, 173–181.

Dark, J. H., Patterson, G. A., Al-Jilaihawi, A. N., Hsu, H., Egan, T. and Cooper, J. D. (1986). Experimental en bloc double-lung transplantation. *Ann. Thorac. Surg.* **42**, 394–398.

Derom, F., Barbier, F., Ringoir, S., Versieck, J., Rolly, G., Berzsenyi, G., Vermeire, P. and Vrints, L. (1971). Ten month survival after lung homotransplantation in man. *J. Thorac. Cardiovasc. Surg.* **61**, 835–846.

Dubois, P., Choiniere, L. and Cooper, J. D. (1984). Bronchial omentopexy in canine lung allotransplantation. *Ann. Thorac. Surg.* **38**, 211–214.

Goldberg, M., Lima, O., Morgan, E., Ayabe, H. A., Luk, S., Ferdman, A., Peters, W. J. and Cooper, J. D. (1983). A comparison between cyclosporin A and methylprednisolone plus azathioprine on bronchial healing following canine lung autotransplantation. *J. Thorac. Cardiovasc. Surg.* **85**, 821–826.

Hardin, C. A. and Kittle, C. F. (1954). Experiences with transplantation of the lung. *Science* **119**, 97–98.

Hardy, J. D., Webb, W. R., Dalton, M. L. and Walker, G. R. (1963). Lung homotransplantation in man. *J. Am. Med. Ass.* **186**, 1065–1074.

Haverich, A., Scott, W. C. and Jamieson, S. W. (1985). Twenty years of lung preservation — a review. *Heart Transplant.* **4**, 234–240.

Lima, O., Cooper, J. D., Peters, W. J., Ayabe, H., Townsend, E., Luk, S. C. and Goldberg, M. (1981). Effects of methylprednisolone and azathioprine on bronchial healing following lung autotransplantation. *J. Thorac. Cardiovasc. Surg.* **82**, 211–215.

Medawar, P. B. (1944). The behaviour and fate of skin autografts and skin homografts in rabbits. *J. Anat.* **78**, 176–199.

Metras, H. (1950). Note preliminaire sur la greffe totale du poumon chez le chien. *Fr. Acad. Sci.* 30 Oct., 1176–1177.

Morgan, W. E., Lima, O., Goldberg, M., Ayabe, H., Ferdman, A. and Cooper, J. D. (1983). Improved bronchial healing in canine left lung reimplantation using omental pedicle wrap. *J. Thorac. Cardiovasc. Surg.* **85**, 134–139.

Nelems, J. M., Rebuck, A. S., Cooper, J. D., Goldberg, M., Halloran, P. F. and Vellend, H. (1980). Human lung transplantation. *Chest.* **78**, 569–573.

Patterson, G. A., Coppper, J. D., Goldman, B., Weisel, R. D., Pearson, F. G., Waters, P. F., Todd, T. R., Scully, H., Goldberg, M. and Ginsberg, R. J. (1988). Technique of successful clinical double lung transplantation. *Ann. Thorac. Surg.* (in press).

Reitz, B. A., Wallwork, J. L., Hunt, S. A., Pennock, J. L., Billingham, M. E., Oyer, P. E., Stinson, E. B. and Shumway, N. E. (1982). Heart–lung transplantation: successful therapy for patients with pulmonary vascular disease. *N. Engl. J. Med.* **306**, 557–564.

Saunders, N. R., Alpert, H. M. and Cooper, J. D. (1985). Sequential bilateral lung transplantation for paraquat poisoning: a case report. *J. Thorac. Cardiovasc. Surg.* **89**, 734–742.

Todd, T. R., Goldberg, M., Koshal, A., Menkis, A., Boychuk, J., Patterson, G. A. and Cooper, J. D. (1988). Separate extraction of cardiac and pulmonary grafts from a single organ donor. *Ann. Thorac. Surg.* (submitted).

Vanderhoeft, P., Dubois, A., Lauvan, N., de Francquen, P. H., Carpentier, Y., Rocmans, P., Nelson, R., Kaufman, S., Brickman, L., Gyhra, A. and Ectars, P. (1972). Block allotransplantation of both lungs with pulmonary trunk and left atrium in dogs. *Thorax* **27**, 415–419.

Bartley P. Griffith

26

Detection of Rejection in the Transplanted Lungs and Immunology

INTRODUCTION

Since the reintroduction of cardiopulmonary transplantation by Reitz *et al.* (1980), close to 200 procedures have been performed worldwide, including 48 in Pittsburgh (Reitz *et al.*, 1980, 1982; Griffith *et al.*, 1987a). Much has been learned about the patterns of allograft rejection. It has been determined that isolated rejection of the lung occurs most frequently and that the endomyocardial biopsy can be misleading.

Open biopsy of the lung is the only reliable method for providing tissue for a definitive diagnosis of rejection, but it is impractical to perform as a routine procedure because of its attendant morbidity. Bronchoscopy has been useful in the early postoperative period to clear secretions, but visual inspections of the airways during episodes of rejection have not revealed a suspicious mucosal appearance. Biopsy of the mucosa has consistently shown mild non-specific inflammatory changes from the early postoperative period (Reitz *et al.*, 1982; Baldwin *et al.*, 1985; Griffith *et al.*, 1987a). Transbronchial biopsies have been rarely performed, because they had been found to be unhelpful in canine experiments, and exposed the patient to significant risk of bleeding and pneumothorax (Veith, 1978). Early in our experience, open biopsy of the lung helped to define the histology of pulmonary rejection and alerted us to its presence in the absence of cardiac rejection. Cyto-immunological studies based upon peripheral and intra-alveolar lymphocytes hold promise for the future (Emeson, 1983; Duquesnoy *et al.*, 1985; Ertel *et al.*, 1985; Fung *et al.*, 1985; Gryzan *et al.*, 1985; Zeevi *et al.*, 1985;

Kirby *et al.*, 1986). At present, the diagnosis of acute rejection of the lung is based upon a typical opacified appearance of the chest radiograph and its rapid resolution following augmented immunosuppression (Griffith, 1987b). The accuracy of this clinically applied method has improved with experience and with analysis of fluid returned from the lung by bronchoalveolar lavage.

Although the radiograph of the chest is the touchstone for acute pathology in the allograft, it is not helpful in assessing late obliterative changes in the small airways. Diagnosed as a form of bronchiolitis obliterans, the process is probably related to a chronic form of rejection. It is suspected from the results of spirometric investigations, and confirmed by open biopsy of the lung (McGregor *et al.*, 1986).

The purpose of this chapter is to demonstrate the histology and radiography of pulmonary rejection based upon clinical experience, and to describe clinical methods helpful in detection and in treatment. While much of the process remains empirical, it can be expected that, with increasing experience and pursuit of discriminating techniques, our diagnostic acumen will improve.

OPEN BIOPSY OF THE LUNG

Most of the information available about the histology of pulmonary rejection has been learned from canine experiments. Veith and co-workers postulate that rejection in the lung can be manifest in two ways (Veith, 1978). In the more common form, perivascular cuffs of lymphocytes and alveolar exudates made up of desquamated pneumocytes and inflammatory cells, including lymphocytes, are seen. The second form has been termed alveolar rejection, because fibrinous exudates occur with a paucity of round cells, and without perivascular inflammation. Although both forms are associated with radiographic opacification of the allograft and decreased ventilation, the alveolar form lacks a corresponding reduction in blood flow as assessed by nuclear scans. Further studies of unmodified rejection (Veith *et al.*, 1972), including that occurring in xenografts (Veith *et al.*, 1981), have shown progressive perivascular, peribronchial and parenchymal infiltrates of mononuclear cells, thickening of alveolar septa, and alveolar exudates containing fibrin, oedema, inflammatory cells and denuded pneumocytes. Ultimately, the process of rejection causes intimal proliferation, parenchymal haemorrhage and fibrinoid degeneration. A microscopic grading system has been suggested based upon experimental studies (Veith *et al.*, 1981) (Table 26.1).

The histology of the human process is less well established because there have been fewer recipients, due to the morbidity associated with open

TABLE 26.1
*Microscopic Grading System**

MILD REJECTION	Mononuclear cells are present in perivascular cuffs around the small pulmonary arteries and veins, with occasional round cell infiltrates in the intra-alveolar spaces. Such changes are scattered among large areas of completely normal lung
MODERATE REJECTION	Perivascular mononuclear cell cuffing involves most of the pulmonary vasculature. The alveoli contain some oedema fluid, fibrinous exudate, and round cell infiltrates containing polymorphonuclear leucocytes and desquamated pneumocytes. The bronchioles also show cuffing and have round cells and some oedema fluid in their lumina
MODERATELY ADVANCED REJECTION	The mononuclear cellular infiltration encompasses nearly the entire xenograft vasculature and all bronchioles. There is marked vascular intimal hyperplasia and occlusion of alveolar spaces by fibrinous exudate containing inflammatory cells and sloughed pneumocytes. There is early necrosis of alveolar septa
ADVANCED REJECTION	The pulmonary architecture is replaced by necrotic alveolar and vascular tissue. Masses of erythrocytes and fibrin denote pulmonary infarction

* After Veith, F. J. (1972). *J. Thorac. Cardiovasc. Surg.*, **63**, 509–520.

biopsy, and because infection, which is often coexistent, confuses the interpretation (Kamholtz *et al.*, 1983). Five of our patients underwent biopsy when isolated rejection was suspected. While no patient died or developed a persistent air leak as a consequence of biopsy, one patient developed an aspiration pneumonia, and all complained of significant post-thoracotomy pain. These biopsies showed variable degrees of hyperplasia of the alveolar lining and alveolar spaces containing dequamative pneumocytes, macrophages and fibrinous debris (Fig. 26.1). Alveolar septa contained variable numbers of round cells and polymorphonuclear cells. The interstitium usually was oedematous with accumulations of fibrin and histiocytes. Peribronchial and perivascular oedema and infiltration by round cells were present focally (Fig. 26.2). Frequently, many areas displayed non-specific changes common to the response of the lung to any injury. Therefore, an effort is made to sample ample tissue from a radiographically suspicious area. Open biopsy is now considered only when a radiographic abnormality does not resolve rapidly after intravenous pulses of steroid, and when co-existing infection or sepsis increases the risk of empirically augmented immunosuppression.

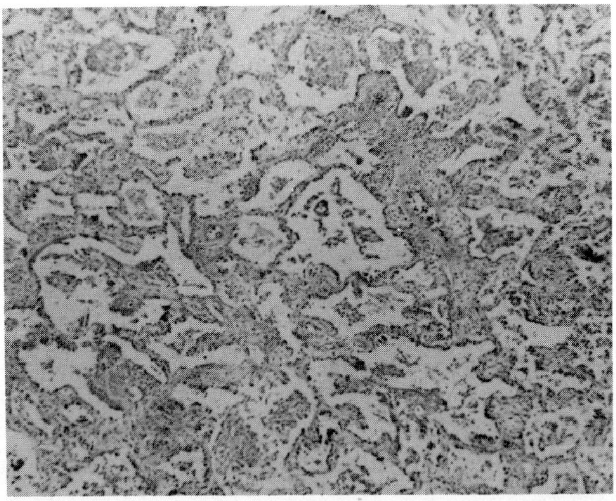

Fig. 26.1. *Open lung biopsy showing hyperplasia of the alveolar lining, and alveolar spaces containing desquamated pneumocytes, macrophages and lymphocytes, and fibrinous debris. Septa are oedematous and contain inflammatory cells. H&E ×50.*

RADIOGRAPH OF THE CHEST

Subhuman primate experiments and the initial experience in humans suggested that rejection of the heart and lungs occurs synchronously and that the endomyocardial biopsy adequately diagnoses the process in both organs

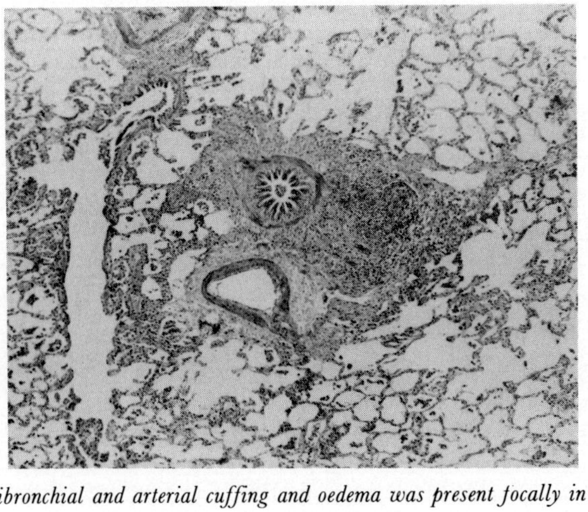

Fig. 26.2. *Peribronchial and arterial cuffing and oedema was present focally in most specimens. H&E ×45.*

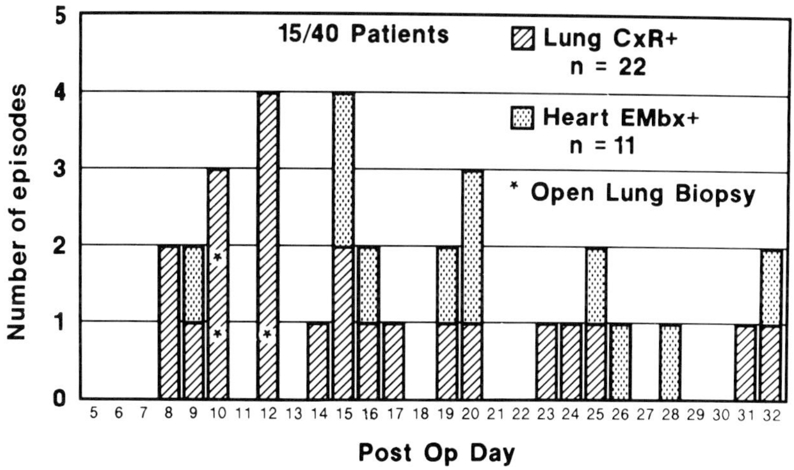

Fig. 26.3. *Asymmetrical pattern of rejection after heart–lung transplantation. Rejection was frequent in the pulmonary allograft between 7 and 32 days. Lung CxR+, radiographic signs of rejection; heart EMbx+, rejection diagnosed by endomyocardial biopsy. (From Griffith, B. P. (1978b) Transplant. Proc.,* ***19****.)*

(Reitz *et al.*, 1983). This conferred a potentially great advantage on combined transplantation of heart and lungs because it was presumed that an abnormal chest radiograph in the absence of cardiac rejection would be due to an infectious process. Unfortunately, the endomyocardial biopsy is now known to be useful only in that it sometimes confirms the clinical impression of pulmonary rejection. Significant myocyte necrosis is rarely, if ever, found in the absence of an abnormal chest radiograph, and in fact myocardial necrosis has been extremely uncommon. However, rejection of the lung is found to occur frequently without significant abnormalities in the endomyocardial biopsy (Griffith *et al.*, 1985; McGregor *et al.*, 1985) (Fig. 26.3). Rejection of the lung, as defined by an abnormal chest radiograph and its favourable response to treatment, occurs most commonly between 7 and 14 days postoperatively and has been diagnosed in more than half of our survivors (Griffith *et al.*, 1987b). It has been controlled in all but one recipient, who developed a fatal mediastinitis caused by *Staphylococcus aureus*. Interestingly, acute rejection has not been observed after the fifth postoperative week, and all subsequent radiographic abnormalities have been related to an infectious process.

The most common radiographic abnormality associated with pulmonary rejection has been the gradual onset over 12–36 h of a homogeneous opacification of the parenchyma. Early, the opacification often has an intra-alveolar pattern or 'popcorn' appearance which, if untreated, progresses to a more consolidated, diffuse pattern over 24 h. The process is usually bilat-

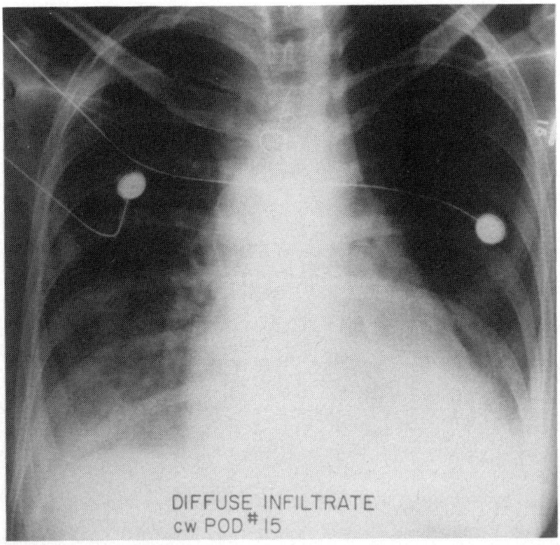

Fig. 26.4(a). *Typical radiographic opacification of the pulmonary allograft due to rejection, proven in this instance by open biopsy of the lung.*

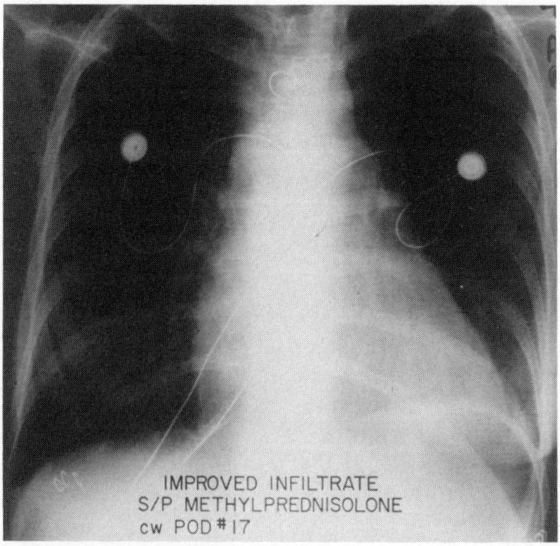

Fig. 26.4(b). *Rapid clearing of radiograph following augmented immunsuppression.*

eral, but in our experience the right lung and the lower lobes have been more obviously affected. Pleural effusions frequently co-exist, but are small and have not occurred as the sole radiographic abnormality (Fig. 26.4). Rapid improvement within 12 h and clearing within 48–72 h after daily doses of intravenous methylprednisolone (1 g) has been the rule (Fig. 26.5). Since rejection is associated with radiological opacification caused by inflammation and oedema of the interstitium and alveolar spaces, it is not surprising that identical changes have been noted after transplantation from inadequate *ex vivo* or *in vivo* preservation of the organs of the donor, from a response to reimplantation, and more importantly from infections. In these situations, the chest radiograph is not discriminating. Pneumonia caused by bacteria, viruses, protozoa and fungi is common, and its differentiation from a process of rejection is critical to the choice of life-saving therapy. On one occasion, a recipient was readmitted to the hospital on the 26th postoperative day with fever and a diffuse pulmonary infiltrate. Bronchoalveolar lavage (BAL) failed to reveal infection, and methylprednisolone was given daily for 3 days. Mild improvement was evanescent, and the patient expired from cytomegalic viral pneumonia (Fig. 26.6a–c).

BRONCHOALVEOLAR LAVAGE

A unique diagnostic aid in transplantation of the lung, BAL is a source of immunocompetent cells, and is performed at least once during the first month after transplantation, at 2–3-month intervals thereafter, and whenever an episode of infection or rejection is suspected.

The analysis of the cells recovered by BAL provides useful information regarding infection and may help to elucidate the allogenic response and permit a differential diagnosis of rejection (Griffith *et al.*, 1987a). Cellular profiles of rejection have shown a total cell count of $72 \pm 39 \times 10^6$ cells, composed of $43 \pm 10 \times 10^6$ macrophages, $6 \pm 2.1 \times 10^6$ lymphocytes and $23 \pm 27 \times 10^6$ polymorphonuclear cells. The increase in the total cell count from the $28 \pm 9 \times 10^6$ cells counted in recipients devoid of infection or rejection, has been significant. These recipients had lower numbers of macrophages ($22 \pm 9 \times 10^6$) and of polymorphonuclear cells ($3 \pm 5 \times 10^6$). Bacterial pneumonia has been distinguished by a rise in polymorphonuclear cells to $182 \pm 21 \times 10^6$, and infection with *Pneumocystis carinii* by a rise in macrophages to $34 \pm 23 \times 10^6$ and lymphocytes to $38 \pm 20 \times 10^6$. Cytomegalic viral infections have been associated with similar increases in macrophages and lymphocytes. All infections of the lung are associated with elevated total cell counts.

It was hoped initially that the cell profiles alone would provide ready discrimination between the multiple causes of parenchymal opacification of

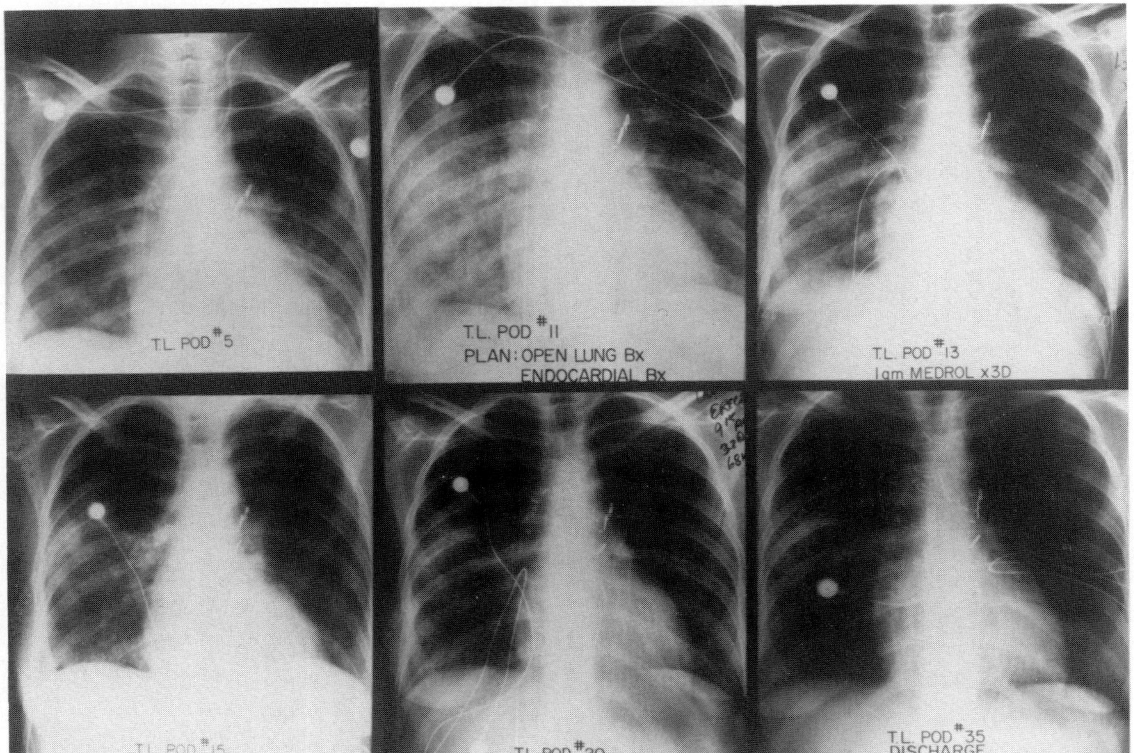

Fig. 26.5. *Isolated rejection of the lung that cleared following intravenous methylprednisolone. (From Griffith, B. P. (1985) Ann. Thorac. Surg.* ***40****, 488.)*

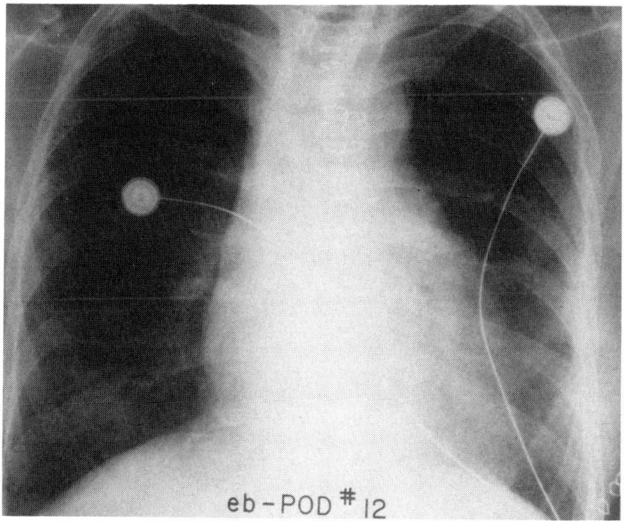

Fig. 26.6(a). *Normal radiograph 12 days after transplantation.*

the transplanted lung, including rejection, viral pneumonia, respiratory distress syndromes, and even difficult-to-diagnose diffuse protozoan and bacterial infections. As previously described, misdiagnosis of the causes has resulted in death (Fig. 26.6a–c). While many data have been obtained by

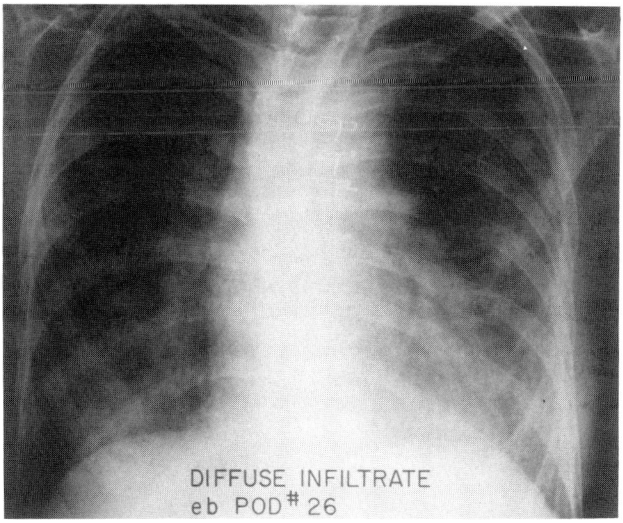

Fig. 26.6(b). *Radiograph of patient upon readmission on the 26th postoperative day. Clinical and radiographic picture suggesting rejection.*

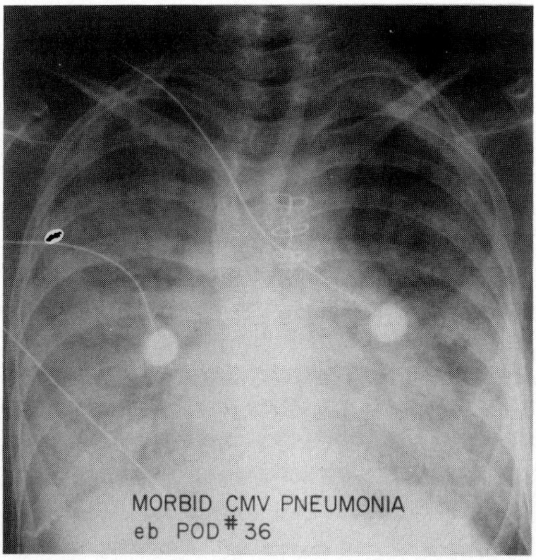

Fig. 26.6(c). *Unfortunately, a misdiagnosis of rejection was made and after initial improvement in the radiograph the patient's condition worsened and he died with an infection from cytomegalovirus.*

BAL in heart–lung recipients, too few patients have been studied prior to treatment for rejection to permit more than a broad range of cellular profiles to be included in the category of rejection, and unfortunately there is an overlap into categories of infection.

The current clinical role of BAL is the exclusion of infection by microscopy and culture. Staining of the lavage fluid has been useful for the diagnosis of *P. carinii* infection, but cytomegalic viral pneumonia has been missed (Dummer *et al.*, 1985). However, indirect immunoperoxidase staining of monoclonal antibodies against cytomegalovirus has recently shown promise as a sensitive early assay for active infection.

Functional analysis of cells has shown that lymphocytes exhibit significant spontaneous proliferation and interleukin-2 response. The lymphocytes are far more likely than peripheral blood lymphocytes to express high levels of cell-mediated lympholysis (CML activity) during episodes of rejection. Cytological immune monitoring of lymphoblasts from peripheral blood has not been of value in our experience, but has been useful for others (Ertel *et al.*, 1985).

The results of HLA phenotyping of BAL lymphocytes and macrophages reveal that during the first 6 weeks after transplantation, transplanted cells of the donor are incompletely replaced by those of the recipient, suggesting a reason for the high incidence of early rejection.

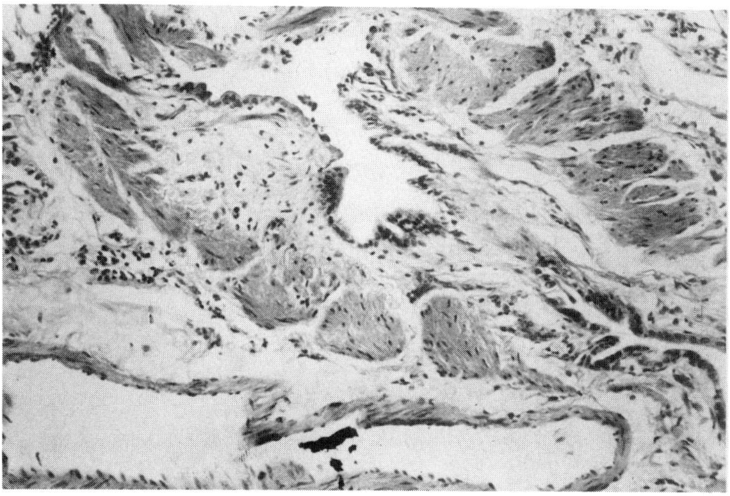

Fig. 26.7. *Bland submucosal infiltrate and occluding fibrosis in a small airway in a patient with progressive loss of forced expiratory volumes.* × *20.*

LONG-TERM ALLOGRAFT FUNCTION

In our experience a moderate restrictive defect and a mild impairment of the diffusing capacity has been present after 1.5 months. After the first 6 months only a mild, restrictive defect remains, and most recipients have a normal capacity for exercise. There is a significant improvement in the diffusing capacity over the first 12 months. Function of the airway (FEV_1, FVC and FEF_{25-75}), which is normal after 1.5 months, does decline with time, but this change generally has been minimal and significant in only 3 patients. Two have developed chronic bronchitis with *Pseudomonas aeruginosa*, and 1 patient has bronchiolitis obliterans.

Histological study of the patient with bronchiolitis showed focal submucosal fibrosis of the bronchioles with occasional areas of round-cell inflammation consistent with bronchiolitis obliterans (Fig. 26.7). This finding has been noted by others and raises concerns regarding the long-term benefit of lung transplantation (McGregor *et al.*, 1985). Unfortunately, over the past 18 months the obstructive defect has been increasing slowly and the patient has an FEV_1 of 1 litre. BAL has shown an increased activity of lymphocytes by primed lymphocyte testing prior to each deterioration in airway function.

The cause of bronchiolitis after heart–lung transplantation is probably chronic rejection, but other factors, such as inefficient cough and mucociliary clearance, and ischaemia of the airway devoid of bronchial collateral circulation, might contribute. Bronchiolitis obliterans has been observed in various autoimmune disorders and as a manifestation of graft-versus-host disease after transplantation of bone marrow. At present, heart–lung recipients are maintained on an augmented triple drug regimen of prednisone, cyclosporin and azathioprine in the hope that the incidence of chronic airway disease will decrease. The onset of a productive cough without infection and evidence of progressive obstruction of the airway is an indication for increased immunosuppression.

CLINICAL APPROACH TO THE DIAGNOSIS OF REJECTION

The recipients of heart–lung allografts have established certain patterns that allow a reasonable approach to the diagnosis of rejection. The endomyocardial biopsy has not been helpful, and in fact may not be needed as a routine procedure, since isolated cardiac rejection has not occurred with any frequency. When the endomyocardial biopsy demonstrates myocardial inflammation, an infectious process responsible for an opacification of the lung must be excluded. It is unlikely that survivable rejection will occur prior to the end of the first postoperative week, as the earliest the diagnosis was made in our series was 7 days. Prior to 7 days, the chest radiograph often shows opacifications related in some combination to pre-existing injury in the donor, operative trauma, inadequate preservation, infection, and perhaps the elusive re-implantation response. Usually, considerable clearing of early opacification occurs and changes associated with later-occurring cell-mediated rejection can be recognized.

It is probable that the changes associated with rejection occur over 12–24 h. Frequent radiographic studies are indicated between 7 and 21 days in order that the process can be diagnosed in its reversible, early stages. Early rejection has rarely been associated with clinical symptoms such as shortness of breath, cough, and deterioration of arterial blood gases. Because of concern about the deleterious effects of steroids upon healing and infection, pulse therapy with methylprednisolone is initiated only when a number of observers agree about a change in the radiograph and only after infection has been excluded to a near certainty, usually by analysis of bronchoalveolar lavage fluid. At present, we would not hesitate to use augmented immunosuppression when the profile of cells from the lavage is atypical, so long as infection has been excluded. We have confidence that, with additional clinical and experimental experience, the BAL will be a discriminating diagnostic aid.

Acute rejection will not often occur after 4 weeks, and any late changes should strongly suggest an infectious aetiology. Bacterial pneumonias are most common early, but can occur at any time and are relatively easy to detect by culture and clinical presentation. Fungal, viral and protozoan infections are more difficult and continue to challenge. Fungal infections plague transplant recipients, and usually occur during treatment of bacterial infection with antimicrobials. The radiographic changes seen in pneumonia from CMV and *P. carinii* infections have been indistinguishable from those of rejection. The earliest CMV pneumonia which has occurred has been during the fifth postoperative week, and the diagnosis of late rejection was made initially. *Pneumocystis carinii* infections have been common, but generally are not seen until after the third month.

Frequent spirometry and follow-up are necessary to detect early bronchitis and bronchiolitis obliterans. It is likely that these chronic problems will respond to augmented maintenance immunosuppression. Additional research must be completed to clarify the role of the allogenic response in this chronic process and to elucidate appropriate and, we hope, preventive therapy.

Although much of our current method is empirical, it is based upon hard-learned experiences and is providing a reasonable outcome for our patients. It is hoped that future development in the analysis of the fluid from the bronchoalveolar lavage will provide us with a tool that would have an impact similar to that of endomyocardial biopsy for cardiac transplantation.

REFERENCES

Baldwin, J. C., Jamieson, S. W., Oyer, P. E., Stinson, E. B., Billingham, M. E., Shumway, N. E. and Mark, J. B. (1985). Bronchoscopy after cardiopulmonary transplantation. *J. Thorac. Cardiovasc. Surg.* **89**, 1–7.

Dummer, J. S., White, L. T., Ho, M., Griffith, B. P., Hardesty, R. L. and Bahnson, H. T. (1985). Morbidity of cytomegalovirus infection in recipients of heart and heart–lung transplantation who received cyclosporine. *J. Infect. Dis.* **152**(6), 1182–1191.

Duquesnoy, R. J., Zeevi, A., Fung, J., Paradis, I., Dauber, J., Griffith, B. and Hardesty, R. L. (1985). Functional characterization of lymphocytes in bronchoalveolar lavage from heart lung transplant patients. *Heart Transplant.* **4**, 135.

Emeson, E. E., Norin, A. J., Kamholtz, S. L., Pinsker, K. L. and Veith, F. J. (1983). Cytotoxic T-cells and suppressor macrophages in bronchoalveolar lavage: an index to lung allograft rejection in cyclosporin A-treated dogs. *Transplant. Proc.* **15**, 550.

Ertel, W., Reichenspurner, H., Lersch, C., Hammer, C., Plahl, M., Lehmann, M., Kemkes, B. M., Osterholzer, G., Reble, B., Reichart, B. and Brendel, W. (1985). Cytoimmunologic monitoring in acute rejection and viral, bacterial, or fungal infection following transplantation. *Heart Transplant.* **4**, 390–394.

Fung, J. J., Zeevi, A., Kaufman, C., Paradis, I. L., Dauber, J. H., Hardesty, R. L., Griffith, B. and Duquesnoy, R. J. (1985). Interactions between bronchoalveolar lymphocytes and macrophages in heart–lung transplant recipients. *Human Immunol.* **14**, 287–294.

Griffith, B. P., Hardesty, R. L., Trento, A., Paradis, I. L., Duquesnoy, R. J., Zeevi, A., Dauber, J. H., Dunner, J. S., Thompson, M. E., Gryzan, S. and Bahnson, H. T. (1987a). Heart–lung transplantation: lessons learned and future hopes. *Ann. Thorac. Surg.* **43**, 6–17.

Griffith, B. P., Hardesty, R. L., Trento, A. and Bahnson, H. T. (1985). Asynchronous rejection of heart and lungs following cardiopulmonary transplantation. *Ann. Thorac. Surg.* **40**, 488–493.

Griffith, B. P., Durham, S. J., Hardesty, R. L., Trento, A., and Paradis, I. L. (1987b). Acute rejection of the heart–lung allograft and methods of its detection. *Transplant. Proc.* **19**, (1, pt 3), 2527–2530.

Gryzan, S., Paradis, I. L., Hardesty, R. L., Griffith, B. P. and Dauber, J. H. (1985). Bronchoalveolar lavage in heart–lung transplantation. *Heart Transplant.* **4**, 414–416.

Kamholtz, S. L., Veith, F. J., Mollenkopf, F. P., Pinsker, K. L., Kaleya, R. R., Norin, A. J., Gliedman, M. L., Emeson, E. E., Merav, A. D., Brodman, R., Fell, S. C., Sheldon, M. and Montefusco, C. M. (1983). Single lung transplantation with cyclosporin immunosuppression. Evaluation of canine and human recipients. *J. Thorac. Cardiovasc. Surg.* **86**, 537–542.

Kirby, J. A., Pepper, J. R., Reader, J. A., Corbishley, C. M. and Hudson, L. (1986). Precursor frequency of donor-specific lymphocytes recovered from canine lung transplants. *Clin. Exp. Immunol.* **63**, 334–342.

McGregor, C. G. A., Baldwin, J. C., Jamieson, S. W., Billingham, M. E., Yousem, S. A., Burke, C. M., Oyer, P. E., Stinson, E. B. and Shumway, N. E. (1985). Isolated pulmonary rejection after combined heart–lung transplantation. *J. Thorac. Cardiovasc. Surg.* **90**, 623–626.

McGregor, C. G. A., Jamieson, S. W., Baldwin, J. C., Burke, C. M., Dawkins, K. D., Stinson, E. B., Oyer, P. E., Billingham, M. E., Zusman, D. R., Reitz, B. A., Morris, A., Yousem, S., Hunt, S. A. and Shumway, N. E. (1986). Combined heart and lung transplantation for end-stage Eisenmenger's syndrome. *J. Thorac. Cardiovasc. Surg.* **91**, 443–450.

Reitz, B. A., Burton, N. A., Jamieson, S. W., Bieber, C. P., Pennock, J. L., Stinson, E. B. and Shumway, N. E. (1980). Heart and lung transplantation. *J. Thorac. Cardiovasc. Surg.* **80**, 360–372.

Reitz, B. A., Gaudiani, V. A., Hunt, S. A., Wallwork, J., Billingham, M. E., Oyer, P. E., Baumgartner, W. A., Jamieson, S. W., Stinson, E. B. and Shumway, N. E. (1983). Diagnosis and treatment of allograft rejection in heart–lung transplant recipients. *J. Thorac. Cardiovasc. Surg.* **85**, 354–361.

Reitz, B. A., Wallwork, J., Hunt, S. A., Pennock, J. L., Billingham, M. E., Oyer P. E., Stinson, E. B. and Shumway, N. E. (1982). Heart–lung transplantation: successful therapy for patients with pulmonary vascular disease. *New Engl. J. Med.* **306**, 557–564.

Veith, F. J. (1978). Lung transplantation. *Surg. Clin. N. Am.* **58**, 357.

Veith, F. J., Richards, K. U., Hagstrom, J. W. C. and Montefusco, C. M. (1981). Intrafamilial lung xenografts from fox to dog. *J. Thorac. Cardiovasc. Surg.* **81**, 546–552.

Veith, F. J., Sinha, S. B. P., Blümcke, S., Dougherty, J. C., Becker, N. H., Siegelman, S. S. and Hagstrom, J. W. C. (1972). Nature and evolution of lung allograft rejection with and without immunosuppression. *J. Thorac. Cardiovasc. Surg.* **63**, 509–520.

Zeevi, A., Fung, J. J., Paradis, I. L., Dauber, J. H., Griffith, B. P., Hardesty, R. L. and Duquesnoy, R. J. (1985). Lymphocytes of bronchoalveolar lavages from heart–lung transplant recipients. *Heart Transplant.* **4**, 417–421.

Tim Higenbottam and Susan Stewart

27

Transbronchial Lung Biopsy in the Diagnosis of Rejection of the Transplanted Lungs

INTRODUCTION

The initial belief that, by combining heart and lung transplantation, rejection of the lungs could be monitored by endomyocardial biopsy (Reitz *et al.*, 1983) has proved to be illusory. Experimentally (Cooper *et al.*, 1986) and clinically (McGregor *et al.*, 1985), lung rejection develops before cardiac rejection and independently from it. Moreover, lung rejection manifests itself more aggressively than cardiac rejection in these patients.

The inadequacy of non-invasive clinical methods to distinguish between infection and rejection of the lungs has probably contributed to the reported high prevalence of chronic rejection, obliterative bronchiolitis (Burke *et al.*, 1984; Tazelaar *et al.*, 1987) and of opportunistic infection (Dummer, 1986). What has been lacking is an effective and *repeatable* method of obtaining lung tissue for histology.

Lung tissue can be obtained repeatedly via a fibre-optic bronchoscope using the technique of transbronchial biopsy (TBB) (Levin, Weiss and Ellis, 1974). This method has previously been used effectively to diagnose certain forms of diffuse lung disease, particularly sarcoidosis, and some opportunistic infections (Feldman, Pennington and Ehrie, 1977; Abe *et al.*, 1984; Swuer *et al.*, 1984).

In other forms of lung disease this method of biopsy is less reliable and recourse to open lung biopsy may be necessary. Clinical use in lung transplantation has not been systematic (Burke *et al.*, 1984). It should be emphasized that in sarcoidosis at least four biopsies need to be taken (Murray and Wang, 1980). In dogs, Koerner found that TBBs were inadequate (Koerner, Hagstrom and Veith, 1976), and with the introduction of 'alligator' forceps it is possible to obtain larger specimens. However, fluoroscopic guidance is needed in addition, to position the open forceps correctly in the periphery of the lung.

USE OF TRANSBRONCHIAL BIOPSY IN THE MANAGEMENT OF REJECTION

Heart–lung transplant patients appear to be particularly sensitive to changes in lung function. Early in the onset of lung disease, they complain of breathlessness and chest tightness. The physical signs of crackles and wheezes are heard before the chest radiograph changes.

At Papworth, spirometry is performed regularly and if the FEV_1 falls in association with symptoms and physical signs a TBB is performed (see Chapter 28).

A total of 40 biopsies have been undertaken in 21 patients (Higenbottam *et al.*, 1987). In 8 patients an opportunistic infection was diagnosed from 16 biopsies; these were, 1 case of tuberculous empyema, 5 patients with cytomegalovirus (CMV) pneumonitis and 2 patients with *Pneumocystis carinii* pneumonia. Eleven patients experienced some 20 'episodes' of rejection. These were associated with a fall in spirometry which recovered with augmented immunosuppression on 19 occasions.

In 19 'episodes' of rejection, TBBs were taken — at least 4 specimens from one lung under fluoroscopic control. One patient was diagnosed clinically. Five sets of biopsies were also taken when patients were well, 3 of these after recovery from rejection.

All biopsies were fixed in 10% neutral buffered formaline solution and processed in a Shandon Hypercentre either overnight or within 2 h according to urgency. Initially, biopsies were cut at several levels, 5 μm apart, but the patchy distribution of abnormalities has led to serial sectioning of all material. Sections were routinely stained with haematoxylin and eosin, methyl green pyronine, Perl's/elastic Van Gieson, periodic acid Schiff and Grocott's methenamine silver method. In addition, Ziehl–Nielsen staining for acid-fast bacillus was performed where indicated. Accompanying bronchial aspirates were stained by Papanicolaou's method, with Grocott preparations as necessary.

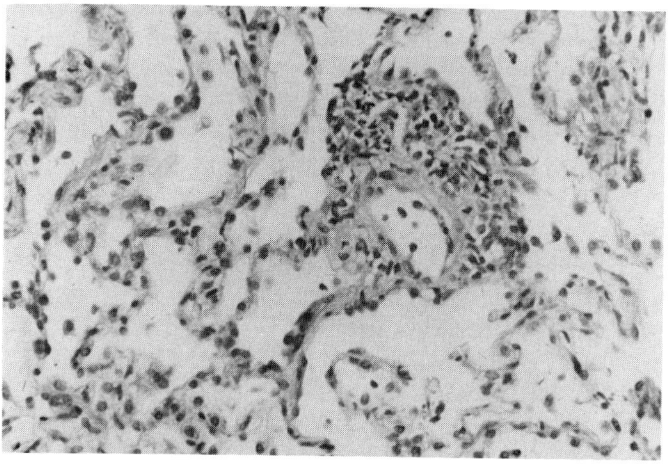

Fig. 27.1. *Perivascular lymphocytic infiltrate.* × *105.*

HISTOLOGICAL APPEARANCE OF REJECTION ON TRANSBRONCHIAL BIOPSY

The commonest pattern of rejection seen in TBBs is scattered foci of perivascular pyroninophilic mononuclear lymphoid cells with minimal infiltration of alveolar walls. The circumscribed infiltrate is usually densely cellular, and may be associated with mild oedema of the vessel wall (Fig. 27.1). Subendothelial lymphocytic infiltration has not been seen on biopsy. These observations are similar to the changes of acute rejection in animal studies and from clinical studies at open lung biopsy and post mortem in rejection (Veith *et al.*, 1972, 1983; Burke *et al.*, 1984; Prop, Wildevuur and Nieuwenhuis, 1985). Other abnormalities seen with perivascular infiltrates are rather non-specific and include focal intra-alveolar oedema or haemorrhage, desquamated pneumocytes and haemosiderin-laden macrophages. Focal alveolar cell hyperplasia is also commonly seen.

Most TBBs have accompanying airway mucosa and submucosa which show in rejection active acute or chronic inflammation involving the epithelial surface, and mucosa-associated lymphoid tissue (Fig. 27.2). This inflammation of the mucosa, in the absence of altered sputum bacteriology, is a very useful indicator of rejection and is readily recognized even in detached strips of mucosa. Some areas show prominent numbers of eosinophils in the acute inflammatory infiltrate, but these do not correlate with severity of rejection. Squamous metaplasia is seen in some mucosal biopsies showing active rejection.

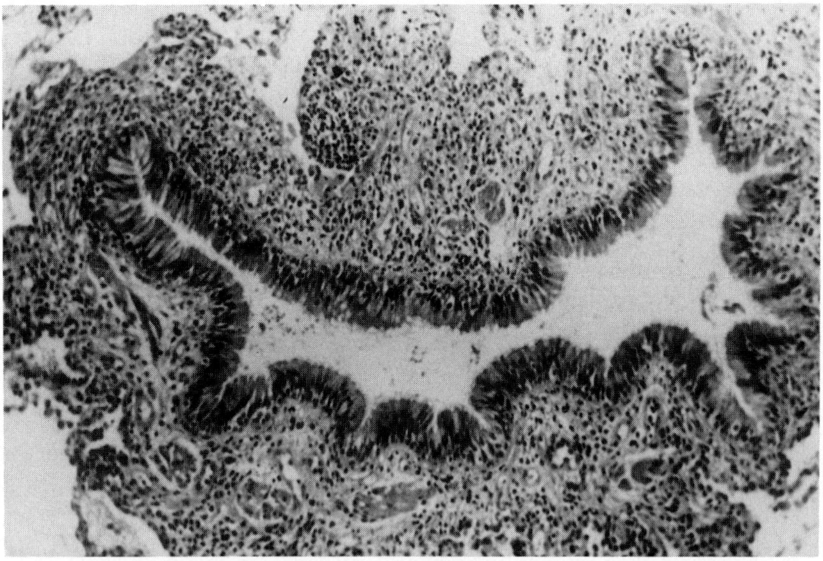

Fig. 27.2. *Mixed cell inflammation of the bronchiolar mucosa and epithelium.* × *60.*

In addition to inflammation of the mucosa of large airways, active bronchiolitis is a striking feature of acute rejection and is often present in TBBs. The inflammatory cell infiltrate varies in density and pyroninophilia (Fig. 27.3). The bronchioles may contain mucopurulent debris and may show

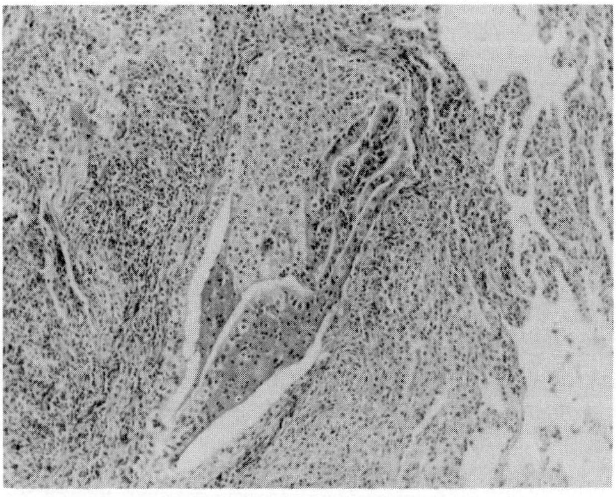

Fig. 27.3. *Mucopurulent material in an intensely inflamed bronchiolar mucosa.* × *70.*

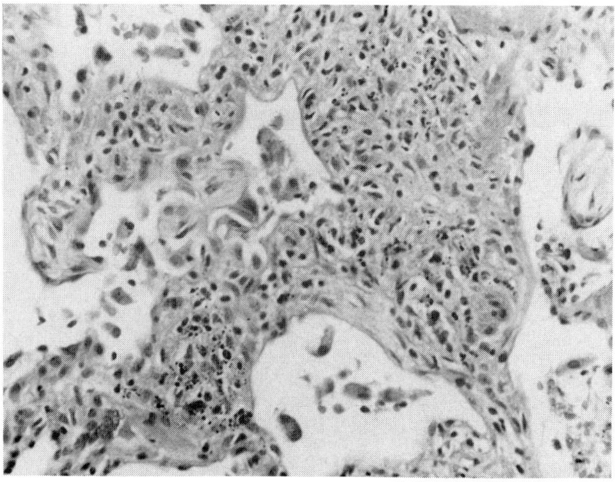

Fig. 27.4. *Inflammatory infiltration of alveolar walls in advanced lung rejection.* × *105.*

complete sloughing of the epithelium in acute episodes. We have seen 2 cases in which large numbers of plasma cells were associated with active bronchiolitis. The histological appearances of the different fragments of lung parenchyma obtained transbronchially may differ considerably, as the perivascular infiltration and bronchiolitis can be very patchy. In association with acute bronchiolitis and vascular rejection, we have noted loose fibromyxoid connective tissue, often with central plasma cells, in bronchioles and alveolar spaces, consistent with the early stages of obliterative bronchiolitis. Dense collagen fibrosis is not seen at this stage, implying reversibility with increased immunosuppression. We have obtained normal TBBs in 3 patients after treated rejection episodes.

More advanced pulmonary rejection is revealed as greater mucosal necrosis and extension of pyroninophilic perivascular mononuclear cells into alveolar walls with consequent thickening. The alveolar spaces show more extensive desquamation of pneumocytes and more diffuse type 2 cell hyperplasia. The TBBs usually still show some relatively normal alveolar tissue with focal perivascular infiltrates, pointing to rejection as the cause of the abnormalities (Fig. 27.4). All our patients have been immunosuppressed with cyclosporin, and severe pulmonary rejection with haemorrhagic necrosis has not been seen. A classification of microscopic grades of rejection has been suggested in Chapter 26 on the basis of Veith's observations in the 1970s. This is analogous to Billingham's grading system for cardiac rejection, and would seem to be applicable, with modification, to TBBs of pulmonary grafts. As much of the earlier work concentrated on open lung or transthoracic needle biopsies, the inflammatory changes in the large airways have not been studied in such detail, but should now be included in a grading system for TBBs. As the rejection becomes more severe, so does the degree of mucosal necrosis and the extent of interstitial infiltration in the lung samples.

RESULTS OF TRANSBRONCHIAL BIOPSIES IN LUNG REJECTION

From the 19 episodes of rejection, finally diagnosed by improvement of FEV_1 and symptoms with augmented immunosuppression, 16 sets of biopsies showed perivascular infiltration, and 12 active mucosal inflammation. One biopsy was normal in a patient who died and who at necropsy was found to have extensive pulmonary fibrosis and end-stage obliterative bronchiolitis. Two early biopsies were minimally abnormal, with alveolar exudate but no perivascular infiltrate (Prop, Wildenuir and Nieuwenhuis). This gives an overall sensitivity of 84% (Higenbottam *et al.*, 1987).

In the 5 sets of biopsies obtained when patients were well, 3 after an episode of rejection, a normal histological appearance was observed. In 2 sets there were single perivascular infiltrates, being quantitatively far less than in patients with overt rejection. These may represent minimal rejection.

The biopsies obtained from patients with opportunistic infections did not show the circumscribed perivascular infiltration so characteristic of rejection. The cases of cytomegalovirus pneumonitis with diagnostic 'owl's eye' inclusions showed more diffuse inflammatory infiltrate involving alveolar spaces and walls often with hyaline membranes. This infiltrate included focal collections of polymorphonuclear leucocytes in addition to variable pyronino philic lymphoid cells. Alveolar cell hyperplasia was more pronounced and diffuse than in cases of rejection, including those biopsies without diagnostic viral inclusions. The histological picture of diffuse alveolar damage with interstitial and alveolar polymorphs, intra-alveolar fibrin and enlarged alveolar lining cells was readily distinguished from all the degrees of rejection seen on TBBs. In the clinical setting of a donor/recipient CMV mismatch, a biopsy showing these features was considered sufficiently suggestive of CMV pneumonitis to begin appropriate therapy. The vascular abnormalities in both the pre-inclusion CMV and diagnostic CMV biopsies were mural oedema, loosely aggregated acute and chronic inflammatory cells and endothelial cell enlargement. Only one patient with primary CMV transmitted by donor organs has shown a focus of dense perivascular infiltrate in an early biopsy, in association with an active alveolitis and endothelial hyperplasia. A subsequent biopsy confirmed CMV pneumonitis, and it is possible that the original biopsy represented concomitant rejection and CMV infection.

The other opportunistic infection encountered in two patients was *Pneumocystis carinii*. In one case the histological appearances were quite distinct from those of rejection with a granulomatous reaction to foamy exudate 'silver-staining' pneumocystis and no evidence of a perivascular distribution of mononuclear cells. We have not seen granulomas in allograft rejection. The second case had occasional perivascular inflammatory foci related to 3 previous biopsy-proven rejection episodes, but most of the biopsy showed non-specific mild interstitial inflammation together with typical foamy intra-alveolar exudate.

COMPARISON OF TRANSBRONCHIAL BIOPSIES WITH OTHER TECHNIQUES OF DIAGNOSING REJECTION

The chest radiographs were abnormal in 8 out of 20 episodes of rejection. This gives a sensitivity of only 40%. The commonest finding was diffuse bilateral shadowing. This appearance was similar in both CMV pneumonitis and *P. carinii* pneumonia (Higenbottam *et al.*, 1987)

One hundred and six endomyocardial biopsies were obtained from the 21 patients and only one showed evidence of significant rejection. This was a single focus of moderate rejection and was not treated. Five myocardial biopsies were performed concurrently with TBBs which showed lung rejection. None of these myocardial biopsies was significantly abnormal.

In one patient an open lung biopsy confirmed the TBB result of 3 weeks earlier, showing obliterative bronchiolitis, perivascular and septal mononuclear cell infiltration. Autopsy 20 months later revealed extensive obliterative bronchiolitis, intra-alveolar and interstitial fibrosis with minimal cellular infiltration.

THE PLACE OF TRANSBRONCHIAL BIOPSY IN LUNG REJECTION

From our early experience of TBB, it would seem to have a very important place in the diagnosis and management of rejection. Not only does the technique help to exclude the opportunistic infection, where the chest radiograph is unhelpful, but it appears sensitive in detecting rejection.

At present, we advocate regular spirometry, and if the FEV_1 falls in association with symptoms, even when the chest radiograph is normal, TBB is performed. Histology combined with clinical investigation offers an early diagnosis of rejection.

Further work is necessary to allow prediction of the stage of development of rejection. However, as the method is easily repeatable, this information will soon be forthcoming.

Open lung biopsy should be reserved for cases for whom re-transplantation is considered, when extensive disease is present.

REFERENCES

Abe, S., Munakata, M., Nishimura, M., Tsuneta, Y., Terai, T., Nakano, I., Oshaki, Y. and Kawakami, Y. (1984). Gallium 67 scintigraphy, bronchoalveolar lavage and pathologic changes in patients with pulmonary sarcoidosis. *Chest* **85**, 650–655.

Burke, C. M., Theodore, J., Dawkins, K. D., Yousem, S. A., Blank, N., Billingham, M. E., Van Kessel, A., Jamieson, S. W., Oyer, P. E., Baldwin, J. C., Stinson, E. B., Shumway, N. E. and Robin, E. D. (1984). Post-transplant obliterative bronchiolitis and other late lung sequelae in human heart–lung transplantation. *Chest* **86**, 824–829.

Cooper, D. A. C., Novitzky, D., Rose, A. G. and Reichart, B. A. (1986). Acute pulmonary rejection precedes cardiac rejection following heart–lung transplantation in a primate model. *J. Heart Transplant.* **5**, 129–131.

Dummer, J. S. (1986). Infections in heart–lung transplant recipients. *Transplantation* **41**, 725–729.

Feldman, N. T., Pennington, J. E. and Ehrie, M. G. (1977). Transbronchial lung biopsy in the immunocompromised host. *J. Am. Med. Ass.* **238**, 1377–1379.

Higenbottam, T. W., Stewart, S., Penketh, A. R. L. and Wallwork, J. (1987). The diagnosis of lung rejection and opportunistic infection by transbronchial lung biopsy. *Transplant Proc.* **19**, 3777–3778.

Koerner, S. K., Hagstrom, J. W. C. and Veith, F. J. (1976). Transbronchial biopsy for the diagnosis of lung transplant rejection: comparison with needle and open biopsy techniques in canine lung allograft. *Am. Rev. Resp. Dis.* **114**, 575–579.

Levin, D. C., Weiss, A. B. and Ellis, J. H. (1974). Transbronchial lung biopsy via the fibreoptic bronchoscope. *Am. Rev. Resp. Dis.* **110**, 4–12.

McGregor, C. G. A., Baldwin, J. C., Jamieson, S. W., Billingham, M. E., Yousem, S. A., Burke, C. M., Oyer, P. E., Stinson, E. B. and Shumway, N. E. (1985). Isolated pulmonary rejection after combined heart–lung transplantation. *J. Thorac. Cardiovasc. Surg.* **90**, 623–626.

Murray, J. G. and Wang, K. P. (1980). Transbronchial lung biopsy in sarcoidosis: an approach to determine the optimal number of biopsies. *Am. Rev. Resp. Dis.* **122**, 721–724.

Prop, J., Wildevuur, C. R. and Nieuwenhuis, P. (1985). Lung allograft rejection in the rat. III. Corresponding morphological rejection phases in various rat strain combinations. *Transplantation* **40**, 132–136.

Reitz, B. A., Guadiani, V. A., Hunt, S. A., Wallwork, J., Billingham, M. E. Oyer, P. E., Baumgartner, W. A., Jamieson, S. W., Stinson, E. B. and Shumway, N. E. (1983). Diagnosis and treatment of allograft rejection in heart–lung transplant recipients. *J. Thorac. Cardiovasc. Surg.* **85**, 354–361.

Swuer, D. E., Stover, D. E., White, D. A., Romana, P. A. and Gellen, R. A. (1984). Diagnosis of pulmonary disease in AIDS: role of bronchoscopy and broncho-alveolar lavage. *Am. Rev. Resp. Dis.* **130**, 659–662.

Tazelaar, H. D., Prop, J., Nieuwenhuis, P., Billingham, M. E. and Wildevuur, C. R. H. (1987). Obliterative bronchiolitis in the transplanted rat lung. *Transplant. Proc.* **xix**, 1052.

Veith, F. J., Kamholz, S. L., Mollenkopf, F. P. and Montefusco, C. M. (1983). Lung transplantation. *Transplantation* **35**, 271–278.

Veith, F. J., Sinha, S. B. P., Blümcke, S., Doughery, J. C., Becker, N. H., Siegelman, S. S. and Hagstrom, J. W. C.R (1972). Nature and evolution of lung allograft rejection with and without immunosuppression. *J. Thorac. Cardiovasc. Surg.* **63**, 509–520.

Tim Higenbottam

28

Physiology of the Transplanted Lungs and the Results

INTRODUCTION

It is surprising that the lungs continue to function so well after transplantation. The lung volume depends not only upon its own 'elastic' supporting structure, but also upon the integrity of the surrounding rib-cage and diaphragm (Mead, Takishara and Leith, 1970; Fung, 1977). The disturbance to both factors could pose enormous problems for early postoperative function. The established view of the control of breathing is that the timing and the volume of each breath depend upon afferent information from the lung travelling via the vagus nerve to the central pattern generator of respiration in the medulla (Euler, 1983). Transplantation, by causing total denervation of the lungs, should lead to a disordered pattern of breathing. In man, however, none of these factors appears to impede normal function of the transplanted lung (Theodore *et al.*, 1984).

The physiology of the lungs is well understood. A number of straightforward and reproducible tests is available to describe accurately and sensitively not only airway function but also gas exchange. These provide simple and non-invasive methods of monitoring the function of the transplanted lungs.

The purpose of this chapter is to review these issues and to illustrate how pulmonary function testing can be used to screen patients for opportunistic infection and rejection of the lung.

SUPPORTING STRUCTURES OF THE LUNGS

The volume which the lung adopts depends upon the balance of forces between those retracting the lungs to the hilum, namely the longitudinal elastic fibres of the airways and blood vessels and those expanding the chest wall (Mead, Takishara and Leith, 1970; Fung, 1977). This system depends upon mechanical coupling between the pleural surfaces.

In transplanting the lungs the most important matching is between the size of the thoracic cavity of the recipient and the volume of the donor lungs. At Papworth Hospital, Cambridge, this is achieved by measuring the total thoracic vertebral height of the donor and matching it to that of the recipient (see Chapter 23). This avoids the problem of attempting to insert lungs which are too large for the thoracic cavity. Where this has happened, atelectasis and right to left intrapulmonary shunting have occurred (Theodore *et al.*, 1984), compromising early postoperative survival.

After median sternotomy for routine cardiac operations, lung volume is reduced (Braun, Birnbaum and Chopra, 1987). It may take up to 6 months for the volume to return to normal. This appears to be the result of the thoracic spine becoming more curved and the ribs adopting an expiratory position (Kenyon, Pedley and Higenbottam, 1987). In heart–lung transplantation, a similar postoperative reduction in lung volume is observed, which appears to return to normal over 6 months (Theodore *et at.*, 1984).

CONTROL OF BREATHING

The established view of the control of breathing is that inspiration is initiated by specialized neurons of the central pattern generator in the medulla (Euler, 1983). The activity of these neurons progressively increases causing increasing activity of the inspiratory muscles, which in turn causes the volume of the lungs to change. A point is reached, at the end of each breath, at which this rising inspiratory neuron activity is 'switched off', and expiration follows (Sears, 1984). This 'switch off' depends upon increasing afferent information instructing the medullary neurons that the lungs have expanded. The afferent information is believed to come from pulmonary stretch receptors, or slowly adapting receptors (SARs) and is relayed in the vagal nerves (Euler, 1983).

Early studies on homologous transplantation of the lungs in non-primate animals showed that respiratory failure developed, the animals failing to sustain adequate ventilation. Characteristically, they exhibited a slowed frequency of breathing with larger breaths or tidal volumes (Nakae *et al.*, 1967; Mattila *et al.*, 1987). A similar pattern is seen following bilateral vagotomy (Favier *et al.*, 1982).

By contrast primates, including man, appear to breath normally after denervation (Nakae *et al.*, 1967; Reitz *et al.*, 1980). This poses a major question as to the importance of the vagus in the regulation of breathing in man. Physiological experiments have suggested that the vagus is important only during the increased ventilation rate of exercise (Winning *et al.*, 1985). However, after transplantation, not only are normal blood gases maintained (Theodore *et al.*, 1984), but during exercise the rate of ventilation responds in a similar pattern to that of normals (Theodore *et al.*, 1986) (Fig. 28.1). Further evidence that the breathing pattern after transplantation is normal comes from studies of rebreathing of carbon dioxide (Higenbottam, Fitzpatrick and Wallwork, 1987a). The increased ventilation which occurs as CO_2 rises in the arterial blood is achieved by progressive increases in tidal volume, the inspiratory timing remaining unchanged. This is exactly the same as is seen in normal individuals (Fig. 28.2). In other words, the pattern of breathing is normal despite the absence of vagal afferent information from the lungs.

These observations support the view that in man inspiratory timing, and also tidal volume, even when ventilation rate is increased, do not depend upon intact vagal innervation of the lungs. Instead, chest wall afferents are probably important, as has been suggested both in animals (Bland *et al.*, 1967) and neonates (Trippenoch, 1985). Effectively, after transplantation patients breathe normally at rest and during exercise.

POSTOPERATIVE LUNG FUNCTION

After transplantation, total lung capacity (TLC), and the forced expired volume in 1 sec (FEV_1) are reduced to a degree similar to that in other patients who undergo cardiopulmonary bypass (Fig. 28.3) (Theodore *et al.*, 1984; Wallwork *et al.*, 1987). The gas transfer for carbon monoxide (D_LCO) is also reduced (Fig. 28.3).

It takes up to 6 months for lung function to return to normal. This is probably the result of the spine and ribs returning to a normal position. The progressive improvement with time is best seen in patients with chronic lung disease who have undergone transplantation (Penketh *et al.*, 1987) (Fig. 28.4).

DETECTION OF REJECTION AND INFECTION IN TRANSPLANTED LUNGS

The major clinical complications occurring in patients after combined heart and lung transplantation are pulmonary and not cardiac in origin (Burke *et*

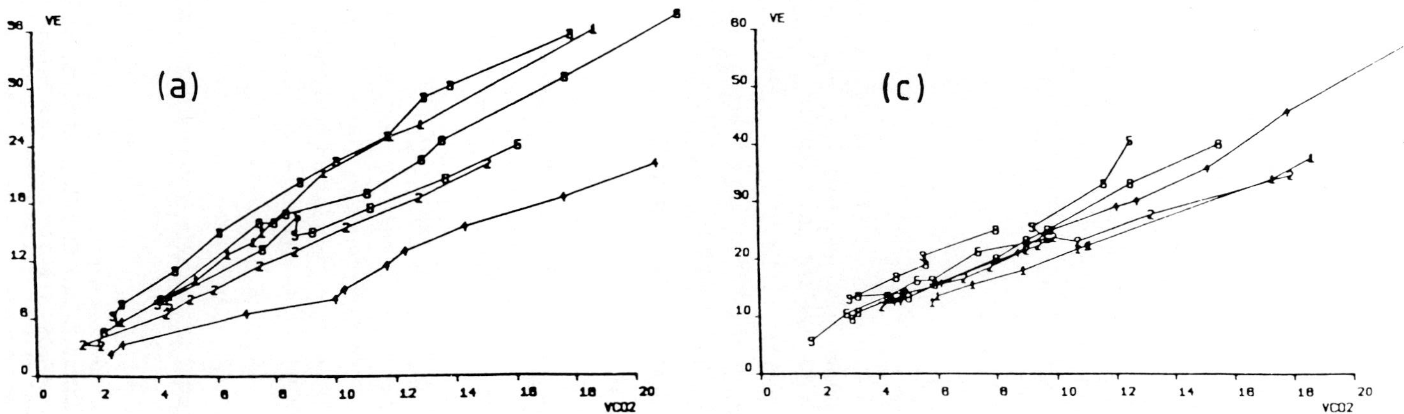

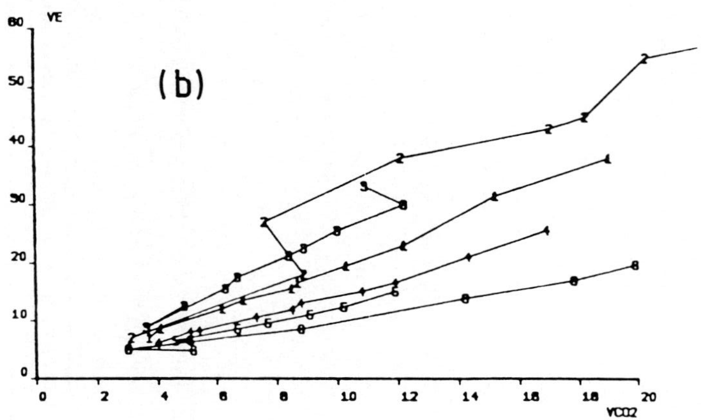

Fig. 28.1. *Ventilation rate during exercise plotted against rate of production of carbon dioxide, as a measure of metabolic rate. The figures show heart transplant patients and normals compared with heart–lung patients. Each patient or subject is shown by a separate number and measurements were made every minute during progressive exercise testing on a treadmill. All three groups show a rise in ventilation as the work of exercise increases. (a, Normals V_E vs. V_{CO_2}; b, heart–lungs V_E vs. V_{CO_2}; c, hearts V_E vs. V_{CO_2}.)*

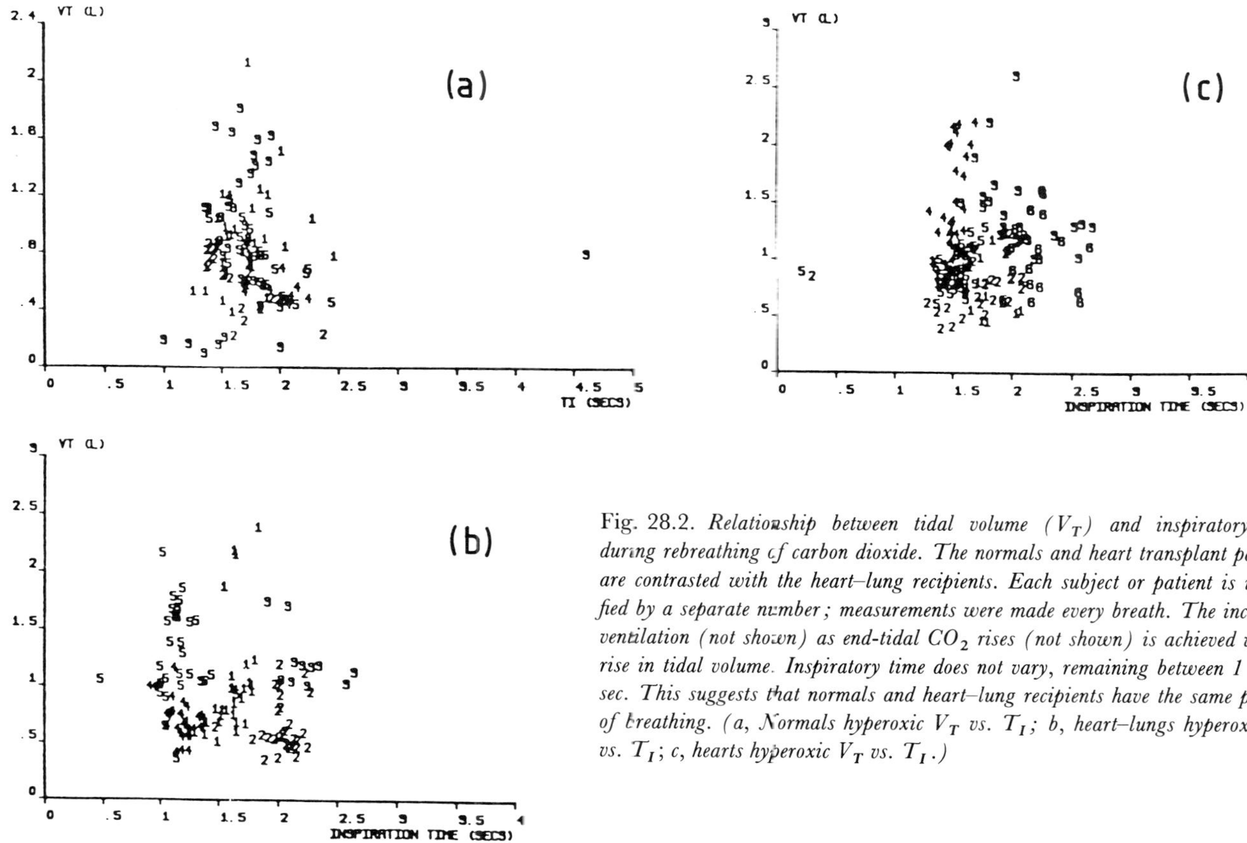

Fig. 28.2. *Relationship between tidal volume (V_T) and inspiratory time during rebreathing of carbon dioxide. The normals and heart transplant patients are contrasted with the heart–lung recipients. Each subject or patient is identified by a separate number; measurements were made every breath. The increased ventilation (not shown) as end-tidal CO_2 rises (not shown) is achieved with a rise in tidal volume. Inspiratory time does not vary, remaining between 1 and 2 sec. This suggests that normals and heart–lung recipients have the same pattern of breathing. (a, Normals hyperoxic V_T vs. T_I; b, heart–lungs hyperoxic V_T vs. T_I; c, hearts hyperoxic V_T vs. T_I.)*

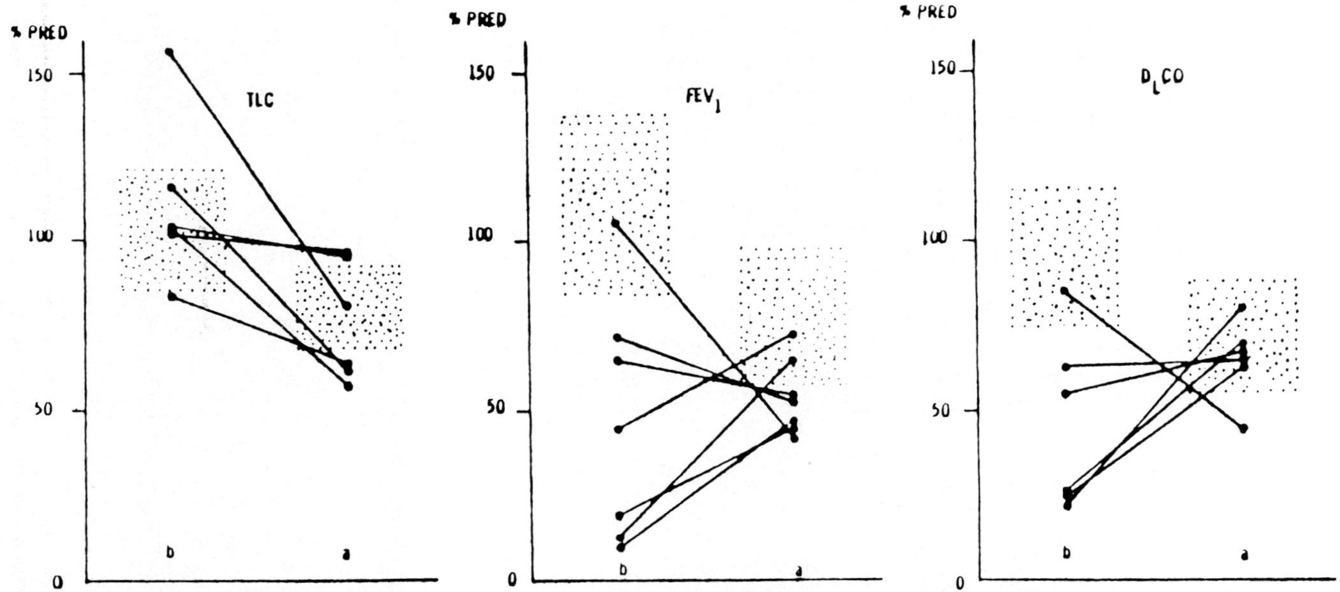

Fig. 28.3. *Total lung capacity TLC, FEV_1 and D_LCO before (b) and after (a) heart–lung transplantation in 7 patients, expressed as % predicted. Stippled areas show comparable pre- and postoperative values (mean ± ISD) for 13 patients who underwent routine coronary artery bypass surgery. The heart–lung transplant recipients behave in a similar way to the routine median sternotomy patients.*

al., 1986). Initially it was believed that rejection could be monitored by means of endomyocardial biopsies (Reitz *et al.*, 1982). However, in clinical practice (McGregor *et al.*, 1985), rejection of the lungs precedes, and is independent of, rejection of the heart.

In vivo studies suggest that in the lungs, in common with other transplanted organs, the major site of rejection is in the small blood vessels. Perivascular lymphocytic infiltrates appear to develop early (Veith *et al.*, 1972).

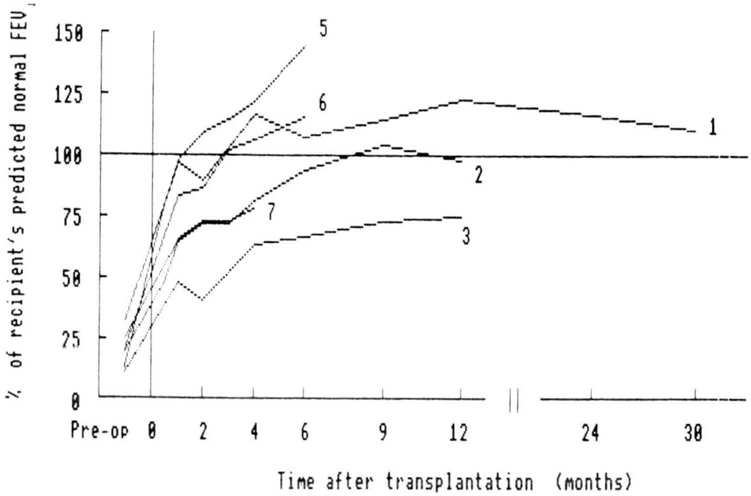

Fig. 28.4. *Progressive rise in FEV_1 from before (pre-op) to after transplantation in 7 patients with chronic end-stage lung disease. The values are expressed as % predicted. Only 1 patient failed to return to normal 6 months after surgery. This was the result of a persisting kyphoscoliosis.*

In man, however, the epithelial surfaces of the airways are also involved in the inflammatory process, causing airway narrowing and obliteration of the bronchioli (Burke *et al.*, 1984). A similar process has been reported in the biliary canaliculi of the liver (Hubscher *et al.*, 1985). The physiological consequence is the development of airflow obstruction (Burke *et al.*, 1984). Early reports suggested that a state of irreversible chronic obliterative bronchiolitis, which is believed to be a result of chronic rejection (Tazelaar *et al.*, 1987), develops in a high proportion of patients. The question has arisen whether the rejection process, if detected early, can be reversed by augmented immunosuppression.

At Papworth we have monitored the FEV_1 as a measure of airflow obstruction. A reduction in value has been used as an indication for transbronchial lung biopsy (Higenbottam *et al.*, 1987b) (see Chapter 27)

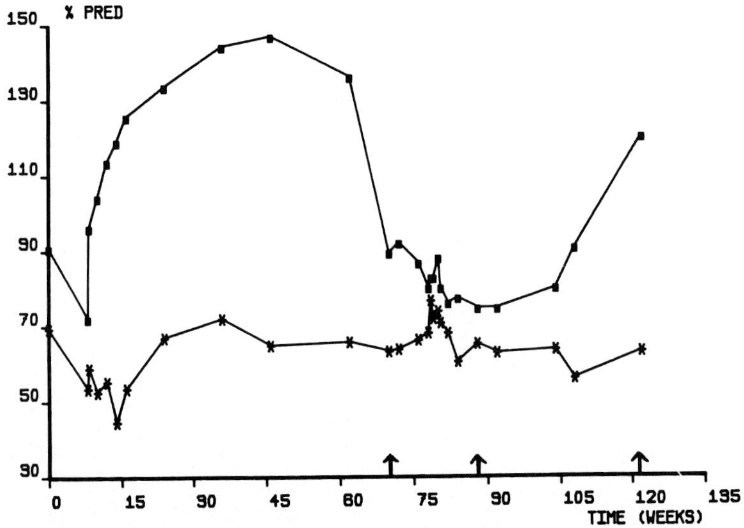

Fig. 28.5. *Change in* FEV_1 *(■) and* D_LCO *(∗)(% predicted) in a patient with recurrent rejection. Arrows denote when biopsies of the lungs were performed. The first two showed rejection, but the last biopsy performed after return to near normal function was quite normal. Augmented immunosuppression was maintained throughout the period of reduction of* FEV_1.

(Figs 28.5 and 28.6). Augmented immunosuppression appears to reverse the fall in FEV_1, provided that it is given early enough (Fig. 28.5), although sustained augmented immunosuppressive therapy may be required to reverse the process fully. Once severe airflow limitation has occurred, it does not appear possible to reverse it (Fig. 28.6). At this time, the gas transfer for carbon monoxide also becomes reduced.

The D_LCO in the early stages of rejection is variably affected. This is not the case in opportunistic infections, for example cytomegalovirus (CMV) pneumonitis and *Pneumocystis carinii* pneumonia (PCP) where the D_LCO is reduced (Fig. 28.7). Although a fall in D_LCO has been used to detect opportunistic infection in the immunosuppressed patient (Fanta and Pennington, 1981), information is still too scarce in heart–lung recipients to allow a decision as to whether lung function is sufficiently specific to be diagnostic. At present, lung function is used simply as an indication of when to biopsy the lungs.

Lung function testing is simple and accurate. As lung recipients appear to sense disturbance of lung mechanics early, complaining of breathlessness, testing offers immediate confirmation that disturbance has occurred. Such a change in function precedes radiological abnormalities and provides adequate grounds to undertake transbronchial biopsy (see Chapter 27).

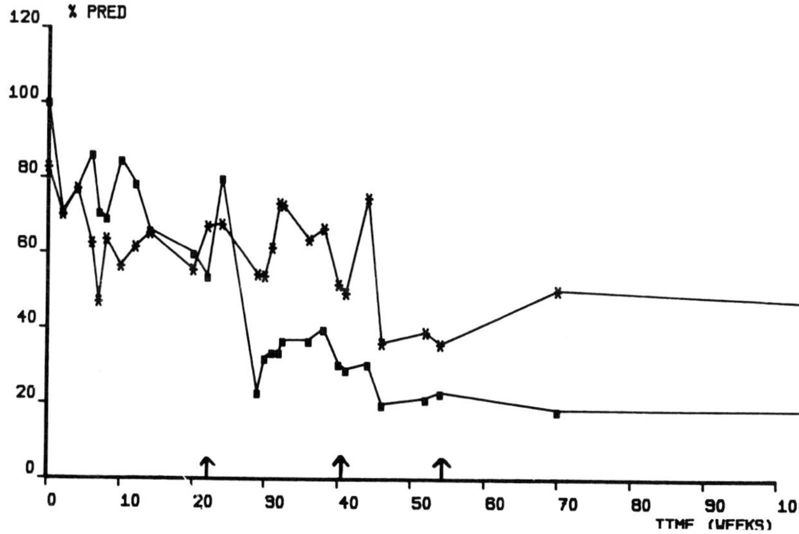

Fig. 28.6. *Change in* FEV_1 *(■) and* D_LCO *(∗) (% predicted) in a patient who developed obliterative bronchiolitis. Arrows denote when biopsies were taken. The last biopsy, an open lung biopsy, confirmed the findings of the transbronchial biopsy. This patient, in contrast to the last, only received a 10-day course of prednisolone.*

LONG-TERM CONSEQUENCES OF LUNG DENERVATION

Although the vagus nerve appears to be unimportant in the regulation of breathing, denervation of the lungs does result in disturbances of airway function. To understand this consequence of denervation, it is necessary to consider the pathophysiology of asthma. The airways of asthmatics appear to be hyper-responsive to a wide range of inhaled non-specific irritants. Asthmatics respond with bronchoconstriction when inhaling low concentrations of histamine, methacholine and ultrasonically nebulized distilled water (Foresi *et al.*, 1986). This is believed to be a result of airway inflammation.

After heart–lung transplantation, patients show enhanced responsiveness to methacholine but not to histamine (Banner *et al.*, 1987) or to nebulized distilled water (Jackson *et al.*, 1987). Both the latter stimuli can act upon pulmonary afferent nerves. In other words, only methacholine hyper-responsiveness is seen. This does not appear to be a result of lung inflammation (Jackson *et al.*, 1987). Instead, it has been suggested that loss of vagal innervation leads to an up-regulation of airway smooth muscle muscarinic receptors. Whether there is a pathological consequence remains uncertain, but this does demonstrate how much physiological knowledge can be gained as a result of lung transplantation programmes.

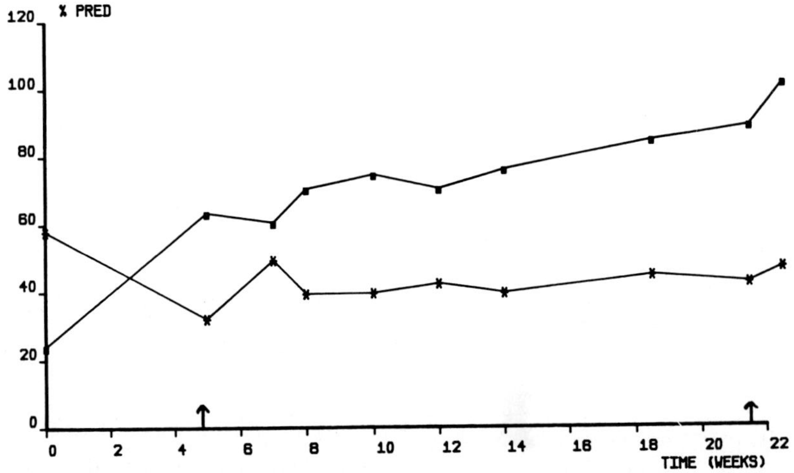

Fig. 28.7. *Change in* FEV_1 *(■) and* D_LCO *(*) (% predicted) in a patient who developed CMV pneumonitis. First arrow shows when the transbronchial biopsy was performed and treatment with sulphadimidine and trimethoprim was started. A normal biopsy (shown by second arrow) was obtained when the patient had recovered.*

REFERENCES

Banner, N. R., Hollingshead, L., Dear, L., Heaton, R., Guz, A. and Jacoub, M. H. (1987). Increased bronchial reactivity to methacholine following combined heart–lung transplantation (Abstract). *Thorax* **42**, 239–240.

Bland, S., Laserov, L., Dyck, G. and Cherniack, R. M. (1967). The influence of the chest wall on respiratory rate and depth. *Resp. Phys.* **3**, 47–54.

Braun, S. R., Birnbaum, M. L. and Chopra, P. S. (1987). Pre and post operative pulmonary function abnormalities in coronary artery revascularization surgery. *Chest* **73**, 316–320.

Burke, C. M., Theodore, J., Baldwin, J. C., Tazelaar, H. D., Morris, A. J., McGregor, C., Shumway, N. E., Robin, E. D. and Jamieson, S. W. (1986). Twenty eight cases of human heart–lung transplantation. *Lancet* **i**, 517–519.

Burke, C. M., Theodore, J., Dawkins, K. D., Yousem, S. A., Blank, N., Billingham, M. E., Van Kessel, A., Jamieson, S. W., Oyer, P. E., Baldwin, J. C., Stinson, G. B., Shumway, N. E. and Robin, E. D. (1984). Post-transplant obliterative bronchiolitis and other late lung sequelae in human heart–lung transplantation. *Chest* **86**, 824–829.

Euler, C. Von. (1983). On the central pattern generator for the basic breathing rhythmicity. *J. Appl. Phys.* **55**, 1647–1659.

Fanta, C. H. and Pennington, J. E. (1981). Fever and new lung infiltrates in the immunocompromised host. *Clin. Chest. Med.* **2**, 19–39.

Favier, G., Kepenekian, D., Desplanches, S. and Flandrois R. (1982). Effects of chronic lung denervation on breathing pattern and respiratory gas exchange during hypoxia, hypercapnia and exercise. *Resp. Phys.* **47**, 107–119.

Foresi, A., Mattoli, S., Corbo, G. M., Polidori, G. and Ciappi, G. (1986). Comparison of bronchial responses to ultrasonically nebulized distilled water, exercise and methacholine in asthma. *Chest* **90**, 822–826.

Fung, Y. C. (1977). Stress, deformation and atelectasis of the lung. *Circ. Resp.* **37**, 481–503.

Higenbottam, T. W., Fitzpatrick, M. E. and Wallwork, J. (1987a). Pattern of ventilatory response to CO_2 after heart or heart and lung transplantation (Abstract). *Thorax* **42**, 236.

Higenbottam, T. W., Stewart, S., Penketh, A. and Wallwork, J. (1987b). Transbronchial lung biopsy in the diagnosis of infection and rejection in heart–lung transplantation (Abstract). *Am. Rev. Resp. Dis.* (in press).

Hubscher, S. G., Clements, D., Elias, E. and McMaster, P. (1985). Biopsy findings in cases of rejection of liver allograft. *J. Clin. Path.* **38**, 1366–1373.

Jackson, M., Rashdi, T., Wallwork, J. and Higenbottam, T. W. (1987). Bronchial muscarinic receptor hypersensitivity after heart–lung transplantation (HLT) (Abstract). *Thorax.* (in press).

Kenyon, C. M., Pedley, T. and Higenbottam, T. W. (1987). Changes in chest wall configuration following medium sternotomy (Abstract). *Clin. Sci.* (in press).

Mattila, S. P., Mattila, P., Viljanen, B. C. and Viljanen, A. A. (1987). Cardiopulmonary transplantation and regulation of breathing. *Transplant. Proc.* **xix**, 1043–1044.

McGregor, C. G. A., Baldwin, J. C., Jamieson, S. W., Billingham, M. E., Yousem, S. A., Burke, C. M., Oyer, P. E., Stinson, E. B. and Shumway, N. E. (1985). Isolated pulmonary rejection after combined heart–lung transplantation. *J. Thorac. Cardiovasc. Surg.* **90**, 623–626.

Mead, J., Takishara, T. and Leith, D. (1970). Stress distribution in lungs: a model of pulmonary elasticity. *J. Appl. Phys.* **28**, 596–602.

Nakae, A., Webb, W. R., Theodorides, T. and Sugg, W. L. (1967). Respiratory function following cardiopulmonary denervation in dog, cat and monkey. *Surg. Gynec. Obst.* **62**, 1285–1292.

Penketh, A., Higenbottam, T., Hakim, M. and Wallwork, J. (1987). Heart and lung transplantation in patients with end-stage lung disease. *Br. Med. J.* **295**, 311–314.

Reitz, B. A., Burton, N. A., Jamieson, S. W., Bieber, C. P., Pennock, J. L., Stinson, E. B. and Shumway, N. E. (1980). Heart and lung transplantation. *J. Thorac. Cardiovasc. Surg.* **80**, 360–372.

Reitz, B. A., Wallwork, J., Hunt, S. A., Pennock, J. L., Billingham, M. E., Oyer, P. E., Stinson, E. B. and Shumway, N. E. (1982). Heart–lung transplantation: a successful therapy for patients with pulmonary vascular disease. *New Engl. J. Med.* **306**, 557–564.

Sears, T. A. (1984). Spinal integration and rhythm generation in breathing. *Clin. Resp. Phys.* **20**, 399–401.

Tazelaar, H. D., Prop, J., Nieuwenhais, P, Billingham, M. E. and Wildevuur, C. R. H. (1987). Obliterative bronchiolitis in the transplanted rat lung. *Transplant. Proc.* **xix**, 1052.

Theodore, J., Jamieson, S. W., Burke, C. M., Reitz, B. A., Stinson, E. B., Van Kessel, A., Dawkins, K. D., Herran, J. J., Oyer, P. E., Hunt, S. A., Shumway, N. E. and Robin, E. D. (1984). Physiologic aspects of human heart–lung transplantation: pulmonary function status of the post-transplanted lung. *Chest* **86**; 349–357.

Theodore, J., Robin, E. D., Morris, A. J., Burke, C. M., Jamieson, S. W., Van Kessel, A., Stinson, E. B. and Shumway, N. E. (1986). Augmented ventilatory response to exercise in pulmonary hypertension. *Chest* **89**, 39–44.

Trippenoch, T. (1985). Chest wall reflexes in the newborn. *Clin. Resp. Phys.* **21**, 115–122.

Veith, F. J., Sinha, S. B. P., Blümcke, S., Dougherty, J. C., Becker, N. H., Siegelman, S. S. and Hagstrom, J. W. C. (1972). Nature and evolution of lung allograft rejection with and without immunosuppression. *J. Thorac. Cardiovasc. Surg.* **63**, 509–520.

Wallwork, J., Jones, K., Cavarrocchi, N., Hakim, M. and Higenbottam, T. W. (1987). Distant procurement of organs for clinical heart–lung transplantation using a single-flush technique. *Transplantation* (in press).

Winning, A. J., Hamilton, R. D., Sheu, S. A., Knott, C. and Guz, A. (1985). The effect of airway anaesthesia on the control of breathing and the sensations of breathlessness in man. *Clin. Sci.* **68**, 215–225.

Index